Principles and Practice of Medical Genetics

Principles and Practice of Medical Genetics

Edited by Ellie Peyton

AMERICAN
MEDICAL PUBLISHERS
www.americanmedicalpublishers.com

American Medical Publishers,
41 Flatbush Avenue,
1st Floor, New York,
NY 11217, USA

Visit us on the World Wide Web at:
www.americanmedicalpublishers.com

ISBN: 978-1-63927-258-7

Cataloging-in-Publication Data

Principles and practice of medical genetics / edited by Ellie Peyton.
p. cm.
Includes bibliographical references and index.
ISBN 978-1-63927-258-7
1. Medical genetics. 2. Human genetics. 3. Genetic disorders. I. Peyton, Ellie.
RB155 .P75 2022
616.042--dc23

Table of Contents

Preface

Medicinal genetics is a field of medicine that focuses on the diagnosis and management of hereditary disorders. It is concerned with the application of genetics to medical care that includes researching the causes of genetic disorders as well as management, diagnosis and counseling of the people suffering from these disorders. It also includes areas such as personalized medicine, gene therapy and predictive medicine. Some of the techniques used in this field are fluorescence in-situ hybridization, Southern blotting, DNA sequencing, comparative genomic hybridization, etc. Conditions such as birth defects, autism, skeletal dysplasia, connective tissue disorders, cancer genetics and prenatal diagnosis are studied and treated under this domain. This book contains some path-breaking studies in the field of medical genetics. It presents researches and studies performed by experts across the globe. It will serve as a valuable source of reference for graduate and post graduate students.

This book is a comprehensive compilation of works of different researchers from varied parts of the world. It includes valuable experiences of the researchers with the sole objective of providing the readers (learners) with a proper knowledge of the concerned field. This book will be beneficial in evoking inspiration and enhancing the knowledge of the interested readers.

In the end, I would like to extend my heartiest thanks to the authors who worked with great determination on their chapters. I also appreciate the publisher's support in the course of the book. I would also like to deeply acknowledge my family who stood by me as a source of inspiration during the project.

Editor

1

'Sifting the significance from the data' - the impact of high-throughput genomic technologies on human genetics and health care

Angus J Clarke[1*], David N Cooper[1], Michael Krawczak[2], Chris Tyler-Smith[3], Helen M Wallace[4], Andrew O M Wilkie[5], Frances Lucy Raymond[6], Ruth Chadwick[7], Nick Craddock[8], Ros John[9], John Gallacher[10] and Mathias Chiano[11]

Abstract

This report is of a round-table discussion held in Cardiff in September 2009 for Cesagen, a research centre within the Genomics Network of the UK's Economic and Social Research Council. The meeting was arranged to explore ideas as to the likely future course of human genomics. The achievements of genomics research were reviewed, and the likely constraints on the pace of future progress were explored. New knowledge is transforming biology and our understanding of evolution and human disease. The difficulties we face now concern the interpretation rather than the generation of new sequence data. Our understanding of gene-environment interaction is held back by our current primitive tools for measuring environmental factors, and in addition, there may be fundamental constraints on what can be known about these complex interactions.

Introduction

The advent of 'high throughput' or 'next generation' genomic sequencing technologies has raised expectations of what laboratory genetics has, and will have, to offer to both the clinician and the patient. Our greatly increased ability to generate nucleic acid sequence data raises the question of how this rapidly accumulating mass of new genomic information will be interpreted and when this will become feasible in general clinical practise. How much sense will have been made of the new data within the next 10 to 15 years? What new questions will it be possible for us to pose once these new technologies are readily available to provide the information upon which biologically meaningful answers to these questions can be based? The extended lag time between generating a basic understanding of the pathogenesis of many single gene (Mendelian) disorders and devising effective remedies has long been acknowledged. In the context of complex disorders and the many known quantitative (non-disease) traits, will the lag time between data collection and its interpretation be shortened?

Such questions were addressed at a round-table discussion held in Cardiff in September 2009. This was arranged as part of the work programme of Cesagen, a joint research centre at the Universities of Cardiff (Wales) and Lancaster (England) established by the UK's Economic and Social Research Council as part of its Genomics Network. Cesagen studies the societal impact of developments in genetics and genomics; the meeting was arranged to explore and discuss ideas as to the likely future course of human genomics. Such technologies will permit researchers to ask new questions of theoretical (biological, e.g. evolutionary) significance and practical (medical and other) application.

The starting point for the discussion was the recent leap in DNA sequencing capability developed by several different commercial enterprises. There was no need to dwell upon the specifics of the technologies; rather, the point was to address the potential benefits for the sciences and clinical medicine of having large volumes of genomic sequence data available, effectively without major constraints of time or cost and alongside an emerging capacity to determine the CpG methylation status of the corresponding nucleotide sequences, the 'methylome', and other modifications of chromatin [1]. Several short presentations were made during the round-table

* Correspondence: clarkeaj@cardiff.ac.uk
[1]Institute of Medical Genetics, School of Medicine, Cardiff University, Cardiff, Wales CF14 4XN, UK
Full list of author information is available at the end of the article

sessions, but the emphasis of the meeting was on open discussion among the 20 participants, who have backgrounds in human and evolutionary genetics, clinical medicine, social science and philosophy. The perspectives developed at the meeting have been refined 'virtually' since then through multiple cycles of e-mail exchanges.

Experience of exomics

Useful insights had already been obtained through two large studies: the Genetics of Learning Disability (GOLD) study with complete X chromosomal 'exome' sequences from >200 patients with sex-linked cognitive impairment [2] and the description of the full exomes of 12 selected individuals [3]. Frances Lucy Raymond (Cambridge, England) was able to draw a number of general lessons from the GOLD study:

- Sample quality is critical for obtaining reliable DNA sequence data; poor sample quality generates multiple sequence variants per sample, making it difficult to distinguish real sequence from experimental artefact; the assumption that poor quality samples would not amplify was false.
- Truncating sequence variants - termed nulls - are found in approximately 1% of genes on the X chromosome but are nevertheless compatible with normal life in the hemizygous male.
- Missense variants are common, with an average of four unique single nucleotide non-synonymous variants per family with X-linked intellectual disability.
- Data access remains a sensitive issue; there is a need to publish variants and allele frequencies while preserving the anonymity of research participants. This would generally entail publishing aggregate data and new variants rather than individual-specific haplotype information.

These findings emphasise what is already well known, that a disrupted gene need not necessarily lead to a clinically overt disease state, i.e. many genes are dispensable, and even for inactivated essential genes, penetrance will often be incomplete [4,5]. The difficulties inherent in this analysis with regard to the interpretation of previously unreported variants - mutations that may be of pathogenic significance - will be even more substantial when we consider autosomal loci, of which (almost) everyone will have two copies [6]. Additional new approaches to determine the functional significance of genomic variation will be required if any coherent interpretation of the approaching deluge of data is to be feasible [7].

Epigenetics

Epigenetic influences together introduce an additional layer of complexity over and above the functionality of genomic DNA sequences [4]. The inter-relationship of DNA sequence and DNA sequence modification has not yet been adequately addressed in either theory or experiment; it should, however, be noted that this relationship is likely to be bi-directional with certain polymorphic variants influencing methylation status and the methylation status in turn influencing mutability. Ros John (Cardiff, Wales) introduced this topic and its relationship to known imprinting phenomena, referring to both epidemiological and experimental work, *viz.* records of the Dutch famine at the end of World War II [8] and contemporary work with the agouti mouse [9]. The term 'epigenetics' includes the study of both conventional gene-gene (GxG) interactions, long recognised in principle but in practise exceedingly difficult to measure in humans, and the still under-researched area of 'predictive adaptive responses'. The latter has been elaborated theoretically [10], triggering very interesting - but so far perhaps more tantalising than illuminating - laboratory work on the possible influence of early life experiences (before or soon after birth) on patterns of DNA methylation and subsequent disease susceptibility in the face of dietary challenges and other environmental circumstances.

Our understanding of the intricate role of the epigenome in directing differentiation, communicating cell fate and mediating adaptive response will be informed by comprehensive surveys of epigenetic marks across space (cell type/state) and time (development and ageing), and in response to environmental challenges (diet, stress). To this end, a number of ingenious genome-wide, high-throughput technologies have been developed. Some are based on the ability to selectively capture methylated fragments of the genome using methyl-binding proteins and then sequencing these fragments. MeDIP-seq, MBD-seq and MethylCap-seq have all been applied successfully, although with differences in selectivity for specific sequences [11,12]. A readout of the whole genome methylation status can also be obtained by applying a bisulfite-sequencing technique, whereby genomic DNA is exposed to HSO_3^-, which deaminates only the unmethylated (and, hence, unprotected) cytosine residues resulting in a change in the DNA sequence. This technique may provide greater coverage of the genome [13]. The genome-wide assessment of histone modifications is a more complex task since these modifications are numerous, and activating and silencing marks are not necessarily mutually exclusive [14]. Chromatin immunoprecipitation followed by high-throughput sequencing is the preferred technique for determining the genome-wide locations of specific histone modifications [15,16]. Although there are still issues, in particular, the biassed representation of certain sequences, computational analyses and further technical refinements will undoubtedly increase the sensitivity of these techniques and further reduce the costs.

One potentially very important aspect of GxG and gene-environment (GxE) interactions that may limit their importance, or at least our ability to detect them, is the small effective population size (N_e in population genetic notation) of humans [17]. Another important question is the extent to which the assessment of CpG methylation can serve as an adequate biomarker for the full range of epigenetic influences. A systems biology approach to the recognition of biological networks may be one way of addressing GxG and GxE interactions in humans [18,19], given that the types of breeding experiments pioneered in *Drosophila* species are clearly ruled out in humans, not only on ethical grounds but also by the restrictions of time-scale available to researchers. The collection of biological samples and data on the large Helmholtz cohort in Germany is intended to address some of these issues.

Behaviour and psychiatry

When one turns to consider human behaviour and psychiatric disorders, rather than the (relatively) simple phenotypes associated with human growth or with metabolic and developmental disorders, additional layers of complexity become evident in the GxE interactions. As Anita Thapar (Cardiff, Wales) made clear, there is a pressing need for good measures of both the environmental factors and the behavioural phenotypes of potential interest. The GxE interactions can be looked at as purely statistical phenomena or, more interestingly and perhaps more importantly, as phenomena of potential biological meaning. Here more than anywhere, and in deference to the great David Hume, it is essential to avoid the all-too-easy slide from the observation of an association into unwarranted assumptions about causation. Thus, if one observed an association between attention deficit hyperactivity disorder in children and maternal cigarette smoking, what causal influences might have been at work, - e.g. an environmental effect of smoking in pregnancy or a common genetic basis to both behaviours? One opportunity to clarify such questions, although difficult to establish, would be longitudinal studies of children born following conception by IVF. Some of these questions are profound, touching our very humanity; for instance, how (through what process) does the early maltreatment of children result in later antisocial behaviour? How may social interventions be designed effectively to interrupt such pathogenetic linkages, for the long-term benefit of society as a whole? The Bradford-Hill criteria [20] address this problem of causation but have yet to be fully tested in the genomic era.

Improved methods of measuring environmental factors and their behavioural correlates are clearly required for the full benefits of the progress in genome sequencing to be attained; these measurements should be made without lapsing into implicitly deterministic assumptions.

Common disease genetics

Michael Krawczak (Kiel, Germany) challenged the assumptions underlying much 'common disease genetics' - especially the limitations of its most influential models. He expanded upon three critical underlying assumptions made by Reich and Lander [21,22]:

- The allelic spectrum of common disease genes is simple.
- There was a single, sudden expansion event of the human population (at least, the out-of-Africa population) from 10,000 members to its modern size.
- The part played by selection in the spread of alleles predisposing to common diseases was relatively small.

This model has led to the neglect of new mutants arising from existing variants during the turnover of the allelic spectrum of common disease. Krawczak explained why these assumptions are highly implausible and what effect this is likely to have had on the current allelic spectrum of genetic predisposition to complex disease. In particular, as is apparent both when other modelling approaches, such as coalescence theory, are used and from the data currently accumulating:

- The allelic spectrum of complex disorders, like that of Mendelian disorders, is likely to be diverse.
- There may be only a weak correlation between the risk of disease and the population frequency of risk alleles.
- The functional effects of predisposing alleles may be weakly or even inversely related to the associated disease risk (some predisposing alleles may even, counter-intuitively and due to stochastic processes, be more frequent in unaffected than affected individuals).
- The mutational load in unaffected individuals may be particularly high for common diseases.

Mapping the 'polygenes'

Krawczak also discussed the limitations of the available strategies for mapping the loci which contribute to the common, complex disorders. The power of the affected sib pair (ASP) linkage approach has been regarded as low [21] in comparison to association studies employing the transmission disequilibrium test (TDT), not a case–control design, but that view also had shortcomings:

- The paper assumed knowledge of the risk allele when assessing the TDT but not when assessing the ASP method.
- The relative risks invoked were unrealistically high.
- The association approach was found to be advantageous for studies of candidate genes (or

regions) but not necessarily for genome-wide methods exploiting linkage disequilibrium, such as genome-wide association studies (GWAS).

There are good grounds for using both family studies and GWAS to utilise all the available evidence [23]. Family-based approaches that could be used with whole-genome sequencing (potential scenarios) include:

- sequencing the index patients and evaluating the inheritance pattern of 'interesting' genes or gene regions in their families
- sequencing the parents of the patient, comparing the results to population controls, and using TDT on 'promising' alleles
- assessing the co-inheritance pattern of unlinked genes in families to derive candidate regions for GxG interactions
- defining and assessing pre-disease or sub-clinical disease states in genetically-defined high-risk individuals identified in families.

Andrew O M Wilkie (Oxford, England) mentioned that the supposed 'triumphs' of the common disease/common variants (CD/CV) model conveniently ignore the fact that the relative risks conferred by susceptibility alleles cluster much more closely around 1.0 than anyone envisaged two decades ago; relative risks above 2.0 are decidedly unusual. Hence, the majority of heritability remains unexplained, and useful personalised prediction in healthy individuals (largely based on family history) has hardly improved over this time.

Additional challenges to our understanding include the greater heritability of diseases (e.g. schizophrenia, as presented by Nick Craddock of Cardiff, Wales) than would be expected given the CD/CV model of disease causation and the greater difficulty of interpreting any estimates of heritability when the disease phenotype results from the joint action of several predisposing genes (as Helen M Wallace (Buxton, UK) reminded us). Whether these insights into pathogenesis will eventually convert to promised improvements in human health remains to be seen.

There was discussion about the possible 'replication' of the results of GWAS, led by Mathias Chiano (Stevenage, England). Even the question of what exactly 'replication' would entail needs to be clarified, as when specifying the population(s) from which study participants are drawn. If an attempt is made to replicate a given study in a different population, the meaning of a negative result will be unclear because the relevant genetic factors may differ between this and the original population; there are no easy answers in relation to population differences.

Selection

Chris Tyler-Smith (Hinxton, England) continued with the theme of human history and the contemporary traces of past selection. Selection can take many forms but the presence of high levels of polymorphism suggests either an ancient origin for neutral mutations or the maintenance of polymorphism by fluctuating or balancing selection. Recognising past selection is possible by (i) counting offspring, (ii) looking for patterns of DNA variation in populations that depart from neutrality (such as long haplotypes, skewed allele frequency spectra, large differences between populations), and (iii) functional studies. Recent genomic studies comparing populations have drawn upon the second category of evidence that detects the net effects of positive selection over millennia, but these have mostly been based on simple models of selection and are less able to detect phenomena such as heterozygote advantage, frequency-dependent selection, disruptive selection - selection for both homozygotes - or antagonistic but stabilising selection with contrary effects at different stages of the life cycle in the two sexes or in different environments.

While there are grounds for thinking that selective 'sweeps' have been uncommon in recent human evolution [24], the role of selection in maintaining substantial levels of polymorphism remains less clear. Although a biological (natural selection-based) account for many genetic observations consistent with selection remains elusive, this could be the result of the challenging nature of such studies. The persistence of polymorphism without a clear genomic signature may result from changes in the strength and direction of selection. Despite these complexities, there are widely accepted examples of positive selection, including disease-associated variants and those influencing visible traits such as skin colour or hair, where sexual selection through gene-culture interaction may have been relevant [25,26].

Human genetic variation: the 1000 Genomes Project

Results from the 1000 Genomes Project [27] and other studies indicate that, despite the low level of genetic variation in humans compared with other apes, there are still enormous inter-individual differences in genome sequence, which can now be identified in a comprehensive way at the level of CNVs, indels and SNPs. Notably, there are on average 250 to 300 loss-of-function variants such as 'nonsense' or splicing SNPs in the genome of the average 'healthy' person, 50 to 100 previously implicated, disease-associated variants and approximately 80 genes that vary in copy number. As suggested by the GOLD study (*op cit*), this greatly complicates the clinical interpretation of an individual's genome sequence.

The first goal of the 1000 Genomes Project has been to capture important data about background human genetic variation which will be essential in studies of both inherited and acquired disease. The samples being studied:

- were initially drawn from urban populations in four countries (HapMap Nigerian, Japanese, Chinese, and families with European ancestry from the USA) but additional samples will be drawn from elsewhere, including South Asia
- were from anonymous individuals with no phenotypic information provided (except sex, population of origin and that they are adults competent to provide consent), but do have consent for free web release of the sequence data, and are available as cell-lines to researchers
- because full × 30-depth sequencing to detect heterozygous variants in a single individual effectively would be too costly, low coverage sequencing of samples from many individuals is being used to capture the variants shared between individuals; the full project aims to detect essentially all polymorphic variants (i.e. those at >1% frequency) in the geographical areas investigated that lie in the accessible part of the genome.

1000 Genomes pilot studies

- Samples (179) at depth × 2-4 should identify most variants present at >5% - so far, 17.2 million SNPs have been found, of which >50% were novel.
- Two trios sequenced at × 30-60 revealed many 'new' (*de novo*) mutation events (see below)
- Approximately 1,000 genes were sequenced deeply in samples from 700 volunteers.

The next task: it will be necessary to draw upon large population studies to seek evidence of variable mutation penetrance.

Mosaicism and foetal DNA in the maternal circulation

High-throughput sequencing is also opening up the detection of mosaicism, which is likely to have many biological consequences in addition to neoplasia [28]. With a read depth of × 30, it is difficult to detect mosaicism at or below the level of 5% because of the 1% error in typing each nucleotide position. This could have applications in the study of cancers, e.g. the evolution of individual tumours as reflected in tumour-specific DNA [29], and in prenatal diagnosis, where free foetal DNA is currently used to look for alleles not present in the mother, such as Rhesus or Y chromosome sequences, but is likely soon to be applicable to population screening, especially for trisomy 21 [30-32]. Greater read depths will be required for clinically important applications reliant upon the detection of low levels of mosaicism [33].

Phenotypes and taxonomy

Craddock led a discussion on disease phenotypes and their relation to disease taxonomy, especially in relation to psychiatric disorders. The definition of a phenotype is crucial as it may be influenced by numerous factors including 'culture' and tradition, established or desired patterns of health service utilisation, interacting environmental variables and previously accepted models of disease causation.

There has been a growing awareness that the specific single genes in which mutations cause a few rare disorders may also be (more loosely) associated with disease predispositions apparent in GWAS. Thus, rare mutations in the *CACNA1C* gene can result in a multisystem disorder, manifesting as cardiac dysrhythmias, epilepsy, autism, cognitive impairment and abnormal physical features, whereas variation in the same gene is more weakly associated with bipolar disease, schizophrenia and unipolar depression, as evidenced by GWAS. The benefits of identifying specific genes in which variation contributes to disease susceptibility include understanding the pathogenesis, establishing a diagnosis, devising new therapies and selecting the most appropriate treatment for the individual patient.

Following the course of human genetics research over the past 15 years, one may perceive a shift in focus from rare to common diseases and from genes of large effect in which mutations cause disease to genes of small effect in which variants merely modify the risk of disease. Mutations in genes of large effect are usually accepted unequivocally as important causal factors; the modifying genes of lesser effect can, however, also provide insights into pathogenesis when several loci in the same developmental or functional pathway interact to contribute to a specific disease. It is also clear that defining the phenotype is, itself, an iterative process, taking the researcher back and forth between the phenotype and the genotype. The researcher can use different values of a given parameter in order to establish which yields the clearest discrimination between individuals with and without disease.

The finding that sequence variation at some of the same loci influence both schizophrenia and bipolar disease has cast doubt on the validity of the Kraepelinian dichotomy of the psychoses into these categories [34,35]. The exclusion of 'intermediate' categories of patients from much previous research had in effect prevented this dogma from being challenged in the past - it became a closed 'view of the world' (a prophecy that was both dogmatic and self-fulfilling).

More recently still, it has become clear that new mutations at many loci contribute very substantially to schizophrenia, confirming the indications from studies of *de novo* CNVs that *de novo* rare mutations contribute importantly to this relatively common disease [36,37] and demonstrating that the reservations of Krawczak and others about the CD/CV model were warranted.

Mutation and selection at single loci

There is still much to be learned from the detailed study of single loci, in addition to genome-wide research that does not assume the applicability of the CD/CV model of complex disorders. As an example, Wilkie presented information from his long term studies of the fibroblast growth factor receptor (*FGFR*) genes.

As background to the *FGFR* studies, germline mutation rates have been estimated to be about 2.5×10^{-8} [38] or 1.8×10^{-8} [39] - equivalent to approximately 120 nucleotide substitutions per birth. The fitness of amino acid substitutions has been estimated [40,41], and purifying selection is thought to act on 2.5% to 5% of the genome (of which 1% will be coding sequence). This will lead to 1 to 3 harmful amino acid substitutions per birth, plus a similar number from each previous generation. Recent data from the 1000 Genomes Project suggest a slightly lower rate of new mutations, closer to 10^{-8} per base pair per generation, and that the influence of purifying selection can be detected through a reduction in genetic variation at distances of up to 100 kb from genes, implying that few parts of the genome are entirely unaffected by such selection. Similarly low rates of mutation have been found by others [42].

Wilkie described how he set out to explain the apparently very high levels of mutation in specific genes using the *FGFR* genes as a model. The most frequent transition mutation in the human germline is the *FGFR3* mutation that causes achondroplasia, but Wilkie chose to study the Apert syndrome mutation 755 C > G in *FGFR2*, which is the most common transversion mutation in humans. The mutations originate exclusively from the healthy fathers of the affected individuals, who tend to be older than average for the population (paternal age effect). From the analysis of normal sperm and testes, it can be deduced that the positions that mutate in *FGFR* genes are not true mutation hotspots; rather, there is positive selection for spermatogonia carrying the mutation because the mutation confers gain-of-function properties upon the encoded protein [43-45]. Wilkie looked for these mutations in an uncommon testicular tumour - spermatocytic seminomas - and a comparable spectrum of mutations was found here as in congenital disorders and in bladder tumours: they all act on the Ras/MAPK pathway, which plays a central role in regulating proliferation and other critical cellular processes. The testis may be viewed as a 'bioreactor' for selfish mutations that promote the clonal growth of spermatogonia harbouring one of these growth-promoting mutations [46]. The effects of each mutation vary with the degree to which it is activating:

1) highly activating mutations: lethal disorders or testicular tumours
2) moderately activating mutations: congenital malformation syndromes exhibiting a paternal age effect
3) weakly activating mutations: rare sequence variants that may predispose to a wide spectrum of disorders, involving for example neurodevelopment and cancer predisposition

It should be noted that the latter category of mutations will be undetectable by GWAS, and so may contribute to missing heritability [47].

The paternal age effect for schizophrenia may occur through a similar mechanism. It should be remembered that more than 1% individuals with schizophrenia have a *de novo* CNV, often a rare but recurrent CNV [48], while CNVs have been shown to be much more common in cases of schizophrenia than in controls (5% of controls, 15% to 20% of cases) [49] and, interestingly, to overlap with the CNVs found in attention deficit hyperactivity disorder [50]. However, the frequency of *de novo* CNVs is high enough in controls that such *de novo* events cannot be taken as *ipse facto* proof of pathogenicity.

Pharmacogenetics

Chiano led a discussion on pharmacogenetics and medical practice. Genetics is just one of the factors that influence the safety and efficacy of particular drugs. These factors include dosage, 'the environment', compliance, other drugs, diet, age and the co-occurrence of other diseases. Efficacy can vary from 80% for COX-2 inhibitors to 25% for cancer chemotherapy. The abacavir-associated hypersensitivity reaction can occur in 5% to 8%; there is a major susceptibility locus in the HLA region [51,52]. Proponents have been disappointed at the slow pace of introduction of pharmacogenetic testing into clinical practice. Meanwhile, somatic genetic tests are proving to be helpful in guiding the treatment of some malignancies but have been slower to enter regular clinical practice for a wider set of indications despite the longstanding recognition of the relevant pharmacogenetic phenomena: additional criteria of utility and cost-effectiveness also need to be fulfilled [53].

Privacy and consent

Ruth Chadwick (Cardiff, Wales) led a discussion on issues of privacy and consent in genomic research. It is becoming impossible for medical researchers to guarantee privacy to the research participants they recruit - especially with the pressure from funding agencies who insist upon open-access archiving of genomic sequence data, as these data inevitably contain potentially identifying information. Indeed, it would now be misleading to promise privacy of personal genome information to research participants in exchange for consent to donate samples.

There are difficulties at the level of the technology (sample collection and storage, and data generation, storage and access) and the interpretation of information collected. It has been argued that the very concept of privacy will have to be renegotiated in the context of the rationale(s) for data sharing, especially at international level. Indeed, there has been a move from 'traditional' notions of informed consent to one of a broad consent and then to open consent. One must either strengthen the traditional practises of consent - ensuring that participants understand the difficulties of ensuring privacy before giving consent (while at the same time pursuing the data protection strategies that are possible) - or rethink the whole notion of privacy [54]. In clinical practice, there may be recurrent difficulties when molecular studies of a malignancy, designed to guide therapeutics, thereby, also yield unwelcome information about prognosis or implications for close relatives [55]. In the context of research, however, new forms of consent (e.g. broad consent taken online) may well be readily accepted [56]. One approach is for the researcher to move from guaranteeing (and so protecting) privacy to practising veracity, explaining to potential participants that their data will be accessed by, and shared with, others; those consenting to research have to be open to this [57].

Those participating in 'personal genomics' would be deluding themselves if they thought that privacy was still possible once their genome sequences became accessible online [58,59]). This is the age of bioinformatics, surveillance, Facebook and Twitter. There is inevitably a risk of personal consequences for research participants when their data are released. These will take different forms under different circumstances. Access to health care may become more difficult in countries without state health care or universal and compulsory health insurance, as when health care is made available through commercial insurance schemes. In addition, if information about other family members becomes available, then biological family relationships might be shown to differ from the pattern of social relationships presented in public (e.g. paternity may have been misattributed).

One perspective reveals a clash of research cultures: molecular scientists (who seek instant open access to all data to maximise the scientific - and perhaps commercial - exploitation of the data) and the clinicians (who are often more insistent upon protecting their patients and more modest in their assessment of the likely short-term benefits to the participants, and other patients, of the research itself).

One key notion is that of the acceptable uses for research data. Participants tend to trust 'the system' to use their data in a 'good' way. The system of research governance is designed (in part) to ensure that such trust is warranted - although the system of governance also serves other, more institutional purposes. The prospect of internet-based marketing corporations using access to research data and to electronic health records as an opportunity to market more products seems both manipulative and cynical.

The concept of 'consent' is also problematic in ways unrelated to the concept of privacy. As Raymond explained, families participating in research studies could allow their genuine altruism to lead them to sign the research consent forms because their thoroughly worthy impulses blinded them to the potential for problems to arise from participation. Such problems might include results of uncertain significance, which may remain difficult to interpret for many years or whose significance might only be clarified through the performance of family studies that could be confusing or distressing; even with such family studies, the significance of the results may remain opaque. If the reasons underlying the importance and relevance of consent to research were explained, then many families might decline participation.

One response to these possibilities has been the suggestion that a solution should be found through information technology itself, with the development of a system of 'data enclaves', within which researchers can utilise data in a predefined analysis but from which they cannot export any data about individuals - only aggregate data and the derived results of analysis.

Limited clinical utility of genetic association

Wallace set out her answer to the important question, 'What are the (biological) limits to the predictive value and clinical utility of the 'predict and prevent' strategy?' An early approach to this led to the conclusion that environmental interventions targeted by genotype might significantly reduce the incidence of some diseases [60], dependent on the magnitude of gene-environment interactions (in the statistical sense of their influence on risk at a population level). However, there was an error in the measure of clinical utility used in this paper, and in addition, it took no account of the proportion of the population in the high-risk group (thus, erroneously suggesting that a genetic test which identified the whole population as at high risk would have high clinical utility). Further, the aetiology of a given disease will place constraints on the potential magnitude of both the genetic component of a disease and of any gene-environment interaction. Wallace set out her approach to assessing clinical utility in the context of genetic testing [61].

Utility, U_{GE} = population impact – gamma, where gamma is the fraction of the population classified as at high genotypic risk, and the population impact is the avoidable proportion of disease occurring in this fraction of the population, compared to the population as a whole.

Utility is larger if gamma is small, and targeting is only effective in the presence of GxE interactions. If there is no GxE interaction, genotyping performs no better than random selection in terms of reducing the incidence of the disease in a population. If high-risk individuals have less to gain from intervention than the low-risk group, then targeting has negative utility. There is a range of solutions for any given disease, which can be mapped out if data on relative risks from both twin and family studies, plus environmental data, is known. Each solution depends on the model that is assumed for gene-gene and gene-environment interactions. Because of the number of alternative models, the sample sizes required to evaluate or validate risk predictions may be too high, and it could be impossibly difficult to generate good association (GWAS) data and integrate it with environmental information [62]. The model also confirms earlier findings that heritability estimates can be high even in the complete absence of any genetic component to a disease [63] and that gene-gene and gene-environment interactions, as well as the equal environments assumption, may account for some (or even all) of the 'missing heritability' of complex diseases.

It should be noted that recent modelling of heritability and GWAS data suggest that a much greater fraction of the heritability of quantitative traits can be accounted for by GWAS data than had been found previously, once allowance is made for the incomplete linkage disequilibrium between the genotyped SNPs and the 'true' causal factors [64-66]. However, such modelling is still unable to identify the factors involved and cannot deliver improved capacity to predict disease. Furthermore, only a small proportion of the calculated heritability has yet been identified for any common disease [67].

Conclusion

The space provided by this workshop and the subsequent e-mail exchanges has served to clarify our thoughts and allowed several modest conclusions to emerge, although unanimity was not achieved on all issues. Four points, in particular, became progressively clearer during these discussions.

First, the new insights derived from the application of high throughput sequencing are likely to transform our understanding of human biology, especially in the context of human genetic disease and evolution. Clinical applications of human genome sequencing are emerging in oncology and reproductive genetics and are beginning to impact upon other clinical areas and disciplines. The old debates about nature vs. nurture are likely to re-emerge in new guises, and great care will be needed in case fruitless debate consumes too much energy or misconceived arguments lead to the inappropriate application of theory in policy and practise across various walks of life, most especially psychiatry, education and the law.

Second, and despite a full acceptance of this first point, major problems remain in moving from the rapidly accumulating raw sequence data and catalogues of genetic variation to warranted conclusions in their interpretation. These problems include questions relating to the clinical utility of conclusions drawn on the basis of genetic association studies that lack a plausible pathogenic mechanism underlying the observed association. There will inevitably be uncertainties in the face of a morass of interacting variables, but some of the difficulties should be resolved over time - although perhaps on a timescale of decades rather than months. In addition, our current measures of environmental factors are primitive, and our ability to record the variation in such factors over a lifetime of many years is still crude.

Finally, and despite the continuing advances in information technologies, the accumulation of both genomic and environmental data may outstrip the capacity of our information systems to store and analyse the data [68]. These limits to computability may not be merely practical in nature - to be overcome once technology has moved on - but may represent constraints as to what can be known or calculated even in principle, given limits to global population size, the nonrandom distribution of genotypes and the exponentially increasing number of statistical comparisons that can be made; how can one correct adequately for such astronomical numbers of comparisons? Deductive, hypothesis-driven research on the basis of such data will be challenging!

Acquiring the necessary genome sequence data appears now to be almost the easy step by comparison with the quantification of environmental factors and of human phenotypes, the physical limits to data storage and constraints in principle to computability and interpretation.

Competing interests

The authors declare that they have no competing interests.

Authors' contributions

AC initiated the project and led the writing of this report. RC ensured the fit between the project and the scope of Cesagen/ESRC support. All authors participated in the discussion and the development of the report into this article and then read and approved the final manuscript.

Acknowledgements

The support of the Economic and Social Research Council (ESRC) is gratefully acknowledged. The work is part of the research programme of the ESRC Genomics Network at Cesagen (website: http://www.genomicsnetwork.ac.uk/cesagen/). CT-S, FLR and AOMW wish to thank The Wellcome Trust for support. We thank the other participants for their contributions to the discussion: Hana Lango Allen (Exeter University), Michael Arribas-Ayllon (Cesagen, Cardiff, Wales), Ian Frayling (All Wales Medical Genetics Service, Cardiff, Wales), Andrew Fry (All Wales Medical Genetics Service, Cardiff, Wales), Peter Harper (Medical Genetics, Cardiff University, Wales), Adam

Hedgecoe (Cesagen, Cardiff, Wales), Ruth McNally (Cesagen, Lancaster, England), Anita Thapar (Psychological Medicine, Cardiff University, Wales).

Author details
[1]Institute of Medical Genetics, School of Medicine, Cardiff University, Cardiff, Wales CF14 4XN, UK. [2]Institute of Medical Informatics and Statistics, Christian-Albrechts University Kiel, Brunswiker Straße 10, Kiel 24105, Germany. [3]The Wellcome Trust Sanger Institute, Wellcome Trust Genome Campus, Hinxton, Cambridgeshire CB10 1SA, UK. [4]GeneWatch UK, 60 Lightwood Rd, Buxton SK17 7BB, UK. [5]Weatherall Institute of Molecular Medicine, John Radcliffe Hospital, University of Oxford, Headington, Oxford OX3 9DS, UK. [6]Department of Medical Genetics, Cambridge Institute for Medical Research, University of Cambridge, Cambridge CB2 0XY, UK. [7]Cesagen, 6 Museum Place, Cardiff University, Cardiff, Wales CF10 3BG, UK. [8]Department of Psychological Medicine, Cardiff University School of Medicine, Heath Park, Cardiff CF14 4XN, UK. [9]Cardiff School of Biosciences, Cardiff University, Cardiff, Wales CF10 3AX, UK. [10]Clinical Epidemiology, School of Medicine, Cardiff University, Cardiff, Wales CF14 4XN, UK. [11]GlaxoSmithKline Medicines Research Centre, Gunnels Wood Road, Stevenage, Hertfordshire SG1 2NY, UK.

References

1. Ernst J, Kheradpour P, Mikkelsen TS, Shoresh N: **Mapping and analysis of chromatin state dynamics in nine human cell types.** *Nature* 2011, **473**:43–49.
2. Tarpey PS, Smith R, Pleasance E, Whibley A, Edkins S, Hardy C, O'Meara S, Latimer C, Dicks E, Menzies A, Stephens P, Blow M, Greenman C, Xue Y, Tyler-Smith C, Thompson D, Gray K, Andrews J, Barthorpe S, Buck G, Cole J, Dunmore R, Jones D, Maddison M, Mironenko T, Turner R, Turrell K, Varian J, West S, Widaa S, *et al*: **A systematic large-scale resequencing screen of X-chromosome coding exons in mental retardation.** *Nat Genet* 2009, **41**:535–543.
3. Ng SB, Turner EH, Robertson PD, Flygare SD, Bigham AW, Lee C, Shaffer T, Wong M, Bhattacharjee A, Eichler EE, Bamshad M, Nickerson DA, Shendure J: **Targeted capture and massively parallel sequencing of 12 human exomes.** *Nature* 2009, **461**:272–276.
4. Cooper DN, Chen JM, Ball EV, Howells K, Mort M, Phillips AD, Chuzhanova N, Krawczak M, Kehrer-Sawatzki H, Stenson PD: **Genes mutations, and human inherited disease at the dawn of the age of personalized genomics.** *Hum Mutat* 2010, **31**:631–655.
5. MacArthur DG, Tyler-Smith C: **Loss-of-function variants in the genomes of healthy humans.** *Hum Mol Genet* 2010, **19**:R125–R130.
6. Raymond FL, Whibley A, Stratton MR, Gecz J: **Lessons learnt from large-scale exon re-sequencing of the X chromosome.** *Hum Mol Genet* 2009, **18**: R60–R64.
7. Freedman ML, Monteiro AN, Gayther SA, Coetzee GA, Risch A, Plass C, Casey G, De Biasi M, Carlson C, Duggan D, James M, Liu P, Tichelaar JW, Vikis HG, You M, Mills IG: **Principles for the post-GWAS functional characterization of cancer risk loci.** *Nat Genet* 2011, **43**:513–518.
8. Schulz LC: **The Dutch Hunger Winter and the developmental origins of health and disease.** *Proc Natl Acad of Sci USA* 2010, **107**:16757–16758.
9. Morgan HD, Sutherland HG, Martin DI, Whitelaw E: **Epigenetic inheritance at the agouti locus in the mouse.** *Nat Genet* 1999, **23**:314–318.
10. Gluckman P, Hanson M: *The Fetal Matrix. Evolution, Development and Disease.* Cambridge: Cambridge University Press; 2005.
11. Down TA, Rakyan VK, Turner DJ, Flicek P, Li H, Kulesha E, Gräf S, Johnson N, Herrero J, Tomazou EM, Thorne NP, Bäckdahl L, Herberth M, Howe KL, Jackson DK, Miretti MM, Marioni JC, Birney E, Hubbard TJ, Durbin R, Tavaré S, Beck S: **A Bayesian deconvolution strategy for immunoprecipitation-based DNA methylome analysis.** *Nat Biotechnol* 2008, **26**:779–785.
12. Harris RA, Wang T, Coarfa C, Nagarajan RP, Hong C, Downey SL, Johnson BE, Fouse SD, Delaney A, Zhao Y, Olshen A, Ballinger T, Zhou X, Forsberg KJ, Gu J, Echipare L, O'Geen H, Lister R, Pelizzola M, Xi Y, Epstein CB, Bernstein BE, Hawkins RD, Ren B, Chung WY, Gu H, Bock C, Gnirke A, Zhang MQ, Haussler D, *et al*: **Comparison of sequencing-based methods to profile DNA methylation and identification of monoallelic epigenetic modifications.** *Nat Biotechnol* 2010, **28**:1097–1105.
13. Bock C, Tomazou EM, Brinkman AB, Müller F, Simmer F, Gu H, Jäger N, Gnirke A, Stunnenberg HG, Meissner A: **Quantitative comparison of genome-wide DNA methylation mapping technologies.** *Nat Biotechnol* 2010, **28**:1106–1114.
14. Bernstein BE, Mikkelsen TS, Xie X, Kamal M, Huebert DJ, Cuff J, Fry B, Meissner A, Wernig M, Plath K, Jaenisch R, Wagschal A, Feil R, Schreiber SL, Lander ES: **A bivalent chromatin structure marks key developmental genes in embryonic stem cells.** *Cell* 2006, **125**:315–326.
15. Barski A, Cuddapah S, Cui K, Roh TY, Schones DE, Wang Z, Wei G, Chepelev I, Zhao K: **High-resolution profiling of histone methylations in the human genome.** *Cell* 2007, **129**:823–837.
16. Mikkelsen TS, Ku M, Jaffe DB, Issac B, Lieberman E, Giannoukos G, Alvarez P, Brockman W, Kim TK, Koche RP, Lee W, Mendenhall E, O'Donovan A, Presser A, Russ C, Xie X, Meissner A, Wernig M, Jaenisch R, Nusbaum C, Lander ES, Bernstein BE: **Genome-wide maps of chromatin state in pluripotent and lineage-committed cells.** *Nature* 2007, **448**:553–560.
17. Charlesworth B: **Effective population size and patterns of molecular evolution and variation.** *Nat Rev Genet* 2009, **10**:195–205.
18. Flint J, Mott R: **Applying mouse complex-trait resources to behavioural genetics.** *Nature* 2008, **456**:724–727.
19. Emily M, Mailund T, Hein J, Schauser L, Schierup MH: **Using biological networks to search for interacting loci in genome-wide association studies.** *Eur J Hum Genet* 2009, **17**:1231–1234.
20. Bradford-Hill A: **The environment and disease: association or causation?** *Proc R Soc Med* 1965, **58**:295–300.
21. Reich DE, Lander ES: **On the allelic spectrum of human disease.** *Trends in Genetics* 2001, **17**:502–510.
22. Risch N, Merikangas K: **The future of genetic studies of complex human diseases.** *Science* 1996, **273**:1516–1517.
23. Clerget-Darpoux F, Elston RC: **Are linkage analysis and the collection of family data dead? Prospects for family studies in the age of genome-wide association.** *Hum Hered* 2007, **64**:91–96.
24. Hernandez RD, Kelley JL, Elyashiv E, Melton SC, Auton A, McVean G, 1000 Genomes Project, Sella G, Przeworski M: **Classic selective sweeps were rare in recent human evolution.** *Science* 2011, **331**:920–924.
25. Xue Y, Zhang X, Huang N, Daly A, Gillson CJ, Macarthur DG, Yngvadottir B, Nica AC, Woodwark C, Chen Y, Conrad DF, Ayub Q, Mehdi SQ, Li P, Tyler-Smith C: **Population differentiation as an indicator of recent positive selection in humans: an empirical evaluation.** *Genetics* 2009, **183**:1065–1077.
26. Laland KN, Odling-Smee J, Myles S: **How culture shaped the human genome: bringing genetics and the human sciences together.** *Nat Rev Genet* 2010, **11**:137–148.
27. The 1000 Genomes Consortium: **A map of human genome variation from population-scale sequencing.** *Nature* 2010, **467**:1061–1073.
28. De S: **Somatic mosaicism in healthy human tissues.** *Trends in Genetics* 2011, **27**:217–223.
29. Shah SP, Morin RD, Khattra J, Prentice L, Pugh T, Burleigh A, Delaney A, Gelmon K, Guliany R, Senz J, Steidl C, Holt RA, Jones S, Sun M, Leung G, Moore R, Severson T, Taylor GA, Teschendorff AE, Tse K, Turashvili G, Varhol R, Warren RL, Watson P, Zhao Y, Caldas C, Huntsman D, Hirst M, Marra MA, Aparicio S: **Mutational evolution in a lobular breast tumour profiled at single nucleotide resolution.** *Nature* 2009, **461**:809–813.
30. Sehnert AJ, Rhees B, Comstock D, de Feo E, Heilek G, Burke J, Rava RP: **Optimal detection of fetal chromosomal abnormalities by massively parallel DNA sequencing of cell-free fetal DNA from maternal blood.** *Clin Chem* 2011, **57**:1042–1049.
31. Kinde I, Wu J, Papadopoulos N, Kinzler KW, Vogelstein B: **Detection and quantification of rare mutations with massively parallel sequencing.** *Proc Natl Acad Sci USA* 2011, **108**:9530–9535.
32. Chiu RWK, Akolekar R, Zheng YW, Leung TY, Sun H, Chan KC, Lun FM, Go AT, Lau ET, To WW, Leung WC, Tang RY, Au-Yeung SK, Lam H, Kung YY, Zhang X, van Vugt JM, Minekawa R, Tang MH, Wang J, Oudejans CB, Lau TK, Nicolaides KH, Lo YM: **Non-invasive prenatal assessment of trisomy 21 by multiplexed maternal plasma DNA sequencing: large scale validity study.** *British Medical Journal* 2011, **342**. doi:10.1136/bmj.c7401.
33. Lo YM, Chan KC, Sun H, Chen EZ, Jiang P, Lun FM, Zheng YW, Leung TY, Lau TK, Cantor CR, Chiu RW: **Maternal plasma DNA sequencing reveals the genome-wide genetic and mutational profile of the fetus.** *Science Translational Medicine* 2010, **2**:61–91.
34. Williams HJ, Craddock N, Russo G, Hamshere ML, Moskvina V, Dwyer S, Smith RL, Green E, Grozeva D, Holmans P, Owen MJ, O'Donovan MC: **Most genome-wide significant susceptibility loci for schizophrenia and bipolar disorder reported to date cross-traditional diagnostic boundaries.** *Hum Mol Genet* 2011, **20**:387–391.

35. Green EK, Grozeva D, Jones I, Jones L, Kirov G, Caesar S, Gordon-Smith K, Fraser C, Forty L, Russell E, Hamshere ML, Moskvina V, Nikolov I, Farmer A, McGuffin P, Wellcome Trust Case Control Consortium, Holmans PA, Owen MJ, O'Donovan MC, Craddock N: **The bipolar disorder risk allele at CACNA1C also confers risk of recurrent major depression and of schizophrenia.** *Molecular Psychiatry* 2010, **15:**1016–1022.

36. Girard SL, Gauthier J, Noreau A, Xiong L, Zhou S, Jouan L, Dionne-Laporte A, Spiegelman D, Henrion E, Diallo O, Thibodeau P, Bachand I, Bao JY, Tong AH, Lin CH, Millet B, Jaafari N, Joober R, Dion PA, Lok S, Krebs MO, Rouleau GA: **Increased exonic de novo mutation rate in individuals with schizophrenia.** *Nat Genet* 2011, **43:**860–863.

37. Xu B, Roos JL, Dexheimer P, Boone B, Plummer B, Levy S, Gogos JA, Karayiorgou M: **Exome sequencing supports a de novo mutational paradigm for schizophrenia.** *Nat Genet* 2011, **43:**864–868.

38. Nachman MW, Crowell SL: **Estimate of the mutation rate per nucleotide in humans.** *Genetics* 2000, **156:**297–304.

39. Kondrashov AS: **Direct estimates of human per nucleotide mutation rates at 20 loci causing Mendelian diseases.** *Hum Mutat* 2003, **21:**12–27.

40. Ponting CP, Lunter G: **Signatures of adaptive evolution within human non-coding sequence.** *Hum Mol Genet* 2006, **15:**R170–175.

41. Eyre-Walker A, Keightley PD: **The distribution of fitness effects of new mutations.** *Nat Rev Genet* 2007, **8:**610–618.

42. Roach JC, Glusman G, Smit AF, Huff CD, Hubley R, Shannon PT, Rowen L, Pant KP, Goodman N, Bamshad M, Shendure J, Drmanac R, Jorde LB, Hood L, Galas DJ: **Analysis of genetic inheritance in a family quartet by whole-genome sequencing.** *Science* 2010, **328:**636–639.

43. Goriely A, McVean GA, Röjmyr M, Ingemarsson B, Wilkie AO: **Evidence for selective advantage of pathogenic *FGFR2* mutations in the male germ line.** *Science* 2003, **301:**643–646.

44. Goriely A, McVean GA, van Pelt AM, O'Rourke AW, Wall SA, de Rooij DG, Wilkie AO: **Gain-of-function amino acid substitutions drive positive selection of *FGFR2* mutations in human spermatogonia.** *Proc Natl Acad Sci USA* 2005, **102:**6051–6056.

45. Qin J, Calabrese P, Tiemann-Boege I, Shinde DN, Yoon SR, Gelfand D, Bauer K, Arnheim N: **The molecular anatomy of spontaneous germline mutations in human testes.** *Public Library of Science Biology* 2007, **5:**e224.

46. Goriely A, Hansen RM, Taylor IB, Olesen IA, Jacobsen GK, McGowan SJ, Pfeifer SP, McVean GA, Rajpert-De Meyts E, Wilkie AO: **Activating mutations in *FGFR3* and HRAS reveal a shared genetic origin for congenital disorders and testicular tumors.** *Nat Genet* 2009, **41:**1247–1252.

47. Goriely A, Wilkie AOM: **Missing heritability: paternal age effect mutations and selfish spermatogonia.** *Nat Rev Genet* 2010, **11:**589.

48. Stefansson H, Rujescu D, Cichon S, Pietiläinen OP, Ingason A, Steinberg S, Fossdal R, Sigurdsson E, Sigmundsson T, Buizer-Voskamp JE, Hansen T, Jakobsen KD, Muglia P, Francks C, Matthews PM, Gylfason A, Halldorsson BV, Gudbjartsson D, Thorgeirsson TE, Sigurdsson A, Jonasdottir A, Jonasdottir A, Bjornsson A, Mattiasdottir S, Blondal T, Haraldsson M, Magnusdottir BB, Giegling I, Möller HJ, Hartmann A, *et al*: **Large recurrent microdeletions associated with schizophrenia.** *Nature* 2008, **455:**232–236.

49. Walsh T, McClellan JM, McCarthy SE, Addington AM, Pierce SB, Cooper GM, Nord AS, Kusenda M, Malhotra D, Bhandari A, Stray SM, Rippey CF, Roccanova P, Makarov V, Lakshmi B, Findling RL, Sikich L, Stromberg T, Merriman B, Gogtay N, Butler P, Eckstrand K, Noory L, Gochman P, Long R, Chen Z, Davis S, Baker C, Eichler EE, Meltzer PS, *et al*: **Rare structural variants disrupt multiple genes in neurodevelopmental pathways in schizophrenia.** *Science* 2008, **320:**539–543.

50. Williams NM, Zaharieva I, Martin A, Langley K, Mantripragada K, Fossdal R, Stefansson H, Stefansson K, Magnusson P, Gudmundsson OO, Gustafsson O, Holmans P, Owen MJ, O'Donovan M, Thapar A: **Rare chromosomal deletions and duplications in attention-deficit hyperactivity disorder: a genome-wide analysis.** *Lancet* 2010, **376:**1401–1408.

51. Mallal S, Nolan D, Witt C, Masel G, Martin AM, Moore C, Sayer D, Castley A, Mamotte C, Maxwell D, James I, Christiansen FT: **Association between presence of HLA-B*5701 HLA-DR7, and HLA-DQ3 and hypersensitivity to HIV-1 reverse-transcriptase inhibitor abacavir.** *Lancet* 2002, **359:**727–732.

52. Mallal S, Phillips E, Carosi G, Molina JM, Workman C, Tomazic J, Jägel-Guedes E, Rugina S, Kozyrev O, Cid JF, Hay P, Nolan D, Hughes S, Hughes A, Ryan S, Fitch N, Thorborn D, Benbow A, PREDICT-1 Study Team: **HLA-B*5701 screening for hypersensitivity to abacavir.** *N Engl J Med* 2008, **358:**568–578.

53. Furness P, Zimmern R, Wright C, Adams M: *The Evaluation of Diagnostic Laboratory Tests and Complex Biomarkers.* Cambridge and The Royal College of Pathologists, London: Public Health Genetics Foundation; 2008.

54. Manson N, O'Neill O: *Rethinking Informed Consent in Bioethics.* Cambridge, England: Cambridge University Press; 2007.

55. Lobb EA, Barlow-Stewart K, Suthers G, Hallowell N: **Treatment-focused DNA testing for newly diagnosed breast cancer patients: some implications for clinical practice.** *Clin Genet* 2010, **77:**350–354.

56. Wood F, Kowalczuk J, Elwyn G, Mitchell C, Gallacher J: **Achieving online consent to participation in large-scale gene-environment studies: a tangible destination.** *Journal of Medical Ethics* 2011, **37:**487–492.

57. Lunshof J, Chadwick R, Vorhaus D, Church G: **From genetic privacy to open consent.** *Nat Rev Genet* 2008, **9:**406–411.

58. Knoppers BM: **Consent to 'personal' genomics and privacy.** *European Molecular Biology Reports* 2010, **11:**416–419.

59. Ashley EA, Butte AJ, Wheeler MT, Chen R, Klein TE, Dewey FE, Dudley JT, Ormond KE, Pavlovic A, Morgan AA, Pushkarev D, Neff NF, Hudgins L, Gong L, Hodges LM, Berlin DS, Thorn CF, Sangkuhl K, Hebert JM, Woon M, Sagreiya H, Whaley R, Knowles JW, Chou MF, Thakuria JV, Rosenbaum AM, Zaranek AW, Church GM, Greely HT, Quake SR, *et al*: **Clinical assessment incorporating a personal genome.** *Lancet* 2010, **375:**1525–1535.

60. Khoury MJ, Wagener DK: **Epidemiological evaluation of the use of genetics to improve the predictive value of disease risk factors.** *Am J Hum Genet* 1995, **56:**835–844.

61. Wallace HM: **Model of gene-gene and gene-environment interactions and its implications for targeting environmental interventions by genotype.** *Theoretical Biology and Medical Modelling* 2006, **3:**35.

62. Terwilliger JD, Weiss KM: **Confounding ascertainment bias, and the blind quest for a genetic 'fountain of youth'.** *Annals of Medicine* 2003, **35:**532–544.

63. Guo S: **The behaviors of some heritability estimators in the complete absence of genetic factors.** *Hum Hered* 1999, **49:**215–228.

64. Yang J, Benyamin B, McEvoy BP, Gordon S, Henders AK, Nyholt DR, Madden PA, Heath AC, Martin NG, Montgomery GW, Goddard ME, Visscher PM: **Common SNPs explain a large proportion of the heritability for human height.** *Nat Genet* 2010, **42:**565–569.

65. Visscher PM, Yang J, Goddard ME: **A commentary on 'common SNPs explain a large proportion of the heritability for human height' by Yang et al (2010).** *Twin Research and Human Genetics* 2010, **13:**517–24.

66. Lanktree MB, Guo Y, Murtaza M, Glessner JT, Bailey SD, Onland-Moret NC, Lettre G, Ongen H, Rajagopalan R, Johnson T, Shen H, Nelson CP, Klopp N, Baumert J, Padmanabhan S, Pankratz N, Pankow JS, Shah S, Taylor K, Barnard J, Peters BJ, Maloney CM, Lobmeyer MT, Stanton A, Zafarmand MH, Romaine SP, Mehta A, van Iperen EP, Gong Y, Price TS, *et al*: **Meta-analysis of Dense Genecentric Association Studies reveals common and uncommon variants associated with height.** *Am J Hum Genet* 2011, **88:**6–18.

67. So HC, Li M, Sham PC: **Uncovering the total heritability explained by all true susceptibility variants in a genome-wide association study.** *Genetic Epidemiology* 2011, **35:**447–456.

68. Kahn SD: **On the future of genomic data.** *Science* 2011, **331:**728–729.

2

A hypomorphic inherited pathogenic variant in DDX3X causes male intellectual disability with additional neurodevelopmental and neurodegenerative features

Georgios Kellaris[1,2], Kamal Khan[1,3], Shahid M. Baig[3], I-Chun Tsai[1], Francisca Millan Zamora[6], Paul Ruggieri[4], Marvin R. Natowicz[5] and Nicholas Katsanis[1,4*]

Abstract

Background: Intellectual disability (ID) is a common condition with a population prevalence frequency of 1–3% and an enrichment for males, driven in part by the contribution of mutant alleles on the X-chromosome. Among the more than 500 genes associated with ID, *DDX3X* represents an outlier in sex specificity. Nearly all reported pathogenic variants of *DDX3X* are de novo, affect mostly females, and appear to be loss of function variants, consistent with the hypothesis that haploinsufficiency at this locus on the X-chromosome is likely to be lethal in males.

Results: We evaluated two male siblings with syndromic features characterized by mild-to-moderate ID and progressive spasticity. Quad-based whole-exome sequencing revealed a maternally inherited missense variant encoding p.R79K in *DDX3X* in both siblings and no other apparent pathogenic variants. We assessed its possible relevance to their phenotype using an established functional assay for DDX3X activity in zebrafish embryos and found that this allele causes a partial loss of DDX3X function and thus represents a hypomorphic variant.

Conclusions: Our genetic and functional data suggest that partial loss of function of *DDX3X* can cause syndromic ID. The p.R79K allele affects a region of the protein outside the critical RNA helicase domain, offering a credible explanation for the observed retention of partial function, viability in hemizygous males, and lack of pathology in females. These findings expand the gender spectrum of pathology of this locus and suggest that analysis for *DDX3X* variants should be considered relevant for both males and females.

Background

Intellectual disability (ID) is a common (estimated prevalence of 1–3% [1–3]), clinically variable phenotype, defined by impairment in both intellectual function and adaptive behavior, with onset during the developmental period [4, 5]. ID is clinically and etiologically heterogeneous, with varying disability of the two aspects of the condition [6]. In addition, ID can occur as an isolated trait but is accompanied frequently by one or more comorbidities; these can include seizures or other neurological involvement [7], microcephaly or macrocephaly [8], dysmorphic features, and structural and/or functional abnormalities in organ systems other than the brain [9].

ID is more prevalent in males than females with a ratio of 1.3–1.4:1 [10], a gender bias partially reflective of the observation that numerous genes on the X-chromosome contribute to ID under an X-linked recessive paradigm [10]. Indeed, substantial gene discovery efforts have focused on male-enriched or male-specific cohorts as a means to accelerate the discovery of ID-associated genes and mutational mechanisms [10]. Genetic and genomic

* Correspondence: natowim@ccf.org; nicholas.katsanis@duke.edu
[1]Center for Human Disease Modeling, Duke University, 300 North Duke Street, Durham, NC 27701, USA
[4]Imaging Institute, Cleveland Clinic, 9500 Euclid Avenue, Cleveland, OH 44195, USA
Full list of author information is available at the end of the article

studies of individuals, families, and populations with ID have led to the identification of more than 500 mutated genes, with some estimates predicting that number to exceed 1000, possibly reflective of the large number of transcripts expressed in and necessary for the development and maintenance of the central nervous system [10, 11]. In several instances, female carriers are protected by virtue of functional mosaicism due to random X-inactivation or by X-inactivation that favors the wild-type allele [12]. Further phenotypic analyses have also led to the appreciation of subtle phenotypic defects under a dosage model, in which males manifest the extreme range of pathology and females are partially protected [13].

The *DDX3X* locus on Xp11.4 represents an exception to the male specificity paradigm. To date, *DDX3X* pathogenic variants have been reported in 35 females with ID [3, 14], all of which were de novo. As of September 2017, 52 cases have been deposited in Decipher: 49 females, all but one of whom have de novo alleles (the 50th was inherited from a mosaic father) and three males, two harbor de novo mutations and one whose mutation is of unknown origin [15]. Consistent with the intolerance of the locus to variation [3], there are no null alleles found in control populations of either gender and a concomitant depletion of missense variants as well [16].

Herein, we report our investigation of two adult male siblings with ID, born to parents of normal intelligence. Whole-exome sequencing (WES) identified a rare, nonsynonymous, maternally transmitted variant in *DDX3X* as a likely driver of their phenotype. DDX3X is necessary for canonical *Wnt* signaling [17], an observation utilized previously to develop an in vivo ventralization assay in zebrafish embryos as a means to assess the pathogenic potential of alleles [3]. Using this assay, we found that the *DDX3X* variant results in reduced DDX3X function, reinforcing the genetic hypothesis. Together, our data support the notion that partial loss of function in *DDX3X* can lead to ID in males and reinforce a gradient of severity model that is dependent on the strength of the mutation as it pertains to residual protein function.

Materials and methods

Subjects

We studied a pedigree with two affected male siblings. Diagnostic testing of subjects was done as part of their clinical evaluations with informed consent from the mother and assent of the two cases. Research-based testing protocols were approved by the Cleveland Clinic Institutional Review Board.

Whole-exome sequencing

WES was carried out at GeneDx, Inc. subsequent to informed consent of the parents and assent of the affected individuals. Using genomic DNA from the ID cases and their parents, the exonic regions and flanking splice junctions of the genome were captured using the Clinical Research Exome kit (Agilent Technologies, Santa Clara, CA). Massively parallel (NextGen) sequencing was done on an Illumina system with 100 bp paired-end reads. The percent coverage at 10X or greater in the two brothers and their two parents ranged from 97.14 to 97.49%; the younger brother had 97.18% coverage that was at least 10X and the older brother had 97.49% coverage at least at 10X. The mean coverage in the younger brother was 132X and in the older brother 197X. The mean coverage in the father and the mother was 134.29X and 222.05X, respectively.

Data analysis

Reads were aligned to human genome build GRCh37/UCSC hg19 and were analyzed for sequence variants using a custom-developed analysis tool. Additional sequencing technology and variant interpretation protocols have been described [18]. The general assertion criteria for variant classification are available on the GeneDx ClinVar submission page (http://www.ncbi.nlm.nih.gov/clinvar/submitters/26957/). Variants of possible clinical significance relative to the phenotype of interest were confirmed by Sanger sequencing. Variants were named according to the following GenBank identifiers: *DDX3X* (NM_001356) and *SPG7* (NM_003119).

In vivo complementation studies in zebrafish

We obtained a plasmid containing the wild-type (wt) human open reading frame (ORF) of *DDX3X* and *WNT3A* from Ultimate ORF Collection (LifeTechnologies; clone ID *DDX3X*: IOH13891; *WNT3A*: IOH80731). Both plasmids were sequence-confirmed and cloned into the pCS2+ vector using Gateway LR clonase II-mediated recombination (LifeTechnologies) as described [19]. For *WNT3A*, a stop codon was introduced by site-directed mutagenesis using primer (5′-ctgcaaggccgccaggcacTAG GGTGGGCGCGCCGA-3′ and its reverse complement). To generate the mutant constructs for the ID-associated variant c.236 G>A (p.R79K) along with the positive control female variant c.641T>C (p.I214T) and a negative control male variant c.898G>T (p.V300F), we conducted site-directed mutagenesis using primers (c.641T>C: 5′-CTATTCCTATTACCAAAGAGAAAAG-3′, c.898G>T: 5′CTAGAGTTCGTCCTTGCGTGTTT TATGGTGGTGCCGATATT-3′, and c.236 G>A G: 5′-TTGGATCTCGTAGTGATTCAAAAGGGAAGTCTAG CTTC-3′ and their reverse complements). We then generated capped mRNA from linearized wt-*DDX3X* and *WNT3A* pCS2+ constructs as well as for *DDX3X* variants with the mMessage mMachine SP6 kit (ThermoFisher). Injections were conducted with wt (ZDR) embryos, and resulting embryos were phenotyped at 48 hpf for eye phenotypes according to established criteria (class I: hypoplasia of the eye and class II: absence of one or both eyes; [3]. The mRNAs (wt-*WNT3A*, wt-*DDX3X*, and *DDX3X* variants) were injected in the yolk of the embryos at 1–4 cell stage as described [20]. We acquired lateral and dorsal images with an AZ100 florescent microscope (Nikon), digital sight black and white camera (Nikon), and NIS Elements software (Nikon) at × 4 magnification. We determined statistical differences between pairs of batches with an unpaired *t* test.

Results

Clinical evaluations

We evaluated two affected male siblings from a non-consanguineous family (Fig. 1; Table 1; for full clinical descriptions, see Additional file 1). The eldest affected, currently 29 years old, was diagnosed with ID, macrocephaly, dysarthria, progressive spastic paraparesis, and decreased lower extremity strength. He presented for clinical evaluation at 2 years of age; he had reduced speech output for age and was easily agitated and hyperactive. He walked at 15 months, said his first words at 1–2 years, talked in sentences at 3–4 years, and was toilet-trained at 3 years. Developmental assessment at 6.5 years showed nonverbal cognitive function and composite mental processing at 5 and 3 percentiles, respectively, and adaptive behavior functions ranging from 0.3 to 3%. At age 9.5 years, he showed verbal, performance, and full-scale IQ scores of 71, 80, and 73, respectively. Assessment of communication function showed receptive and expressive language function at about 0.5 and 0.04 percentiles, while adaptive behavior assessment showed communication, daily living, and socialization functions at 1, 2, and 10 percentiles, respectively.

At 14 years of age, he developed a stiff gait. Exam at 15 years showed an acquired macrocephaly, an asymmetric spastic gait, lower extremity hyperreflexia, and tight heel cords. He began treatment with oral baclofen for spasticity at 17 years of age. He had an adjusted curriculum during high school, graduated at 19 years, and has worked part-time afterwards in a supported workplace. His gait slowly worsened and he was last able to ambulate independently at 21 years. On neurological exam at 23 years, there was a slow, spastic gait, decreased lower extremity strength, especially with hip flexion, markedly increased the tone of the lower extremities, lower extremity hyperreflexia, and slowed fine finger and rapid alternating movements. At 29 years of age, he has progressive lower extremity and hand weakness and decreased fine motor function.

Brain MRI scan at 16 years of age (Fig. 1i) showed mildly prominent lateral ventricles and cortical sulci, atrophy of the entire corpus callosum that was accentuated in the anterior body and genu, and mild, symmetric, confluent T2-hyperintensity in the supratentorial periventricular white matter. The follow-up study 2 years later demonstrated further interval enlargement of the lateral ventricles and periventricular white matter T2-hyperintensity, suggesting progression of central white matter volume loss. Myelination was otherwise within normal limits (Fig. 1ii). Cerebrospinal fluid analyses at 19 years showed a normal cell count, CSF glucose, and protein levels and normal CSF IgG synthesis and index. Metabolic testing included increased CSF alanine and intermittent mildly increased urinary lactate (Additional file 2: Table S1).

The younger affected brother, 25 years old, has progressive spastic paraparesis and tremor and learning disability/mixed expressive-receptive language disorder (Fig. 1; Table 1). The first concern about his neurodevelopmental status was when he was about 2 years old and had mildly delayed speech development; he spoke in sentences at 3 years and began speech therapy at that time. He developed an intentional hand tremor at about 6 years that worsened over time. Developmental assessment at 5.6 years showed normal development in all areas except for mild receptive and expressive language delay. Re-evaluation at 6 years showed receptive and expressive language skills at 39 and 16 percentiles, with weaknesses in auditory memory, interpreting directions, and categorizing words. Assessment at 7 years showed verbal, performance, and full-scale IQ scores of 84, 81, and 81, respectively. Academic achievement testing showed basic reading, reading comprehension, mathematics calculation, mathematics reasoning, and written expression at 1, 5, 16, 9, and 23 percentiles, respectively; receptive and expressive language tested at 37 and 16 percentiles. He did not have significant behavioral issues.

Examination at 15 years old, for worsening hand tremors, showed a non-dysmorphic male with lower extremity hyperreflexia and tremor; the gait and motor tone were normal. At 17 years, he was noted to have a mild spastic gait and bilateral Babinski signs. At 18 years, he was noted to have a worsening asymmetric spastic paretic gait and bilateral hip flexor weakness. Schooling involved an adjusted curriculum with training in service occupations, and he graduated from high school at 18 years of age, subsequently working part-time and requiring supports in complex daily living tasks.

His diagnostic evaluation included an abnormal brain MRI scans at 15, 16, and 17 years of age showing mild, diffuse prominence of the cortical sulci suggesting mild cortical volume loss and mild enlargement of the lateral ventricles, generalized volume loss in the corpus callosum that was more prominent in the genu and anterior body, and mild symmetric confluent periventricular T2-

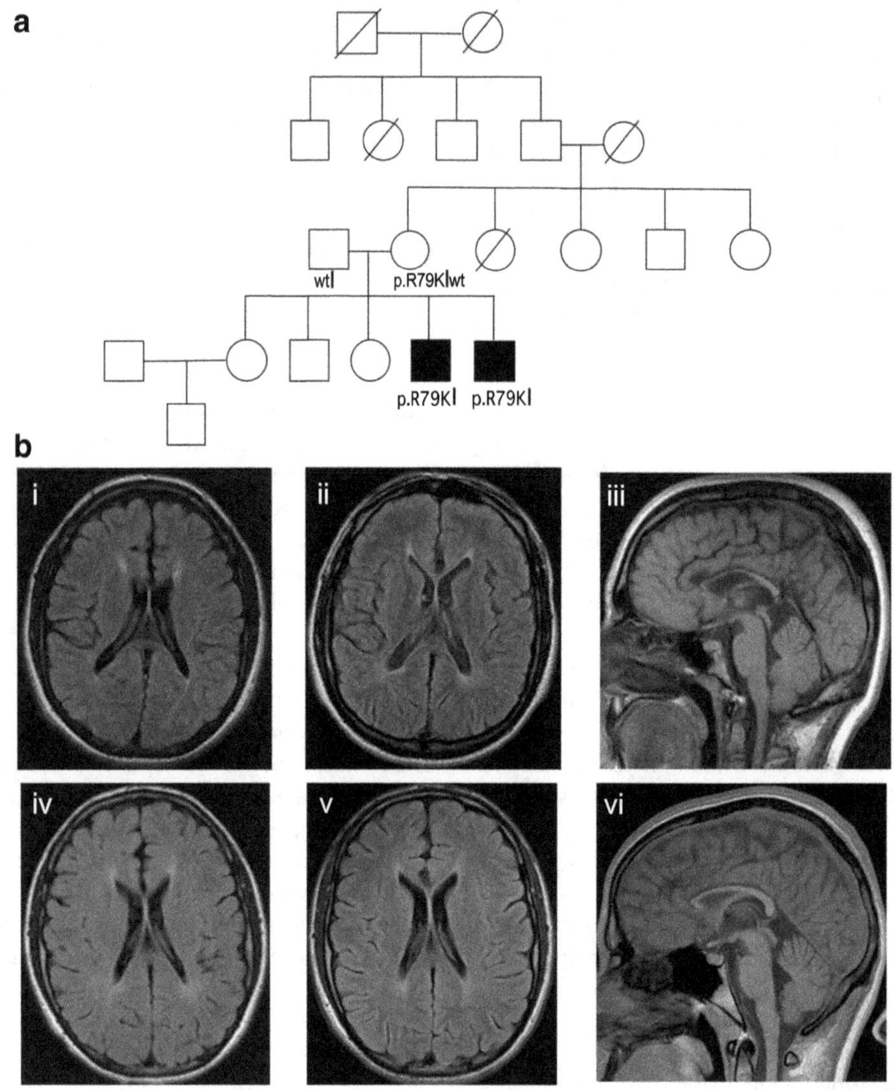

Fig. 1 Brain MRI of both affected syndromic ID cases. **a** Family pedigree showing the two affected brothers and the family pedigree. **b** (i) Axial T2 FLAIR of sibling 1 at age 16 demonstrates mild enlargement of the lateral ventricles and mild confluent hyperintensity in the adjacent white matter. (ii) Axial T2 FLAIR of sibling 1 2 years later demonstrates interval enlargement of the lateral ventricles and mild progression of the confluent hyperintensity in the adjacent white matter suggesting progressive damage to the central white matter and volume loss. (iii) Sagittal T1 demonstrates generalized volume loss in the corpus callosum that is more prominent in the genu and anterior body, further supporting central white matter volume loss that is more severe anteriorly. (iv) Axial T2 FLAIR of sibling 2 at age 15 demonstrates mild enlargement of the lateral ventricles and mild, symmetric hyperintensity in the adjacent white matter, suggesting central white matter volume loss and gliosis. (v) Axial T2 FLAIR of sibling 2 2 years later demonstrates mild interval increase in size of the lateral ventricles suggesting mild progression of central white matter volume loss, but no significant change in the periventricular hyperintensity. (vi) Sagittal T1 image is also comparable in appearance to his sibling, with prominent volume loss in the corpus callosum that is more striking anteriorly

hyperintensity within the supratentorial periventricular white matter suggesting central white matter volume loss that was more prominent in the frontal lobes (Fig. 1iv–vi). There was also slight further enlargement of the lateral ventricles without significant change in the T2-hyperintensity or the corpus callosum over the 2-year period. The MRI of the entire spinal cord was normal in caliber and signal intensity. CSF analyses showed normal cellular CSF and normal levels of CSF glucose and protein, normal CSF IgG synthesis and IgG index, normal levels of CSF lactate and pyruvate, and increased CSF alanine. Plasma amino acid analyses consistently showed mildly moderately increased levels of alanine and, sometimes, increased levels of proline and glycine (Additional file 2: Table S1).

Genomic analysis

A host of known genetic and metabolic etiologies of ID and of spasticity were ruled-out in the two cases

Table 1 Summary of clinical findings in the two subjects. Human phenotype ontology (HPO) terms and codes are shown

Phenotype	HPO code	Case 1	Case 2
Intellectual disability or related neurodevelopmental disability	HP:0001256	+	+
Macrocephaly	HP:0000256	+	+
Dysarthria	HP:0001260	+	+
Tight heel cords		+	+
Progressive spastic paraparesis	HP:0007199	+	+
Tremor	HP:0002322	–	+
Hand weakness	HP:0030237	+	–
Proximal leg weakness	HP:0007340	+	+
Brain MRI with abnormal periventricular T2 intensity	HP:0002518	+	+
Ventriculomegaly	HP:0002119	+	+
Atrophy of corpus callosum, esp. the genu and anterior body of corpus callosum	HP:0006989	+	+
Increased cerebrospinal fluid alanine level	n/a	+	+

n/a not applicable

(Additional file 2: Table S1). Consequently, given that both parents are of normal intelligence, we undertook quad-based WES analysis hypothesizing either a recessive or an X-linked paradigm of disease inheritance. Under a rare variant hypothesis, the WES data were evaluated for alleles shared among the two affected siblings that are rare (minor allele frequency < 1%) and affect coding residues or canonical splice sites. We identified several variants of potential interest (Additional file 3: Table S2), but only a single, maternally inherited variant fulfilled our stringent criteria: a c.236G>A change encoding p.R79K in *DDX3X* was identified (Fig. 2a, b). The *DDX3X* locus has been implicated previously in ID and, sometimes, other features in females; however, nearly all published variants described to date are de novo, which has led to the hypothesis that haploinsufficiency of *DDX3X* in males might be incompatible with life [3]. Nonetheless, multiple sequence alignment across vertebrates showed the p.R79 position to be conserved (Fig. 2b). Prediction algorithms were discordant: PolyPhen2 [21] predicted the allele to be benign, whereas MutationTaster [22] predicted it to be deleterious. Overall, 11 variant prediction algorithms predict this

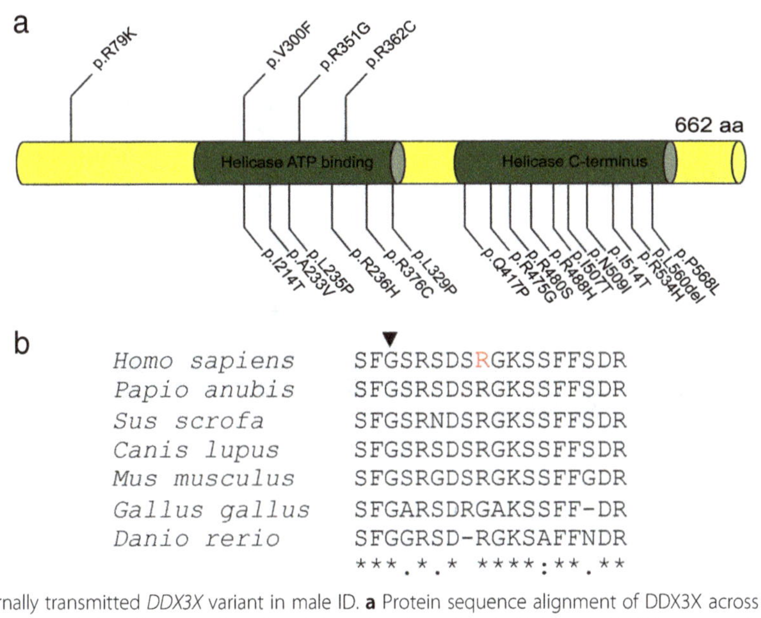

Fig. 2 Discovery of a maternally transmitted *DDX3X* variant in male ID. **a** Protein sequence alignment of DDX3X across vertebrate species; the mutated residue is shown by arrow. **b** Location of all functionally tested amino acid substitutions in DDX3X. Reported male alleles (top); alleles found in females (bottom). The helicase ATP-binding domain and a helicase C-terminal domain are also shown (green)

variant to be damaging to the structure/function of DDX3X out of a total of 21 in silico assessments [23], http://159.226.67.237/sun/varcards/welcome/index). The variant was found only once in heterozygosity, in a female, in > 170,000 control exomes [16]. We note that, in contrast to the majority of described *DDX3X* variants that lie in the helicase domain, the p.R79K variant maps proximal to that region (Fig. 2b). Together, these data raised the hypothesis that, in contrast to previously reported alleles in *DDX3X* that abrogate protein function, p.R79K might be a hypomorph, which could explain its transmission and the phenotypic outcome in this kindred.

Functional testing

We and others have shown that expression of human *DDX3X* mRNA exacerbates the ventralization phenotype induced by the expression of femtogram (fg) quantities of the canonical Wnt ligand *WNT3A* in zebrafish embryos [3]. This phenotype can be binned into two phenotypic classes (class I and class II; Fig. 3a–c) based on previously established and validated morphometric criteria [24]. Using this model system, we tested the functionality of missense *DDX3X* alleles discovered in ID patients and found that DNA sequence variants predicted to cause loss of function of *DDX3X* and which were associated with ID failed to exacerbate WNT3A-driven pathology, whereas benign alleles were indistinguishable in their activity and promoted significant Wnt-dependent pathology [3]. Here, we utilized this assay to test the activity of the p.R79K allele. First, we optimized the in vivo complementation assays to the *ZDR* wt genetic background by injecting progressively increasing doses of wt-*WNT3A*; we found that 550 fg of mRNA was sufficient to induce a modest phenotype (~ 8–15% affected embryos, $n = 50–100$ embryos per clutch, replicated; Fig. 3, Additional file 4: Figure S1, Additional file 5: Figure S2A). On this background sensitization with *WNT3A*, we titrated the amount of human *DDX3X* mRNA required to generate pathology. We found a dose-dependent effect that was maximal at 30 pg mRNA (Additional file 4: Figure S1). Therefore, we selected the 500 fg/30 pg mRNA doses to test the effect of the discovered allele. Next, we co-injected *WNT3A*-sensitized *ZDR* embryos with wt *DDX3X*, *DDX3X* encoding the candidate pathogenic allele p.R79K, the known benign allele p.V300F, and the known pathogenic allele p.I214T. Upon blind scoring to injection cocktail, both the positive and negative controls scored as expected: mRNA encoding p.300F was indistinguishable from wt, whereas p.214T failed to induce any significant pathology exceeding that of *WNT3A* alone, consistent with a null (or near null) allele. The candidate mutation of interest, p.R79K, scored intermediate, with the extent of pathology of the resulting embryos significantly different from both wt and null *DDX3X* ($p < 0.0008$ and $p < 0.01$ respectively; Fig. 3d). In contrast, expression of either wt or mutant *DDX3X* mRNA alone did not induce any appreciable pathologies, likely excluding any dominant negative mechanisms (Additional file 5: Figure S2B). Together with the human genetics and evolutionary conservation, these data suggest that the discovered allele is a likely hypomorph.

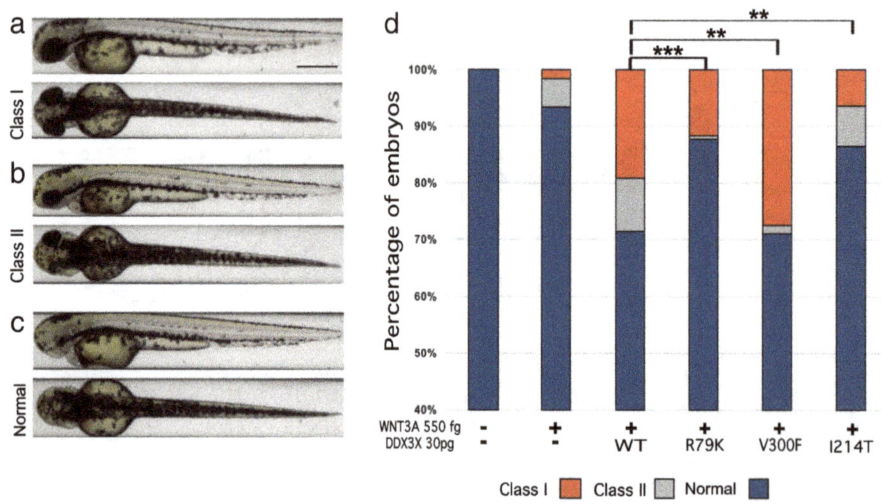

Fig. 3 Functional testing of *DDX3X* variants. **a**–**c** Representative lateral images of zebrafish embryos at 2 dpf that are either uninjected (**a**) or injected with human *WNT3A* without (**b**) or with (**c**) human *DDX3X* show a range of ventralized phenotypes. These were scored according to established criteria as normal, class I, or class II ventralization. No injection condition resulted in severe ventralization (class III or IV) [3]. **d** *DDX3X* variants were tested for their effect on increasing *WNT3A*-mediated ventralization using 550 fg of *WNT3A* mRNA and 30 pg of *DDX3X* mRNA per embryo. *P* values: < 0.0001 (four asterisks); 0.0001 to 0.001 (three asterisks); 0.001 to 0.01 (two asterisks); 0.01 to 0.05 (one asterisk); ≥ 0.05 not significant (ns)

Discussion

Here, we describe the clinical phenotypes of two adult males who have a rare, maternally inherited missense allele of *DDX3X*, a major ID locus that to date has been associated with pathology almost exclusively in females. Both genetics and functional testing support a partial loss of function disease transmission. This notion is consistent with the observation that the mother who transmitted the p.R79K is asymptomatic and that the two affected males have significant neurodevelopmental pathology but have survived. Although the formal possibility remains that the mother might exhibit sub-clinical neuroanatomical findings, careful re-examination revealed no overt neurological concerns. In addition to this notion, it would be important to identify the genotype for the maternal uncle and maternal grandfather, but DNA samples from the individuals were not available. This hypothesis is also supported by recent work in the mouse revealing essential roles of *Ddx3x* in placentation and embryogenesis and the differential phenotypic impacts of inheriting a paternal vs. maternal null allele [25]. Non-lethality of the p.R79K variant in our cases may be due to the maternal, as opposed to paternal, inheritance of the variant. Non-lethality of the p.R79K variant might also be because the location of the amino acid substitution is outside of the critical RNA helicase domain. The DDX3X protein has been investigated extensively [26], but the region of the protein surrounding amino acid residue 79 has only been studied sparingly, although site-directed mutagenesis of several nearby residues resulted in functional impacts [27, 28]. Finally, non-lethality of the p.R79K variant might be explained on the basis of the expected moderate biophysical impact on the structure of DDX3X consequent to the conservative nature of an arginine to lysine substitution.

There is substantial clinical and neuroradiologic overlap between the phenotype in our two cases and those of the females and few males described to date. The most common traits described thus far include ID, microcephaly, hypotonia, movement disorder and/or spasticity, ventricular enlargement, and hypoplasia of the corpus callosum; the subjects reported here have ID, spasticity, ventricular enlargement, and an attenuated corpus callosum. Our two cases also present with features that are distinct from those of other cases with variants in *DDX3X* reported to date; these include progressive spasticity with loss of independent ambulation and, consistent with their clinical courses, evidence of a progressive brain central white matter process including atrophy of the corpus callosum, not hypoplasia. Long-term follow-up of the previously reported cases, some of whom were young children, will be important to determine if any of the neurological findings or developmental disabilities are progressive and if there are ongoing brain white matter changes.

It is also possible that a second clinical process that is distinct from DDX3X may be present in the two subjects reported here. In this regard, both subjects have macrocephaly, as does their father and one sister although the father and the subjects' siblings have clinical phenotypes that are otherwise disparate from the clinical findings in the cases with ID. The finding of increased levels of CSF alanine in both cases and of increased plasma alanine in one case and increased urinary lactate in the other is notable and suggests a disturbance of mitochondrial bioenergetics. No evidence of a primary mitochondrial cytopathy was found, despite considerable investigation, and the relationship of these results to the variant of *DDX3X* is uncertain. In addition, the existence of a clinical process that is/was present in only one of the subjects is likely in view of the variability in neurodevelopmental phenotype between the subjects, although the basis of this process is unknown. Given the reported spasticity in this pedigree, we did evaluate known spastic paraplegia genes for candidate pathogenic variants. We detected a maternally inherited heterozygous variant in *SPG7* in one of the subjects that has been reported to be pathogenic in patients with recessive spastic paraplegia [29]. Although this allele is by itself unable to explain the observed spasticity in our patient, it is possible that it contributes to the phenotype, possibly in epistasis with *DDX3X*; the same might be true for some of the other ultra-rare alleles discovered in this family (Additional file 3: Table S2). For example, it is intriguing that the older brother with the more extensive pathology is also hemizygous for candidate pathogenic variant in *ARGHGAP4*, a gene whose product is required for neuronal migration and which has been reported to be mutated in some patients with ID [30–32]. However, both formal functional testing and delineation of additional patients will be necessary to test this hypothesis.

Conclusions

Overall, our findings suggest that mutational analysis of *DDX3X* in either genetic testing panels or by whole-exome/genome sequencing should not be limited, by testing or interpretation of data, to females. The severity of most discovered *DDX3X* alleles remains consistent with a model of total haploinsufficiency incompatible with life in males. Further studies in expanded cohorts will illuminate this proposed phenotype-genotype correlation further.

Additional files

Additional file 1: Detailed Clinical report.

Additional file 2: Table S1. Clinical Laboratory Diagnostic Evaluations.

Additional file 3: Table S2. Sequence variants identified according to mode of inheritance.

Additional file 4: Figure S1. Co-injection of *DDX3X* and *WNT3A* mRNA produces dose-dependent changes in ventralization. Zebrafish embryos were injected with 550 fg *WNT3A* mRNA without or with wt *DDX3X* mRNA at varying doses. Embryos were scored at 48 h post fertilization for degree of ventralization according to described objective criteria. *P* value: < 0.0001, (****); 0.0001 to 0.001, (***); 0.001 to 0.01, (**); 0.01 to 0.05, (*); ≥ 0.05, not significant (ns).

Additional file 5: Figure S2. Dose-response effect of WNT3A and overexpression of DDX3X variants does not produce alterations in Wnt signaling. (**A**) Injection of WNT3A produces dose-dependent changes in ventralization. Embryos were scored at 48 h post fertilization for degree of ventralization. (**B**) Zebrafish embryos were injected with 100 pg of DDX3X mRNA containing either the wild-type sequence or the non-synonymous variants found in the affected individuals. At 36 h, post-fertilization (hpf) the embryos were phenotyped; no abnormalities could be appreciated.

Acknowledgements
We thank the family for the participation and encouragement of this work. We thank Erica Davis for the critical evaluation of the manuscript and data.

Funding
NK is a Brumley Distinguished Professor of Pediatrics. The study was supported by Core Funding from the Center for Human Disease Modeling at Duke University.

Authors' contributions
GK and KK performed experiments, reviewed and compiled data, and co-wrote the paper. SMB and ICT and NK reviewed and interpreted the data and provided guidance to the work. MRN assessed the family, reviewed and interpreted the WES data, and co-wrote the manuscript. FMZ reviewed and interpreted WES. PR reviewed the brain MRIs. All authors reviewed and commented on the manuscript. All authors read and approved the final manuscript.

Consent for publication
Written informed consent for publication of clinical details and clinical images was obtained from the parent of the probands.

Competing interests
NK is a paid consultant and holds founding stock in Rescindo Therapeutics.

Author details
[1]Center for Human Disease Modeling, Duke University, 300 North Duke Street, Durham, NC 27701, USA. [2]Department of Medical Genetics, University of Athens Medical School, Aghia Sophia Children's Hospital, 11527 Athens, Greece. [3]Human Molecular Genetics Laboratory, Health Biotechnology Division, National Institute for Biotechnology and Genetic Engineering (NIBGE), Faisalabad 38000, Pakistan. [4]Imaging Institute, Cleveland Clinic, 9500 Euclid Avenue, Cleveland, OH 44195, USA. [5]Pathology and Laboratory Medicine and Genomic Medicine Institutes, Cleveland Clinic, Cleveland, OH 44195, USA. [6]GeneDx, 207 Perry Parkway, Gaithersburg, MD 20877, USA.

References
1. Wolfe K, Stueber K, McQuillin A, Jichi F, Patch C, Flinter F, Strydom A, Bass N. Genetic testing in intellectual disability psychiatry: opinions and practices of UK child and intellectual disability psychiatrists. J Appl Res Intellect Disabil. 2017;31(2):273-84.
2. van Bokhoven H. Genetic and epigenetic networks in intellectual disabilities. Annu Rev Genet. 2011;45:81–104.
3. Snijders Blok L, Madsen E, Juusola J, Gilissen C, Baralle D, Reijnders MR, Venselaar H, Helsmoortel C, Cho MT, Hoischen A, et al. Mutations in DDX3X are a common cause of unexplained intellectual disability with gender-specific effects on Wnt signaling. Am J Hum Genet. 2015;97(2):343–52.
4. Harris JC. Intellectual disability: Understanding its development, causes, classification, evaluation, and treatment. New York: Oxford University Press; 2006.
5. Tasse MJ, Luckasson R, Nygren M. AAIDD proposed recommendations for ICD-11 and the condition previously known as mental retardation. Intellect Dev Disabil. 2013;51(2):127–31.
6. American Psychiatric Association. Diagnostic and statistical manual of mental disorders : DSM-5: Fifth edition. Arlington: American Psychiatric Publishing; 2013.
7. McGrother CW, Bhaumik S, Thorp CF, Hauck A, Branford D, Watson JM. Epilepsy in adults with intellectual disabilities: prevalence, associations and service implications. Seizure. 2006;15(6):376–86.
8. de Ligt J, Willemsen MH, van Bon BW, Kleefstra T, Yntema HG, Kroes T, Vulto-van Silfhout AT, Koolen DA, de Vries P, Gilissen C, et al. Diagnostic exome sequencing in persons with severe intellectual disability. N Engl J Med. 2012;367(20):1921–9.
9. Matson JL, Cervantes PE. Comorbidity among persons with intellectual disabilities. Res Autism Spectr Disord. 2013;7(11):1318–22.
10. Vissers LE, Gilissen C, Veltman JA. Genetic studies in intellectual disability and related disorders. Nat Rev Genet. 2016;17(1):9–18.
11. Kochinke K, Zweier C, Nijhof B, Fenckova M, Cizek P, Honti F, Keerthikumar S, Oortveld MA, Kleefstra T, Kramer JM, et al. Systematic phenomics analysis deconvolutes genes mutated in intellectual disability into biologically coherent modules. Am J Hum Genet. 2016;98(1):149–64.
12. Cotton AM, Price EM, Jones MJ, Balaton BP, Kobor MS, Brown CJ. Landscape of DNA methylation on the X chromosome reflects CpG density, functional chromatin state and X-chromosome inactivation. Hum Mol Genet. 2015;24(6):1528–39.
13. Fieremans N, Van Esch H, Holvoet M, Van Goethem G, Devriendt K, Rosello M, Mayo S, Martinez F, Jhangiani S, Muzny DM, et al. Identification of intellectual disability genes in female patients with a skewed X-inactivation pattern. Hum Mutat. 2016;37(8):804–11.
14. Dikow N, Granzow M, Graul-Neumann LM, Karch S, Hinderhofer K, Paramasivam N, Behl LJ, Kaufmann L, Fischer C, Evers C, et al. DDX3X mutations in two girls with a phenotype overlapping Toriello-Carey syndrome. Am J Med Genet A. 2017;173(5):1369–73.
15. Firth HV, Richards SM, Bevan AP, Clayton S, Corpas M, Rajan D, Vooren SV, Moreau Y, Pettett RM, Carter NP. DECIPHER: database of chromosomal imbalance and phenotype in humans using ensembl resources. Am J Hum Genet. 2009;84(4):524–33.
16. Lek M, Karczewski KJ, Minikel EV, Samocha KE, Banks E, Fennell T, O'Donnell-Luria AH, Ware JS, Hill AJ, Cummings BB, et al. Analysis of protein-coding genetic variation in 60,706 humans. Nature. 2016;536:285.
17. Cruciat CM, Dolde C, de Groot RE, Ohkawara B, Reinhard C, Korswagen HC, Niehrs C. RNA helicase DDX3 is a regulatory subunit of casein kinase 1 in Wnt-beta-catenin signaling. Science. 2013;339(6126):1436–41.
18. Tanaka AJ, Cho MT, Millan F, Juusola J, Retterer K, Joshi C, Niyazov D, Garnica A, Gratz E, Deardorff M, et al. Mutations in SPATA5 are associated with microcephaly, intellectual disability, seizures, and hearing loss. Am J Hum Genet. 2015;97(3):457–64.

19. Niederriter AR, Davis EE, Golzio C, Oh EC, Tsai IC, Katsanis N. In vivo modeling of the morbid human genome using Danio rerio. J Vis Exp. 2013;78:e50338.
20. Davis EE, Frangakis S, Katsanis N. Interpreting human genetic variation with in vivo zebrafish assays. Biochim Biophys Acta. 2014;1842(10):1960–70.
21. Adzhubei IA, Schmidt S, Peshkin L, Ramensky VE, Gerasimova A, Bork P, Kondrashov AS, Sunyaev SR: A method and server for predicting damaging missense mutations. In: Nat Methods. 2010;7:248–9.
22. Schwarz JM, Cooper DN, Schuelke M, Seelow D. MutationTaster2: mutation prediction for the deep-sequencing age. Nat Methods. 2014;11:361.
23. Li M, Gong L, Zhao D, Zhou J, Xiang H. The spacer size of I-B CRISPR is modulated by the terminal sequence of the protospacer. Nucleic Acids Res. 2017;45(8):4642–54.
24. Liu YP, Tsai IC, Morleo M, Oh EC, Leitch CC, Massa F, Lee BH, Parker DS, Finley D, Zaghloul NA, et al. Ciliopathy proteins regulate paracrine signaling by modulating proteasomal degradation of mediators. J Clin Invest. 2014;124(5):2059–70.
25. Chen C-Y, Chan C-H, Chen C-M, Tsai Y-S, Tsai T-Y, Wu Lee Y-H, You L-R. Targeted inactivation of murine Ddx3x: essential roles of Ddx3x in placentation and embryogenesis. Hum Mol Genet. 2016;25(14):2905–22.
26. Sharma D, Jankowsky E. The Ded1/DDX3 subfamily of DEAD-box RNA helicases. Crit Rev Biochem Mol Biol. 2014;49(4):343–60.
27. Gu L, Fullam A, Brennan R, Schroder M. Human DEAD box helicase 3 couples IkappaB kinase epsilon to interferon regulatory factor 3 activation. Mol Cell Biol. 2013;33(10):2004–15.
28. Oda S, Schroder M, Khan AR. Structural basis for targeting of human RNA helicase DDX3 by poxvirus protein K7. Structure. 2009;17(11):1528–37.
29. Elleuch N, Depienne C, Benomar A, Hernandez AM, Ferrer X, Fontaine B, Grid D, Tallaksen CM, Zemmouri R, Stevanin G, et al. Mutation analysis of the paraplegin gene (SPG7) in patients with hereditary spastic paraplegia. Neurology. 2006;66(5):654–9.
30. Vogt DL, Gray CD, Young WS 3rd, Orellana SA, Malouf AT. ARHGAP4 is anovel RhoGAP that mediates inhibiotion of cell motility and axonal outgrowth. Mol Cell Neurosci. 2007;36(3):332–42.
31. Liu F, Guo H, Ou M, Hou X, Sun G, Gong W, Jing H, Tan Q, Xue W, Dai Y, Sui W. ARHGAP4 mutated in a Chinese intellectually challenged family. Gene. 2016;578(2):205–9.
32. Huang L, Poke G, Gecz J, Gibson K. A novel contiguous gene deletion of AVPR2 and ARHGAP4 genes in male dizygotic twins with nephrogenic diabetes insipidus and intellectual disability. Am J Med Genet A. 2012;158a(10):2511–8.

3

Clinical application of next-generation sequencing for Mendelian diseases

Saumya Shekhar Jamuar[1,2] and Ene-Choo Tan[2,3*]

Abstract

Over the past decade, next-generation sequencing (NGS) has led to an exponential increase in our understanding of the genetic basis of Mendelian diseases. NGS allows for the analysis of multiple regions of the genome in one single reaction and has been shown to be a cost-effective and efficient tool in investigating patients with Mendelian diseases. More recently, NGS has been successfully deployed in the clinics, with a reported diagnostic yield of ~25 %. However, recommendations on clinical implementation of NGS are still evolving with numerous key challenges that impede the widespread use of genetics in everyday medicine. These challenges include when to order, on whom to order, what type of test to order, and how to interpret and communicate the results, including incidental findings, to the patient and family. In this review, we discuss these challenges and suggest guidelines on implementing NGS in the routine clinical workflow.

Keywords: Next-generation sequencing, Whole exome sequencing, Clinical applications, Mendelian diseases

Introduction

Mendelian diseases, also known as monogenic diseases, are disorders caused by mutations in one gene and include diseases like thalassemia, cystic fibrosis, among others. Mendelian diseases are considered to be rare individually but collectively occur at a rate of 40 to 82 per 1000 live births, with an estimated 7.9 million children being born annually with a serious birth defect of genetic or partially genetic origin [1, 2]. These disorders tend to run in families, although it has been found that a significant number are caused by de novo events [3]. Depending on the pathomechanism, the phenotype is manifested in a dominant (where one allele is mutated) or recessive (where both alleles are mutated) manner [4]. Of the estimated 20,000–25,000 protein-coding genes in the human genome, mutations in 3348 genes have been associated with Mendelian diseases [5].

Sanger sequencing, also known as the dideoxy method [6], has been the gold standard in molecular diagnostics in Mendelian diseases and remains the test of choice for clinical genetic testing; the purpose of which is to confirm a suspected diagnosis and allow more accurate genetic counseling. However, Sanger sequencing can only analyze one DNA segment at a time and is thus laborious and time consuming. For diseases with genetic heterogeneity, like retinitis pigmentosa, cardiomyopathy, and deafness, a gene-by-gene Sanger sequencing approach has not been shown to be economical or efficient [7].

Recent advances over the past decade have allowed for high-throughput sequencing, and these advances are collectively referred to as next-generation sequencing (NGS). NGS has allowed for substantial increase in sequencing content while dramatically reducing the cost of sequencing per base. This allows for simultaneous interrogation of multiple genes through one single reaction and has been proven to be an effective alternative for establishing the genetic basic of Mendelian diseases in the research setting [8–11], and more recently, in the clinical setting [12–16].

In this review, we shall aim to discuss the clinical utility of NGS, including the opportunities and challenges that arise from the clinical standpoint. We will also focus our discussion on ways of implementing NGS in the routine clinical workflow.

* Correspondence: tanec@bigfoot.com

[2]Paediatrics Academic Clinical Programme, SingHealth Duke-NUS Graduate Medical School, Singapore, Singapore

[3]KK Research Centre, KK Women's and Children's Hospital, 100 Bukit Timah Road, 229899 Singapore, Singapore

Full list of author information is available at the end of the article

Next-generation sequencing: brief overview

The process of NGS starts with extraction of DNA of an individual, most commonly from peripheral leukocytes obtained from blood sample but can be from another tissue such as buccal swab or saliva. The DNA is then broken down into short fragments and amplified using polymerase chain reaction (PCR) or hybridization-based approaches. The regions that are amplified could include either a subset of genes (targeted approach) or all the genes in the genome [9]. When sequencing all the genes, if only the protein-coding regions are amplified, the method is referred to as whole exome sequencing (WES). However, if the target is the entire genome, then it is known as whole genome sequencing (WGS).

These amplified products are then sequenced with the use of one of the various sequencing technologies (e.g., Illumina's sequencing by synthesis, Life Technologies' sequencing by ligation, or Ion semiconductor sequencing) to generate millions of short sequence reads. These sequences are then processed bioinformatically. First, they are aligned to a reference genome (assembly) and then compared for similarities and differences at each target position. A list of variants (or differences in the sequence) is then generated, which is then filtered further, to determine the significance of each of the variant. Common filters include rare or previously unreported variants, variants that lead to altered function of the protein, and variants previously reported to cause disease [17]. More recently, algorithms that include the phenotypic information in the variant analysis have been developed that aid the clinician/researcher in narrowing down the candidate gene list [18, 19].

Next-generation sequencing in the clinical setting

Targeted vs whole exome sequencing

One of the biggest challenges clinicians are facing is deciding between using targeted versus whole exome sequencing. As the cost of sequencing continues to decrease, WES appears to be a more cost-effective approach. However, there are certain considerations before embarking on one over the other.

Although exomes are supposed to cover the protein-coding regions of the genome, the overall coverage tends to be between 85–95 % only. This means that a particular gene of interest with respect to a specific phenotype may not be covered, either completely or partially. Reasons include poorly performing capture probes due to high GC content, sequence homology, or repetitive sequences. A targeted approach, on the other hand, has a much higher or even complete coverage of all the phenotype-specific genes by filling in the gaps with complementary technologies such as Sanger sequencing or long range PCR. For example, 4 of the 73 genes in a hearing loss panel are inadequately covered on WES but are completely covered in a targeted panel [20].

Besides offering a more comprehensive coverage of the "known" phenotype-specific genes, a targeted approach also allows for deeper coverage of these genes compared to WES, which provides greater confidence in the variants detected. However, both are still prone to sequencing artifacts, and Sanger sequencing of candidate variants is recommended in both approaches before returning the results to the patients [20].

Lastly, laboratories that offer targeted testing may have expert knowledge for the given phenotype and may be in a better position to prioritize variants detected through NGS. They may also be able to recommend specific evaluations to determine the significance of certain variants; for example, temporal bone evaluation for *SLC26A4* and otoacoustic emission testing for *OTOF* when variants are detected on a targeted hearing loss panel [20].

Indications and clinical usefulness

NGS is currently indicated for the detection of rare variants in patients with a phenotype suspected to be due to a Mendelian disease. This is done either after single gene testing for candidates has returned negative, or as first line, if there exists genetic heterogeneity where multi-gene Sanger sequencing would be costly and time consuming. Diseases could either include a specific phenotype such as cardiomyopathy, deafness, retinitis pigmentosa, intellectual disability, or be part of a multiple congenital anomaly spectrum (where two or more organs are affected) [21].

The clinical usefulness of performing NGS in the clinical setting varies for different disorders. In the majority of cases, the finding does not alter the clinical management, treatment or prognosis. However, it does allow an end to an expensive and stressful diagnostic odyssey. Reaching a molecular diagnosis allows the clinician to allay the guilt that parents face in the absence of a firm diagnosis [13, 17] and helps them to accept the child's condition.

Identification of the causative variant allows for gene-specific prognostication [22, 23], based on cases reported in the literature and, in some cases, family support groups. It can also allow for anticipatory management of other comorbidities that an individual may be susceptible to. These include assessing other organs (such as performing blood tests and imaging to assess the heart and kidneys) for possible complications. In some cases, it may redirect therapy to treat the underlying genetic etiology as illustrated by the case of a 15-month-old child with clinical presentation mimicking Crohn's disease. WES revealed a pathogenic variant in *XIAP*, affecting the proinflammatory response and bacterial sensing, predisposing the individual to developing hemophagocytosis. Based on these findings, the child was successfully treated with hematopoietic bone marrow transplantation which cured him of his gastrointestinal disease as well [24].

More importantly, it facilitates genetic counseling and allows for more accurate estimates of recurrence risk in the family. Identification of the molecular etiology allows the clinician to guide subsequent pregnancies, either through prenatal diagnostics or preimplantation genetic diagnosis. In some situations, it also allows for identification of other at-risk family members and any available treatment can be instituted in the presymptomatic phase [17]. For example, identification of mutation in a gene causing long QT syndrome in the proband can allow identification of other at-risk family members, who can then have regular Holter monitoring and, in some instances, implantation of a cardiac pacemaker before a catastrophic event occurs [25, 26].

Lastly, as our understanding of the molecular pathways and gene-gene interactions improves, it is possible that targeted molecular therapy may be available for a specific genetic mutation that helps to ameliorate the patient's symptoms. For example, in individuals with vascular malformations, somatic mutations in the *AKT3-PI3K-mTOR* pathway have been identified. Some of these patients have been successfully treated with mTOR-inhibitors such as rapamycin [27, 28]. Our ability to offer such targeted therapy will only improve with time as more high-throughput drug screening methods are being deployed.

Gathering information

The process of ordering NGS starts with gathering a detailed family history to determine if there are individuals with similar or related phenotypes within the same family, as well as to assess for possible inheritance pattern. For example, multiple individuals in the same generation and/or history of consanguinity will suggest a recessive pattern, while having affected individuals in each generation would suggest a dominant pattern [4].

The next step is to perform detailed phenotyping of the affected individual(s). These could include evaluations from other subspecialists and/or performing biochemical and/or radiological tests. For example, a child with a limb anomaly would benefit from cardiac, gastrointestinal, renal, and skeletal evaluations. With the phenotype and pedigree information, a systematic review of literature or syndrome database should be performed to exclude rare but established syndromes [17]. This can then guide the clinician on which gene(s) to test. In cases of genetic heterogeneity, targeted NGS may be the preferred approach. On the other hand, if the disease mechanism is unknown, WES may be the test of choice.

Pretest counseling and informed consent

It is imperative that a patient and his/her family are counseled appropriately by a healthcare professional (such as a clinical geneticist or genetic counselor) who is aware of the nuances of the test. It is important to maintain realistic expectations for the patient and his/her family, as it is possible that the testing may not return any positive results. The diagnostic yield would differ on the test being performed. In a targeted approach, it is possible that the causal variant is in a gene that was not in the subset of genes or regions that were targeted. On the other hand, as the coverage in WES tends to be ~85–95 %, it is possible that the causal variant lies in the region that was either poorly covered or resides outside the protein-coding region of the gene (such as the promoter or regulatory region) [17]. The sensitivity and limitations of the specific NGS test must be clearly communicated.

It is also important to emphasize to the families that a positive result may not change treatment or management decisions, and hence, may not alter the prognosis or outcome for the affected individual [17]. But it is also possible that the test may identify targets that may be amenable to certain medications. This has been the case in the field of oncology, where specific molecular targets are used to treat certain subtypes of cancer.

Cost remains an important consideration as clinical targeted NGS or WES can cost between USD 2000 to 10,000 and USD 5000 to 15,000, respectively [17, 20]. Insurance companies may not approve such costly tests, and in self-payer healthcare systems (such as Singapore) where the individual has to bear the cost, this may be prohibitively expensive.

Lastly, the patient should be advised that variants which are not related to the primary phenotype, also referred to as secondary or incidental findings (IFs), may be detected. Detection of IFs is more common with WES and WGS and may be less of an issue with targeted panels. This may have implications not only for the individual, but also his/her family members [17, 20]. For example, WES on a patient with intellectual disability may detect pathogenic variants in *BRCA1*. This mutation could be inherited from the parents, which would mean that the affected parent (and his/her sibling) is at risk of developing cancer and would require surveillance and monitoring. This family may or may not be prepared to receive such information and this should be discussed during the informed consent process. While genetic nondiscrimination act (GINA 2008) protects individuals against discrimination in the USA, similar laws are lacking in other countries [29]. Hence, individuals with a genetic diagnosis, especially those with incidental findings, may face discrimination at work or be denied medical insurance without any avenue for legal redress.

In 2013, the American College of Medical Genetics and Genomics (ACMG) recommended that laboratories performing WES should report on incidental findings detected in a minimum set of 56 genes. These 56 genes represent disorders that are highly medically actionable and include *BRCA1* and *BRCA2* [30]. In 2015, ACMG updated the recommendations allowing patients and/or parents to opt out of such analysis [31]. On the other hand, the European Society of Human Genetics (ESHG) advises for prudent use of WGS-based testing and to restrict testing to regions of the genome linked to the patient's phenotype in order to avoid detection of such incidental findings [32]. Even for exome or whole genome sequencing, it is possible to mask the results of specific genes with a targeted workflow so that they are excluded from subsequent analysis for variant identification. Thus, physicians would not have to make the hard decisions about the reporting of such incidental findings.

Interpretation of results

On average, ~60,000 to 100,000 variants are detected on WES. These variants can be broadly classified into pathogenic, benign, or variants of uncertain significance (VUS). Pathogenic variants are defined as those variants that adversely alter protein function and have either been reported previously in other affected individuals or have been shown to affect protein function in cellular or animal models. These include variants such as nonsense, frameshift, splicing, small insertion-deletions (indels), or nonsynonymous missense variants. Benign variants, also known as polymorphisms, are variants that exist in a significant proportion of the population, including healthy individuals, and account for majority of the variants detected on NGS testing. These include synonymous missense variants, intronic, or intergenic variants [33].

VUS are variants that could possibly affect protein function based on in silico software (such as Polyphen-2 [34] and SIFT [35, 36]) or other similar parameters, but either have not been described in other individuals (affected or unaffected) or do not have any functional analysis in other model systems [33]. As there are genomic variations across different populations and ethnic groups, a database of common variants from healthy individuals is imperative in understanding the significance of a given variant. Such databases include dbSNP, 1000 Genomes project, Exome Aggregation Consortium (ExAC), and Exome Sequencing Project (ESP), but certain ethnicities are underrepresented in these databases. Interpretation of VUS in such instances requires segregation analysis (by analyzing the variant in other family members)—presence of the variant in affected but not in unaffected family members adds further evidence to the possible causal relationship of a given variant. An alternative approach includes testing the variant in cellular and/or animal models, but this is beyond the realms of a clinic or clinical laboratory and may be best addressed through a research laboratory.

There is a wide range of possible outcomes with NGS testing. Using WES, a single pathogenic variant that is likely to be the cause of the disease can be detected about 20–36 % of the time [14–16, 37, 38]. For the remainder of the cases, it is possible to either find multiple candidate variants or none at all. In the event that multiple candidate variants are detected, segregation analysis and/or functional analysis would help to determine the molecular etiology. If no candidate variants are found, possibilities include poor coverage or the mutation residing outside the protein-coding region of the gene or the defect is not due to a simple nucleotide change in a single gene.

Delivery of results

Clinicians should review the results of NGS and correlate the findings with the relevant medical information. When a pathogenic variant is detected in a gene that explains the patient's clinical phenotype, the clinician should review the results as well as relevant clinical information, including inheritance, prognosis, complications, or management, with the patient and his/her family. Testing of at-risk individuals should be offered, when possible.

On other occasions, finding of a particular variant may prompt the clinician to look for additional history or perform tests which may or may not support the conclusion of the NGS test report. For example, in a patient with chronic diarrhea, finding biallelic mutations in *TTC37* may prompt the clinician to review the hair for specific features of trichorrhexis nodosa, suggestive of a diagnosis of tricho-hepato-enteric syndrome [39]. On the other hand, if more than one candidate variant is detected, the clinician will need to perform further evaluation(s) to determine which of the variant is causing the phenotype.

Lastly, if the test results are negative, reasons for this should be discussed with the patient (as discussed in the pretest counseling). In addition, as our understanding of the human genome improves and more similar cases are reported, there may be a possibility of associating the patient's phenotype to a newly described genetic syndrome. This requires reanalysis of the both clinical reports and genetic data at regular intervals. However, regulations regarding who and how to perform reanalysis are currently lacking and remain a challenge for the near future.

Future directions

Although disease-targeted testing may remain useful in the short term, as our knowledge improves, addition of newly identified genes to the panel (which has to be synthesized according to customized order) may take time, may be laborious and may not be cost-effective for the laboratory. Many laboratories have now shifted to performing WES and limiting the analysis to genes associated with phenotype and filling up the gaps with Sanger sequencing. Although the cost may be 2–5 times higher than targeted panel sequencing (which can go as high as USD 3000 depending on the number of genes in the panel), it allows for reanalysis of the data when new gene associations are made. In addition, some commercial companies have developed kits that capture only medically relevant regions of the genomes. These kits eliminate the risk of finding variants in genes whose function is unknown [20].

Currently, clinicians order NGS testing based on detailed phenotyping and after excluding single candidate genes—also referred to as a "phenotype first" approach. As NGS testing becomes more easily available, there will be a tendency for clinicians to perform the testing first and then assess the patient's phenotype to match the genotype—referred to as "genotype first" approach [40].

It is also possible that in the not so distant future, a relatively healthy individual may perform WES first and then consult a clinician for interpretation of the findings and subsequent evaluations. It may not be long before newborns are screened for inherited disorders using WES. However, there are many ethical, medical, and logistical challenges that need to be addressed before this becomes common practice [20, 41].

Finally, there have been recent reports on the role of somatic mutations in Mendelian diseases. This has been advanced by the ability to perform deep-targeted NGS to detect low level mutations in patients with Mendelian disorders, majority of which would have been missed by conventional testing [42]. As our understanding of the role of somatic mutations in other human diseases increases, deep-targeted NGS may be the test of choice in these disorders.

Conclusion

NGS is a useful diagnostic test for the majority of Mendelian disorders and is gaining acceptance in the medical community. However, there remain certain key challenges that need to be addressed before NGS testing becomes part of routine clinical practice.

Competing interests

The authors declare that they have no competing interests.

Authors' contributions

SSJ and ECT participated in the writing of the manuscript. Both authors read and approved the final manuscript.

Acknowledgements

SSJ is supported by the Nurturing Clinician Scientist Scheme, Paediatrics Academic Clinical Programme, SingHealth Duke-NUS Graduate Medical School, Singapore.

Author details

[1]Genetics Service, Department of Paediatrics, KK Women's and Children's Hospital, Singapore, Singapore. [2]Paediatrics Academic Clinical Programme, SingHealth Duke-NUS Graduate Medical School, Singapore, Singapore. [3]KK Research Centre, KK Women's and Children's Hospital, 100 Bukit Timah Road, 229899 Singapore, Singapore.

References

1. Foundation MDBD. Global report on birth defects: the hidden toll of dying and disabled children. March of Dimes: White Plains, NY; 2006.
2. Baird PA, Anderson TW, Newcombe HB, Lowry RB. Genetic disorders in children and young adults: a population study. Am J Hum Genet. 1988;42(5):677–93.
3. Veltman JA, Brunner HG. De novo mutations in human genetic disease. Nat Rev Genet. 2012;13(8):565–75.
4. Chial H. Mendelian genetics: patterns of inheritance and single-gene disorders. Nature Education. 2008;1(1):63.
5. McKusick-Nathans Institute of Genetic Medicine JHUB, MD. Online Mendelian Inheritance in Man, OMIM®. http://www.omim.org (2015). Accessed 15 Feb 2015.
6. Sanger F, Coulson AR. A rapid method for determining sequences in DNA by primed synthesis with DNA polymerase. J Mol Biol. 1975;94(3):441–8.
7. Neveling K, Feenstra I, Gilissen C, Hoefsloot LH, Kamsteeg EJ, Mensenkamp AR, et al. A post-hoc comparison of the utility of Sanger sequencing and exome sequencing for the diagnosis of heterogeneous diseases. Hum Mutat. 2013;34(12):1721–6.
8. Ng SB, Turner EH, Robertson PD, Flygare SD, Bigham AW, Lee C, et al. Targeted capture and massively parallel sequencing of 12 human exomes. Nature. 2009;461(7261):272–6.
9. Bamshad MJ, Ng SB, Bigham AW, Tabor HK, Emond MJ, Nickerson DA, et al. Exome sequencing as a tool for Mendelian disease gene discovery. Nat Rev Genet. 2011;12(11):745–55.
10. Ku CS, Naidoo N, Pawitan Y. Revisiting Mendelian disorders through exome sequencing. Hum Genet. 2011;129(4):351–70.
11. Boycott KM, Vanstone MR, Bulman DE, MacKenzie AE. Rare-disease genetics in the era of next-generation sequencing: discovery to translation. Nat Rev Genet. 2013;14(10):681–91.
12. Shashi V, McConkie-Rosell A, Rosell B, Schoch K, Vellore K, McDonald M, et al. The utility of the traditional medical genetics diagnostic evaluation in the context of next-generation sequencing for undiagnosed genetic disorders. Genet Med. 2014;16(2):176–82.
13. Liew WK, Ben-Omran T, Darras BT, Prabhu SP, De Vivo DC, Vatta M, et al. Clinical application of whole-exome sequencing: a novel autosomal recessive spastic ataxia of Charlevoix-Saguenay sequence variation in a child with ataxia. JAMA Neurol. 2013;70(6):788–91.
14. Yang Y, Muzny DM, Reid JG, Bainbridge MN, Willis A, Ward PA, et al. Clinical whole-exome sequencing for the diagnosis of Mendelian disorders. N Engl J Med. 2013;369(16):1502–11.
15. Lee H, Deignan JL, Dorrani N, Strom SP, Kantarci S, Quintero-Rivera F, et al. Clinical exome sequencing for genetic identification of rare Mendelian disorders. JAMA. 2014;312(18):1880–7.
16. Yang Y, Muzny DM, Xia F, Niu Z, Person R, Ding Y, et al. Molecular findings among patients referred for clinical whole-exome sequencing. JAMA. 2014;312(18):1870–9.
17. Biesecker LG, Green RC. Diagnostic clinical genome and exome sequencing. N Engl J Med. 2014;370(25):2418–25.
18. Singleton MV, Guthery SL, Voelkerding KV, Chen K, Kennedy B, Margraf RL, et al. Phevor combines multiple biomedical ontologies for accurate identification of disease-causing alleles in single individuals and small nuclear families. Am J Hum Genet. 2014;94(4):599–610.
19. Javed A, Agrawal S, Ng PC. Phen-Gen: combining phenotype and genotype to analyze rare disorders. Nat Methods. 2014;11(9):935–7.
20. Rehm HL. Disease-targeted sequencing: a cornerstone in the clinic. Nat Rev Genet. 2013;14(4):295–300.
21. Board ACMG. of Directors. Points to consider for informed consent for genome/exome sequencing. Genet Med. 2013;15(9):748–9.
22. Saunders CJ, Miller NA, Soden SE, Dinwiddie DL, Noll A, Alnadi NA, et al. Rapid whole-genome sequencing for genetic disease diagnosis in neonatal intensive care units. Sci Transl Med. 2012;4(154):154ra135.
23. Bainbridge MN, Wiszniewski W, Murdock DR, Friedman J, Gonzaga-Jauregui C, Newsham I, et al. Whole-genome sequencing for optimized patient management. Sci Transl Med. 2011;3(87):87re83.
24. Worthey EA, Mayer AN, Syverson GD, Helbling D, Bonacci BB, Decker B, et al. Making a definitive diagnosis: successful clinical application of whole exome sequencing in a child with intractable inflammatory bowel disease. Genet Med. 2011;13(3):255–62.

25. Hanninen M, Klein GJ, Laksman Z, Conacher SS, Skanes AC, Yee R, et al. Manlucu J. Krahn AD: Reduced uptake of family screening in genotype-negative versus genotype-positive Long QT Syndrome. J Genet Couns; 2014 [Epub ahead of print].
26. Theilade J, Kanters J, Henriksen FL, Gilsa-Hansen M, Svendsen JH, Eschen O, et al. Cascade screening in families with inherited cardiac diseases driven by cardiologists: feasibility and nationwide outcome in Long QT Syndrome. Cardiology. 2013;126(2):131–7.
27. Hammill AM, Wentzel M, Gupta A, Nelson S, Lucky A, Elluru R, et al. Sirolimus for the treatment of complicated vascular anomalies in children. Pediatr Blood Cancer. 2011;57(6):1018–24.
28. Iacobas I, Burrows PE, Adams DM, Sutton VR, Hollier LH, Chintagumpala MM. Oral rapamycin in the treatment of patients with hamartoma syndromes and PTEN mutation. Pediatr Blood Cancer. 2011;57(2):321–3.
29. Watson MS, Greene CL. Points to consider in preventing unfair discrimination based on genetic disease risk: a position statement of the American College of Medical Genetics. Genet Med. 2001;3(6):436–7.
30. Green RC, Berg JS, Grody WW, Kalia SS, Korf BR, Martin CL, et al. ACMG recommendations for reporting of incidental findings in clinical exome and genome sequencing. Genet Med. 2013;15(7):565–74.
31. Board ACMG. of Directors. ACMG policy statement: updated recommendations regarding analysis and reporting of secondary findings in clinical genome-scale sequencing. Genet Med. 2015;17(1):68–9.
32. van El CG, Cornel MC, Borry P, Hastings RJ, Fellmann F, Hodgson SV, et al. Whole-genome sequencing in health care. Recommendations of the European Society of Human Genetics. Eur J Hum Genet. 2013;21 Suppl 1:S1–5.
33. MacArthur DG, Manolio TA, Dimmock DP, Rehm HL, Shendure J, Abecasis GR, et al. Guidelines for investigating causality of sequence variants in human disease. Nature. 2014;508(7497):469–76.
34. Adzhubei I, Jordan DM, Sunyaev SR. Predicting functional effect of human missense mutations using PolyPhen-2. Curr Protoc Hum Genet. 2013;Chapter 7:Unit7 20.
35. Ng PC, Henikoff S. SIFT: predicting amino acid changes that affect protein function. Nucleic Acids Res. 2003;31(13):3812–4.
36. Flanagan SE, Patch AM, Ellard S. Using SIFT and PolyPhen to predict loss-of-function and gain-of-function mutations. Genet Test Mol Biomarkers. 2010;14(4):533–7.
37. Need AC, Shashi V, Hitomi Y, Schoch K, Shianna KV, McDonald MT, et al. Clinical application of exome sequencing in undiagnosed genetic conditions. J Med Genet. 2012;49(6):353–61.
38. Study DDD. Large-scale discovery of novel genetic causes of developmental disorders. Nature. 2015;519(7542):223–8.
39. Oz-Levi D, Weiss B, Lahad A, Greenberger S, Pode-Shakked B, Somech R, Olender T, Tatarsky P, Marek-Yagel D, Pras E et al. Exome sequencing as a differential diagnosis tool: resolving mild trichohepatoenteric syndrome. Clin Genet 2014, doi: 10.1111/cge.12494. [Epub ahead of print].
40. Stessman HA, Bernier R, Eichler EE. A genotype-first approach to defining the subtypes of a complex disease. Cell. 2014;156(5):872–7.
41. Korf BR, Rehm HL. New approaches to molecular diagnosis. JAMA. 2013;309(14):1511–21.
42. Jamuar SS, Lam AT, Kircher M, D'Gama AM, Wang J, Barry BJ, et al. Somatic mutations in cerebral cortical malformations. N Engl J Med. 2014;371(8):733–43.

4

Eyeing the Cyr61/CTGF/NOV (CCN) group of genes in development and diseases: highlights of their structural likenesses and functional dissimilarities

Izabela Krupska[1,3], Elspeth A. Bruford[2] and Brahim Chaqour[1,3,4*]

Abstract

"CCN" is an acronym referring to the first letter of each of the first three members of this original group of mammalian functionally and phylogenetically distinct extracellular matrix (ECM) proteins [i.e., cysteine-rich 61 (CYR61), connective tissue growth factor (CTGF), and nephroblastoma-overexpressed (NOV)]. Although "CCN" genes are unlikely to have arisen from a common ancestral gene, their encoded proteins share multimodular structures in which most cysteine residues are strictly conserved in their positions within several structural motifs. The CCN genes can be subdivided into members developmentally indispensable for embryonic viability (e.g., CCN1, 2 and 5), each assuming unique tissue-specific functions, and members not essential for embryonic development (e.g., CCN3, 4 and 6), probably due to a balance of functional redundancy and specialization during evolution. The temporo-spatial regulation of the CCN genes and the structural information contained within the sequences of their encoded proteins reflect diversity in their context and tissue-specific functions. Genetic association studies and experimental anomalies, replicated in various animal models, have shown that altered CCN gene structure or expression is associated with "injury" stimuli—whether mechanical (e.g., trauma, shear stress) or chemical (e.g., ischemia, hyperglycemia, hyperlipidemia, inflammation). Consequently, increased organ-specific susceptibility to structural damages ensues. These data underscore the critical functions of CCN proteins in the dynamics of tissue repair and regeneration and in the compensatory responses preceding organ failure. A better understanding of the regulation and mode of action of each CCN member will be useful in developing specific gain- or loss-of-function strategies for therapeutic purposes.

Introduction

The CCN proteins belong to a group of extracellular matrix (ECM)-associated proteins exhibiting a regulatory rather than structural role in the extracellular environment. As such, these molecules have been classified as members of the matricellular protein family which also includes thrombospondins 1 and 2, osteopontin, tenascins C and X, and the SPARC (secreted protein acidic and rich in cysteine)-related proteins, SC1 (SPARCL1) and QR1 [1]. Overall, matricellular proteins are composed of modular motifs found in other ECM proteins. They are different from traditional adhesive proteins such as fibronectin, laminins, and fibrillar collagens, all of which contribute to the structural stability and scaffolding of the tissues [2]. All CCN proteins are expressed in a variety of organisms, and their expression is spatially and temporally regulated during development. In adults, the CCN genes are differentially regulated in tissues that undergo consistent turnover or at sites of injury, repair, and disease [3]. The encoded CCN proteins regulate cell migration, proliferation, cell lineage commitment and tissue specification, morphogenesis, and/or angiogenesis. Several CCN genes are required for embryonic viability although each assumes distinct functions in different tissues and cell types. Matricellular proteins other than CCNs perform similar functions and are co-expressed when tissues undergo events that dictate changes in cell-

* Correspondence: bchaqour@downstate.edu
[1]Department of Cell Biology, Downstate Medical Center, Brooklyn, NY 11203, USA
[3]Department of Ophthalmology, Downstate Medical Center, Brooklyn, NY 11203, USA
Full list of author information is available at the end of the article

matrix or cell-cell contact [4]. Yet, mice with homozygous-null mutations in the thrombospondin 1 *(Thbs1)*, secreted phosphoprotein 1 *(Spp1)*, and tenascin C *(Tnc)* genes are born with no obvious abnormalities, and only some minor anatomical defects (e.g., kinked tail) emerged during postnatal development. Such an anatomical abnormality might be the result of a defect in collagen fibrillogenesis, which is disordered in the *Thbs2*-null and *Sparc*-null mice [5]. Interestingly, the CCN proteins do not play a role in ECM protein organization even though they assume other essential functions in cardiovascular and skeletal development and pathology. Here, we review the key structural and functional attributes of each of the CCN molecules and their relevance in development and diseases.

CCN nomenclature

Although the acronym "CCN" refers to the initials of the first three members of this group of genes [i.e., cysteine-rich 61 (CYR61), connective tissue growth factor (CTGF), and nephroblastoma overexpressed (NOV)], there are three additional related members named Wnt-inducible secreted proteins WISP1, WISP2, and WISP3 based on their induction by Wnt ligands. The acronym CCN followed by a number reflecting the chronology of the discovery of these proteins, as shown in Table 1, has been proposed to unify the disparate names used in publications for this group of proteins and genes in different species [6]. For instance, CCN1 was referred to as Cyr61 in mouse [7], GIG1 in humans, and CEF10 in chicken [8], CTGF was referred to as Nov2 in human and fisp12 [9] in mouse, and WISP1 and 2 were sometimes referred to as ELM1 [10] and COP1 [11], respectively. An attempt by Baxter and Twigg to reclassify these proteins as insulin-like growth factor binding proteins (IGFBPs) was not followed as this classification had neither a functional nor structural basis [12]. Indeed, these proteins have no real IGF binding properties and the affinity of some of them to IGF is 1000-fold poorer than the original IGFBPs [13]. For the same reasons, the use of other appellations such as IGFBP-related proteins (IGFBP-rP) was not deemed appropriate. A phylogenetic analysis by Vilmos et al. further supported the concept that the CCN and IGFBP proteins are separate sets of genes [14].

The unified CCN nomenclature, which has been endorsed by the International CCN Society (http://www.ccnsociety.com), emphasizes the structural relatedness of these molecules and also eliminates any confusion from the multiple names that have previously been given to them. However, note that the root symbol CCN is already in use and approved by the HUGO Gene Nomenclature Committee (HGNC) for the cyclin gene family, and the original gene symbols (*CYR61, CTGF, NOV, WISP1/2/3*) as listed in Table 1 and at the HGNC's "CYR61/CTGF/NOV matricellular proteins" webpage (http://www.genenames.org/cgi-bin/genefamilies/set/1046) are still widely used by many investigators. While the CCN nomenclature is increasingly adopted and accepted in the literature, and will be used hereafter in the present review, the approved gene symbols will be used when a specific gene is explicitly discussed.

Interestingly, the CCN genes can further be subdivided into members that are indispensable for embryonic viability (i.e., CCN1, CCN2, and CCN5), and other members that are not critical for embryonic development (i.e., CCN3, 4 and 6) as deficiency in mice of these proteins did not compromise fetal development and resulted in a superficially mild or no phenotype [15–17]. Nevertheless, the classification of the CCN proteins as matricellular proteins has held up well, since published data so far continue to lend credence to their matricellular membership and classification. Of note, the matricellular proteins—not included in the CCN family—now include other proteins such as periostin, R-spondins, and the short fibulins including hemicentin, galectins, small leucine-rich proteoglycans, and autotaxin [4]. These proteins are also structurally and functionally diverse, and none of them recapitulate the biological functions of the CCN proteins.

Table 1 Nomenclature and chromosomal location of the genes encoding CCN proteins in the human and mouse genome

Unified nomenclature	Approved gene symbol	Approved gene name	Human		Mouse	
			Chromosome	Chromosome location	Chromosome	Chromosome location
CCN1	CYR61	Cysteine-rich, angiogenic inducer, 61	1	1p22.3	3	70.18 cM
CCN2	CTGF	Connective tissue growth factor	6	6q23.2	10	11.84 cM
CCN3	NOV	Nephroblastoma overexpressed	8	8q24.12	15	21.49 cM
CCN4	WISP1	WNT1 inducible signaling pathway protein1	8	8q24.22	15	29.3 cM
CCN5	WISP2	WNT1 inducible signaling pathway protein 2	20	20q13.12	2	84.49 cM
CCN6	WISP3	WNT1 inducible signaling pathway protein 3	6	6q21	10	20.19 cM

Murine loci are expressed in centimorgans (CM)

CCN gene and protein structure

The primary structure of the CCN genes contains a common intron-exon pattern with most of the family members containing five exons interspersed by four introns (Fig. 1). The gene structure can be further divided into the N-terminus encoded by the first, second, and third exons and the C-terminus encoded by the fourth and fifth exons. The N- and C-termini are separated by a variable hinge region that is sensitive to proteolysis. The first exon corresponds to the signal peptide sequence, followed by four exons that correspond to the four conserved domains with sequence homologies to insulin-like growth factor binding proteins (IGFBPs), von Willebrand factor type C repeat (vWC), thrombospondin type 1 repeat (TSP-1), and a carboxyl domain (CT) that contains a cysteine knot motif [18, 19] present in growth factors including transforming growth factor β (TGFB1), nerve growth factor (NGF), platelet-derived growth factor (PDGFA), and human chorionic gonadotropin [20]. The CT domain is believed to be involved in dimerization and heparin binding [14]. The exception to this shared gene structure is CCN5/*WISP2*, which lacks the last exon encoding the fourth CT module and contains only four exons.

According to Vilmos et al., CCN genes emerged after the divergence of vertebrates and invertebrates [14] and have been characterized from human, mouse, rat, pig, cow, chicken, quail, and frog (Fig. 2). Zebrafish, which is partially tetraploid teleost and possesses orthologous pairs of genes that are found as single copies in mammals, expresses nine genes that have strong homology to the mammalian CCNs; three are paralogs of CCN1, two of CCN2, two of CCN4, one of CCN5, and one of CCN6 [21]. No paralog of CCN3 was found. Their tetra-modular

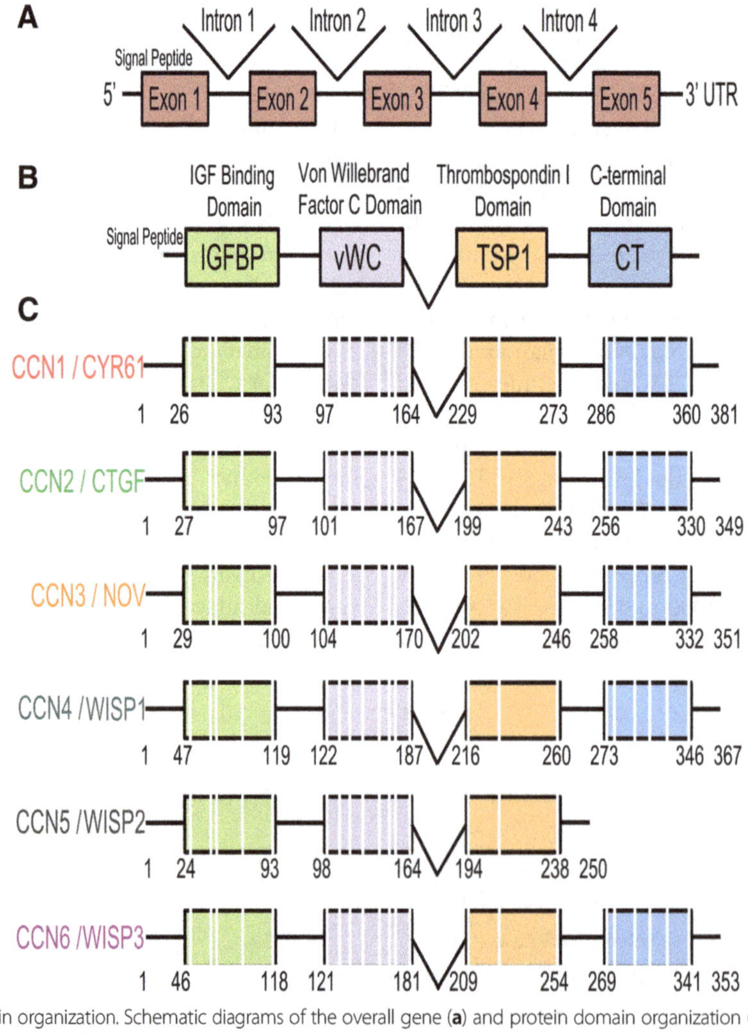

Fig. 1 CCN gene and protein organization. Schematic diagrams of the overall gene (**a**) and protein domain organization (**b**) showing the secretory signal and the homologous domains (*IGFBP* insulin-like growth factor binding protein, *VWC* von Willebrand factor type C repeat, *TSP-1* thrombospondin type 1 repeat, *CT* carboxy-terminal domain). The specific modular organization of each member of this group of genes is shown in **c**. Not to scale

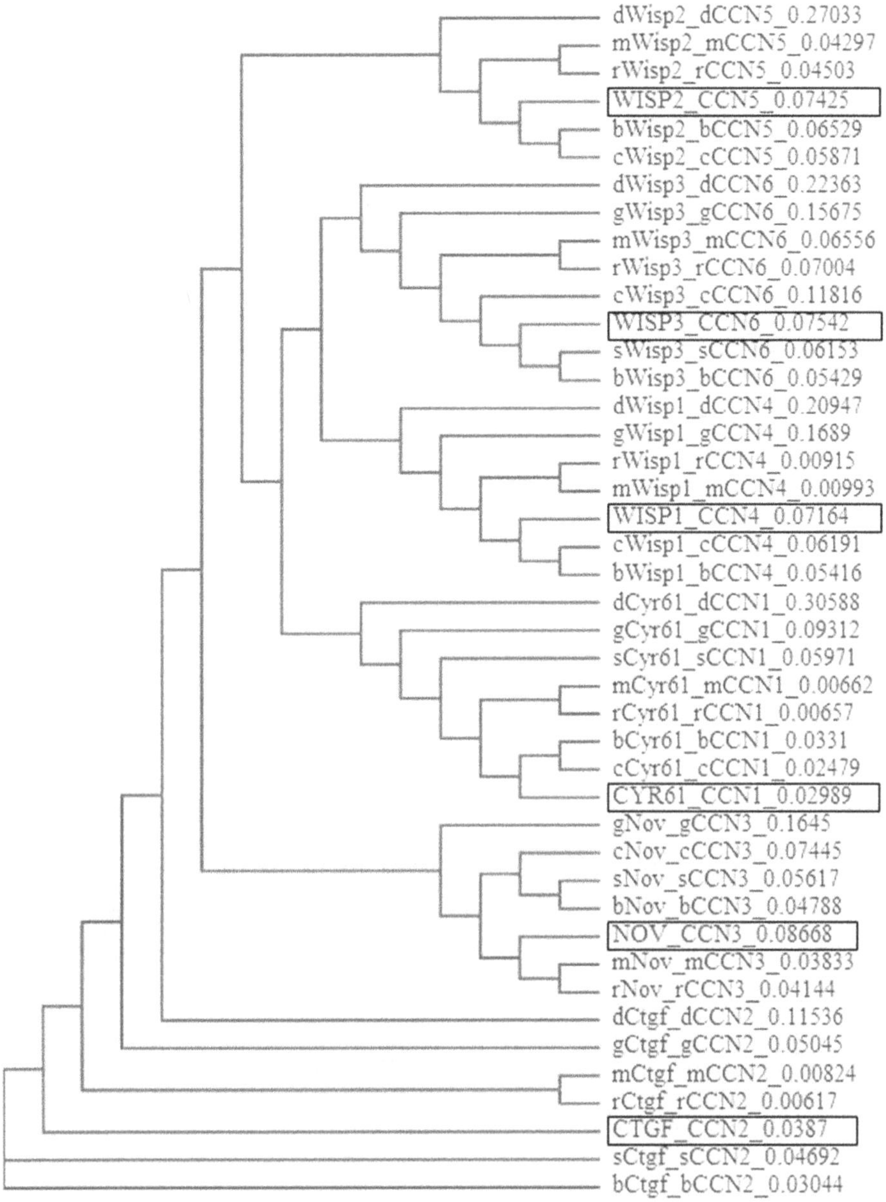

Fig. 2 Dendrogram showing the phylogenetic relations between the genes encoding the CCN proteins. The total number of differences between sequences (i.e., probability of relatedness) is shown to the right. The human genes are framed in the diagram. *m* mus musculus-mouse, *r* rattus norvegicus-rat, *g* gallus gallus-chicken, *b* bos taurus-cow, *s* sus scrofa-pig, *c* canis lupus familiaris-dog, *d* danio rerio-zebrafish

pattern and the shared identity with functional domains of other regulatory proteins suggest that the CCN genes are products of exon shuffling during evolution when multicellular organisms were formed. In this evolutionary process, other recombination mechanisms have also occurred including DNA duplication, deletion, inversion, conversion, and translocation [22]. The evolutionary exon shuffling generated multimodular molecules with four conserved domains and disulfide linkage patterns [23].

The encoded CCN proteins share about 40–60 % similarity in their amino acid sequences including a series of 38 cysteine residues that are strictly conserved in their position and number and form 17 disulfide bonds spread throughout the entire primary sequence of these molecules [19] (Fig. 3). The exceptions are CCN5, which contains only 28 conserved cysteines, and CCN6, which lacks 4 cysteines in the second module [24]. The recombinant remodeling allowed the four domains of each CCN protein to fold into unique three-dimensional structures dictated by the different electrostatic charges on their surfaces. The latter defined their 3D conformation, their

```
                              Signal Peptide
CCN1 ----------MSSRIARA-LALVVT--LLH----L-TRL-------AL------------
CCN2 --------MTAASMGPVR-VAFVV---LLA----LCSRP-------AV------------
CCN3 -----MQSVQSTSFCLRK-QCLCLTFLLLH----LLGQV-------AA------------
CCN4 -----MRWFLPWTLAAVT-AAAASTVLATA----LSPAP-------TTMDFTPAPLEDTS
CCN5 -----------MRGTPKT-HLLAFS--LLC----LLSKV-------R-------------
CCN6 MNKRRLLYPSGWLHGPSDMQGLLFSTLLLAGLAQFCCRVQGTGPLDTTPEGRPGEVSDAP
                              IGFBP domain
CCN1 --S-TCPAACH--CPLEA-PKCAPGVGLVRDGCGCCKVCAKQLNEDCSKTQPCDHTKGLE
CCN2 --GQNCSGPCR--CPDEPAPRCPAGVSLVLDGCGCCRVCAKQLGELCTERDPCDPHKGLF
CCN3 --TQRCPPQCPGRCPATP-PTCAPGVRAVLDGCSCCLVCARQRGESCSDLEPCDESSGLY
CCN4 SRPQFCKWPCE--CPPSP-PRCPLGVSLITDGCECCKMCAQQLGDNCTEAAICDPHRGLY
CCN5 --TQLCPTPCT--CPWPP-PRCPLGVPLVLDGCGCCRVCARRLGEPCDQLHVCDASQGLV
CCN6 QRKQFCHWPCK--CPQQK-PRCPPGVSLVRDGCGCCKICAKQPGEICNEADLCDPHKGLY
                               vWC domain
CCN1 CNFGAS-STALKGICRAQSEGRPCEYNSRIYQNGESFQPNCKHQCTCIDGAVGCIPLCPQ
CCN2 CDFGSP-ANRKIGVCTAK-DGAPCIFGGTVYRSGESFQSSCKYQCTCLDGAVGCMPLCSM
CCN3 CDRSAD-PSNQTGICTAV-EGDNCVFDGVIYRSGEKFQPSCKFQCTCRDGQIGCVPRCQL
CCN4 CDYSGDRPRYAIGVCAQV-VGVGCVLDGVRYNNGQSFQPNCKYNCTCIDGAVGCTPLC-L
CCN5 CQPGAG-PGGRGALCLLAEDDSSCEVNGRLYREGETFQPHCSIRCRCEDGGFTCVPLCSE
CCN6 CDYSVDRPRYETGVCAYL-VAVGCEFNQVHYHNGQVFQPNPLFSCLCVSGAIGCTPL--F

CCN1 ELSLPNLGCPNPRLVKVTGQCCEEWVCDEDSIKDPMEDQDGLLGKELGFDASEVELTRNN
CCN2 DVRLPSPDCPFPRRVKLPGKCCEEWVCDEP-------KDQTVVGPAL-------------
CCN3 DVLLPEPNCPAPRKVEVPGECCEKWICGPD-------EEDSLGGLTL-------------
CCN4 RVRPPRLWCPHPRRVSIPGHCCEQWVCEDDAKRPRKTAPRDTGAFDA-------------
CCN5 DVRLPSWDCPHPRRVEVLGKCCPEWVCGQG--GGLGTQPLPAQGPQF-------------
CCN6 IPKLAGSHCSGAKG----GKKSDQSNCSLE----PLLQQLSTSYKTM-------------
                                             TSP domain
CCN1 ELIAVGKGSSLKRLPVFGMEPRILYNPLQGQKCIVQTTSWSQCSKTCGTGISTRVTNDNP
CCN2 --------AAYRLEDTFGPDPTMI-----RANCLVQTTEWSACSKTCGMGISTRVTNDNA
CCN3 --------AAYRPEATLGVEVSDS-----SVNCIEQTTEWTACSKSCGMGFSTRVTNRNR
CCN4 ----VGEVEAW------------------HRNCIAYTSPWSPCSTSCGLGVSTRISNVNA
CCN5 ----SGLVSSLPP----------------GVPCPEWSTAWGPCSTTCGLGMATRVSNQNR
CCN6 --------PAYRNLPLIW-----------KKKCLVQATKWTPCSRTCGMGISNRVTNENS
                                             CT domain
CCN1 ECRLVKETRICEVRPCGQPVYSSL-K--KGKKCSKTKKSPEPVRFTYAGCLSVKKYRPKY
CCN2 SCRLEKQSRLCMVRPCEADLEENI-K--KGKKCIRTPKISKPIKFELSGCTSMKTYRAKF
CCN3 QCEMLKQTRLCMVRPCEQEPEQPTDK--KGKKCLRTKKSLKAIHLQFKNCTSLHTYKPRF
CCN4 QCWPEQESRLCNLRPCDVDIHTLI-K-AGKKCLAVYQPEASMNFTLAGCISTRSYQPKY
CCN5 FCRLETQRRLCLSRPCPPS---------RGRS----------------------------
CCN6 NCEMRKEKRLCYIQPCDSNILKTI-KIPKGKTCQPTFQLSKAEKFVFSGCSSTQSYKPTF

CCN1 CGSCVDGRCCTPQLTRTVKMRFRCEDGETFSKNVMMIQSCKCNYNCPHANE---AAFPFY
CCN2 CGVCTDGRCCTPHRTTTLPVEFKCPDGEVMKKNMMFIKTCACHYNCPGDNDIF-ESLYYR
CCN3 CGVCSDGRCCTPHNTKTIQAEFQCSPGQIVKKPVMVIGTCTCHTNCPKNNEAFLQELELK
CCN4 CGVCMDNRCCIPYKSKTIDVSFQCPDGLGFSRQVLWINACFCNLSCRNPNDIF-ADLESY
CCN5 ----------PQ-----------------------------------NSAF-------
CCN6 CGICLDKRCCIPNKSKMITIQFDCPNEGSFKWKMLWITSCVCQRNCREPGDIF-SELKIL
```

Fig. 3 Sequence alignments of the CCN proteins. Human sequence alignment was performed using the ClustalW2 multiple sequence alignment program. The sections of the sequences corresponding to each domain are highlighted using a different color. CCN proteins share 38 conserved cysteine residues (in *red*). The exceptions are CCN5 and CCN6, which contain 28 and 34 cysteine residues, respectively

interactivity with other molecules, and their function. Interestingly, the relatively long linker region between the vWC and TSP1 domains and the shorter linkers between IGFBP and vWC and between TSP1 and CT provide both an overall flexibility of the full-length molecule and a local rigidity within the molecule, with the IGFBP and CT domains (at the extreme N- and C-terminal ends, respectively) cocked in almost opposite directions. As shown in recent studies of CCN1, proteolytic cleavage of the protein produces truncated forms of the molecule in which amino acid residues hidden in the compact structure of the intact protein become exposed and readily accessible to receptors and interacting partners [25].

CCN genes in development and diseases

CCN1/CYR61

The human *CYR61* gene encoding CCN1 was mapped to chromosome 1 at band p22.3 (Table 1) [26, 27]. Genetic studies have suggested a relationship between a missense mutation of the *CYR61* gene and patients with severe atrial septal defects [16, 28]. The mutation leads to an exchange of residues with different properties in a highly conserved position in the N-terminal IGFBP module of CCN1. Consistent with these observations, conventional deletion of the *Cyr61* gene in mice caused severe atrioventricular septal defects (AVSD) [16]. AVSDs are characterized by the complete or partial absence of partitioning of the atrioventricular valve (AV) and are common genetic disorders that cause congenital heart disease in humans. CCN1-deficient mice are characterized by early onset of apoptosis in the AV cushion that likely hampers successful fusion between the cushion tissue and the atrial septum. Thus, *CYR61* gene sequence screening may be important in genetic analyses of patients with congenital heart diseases.

During embryonic development, CCN1 is widely expressed in the cardiovascular system [9]. Prominent cardiac expression of CCN1 was seen as early as E8.5 in mice expressing lacZ under the control of the endogenous *Cyr61* promoter. CCN1 expression continued at E10.5 especially in the trunk arteriosus, which later divides to form the aorta and pulmonary trunks [16]. CCN1 expression was also found in all major arteries branching from the heart of the developing fetal circulatory system. These include the aortic and pulmonary trunks which are branches of the aortic arches and the dorsal aorta and the umbilical artery which are of mesodermal origin. The generation of CCN1-deficient mice provided some insights into the vital role of CCN1 during cardiovascular development. A large majority of CCN1 null embryos died of hemorrhage and/or placental defects between E11.5 and E14.5, while a fraction of the embryos died earlier as a result of defects in chorioallantoic fusion [29]. Vascular defects seemed to originate either at the chorioallantoic junction, where the allantois failed to fuse with the placenta resulting in severe undervascularization in the placental labyrinth, or from defects of large vessel bifurcation resulting in a poor vascular coverage of the chorionic plate. Large fetal vessels such as the aorta appeared dilated, similar to large aneurysms. Vascular cells such as endothelial and smooth muscle cells were not confined within their layers and were mislocalized in the media layer of the aorta. Similarly, endothelial-specific deletion of *Cyr61* in mice resulted in the formation of vessels with a large diameter and loss of vessel organization into the arteries, capillaries, and veins [30]. Subsequently, CCN1-deficient embryos suffered from compromised integrity and hemorrhage of arterial vessels and capillaries.

A *Cyr61* promoter-driven reporter gene expressed in transgenic mice further detected *Cyr61* gene expression in a wide range of other tissues including the respiratory system, the embryonic skeletal system including the notochord, sclerotomes, limbs, and developing bone, the developing nervous system including the ventral spinal cord, dorsal root ganglia, parts of the mesencephalon and telencephalon, and the olfactory bulb, the embryonic epidermis, and the inner root sheath of hair follicles [7]. The tissue-specific function of CCN1 during embryonic development has not been established although several laboratories including ours are currently using the Cre-lox system in mice to determine the functional relevance of CCN1 expression in different tissues and cells [30]. At the molecular level, the CCN1 protein seems to act as an adaptor or scaffold that can bring cytokines and growth factors into close proximity to the cell surface by binding integrins, heparan sulfate proteoglycans, and receptor tyrosine kinases [31–33]. Together with the known adhesive and chemotactic functions of the recombinant protein, CCN1 may promote cell migration and guidance during tissue patterning and differentiation. The CCN1-integrin interaction in various cell types activates the RAS signaling pathway axis including MAPK1 and/or AKT1, leading to gene expression of key regulatory proteins that promote cell cycle progression, adhesion and tube formation [34–38]. In addition, CCN1 binds directly to the low-density lipoprotein (LDL) receptor proteins (LRPs) and upregulates Wnt signaling, which activates transcription of targeted genes [39]. Collectively, CCN1 signaling culminates in the upregulation of a broad spectrum of genes that modulate cell growth and differentiation and connective tissue remodeling (e.g., matrix metalloproteinases (MMPs), tissue inhibitor of metalloproteinases (TIMPs), integrins, and VEGF) [40–42].

In the adult, genome-wide scans and association studies have established that the *CYR61* gene showed the third highest mean fold expression differences in a group of obese men with metabolic syndrome as compared with controls [43]. Bouchard et al. further identified up to five polymorphisms within the *CYR61* gene regulatory region and directly linked them to the levels of plasma LDL and HDL cholesterol in a cohort of ~700 obese individuals comprising both men and women [44]. Meanwhile, Schutze et al. further identified a CA polymorphic repeat within the *CYR61* promoter, characteristic of disorders affecting bone metabolism [45]. These observations provide a genetic argument in favor of the involvement of *CYR61* gene regulation in inflammatory disorders. In support of this hypothesis, experimental and clinical data showed that the *CYR61* gene is particularly highly expressed at sites of inflammation and tissue repair. Increased CCN1 levels have been found in a number of chronic inflammatory diseases including colitis [46], rheumatoid arthritis [47], and atherosclerosis [48, 49]. Moreover, analyses of fluids and tissue biopsies from human clinical specimens have shown increased levels of CCN1 in several ocular vascular complications, including proliferative diabetic retinopathy (PDR) and active ophthalmopathy [50, 51]. Similarly, the levels of CCN1 increased in retinal blood vessels in the early stages of diabetes and in late stages of proliferative disorders in mouse models of diabetic and ischemic angiopathies [52, 53]. Whether CCN1 expression under pathological conditions recapitulates biological events characteristic of earlier developmental stages, as many fetal genes do, is unknown. Interestingly, CCN1 expression has been found to be downregulated during tissue involution, in avascular tissues, and under conditions associated with vasoobliteration, which is consistent with a potential role of this protein in vessel formation, stabilization, and integrity [54–56]. In the mouse model of oxygen-induced retinopathy, CCN1 enhanced physiological adaptation of the retinal vasculature to hyperoxia and reduced pathological angiogenesis following ischemia [57]. However, CCN1 protein is a substrate for numerous proteases that are highly expressed and released at sites of inflammation [58]. In particular, vitreal fluid samples from patients with PDR contained CCN1 fragments recognizable by specific antibodies to IGFBP and vWC domains, and only a few samples exhibited an additional product that was also detectable by TSP1-specific antibodies [25]. The truncated forms containing either the partial or complete two-module IGFBP-vWC portion were predominantly represented in PDR fluids along with other proangiogenic and permeability factors such as VEGF and MMP2. Whether and how proteolytic events affect CCN1 function, and whether this defines new cellular responses, is yet to be elucidated.

CCN2/CTGF

The *CTGF* gene encoding CCN2 maps to human chromosome 6q23.1 [59] and to the A3-B1 region of murine chromosome 10 (Table 1) [60]. It is located within a commonly deleted segment of chromosome 6 (q22.1–23.2) in biopsies from patients with abdominal aortic aneurysm (AAA) [61]. Acquired chromosomal aberrations associated with retrotransposon propagation at this location predispose to sporadic AAA. In addition, genes located in this chromosomal region have been implicated in the development of systemic sclerosis and hepatic fibrosis (HF) [62, 63]. Functional single nucleotide polymorphisms (SNPs, rs6918698) implicated CCN2 as a major actor in severe HF in schistosome-infected Chinese, Sudanese, and Brazilian subjects [64]. Another study further confirmed that one *CTGF* gene polymorphism (rs6918698; –945 G/C) is a significant risk factor for the progression of hepatitis C-related chronic liver diseases [65].

Although congenital diseases have, thus far, not been mapped to genetic alterations of the *CTGF* gene, its expression plays an important role in normal embryonic development. The spatial and temporal expression of CCN2 during development is similar to that of CCN1, with high levels present in endothelium and mural cells of the blood vessels, heart, and skeletal tissues such as the cartilage and maturing chondrocytes [66]. This pattern of CCN2 expression during development appears to be largely conserved in vertebrates including fish, frog, and mouse. A loss-of-CCN2 function in zebrafish showed developmental delays and distortion of the notochord [67]. Homozygous *Ctgf* mutant mice were found to have short, misaligned, and inward-bent sterna and kinked ribs, possibly due to decreased growth plate angiogenesis, chondrocyte migration, and matrix degradation, resulting in a visibly reduced thoracic volume [15]. Perinatal lethality ensues as the *Ctgf* mutant mice showed signs of cyanosis and difficulty to breathe, continuously gasping for air. These are the characteristics of numerous human chondrodystrophic pulmonary hypoplasias that frequently prove lethal soon after birth [68]. The lungs of *Ctgf* mutant mice were hypoplastic and seemingly arrested at the canalicular stage of development, with reduced cell proliferation and increased apoptosis [69]. Reduction in lamellar body size in type II pneumocytes, coupled with the great reduction of available alveolar space in the mutant mouse lungs, suggests reduced surfactant production and delayed lung maturity.

In *Ctgf* knockout mice, vascular and skeletal defects begin to emerge at later stages of development [70]. Large vessels in *Ctgf*-null embryos show defects in the organization of tunica media where smooth muscle cells appear less spindle-like, more heterogeneous in size, and not organized into distinct layers when compared to wild-type embryos. In addition, the microvascular endothelium in *Ctgf*-null mice is incompletely covered by pericytes. Loss of CCN2 leads also to diminished expression of vessel maturation markers, such as angiopoietin 1, and elevated expression of immature vasculature markers, such as versican. Furthermore, *Ctgf*-deficient mice exhibit defects in endothelial basement membrane organization where expression of fibronectin and its association with blood vessels is significantly decreased, subsequently leading to discontinuous incorporation of type IV collagen in the basement membrane of the microvasculature. In endothelial cells, CCN2 mediates cell adhesion, directional migration, and proliferation through integrin αvβ3 [71]. CCN2 is also a ligand for integrins α5β1 and α6β1 that are required for endothelial basement membrane formation and vessel stabilization in vitro [72, 73]. However, besides interacting with multiple integrins, CCN2 also modulates the activities of several other ECM components including VEGF, TGF-β, and Wnt signaling [19]. CCN2 has been reported to bind VEGF-A^{165} at two sites through its TSP1 and CT domains [74]. In addition, the TSP1 domain of CCN2 binds to LRP1, which acts as a co-repressor of the Frizzled receptor and downregulates Wnt signaling [75, 76].

In the adult, *Ctgf* mRNA is expressed at high levels in the spleen, ovary, gastrointestinal tract, prostate, heart, and testis and at lower levels in the thymus, placenta, lung, skeletal muscle, kidney, and pancreas [77]. No expression of CCN2 has been detected in the brain, liver, and peripheral leucocytes. Studies of diseased tissues from human clinical specimens and animal models established a correlation between high levels of the CCN2 protein and excessive accumulation and deposition of ECM proteins in fibrotic tissues, suggesting a pathogenic role for CCN2 in fibroproliferative disorders [78]. However, transgenic models of CCN2 overproduction in a number of tissues exhibited various phenotypes, including no fibrotic reaction, mild fibrosis, and clear fibrotic phenotypes depending on the CCN2 levels [79]. Specific thresholds of CCN2 levels are required to induce cell type-specific effects. At the molecular level, CCN2 is able to stimulate the transition of differentiated cells such as tubular epithelial cells, endothelial cells, and fibroblasts to activated myofibroblasts [80–82]. In this transition, proteins that are expressed by differentiated cells, such as E-cadherin in epithelial cells, are lost while proteins expressed by myofibroblasts, such as fibrillar collagens and α-smooth muscle actin, are expressed [83]. There is evidence that anti-CCN2 therapy can successfully attenuate fibrotic reactions in the kidney, liver, and other organs exhibiting fibrotic reactions, suggesting that therapies targeting CCN2 and its signaling pathways may be beneficial for the treatment of the fibrotic diseases [78].

Meanwhile, CCN2 plays an important role in vascular diseases as well. Numerous studies have shown a close correlation in topography and timing between *CTGF* gene expression and spatial distribution and expansion of the blood vessels in response to ischemic injury, as in neovascular diseases of the eye [51]. Examination of the vascular implications of CCN2 expression, or lack thereof, in response to hyperoxic or hyperglycemic injury showed a close correlation between *CTGF* gene expression and blood vessel growth and stabilization [51, 84, 85]. Chintala et al. have shown that CCN2 induces neovascularization through p53-dependent modulation of *MMP2* gene expression, which drives vascular remodeling through degradation of the basement membrane and subsequent formation of new vascular patterns [86]. Interestingly, reduced levels of CCN2 in ischemic retinas correlate with reduced VEGF gradient levels, indicating that coordinated regulation between CCN2 and VEGF indeed exists. CCN2 can bind VEGF and inhibit the angiogenic activity of both molecules when MMPs are not available, forming a negative feedback loop among these angiogenic factors [87].

CCN3/NOV

CCN3 is encoded by the *NOV* gene which maps to human chromosome 8q24.1. CCN3 is expressed during development in derivatives of all three germ layers, with high levels detected in skeletal muscle, smooth muscle of vessel walls, the nervous system, adrenal cortex, and differentiating chondrocytes [88, 89]. CCN3 seems to play a role during myogenesis and in the formation and/or stabilization of adhesion structures specialized in force transmission from the muscle to tendon [90]. However, CCN3-deficient mice developed normally to adulthood and both the males and females were fertile [91]. Similarly, mutant mice in which the protein had lost the vWC domain were in apparent good health although numerous skeletal defects were observed [92]. In particular, development of the appendicular and axial skeleton was affected with enlarged vertebrae, elongated long bones and digits, delayed ossification, increased bone mineralization, and severe joint malformations. In addition, enlargement and abnormal remodeling of the endocardial cushions, associated with septal defects and delayed fusion, were observed in developing embryos. In adults, cardiomyopathy was apparent, with hypertrophy and calcification of the septum and left ventricle dilation. Muscle atrophy was seen by 5 months of age, associated with transdifferentiation to fat. Premature tissue degeneration was also seen in the lens, with cataracts in 6-month-old mice.

CCN3 transgenic mice, in which CCN3 expression was driven by a 2.3-kb *Col1a1* promoter, showed osteopenia compared with wild-type mice [93]. In addition, bone regeneration in *Nov* knockout mice was accelerated compared with that in wild-type mice. CCN3 acts as a selective negative regulator of the expression of osteoblast-related genes, e.g., *Runx2, Sp7, Col1a1, Alpl*, and *Bglap*, and inhibits osteoblastic differentiation [94]. In addition, CCN3 function has been attributed to its functional and physical interactions with many molecules such as integrin, bone morphogenic proteins (BMPs), and Notch [95]. CCN3 was proposed to fine tune the activity of BMPs during bone regeneration by antagonizing BMP effects on its downstream targets such as Noggin, Chordin, and

Gremlin1. BMP inhibition by CCN3 results in the suppression of mesenchymal stem cells differentiating into osteoblasts [39]. Moreover, CCN3 binds to specific epidermal growth factor motifs of the Notch receptor and activates downstream signaling during myogenesis, which underscores the multifaceted activities of this molecule [96].

CCN4/WISP1

CCN4 was initially published as "Wisp1" because, like *WISP2*/CCN5 and *WISP3*/CCN6, it was induced by WNT1 but not by WNT4 [10]. CCN4 was initially identified in the mouse mammary epithelial cell line C57MG transformed by WNT1 [97]. EST database screening further identified *Wisp1* as homologous to *Nov* [98]. CCN4 expression is restricted to osteoblast and osteoblastic progenitor cells during development and bone fracture repair [99]. CCN4 is expressed in several adult tissues including the epithelium, heart, kidney, lung, pancreas, placenta, ovaries, small intestine, spleen, and brain [100].

CCN4 availability is modulated by interactions with decorin and biglycan, two ECM-associated proteoglycans [99]. In addition, CCN4 potentiates the effect of BMP2 on osteoprogenitor cells in the bone marrow and promotes osteoblastic differentiation while repressing chondrocytic differentiation [101, 102]. CCN4 enhances BMP2 signaling through a mechanism involving binding to integrin $\alpha5\beta1$ [102]. This is unlike other CCN proteins like CCN2 and CCN3, which rather inhibit BMP activity in osteoblastic lineage differentiation [103]. CCN4 variant WISP1v lacking the vWC module was reported in a few human gastrointestinal cancer tissues and normal chondrocytes undergoing endochondrial ossification [104]. Indeed, overexpression of WISP1v enhanced the gene expression of alkaline phosphatase, a mineralization marker in chondrocytic cells [105].

Meanwhile, previous studies have identified *WISP1* as an oncogene that accelerates growth and morphological transformation of alveolar epithelial cells and attenuates cell apoptosis in response to DNA damage [106]. CCN4 signaling inhibits cell death following DNA damage by activation of the pro-survival AKT pathway and the anti-apoptotic BCL2L1 (Bcl-XL) [107]. Subsequently, mitochondrial release of the cytochrome c and caspase cascade is suppressed. In a similar way, activation of the AKT kinase pathway in alveolar epithelial type II (ATII) cells treated with CCN4 induces a significant increase in cell proliferation, epithelial-mesenchymal transition (EMT), upregulation of gene expression of pro-fibrotic markers, and production of ECM [108]. These effects were confirmed in both the mouse model of pulmonary fibrosis and patients with idiopathic pulmonary fibrosis, which leads to distortion of normal tissue architecture and a loss of lung function [109]. Most importantly, reduction of CCN4 activity by CCN4-specific antibodies resulted in decreased expression of genes characteristic of fibrosis and significantly attenuated the progression of the lung fibrosis suggesting that CCN4 exhibits antifibrotic activities opposing the profibrotic activities of CCN2 [110].

In primary neuronal cells, CCN4 can avert microglial inflammatory cell death during B-amyloid (Aβ) toxicity and prevent oxidative stress injury [111]. CCN4 promotes neuronal cell survival during oxidative stress by enhancing post-translational phosphorylation of FOXO3a and its sequestration into the cytoplasm of neurons with protein 14-3-3 [112]. CCN4 also minimizes deacetylation of FOXO3a, prevents caspase 1 and 3 activation, and potentiates the neuroprotective potential of SIRT1 activity by preventing SIRT1 caspase degradation. Therefore, CCN4 has a therapeutic potential in fibrotic and neurodegenerative diseases and cancer.

CCN5/WISP2

CCN5 is structurally unique among the CCN family members because it lacks the carboxy-terminal domain that is responsible for the proliferative activity of CCN1 and CCN2 [17]. This suggests that CCN5 is a naturally occurring dominant negative molecule that modulates the effects of other CCN proteins [113].

CCN5 is expressed in nearly all embryonic stages of development, and some level of CCN5 remains present in multiple organs in adult organisms [114]. This widespread expression pattern together with the unique structure of CCN5 suggests that it performs a diverse range of functions during development. CCN5 is expressed as early as E4.5 at the implantation stage of the blastocyst in the uterine wall and continues to be expressed in all three germ layers: endoderm, mesoderm, and ectoderm. It is believed that the antiproliferative activities of CCN5 counterbalance the mitogenic activities of the other CCN family members [114]. Not surprisingly, CCN5-null mice and transgenic mice overexpressing CCN5 die at or before gastrulation due to improper implantation [115]. CCN5 is closely associated with the cell surface, although its presence is also detected in the nucleus in the cells of multiple adult organs including the kidney, ovary, brain, heart, and lung [116]. Particularly, high levels of CCN5 expression are found in the endothelium and smooth muscle of the veins, arteries, and the myocardium of the heart in early embryonic and adult tissues. CCN5 inhibits the proliferation and migration of the smooth muscle in both cell culture and animal models [117, 118]. Consequently, it prevents invasiveness of cells by decreasing the activities of MMPs [119]. Expression of CCN5 is highly upregulated by estrogen, especially in MCF-7 breast cancer lines that express estrogen receptor alpha (*ESR1*), making it an oncogene [120]. *WISP4* knockdown by sh-CCN5 in MCF-7 breast cancer cells leads to an increased expression of the components of the TGFB1 (TGF-β) signaling pathway and induction of breast cancer invasiveness. TGFB1 plays an important role in tumor progression by promoting angiogenesis, EMT, and metastasis [121]. CCN5 attenuates TGFB1 signaling and, by the same token, suppresses the progression of CCN2-mediated fibrogenesis [122]. Concordantly, TGFB1 signaling and cardiac fibrosis are inhibited in CCN5 transgenic mice in contrast to CCN2 transgenic mice. A study by Yoon et al. further demonstrated that deletion of the C-terminal domain of CCN2 transformed CCN2 into a CCN5-like molecule, whereas fusion of the CT domain of CCN2 to the carboxy-terminus of CCN5 transformed CCN5 into a CCN2-like pro-hypertrophic and pro-fibrotic molecule in cardiomyocytes [122].

CCN6/WISP3

CCN6 is an essential protein involved in the maintenance of human articular cartilage [123]. Mutations in human *WISP3* cause progressive pseudorheumatoid dysplasia that manifests itself in early childhood with loss of articular cartilage causing multiple joint and bone abnormalities [124]. Surprisingly, no apparent phenotype was caused by CCN6 deficiency in mice, which made it challenging to understand the functional significance of CCN6 in development and disease. Importantly, CCN6 seems to be involved in gene regulation of proteinases, such as the ADAMTSs and MMPs that cause cartilage matrix degradation found in PPD [123, 125]. Overexpression of CCN6 in immortalized chondrocytic cell lines dramatically reduced the expression of ADAMTS4 and ADAMTS5, while the expression of MMP1 and MMP10 was elevated [123]. On the other hand, *WISP3* knockdown in cytokine-stimulated primary chondrocytes resulted in elevated expression of ADAMTS5 and repression of MMP10. These observations suggest that CCN6 is involved in complex context-dependent control of metalloproteinase expression. However, CCN6 was shown to be downregulated in invasive and metastatic breast cancers, suggesting that it also exerts a tumor suppressive function [126]. In the absence of CCN6, there is activation of the BMP4-induced SMAD-independent MAP3K7 (TAK1)/MAPK14 (p38) pathway that promotes invasion [127]. Conversely, when present, CCN6 protein binds to BMP4 and inhibits the BMP4-mediated activation of MAP3K7/MAPK14 kinases and decreases the invasiveness of breast cancer cells [128]. Thus, CCN6 can be considered as a possible therapeutic target for breast and metastatic cancers.

Conclusion

Taken together, data shows that the CCN proteins regulate development and pathology of different organ systems in various contexts. The requirement of CCN1, CCN2, and CCN5 for embryonic viability indicates their importance in tissue formation, organization, and function. Survival of mice deficient in CCN3, CCN4, or CCN6 suggests that either these molecules are not required for structural integrity and/or function or the existence of a functional redundancy with other molecules. However, all CCN proteins seem to be involved in the physiological and/or pathological responses of tissues and organ systems to injurious stimuli. Whether re-expression of these proteins in disease states recapitulates developmental processes is still unknown. Clearly, the function of all CCN proteins are cell- and tissue-specific and careful consideration of the context in which they are expressed should be taken into consideration when assessing their usefulness as potential markers or therapeutic targets in pathological conditions.

Competing interests
The authors declare that they have no competing interests.

Authors' contributions
IK and BC drafted the manuscript. EAB drafted the gene nomenclature sections, edited the manuscript, and created the HGNC webpage on the CCN genes. All authors read and approved the final manuscript.

Acknowledgements
This work was supported by grants from the National Eye Institute of the National Institutes of Health R01EY022091 to BC and National Human Genome Research Institute (NHGRI) U41HG003345 and Wellcome Trust grant 099129/Z/12/Z to EAB.

Author details
[1]Department of Cell Biology, Downstate Medical Center, Brooklyn, NY 11203, USA. [2]HUGO Gene Nomenclature Committee, European Molecular Biology Laboratory, European Bioinformatics Institute, Wellcome Genome Campus, Hinxton, Cambridge CB10 1SD, UK. [3]Department of Ophthalmology, Downstate Medical Center, Brooklyn, NY 11203, USA. [4]State University of New York (SUNY) Eye Institute Downstate Medical Center, 450 Clarkson Avenue, MSC 5, Brooklyn, NY 11203, USA.

References
1. Bornstein P, Sage EH. Matricellular proteins: extracellular modulators of cell function. Curr Opin Cell Biol. 2002;14:608–16.
2. Kleinman HK, Philp D, Hoffman MP. Role of the extracellular matrix in morphogenesis. Curr Opin Biotechnol. 2003;14:526–32.
3. Chaqour B, Goppelt-Struebe M. Mechanical regulation of the Cyr61/CCN1 and CTGF/CCN2 proteins. FEBS J. 2006;273:3639–49.
4. Murphy-Ullrich JE, Sage EH. Revisiting the matricellular concept. Matrix Biol. 2014;37:1–14.
5. Kyriakides TR, Bornstein P. Matricellular proteins as modulators of wound healing and the foreign body response. Thromb Haemost. 2003;90:986–92.
6. Grotendorst GR, Lau LF, Perbal B. CCN proteins are distinct from and should not be considered members of the insulin-like growth factor-binding protein superfamily. Endocrinology. 2000;141:2254–6.
7. Latinkic BV, Mo FE, Greenspan JA, Copeland NG, Gilbert DJ, Jenkins NA, et al. Promoter function of the angiogenic inducer Cyr61gene in transgenic mice: tissue specificity, inducibility during wound healing, and role of the serum response element. Endocrinology. 2001;142:2549–57.

8. Simmons DL, Levy DB, Yannoni Y, Erikson RL. Identification of a phorbol ester-repressible v-src-inducible gene. Proc Natl Acad Sci U S A. 1989;86:1178–82.
9. Kireeva ML, Latinkic BV, Kolesnikova TV, Chen CC, Yang GP, Abler AS, et al. Cyr61 and Fisp12 are both ECM-associated signaling molecules: activities, metabolism, and localization during development. Exp Cell Res. 1997;233:63–77.
10. Pennica D, Swanson TA, Welsh JW, Roy MA, Lawrence DA, Lee J, et al. WISP genes are members of the connective tissue growth factor family that are up-regulated in wnt-1-transformed cells and aberrantly expressed in human colon tumors. Proc Natl Acad Sci U S A. 1998;95:14717–22.
11. Delmolino LM, Stearns NA, Castellot Jr JJ. COP-1, a member of the CCN family, is a heparin-induced growth arrest specific gene in vascular smooth muscle cells. J Cell Physiol. 2001;188:45–55.
12. Baxter RC, Twigg SM. Actions of IGF binding proteins and related proteins in adipose tissue. Trends Endocrinol Metab. 2009;20:499–505.
13. Kim HS, Nagalla SR, Oh Y, Wilson E, Roberts Jr CT, Rosenfeld RG. Identification of a family of low-affinity insulin-like growth factor binding proteins (IGFBPs): characterization of connective tissue growth factor as a member of the IGFBP superfamily. Proc Natl Acad Sci U S A. 1997;94:12981–6.
14. Vilmos P, Gaudenz K, Hegedus Z, Marsh JL. The Twisted gastrulation family of proteins, together with the IGFBP and CCN families, comprise the TIC superfamily of cysteine rich secreted factors. Mol Pathol. 2001;54:317–23.
15. Ivkovic S, Yoon BS, Popoff SN, Safadi FF, Libuda DE, Stephenson RC, et al. Connective tissue growth factor coordinates chondrogenesis and angiogenesis during skeletal development. Development. 2003;130:2779–91.
16. Mo FE, Lau LF. The matricellular protein CCN1 is essential for cardiac development. Circ Res. 2006;99:961–9.
17. Russo JW, Castellot JJ. CCN5: biology and pathophysiology. J Cell Commun Signal. 2010;4:119–30.
18. Chen CC, Lau LF. Functions and mechanisms of action of CCN matricellular proteins. Int J Biochem Cell Biol. 2009;41:771–83.
19. Holbourn KP, Acharya KR, Perbal B. The CCN family of proteins: structure-function relationships. Trends Biochem Sci. 2008;33:461–73.
20. Bleau AM, Planque N, Lazar N, Zambelli D, Ori A, Quan T, et al. Antiproliferative activity of CCN3: involvement of the C-terminal module and post-translational regulation. J Cell Biochem. 2007;101:1475–91.
21. Fernando CA, Conrad PA, Bartels CF, Marques T, To M, Balow SA, et al. Temporal and spatial expression of CCN genes in zebrafish. Dev Dyn. 2010;239:1755–67.
22. Engel J. Domain organizations of modular extracellular matrix proteins and their evolution. Matrix Biol. 1996;15:295–9.
23. Holbourn KP, Perbal B, Ravi AK. Proteins on the catwalk: modelling the structural domains of the CCN family of proteins. J Cell Commun Signal. 2009;3:25–41.
24. Brigstock DR. The connective tissue growth factor/cysteine-rich 61/ nephroblastoma overexpressed (CCN) family. Endocr Rev. 1999;20:189–206.
25. Choi J, Lin A, Shrier E, Lau LF, Grant MB, Chaqour B. Degradome products of the matricellular protein CCN1 as modulators of pathological angiogenesis in the retina. J Biol Chem. 2013;288:23075–89.
26. Jay P, Berge-Lefranc JL, Marsollier C, Mejean C, Taviaux S, Berta P. The human growth factor-inducible immediate early gene, CYR61, maps to chromosome 1p. Oncogene. 1997;14:1753–7.
27. Martinerie C, Viegas-Pequignot E, Nguyen VC, Perbal B. Chromosomal mapping and expression of the human cyr61 gene in tumour cells from the nervous system. Mol Pathol. 1997;50:310–6.
28. Perrot A, Schmitt KR, Roth EM, Stiller B, Posch MG, Browne EN, et al. CCN1 mutation is associated with atrial septal defect. Pediatr Cardiol. 2015;36:295–9.
29. Mo FE, Muntean AG, Chen CC, Stolz DB, Watkins SC, Lau LF. CYR61 (CCN1) is essential for placental development and vascular integrity. Mol Cell Biol. 2002;22:8709–20.
30. Chintala H, Krupska I, Yan L, Lau L, Grant M, Chaqour B. The matricellular protein CCN1 controls retinal angiogenesis by targeting VEGF, Src homology 2 domain phosphatase-1 and Notch signaling. Development. 2015;142:2364–74.
31. Lau LF. CCN1 and CCN2: blood brothers in angiogenic action. J Cell Commun Signal. 2012;6:121–3.
32. Chen Y, Du XY. Functional properties and intracellular signaling of CCN1/ Cyr61. J Cell Biochem. 2007;100:1337–45.
33. Wolf N, Yang W, Dunk CE, Gashaw I, Lye SJ, Ring T, et al. Regulation of the matricellular proteins CYR61 (CCN1) and NOV (CCN3) by hypoxia-inducible factor-1{alpha} and transforming-growth factor-{beta}3 in the human trophoblast. Endocrinology. 2010;151:2835–45.
34. Grzeszkiewicz TM, Lindner V, Chen N, Lam SC, Lau LF. The angiogenic factor cysteine-rich 61 (CYR61, CCN1) supports vascular smooth muscle cell adhesion and stimulates chemotaxis through integrin alpha(6)beta(1) and cell surface heparan sulfate proteoglycans. Endocrinology. 2002;143:1441–50.
35. Hanna M, Liu H, Amir J, Sun Y, Morris SW, Siddiqui MA, et al. Mechanical regulation of the proangiogenic factor CCN1/CYR61 gene requires the combined activities of MRTF-A and CREB-binding protein histone acetyltransferase. J Biol Chem. 2009;284:23125–36.
36. Kireeva ML, Lam SC, Lau LF. Adhesion of human umbilical vein endothelial cells to the immediate-early gene product Cyr61 is mediated through integrin alphavbeta3. J Biol Chem. 1998;273:3090–6.
37. Kirsch AJ, Macarak EJ, Chaqour B, Quinn T, Zderic S, Flake A, et al. Molecular response of the bladder to obstruction. Adv Exp Med Biol. 2003;539:195–216.
38. Leu SJ, Liu Y, Chen N, Chen CC, Lam SC, Lau LF. Identification of a novel integrin alpha 6 beta 1 binding site in the angiogenic inducer CCN1 (CYR61). J Biol Chem. 2003;278:33801–8.
39. Katsube K, Sakamoto K, Tamamura Y, Yamaguchi A. Role of CCN, a vertebrate specific gene family, in development. Dev Growth Differ. 2009;51:55–67.
40. Si W, Kang Q, Luu HH, Park JK, Luo Q, Song WX, et al. CCN1/Cyr61 is regulated by the canonical Wnt signal and plays an important role in Wnt3A-induced osteoblast differentiation of mesenchymal stem cells. Mol Cell Biol. 2006;26:2955–64.
41. Yang R, Amir J, Liu H, Chaqour B. Mechanical strain activates a program of genes functionally involved in paracrine signaling of angiogenesis. Physiol Genomics. 2008;36:1–14.
42. Zhou D, Herrick DJ, Rosenbloom J, Chaqour B. Cyr61 mediates the expression of VEGF, alphav-integrin, and alpha-actin genes through cytoskeletally based mechanotransduction mechanisms in bladder smooth muscle cells. J Appl Physiol. 2005;98:2344–54.
43. Bouchard L, Tchernof A, Deshaies Y, Marceau S, Lescelleur O, Biron S, et al. ZFP36: a promising candidate gene for obesity-related metabolic complications identified by converging genomics. Obes Surg. 2007;17:372–82.
44. Bouchard L, Tchernof A, Deshaies Y, Lebel S, Hould FS, Marceau P, et al. CYR61 polymorphisms are associated with plasma HDL-cholesterol levels in obese individuals. Clin Genet. 2007;72:224–9.
45. Schutze N, Rucker N, Muller J, Adamski J, Jakob F. 5′ flanking sequence of the human immediate early responsive gene ccn1 (cyr61) and mapping of polymorphic CA repeat sequence motifs in the human ccn1 (cyr61) locus. Mol Pathol. 2001;54:170–5.
46. Choi JS, Kim KH, Lau LF. The matricellular protein CCN1 promotes mucosal healing in murine colitis through IL-6. Mucosal Immunol. 2015.
47. Komatsu M, Nakamura Y, Maruyama M, Abe K, Watanapokasin R, Kato H. Expression profiles of human CCN genes in patients with osteoarthritis or rheumatoid arthritis. J Orthop Sci. 2015.
48. Lee HY, Chung JW, Youn SW, Kim JY, Park KW, Koo BK, et al. Forkhead transcription factor FOXO3a is a negative regulator of angiogenic immediate early gene CYR61, leading to inhibition of vascular smooth muscle cell proliferation and neointimal hyperplasia. Circ Res. 2007;100:372–80.
49. Schober JM, Chen N, Grzeszkiewicz TM, Jovanovic I, Emeson EE, Ugarova TP, et al. Identification of integrin alpha(M)beta(2) as an adhesion receptor on peripheral blood monocytes for Cyr61 (CCN1) and connective tissue growth factor (CCN2): immediate-early gene products expressed in atherosclerotic lesions. Blood. 2002;99:4457–65.
50. Hughes JM, Kuiper EJ, Klaassen I, Canning P, Stitt AW, Van Bezu J, et al. Advanced glycation end products cause increased CCN family and extracellular matrix gene expression in the diabetic rodent retina. Diabetologia. 2007;50:1089–98.
51. Yan L, Chaqour B. Cysteine-rich protein 61 (CCN1) and connective tissue growth factor (CCN2) at the crosshairs of ocular neovascular and fibrovascular disease therapy. J Cell Commun Signal. 2013;7:253–63.
52. Kivela R, Silvennoinen M, Lehti M, Jalava S, Vihko V, Kainulainen H. Exercise-induced expression of angiogenic growth factors in skeletal muscle and in capillaries of healthy and diabetic mice. Cardiovasc Diabetol. 2008;7:13.
53. Zhang X, Yu W, Dong F. Cysteine-rich 61 (CYR61) is up-regulated in proliferative diabetic retinopathy. Graefes Arch Clin Exp Ophthalmol. 2012;250:661–8.
54. Hilfiker-Kleiner D, Kaminski K, Kaminska A, Fuchs M, Klein G, Podewski E, et al. Regulation of proangiogenic factor CCN1 in cardiac muscle: impact of

ischemia, pressure overload, and neurohumoral activation. Circulation. 2004;109:2227–33.
55. Jin Y, Kim HP, Ifedigbo E, Lau LF, Choi AM. Cyr61 protects against hyperoxia-induced cell death via Akt pathway in pulmonary epithelial cells. Am J Respir Cell Mol Biol. 2005;33:297–302.
56. Kubota S, Takigawa M. CCN family proteins and angiogenesis: from embryo to adulthood. Angiogenesis. 2007;10:1–11.
57. Hasan A, Pokeza N, Shaw L, Lee HS, Lazzaro D, Chintala H, et al. The matricellular protein cysteine-rich protein 61 (CCN1/Cyr61) enhances physiological adaptation of retinal vessels and reduces pathological neovascularization associated with ischemic retinopathy. J Biol Chem. 2011;286:9542–54.
58. Butler GS, Dean RA, Morrison CJ, Overall CM. Identification of cellular MMP substrates using quantitative proteomics: isotope-coded affinity tags (ICAT) and isobaric tags for relative and absolute quantification (iTRAQ). Methods Mol Biol. 2010;622:451–70.
59. Martinerie C, Viegas-Pequignot E, Guenard I, Dutrillaux B, Nguyen VC, Bernheim A, et al. Physical mapping of human loci homologous to the chicken nov proto-oncogene. Oncogene. 1992;7:2529–34.
60. Ryseck RP, Macdonald-Bravo H, Mattei MG, Bravo R. Structure, mapping, and expression of fisp-12, a growth factor-inducible gene encoding a secreted cysteine-rich protein. Cell Growth Differ. 1991;2:225–33.
61. Biros E, Moran CS, Rush CM, Gabel G, Schreurs C, Lindeman JH, et al. Differential gene expression in the proximal neck of human abdominal aortic aneurysm. Atherosclerosis. 2014;233:211–8.
62. Dessein A, Arnaud V, He H, Li J, Dessein H, Hou X, et al. Genetic analysis of human predisposition to hepatosplenic disease caused by schistosomes reveals the crucial role of connective tissue growth factor in rapid progression to severe hepatic fibrosis. Pathol Biol (Paris). 2013;61:3–10.
63. Fonseca C, Lindahl GE, Ponticos M, Sestini P, Renzoni EA, Holmes AM, et al. A polymorphism in the CTGF promoter region associated with systemic sclerosis. N Engl J Med. 2007;357:1210–20.
64. Dessein A, Chevillard C, Arnaud V, Hou X, Hamdoun AA, Dessein H, et al. Variants of CTGF are associated with hepatic fibrosis in Chinese, Sudanese, and Brazilians infected with schistosomes. J Exp Med. 2009;206:2321–8.
65. Miyoshi K, Ikebuchi Y, Ishida C, Okamoto K, Murawaki Y. Association between gene polymorphisms of connective tissue growth factor and the progression of chronic liver disease associated with hepatitis C. Intern Med. 2014;53:1461–8.
66. Hall-Glenn F, De Young RA, Huang BL, Van HB, Hofmann JJ, Chen TT, et al. CCN2/connective tissue growth factor is essential for pericyte adhesion and endothelial basement membrane formation during angiogenesis. PLoS One. 2012;7:e30562.
67. Chiou MJ, Chao TT, Wu JL, Kuo CM, Chen JY. The physiological role of CTGF/CCN2 in zebrafish notochond development and biological analysis of the proximal promoter region. Biochem Biophys Res Commun. 2006;349:750–8.
68. Partridge EA, Hanna BD, Panitch HB, Rintoul NE, Peranteau WH, Flake AW, et al. Pulmonary hypertension in giant omphalocele infants. J Pediatr Surg. 2014;49:1767–70.
69. Baguma-Nibasheka M, Kablar B. Pulmonary hypoplasia in the connective tissue growth factor (Ctgf) null mouse. Dev Dyn. 2008;237:485–93.
70. Hall-Glenn F, Aivazi A, Akopyan L, Ong JR, Baxter RR, Benya PD, et al. CCN2/CTGF is required for matrix organization and to protect growth plate chondrocytes from cellular stress. J Cell Commun Signal. 2013;7:219–30.
71. Shi-Wen X, Leask A, Abraham D. Regulation and function of connective tissue growth factor/CCN2 in tissue repair, scarring and fibrosis. Cytokine Growth Factor Rev. 2008;19:133–44.
72. Babic AM, Chen CC, Lau LF. Fisp12/mouse connective tissue growth factor mediates endothelial cell adhesion and migration through integrin alphavbeta3, promotes endothelial cell survival, and induces angiogenesis in vivo. Mol Cell Biol. 1999;19:2958–66.
73. Chen Y, Abraham DJ, Shi-Wen X, Pearson JD, Black CM, Lyons KM, et al. CCN2 (connective tissue growth factor) promotes fibroblast adhesion to fibronectin. Mol Biol Cell. 2004;15:5635–46.
74. Inoki I, Shiomi T, Hashimoto G, Enomoto H, Nakamura H, Makino K, et al. Connective tissue growth factor binds vascular endothelial growth factor (VEGF) and inhibits VEGF-induced angiogenesis. FASEB J. 2002;16:219–21.
75. Gao R, Brigstock DR. Low density lipoprotein receptor-related protein (LRP) is a heparin-dependent adhesion receptor for connective tissue growth factor (CTGF) in rat activated hepatic stellate cells. Hepatol Res. 2003;27:214–20.
76. Segarini PR, Nesbitt JE, Li D, Hays LG, Yates III JR, Carmichael DF. The low density lipoprotein receptor-related protein/alpha2-macroglobulin receptor is a receptor for connective tissue growth factor. J Biol Chem. 2001;276:40659–67.
77. Xu J, Smock SL, Safadi FF, Rosenzweig AB, Odgren PR, Marks Jr SC, et al. Cloning the full-length cDNA for rat connective tissue growth factor: implications for skeletal development. J Cell Biochem. 2000;77:103–15.
78. Leask A, Parapuram SK, Shi-Wen X, Abraham DJ. Connective tissue growth factor (CTGF, CCN2) gene regulation: a potent clinical bio-marker of fibroproliferative disease? J Cell Commun Signal. 2009;3:89–94.
79. Doherty HE, Kim HS, Hiller S, Sulik KK, Maeda N. A mouse strain where basal connective tissue growth factor gene expression can be switched from low to high. PLoS One. 2010;5:e12909.
80. Abu El-Asrar AM, De HG, Van den Eynde K, Alam K, Van RK, Opdenakker G, et al. Myofibroblasts in proliferative diabetic retinopathy can originate from infiltrating fibrocytes and through endothelial-to-mesenchymal transition (EndoMT). Exp Eye Res. 2015;132:179–89.
81. Dockrell ME, Phanish MK, Hendry BM. Tgf-beta auto-induction and connective tissue growth factor expression in human renal tubule epithelial cells requires N-ras. Nephron Exp Nephrol. 2009;112:e71–9.
82. Sonnylal S, Xu S, Jones H, Tam A, Sreeram VR, Ponticos M, et al. Connective tissue growth factor causes EMT-like cell fate changes in vivo and in vitro. J Cell Sci. 2013;126:2164–75.
83. Leask A, Abraham DJ. All in the CCN family: essential matricellular signaling modulators emerge from the bunker. J Cell Sci. 2006;119:4803–10.
84. Gibson DJ, Pi L, Sriram S, Mao C, Petersen BE, Scott EW, et al. Conditional knockout of CTGF affects corneal wound healing. Invest Ophthalmol Vis Sci. 2014;55:2062–70.
85. Pi L, Shenoy AK, Liu J, Kim S, Nelson N, Xia H, et al. CCN2/CTGF regulates neovessel formation via targeting structurally conserved cystine knot motifs in multiple angiogenic regulators. FASEB J. 2012;26:3365–79.
86. Chintala H, Liu H, Parmar R, Kamalska M, Kim YJ, Lovett D, et al. Connective tissue growth factor regulates retinal neovascularization through p53 protein-dependent transactivation of the matrix metalloproteinase (MMP)-2 gene. J Biol Chem. 2012;287:40570–85.
87. Hashimoto G, Inoki I, Fujii Y, Aoki T, Ikeda E, Okada Y. Matrix metalloproteinases cleave connective tissue growth factor and reactivate angiogenic activity of vascular endothelial growth factor 165. J Biol Chem. 2002;277:36288–95.
88. Perbal B. Knock once for yes, twice for no. J Cell Commun Signal. 2015;9:15–8.
89. Su BY, Cai WQ, Zhang CG, Martinez V, Lombet A, Perbal B. The expression of ccn3 (nov) RNA and protein in the rat central nervous system is developmentally regulated. Mol Pathol. 2001;54:184–91.
90. Lafont J, Thibout H, Dubois C, Laurent M, Martinerie C. NOV/CCN3 induces adhesion of muscle skeletal cells and cooperates with FGF2 and IGF-1 to promote proliferation and survival. Cell Commun Adhes. 2005;12:41–57.
91. Shimoyama T, Hiraoka S, Takemoto M, Koshizaka M, Tokuyama H, Tokuyama T, et al. CCN3 inhibits neointimal hyperplasia through modulation of smooth muscle cell growth and migration. Arterioscler Thromb Vasc Biol. 2010;30:675–82.
92. Heath E, Tahri D, Andermarcher E, Schofield P, Fleming S, Boulter CA. Abnormal skeletal and cardiac development, cardiomyopathy, muscle atrophy and cataracts in mice with a targeted disruption of the Nov (Ccn3) gene. BMC Dev Biol. 2008;8:18.
93. Matsushita Y, Sakamoto K, Tamamura Y, Shibata Y, Minamizato T, Kihara T, et al. CCN3 protein participates in bone regeneration as an inhibitory factor. J Biol Chem. 2013;288:19973–85.
94. Minamizato T, Sakamoto K, Liu T, Kokubo H, Katsube K, Perbal B, et al. CCN3/NOV inhibits BMP-2-induced osteoblast differentiation by interacting with BMP and Notch signaling pathways. Biochem Biophys Res Commun. 2007;354:567–73.
95. Wang X, He H, Wu X, Hu J, Tan Y. Promotion of dentin regeneration via CCN3 modulation on Notch and BMP signaling pathways. Biomaterials. 2014;35:2720–9.
96. Sakamoto K, Yamaguchi S, Ando R, Miyawaki A, Kabasawa Y, Takagi M, et al. The nephroblastoma overexpressed gene (NOV/ccn3) protein associates with Notch1 extracellular domain and inhibits myoblast differentiation via Notch signaling pathway. J Biol Chem. 2002;277:29399–405.
97. Wang S, Chong ZZ, Shang YC, Maiese K. WISP1 (CCN4) autoregulates its expression and nuclear trafficking of beta-catenin during oxidant stress with limited effects upon neuronal autophagy. Curr Neurovasc Res. 2012;9:91–101.

98. Sleeman MA, Murison JG, Strachan L, Kumble K, Glenn MP, McGrath A, et al. Gene expression in rat dermal papilla cells: analysis of 2529 ESTs. Genomics. 2000;69:214–24.
99. French DM, Kaul RJ, D'Souza AL, Crowley CW, Bao M, Frantz GD, et al. WISP-1 is an osteoblastic regulator expressed during skeletal development and fracture repair. Am J Pathol. 2004;165:855–67.
100. Katoh M, Katoh M. Comparative genomics on Norrie disease gene. Int J Mol Med. 2005;15:885–9.
101. Inkson CA, Ono M, Kuznetsov SA, Fisher LW, Robey PG, Young MF. TGF-beta1 and WISP-1/CCN-4 can regulate each other's activity to cooperatively control osteoblast function. J Cell Biochem. 2008;104:1865–78.
102. Ono M, Inkson CA, Kilts TM, Young MF. WISP-1/CCN4 regulates osteogenesis by enhancing BMP-2 activity. J Bone Miner Res. 2011;26:193–208.
103. Maeda A, Nishida T, Aoyama E, Kubota S, Lyons KM, Kuboki T, et al. CCN family 2/connective tissue growth factor modulates BMP signalling as a signal conductor, which action regulates the proliferation and differentiation of chondrocytes. J Biochem. 2009;145:207–16.
104. Tanaka S, Sugimachi K, Saeki H, Kinoshita J, Ohga T, Shimada M, et al. A novel variant of WISP1 lacking a Von Willebrand type C module overexpressed in scirrhous gastric carcinoma. Oncogene. 2001;20:5525–32.
105. Yanagita T, Kubota S, Kawaki H, Kawata K, Kondo S, Takano-Yamamoto T, et al. Expression and physiological role of CCN4/Wnt-induced secreted protein 1 mRNA splicing variants in chondrocytes. FEBS J. 2007;274:1655–65.
106. Ono M, Inkson CA, Sonn R, Kilts TM, de Castro LF, Maeda A, et al. WISP1/CCN4: a potential target for inhibiting prostate cancer growth and spread to bone. PLoS One. 2013;8:e71709.
107. Su F, Overholtzer M, Besser D, Levine AJ. WISP-1 attenuates p53-mediated apoptosis in response to DNA damage through activation of the Akt kinase. Genes Dev. 2002;16:46–57.
108. Berschneider B, Konigshoff M. WNT1 inducible signaling pathway protein 1 (WISP1): a novel mediator linking development and disease. Int J Biochem Cell Biol. 2011;43:306–9.
109. Berschneider B, Ellwanger DC, Baarsma HA, Thiel C, Shimbori C, White ES, et al. miR-92a regulates TGF-beta1-induced WISP1 expression in pulmonary fibrosis. Int J Biochem Cell Biol. 2014;53:432–41.
110. Konigshoff M, Kramer M, Balsara N, Wilhelm J, Amarie OV, Jahn A, et al. WNT1-inducible signaling protein-1 mediates pulmonary fibrosis in mice and is upregulated in humans with idiopathic pulmonary fibrosis. J Clin Invest. 2009;119:772–87.
111. Shang YC, Chong ZZ, Wang S, Maiese K. Tuberous sclerosis protein 2 (TSC2) modulates CCN4 cytoprotection during apoptotic amyloid toxicity in microglia. Curr Neurovasc Res. 2013;10:29–38.
112. Wang S, Chong ZZ, Shang YC, Maiese K. WISP1 neuroprotection requires FoxO3a post-translational modulation with autoregulatory control of SIRT1. Curr Neurovasc Res. 2013;10:54–69.
113. Ball DK, Surveyor GA, Diehl JR, Steffen CL, Uzumcu M, Mirando MA, et al. Characterization of 16- to 20-kilodalton (kDa) connective tissue growth factors (CTGFs) and demonstration of proteolytic activity for 38-kDa CTGF in pig uterine luminal flushings. Biol Reprod. 1998;59:828–35.
114. Myers RB, Rwayitare K, Richey L, Lem J, Castellot Jr JJ. CCN5 Expression in mammals. III. Early embryonic mouse development. J Cell Commun Signal. 2012;6:217–23.
115. Jones JA, Gray MR, Oliveira BE, Koch M, Castellot Jr JJ. CCN5 expression in mammals : I. Embryonic and fetal tissues of mouse and human. J Cell Commun Signal. 2007;1:127–43.
116. Gray MR, Malmquist JA, Sullivan M, Blea M, Castellot Jr JJ. CCN5 Expression in mammals. II. Adult rodent tissues. J Cell Commun Signal. 2007;1:145–58.
117. Lake AC, Castellot Jr JJ. CCN5 modulates the antiproliferative effect of heparin and regulates cell motility in vascular smooth muscle cells. Cell Commun Signal. 2003;1:5.
118. Mason HR, Lake AC, Wubben JE, Nowak RA, Castellot Jr JJ. The growth arrest-specific gene CCN5 is deficient in human leiomyomas and inhibits the proliferation and motility of cultured human uterine smooth muscle cells. Mol Hum Reprod. 2004;10:181–7.
119. Banerjee S, Dhar G, Haque I, Kambhampati S, Mehta S, Sengupta K, et al. CCN5/WISP-2 expression in breast adenocarcinoma is associated with less frequent progression of the disease and suppresses the invasive phenotypes of tumor cells. Cancer Res. 2008;68:7606–12.
120. Ray G, Banerjee S, Saxena NK, Campbell DR, Van VP, Banerjee SK. Stimulation of MCF-7 tumor progression in athymic nude mice by 17beta-estradiol induces WISP-2/CCN5 expression in xenografts: a novel signaling molecule in hormonal carcinogenesis. Oncol Rep. 2005;13:445–8.
121. Ferrand N, Gnanapragasam A, Dorothee G, Redeuilh G, Larsen AK, Sabbah M. Loss of WISP2/CCN5 in estrogen-dependent MCF7 human breast cancer cells promotes a stem-like cell phenotype. PLoS One. 2014;9:e87878.
122. Yoon PO, Lee MA, Cha H, Jeong MH, Kim J, Jang SP, et al. The opposing effects of CCN2 and CCN5 on the development of cardiac hypertrophy and fibrosis. J Mol Cell Cardiol. 2010;49:294–303.
123. Baker N, Sharpe P, Culley K, Otero M, Bevan D, Newham P, et al. Dual regulation of metalloproteinase expression in chondrocytes by Wnt-1-inducible signaling pathway protein 3/CCN6. Arthritis Rheum. 2012;64:2289–99.
124. Yu Y, Hu M, Xing X, Li F, Song Y, Luo Y, et al. Identification of a mutation in the WISP3 gene in three unrelated families with progressive pseudorheumatoid dysplasia. Mol Med Rep. 2015;12:419–25.
125. Fang F, Zhao WY, Li RK, Yang XM, Li J, Ao JP, et al. Silencing of WISP3 suppresses gastric cancer cell proliferation and metastasis and inhibits Wnt/beta-catenin signaling. Int J Clin Exp Pathol. 2014;7:6447–61.
126. Leask A. CCN6: a novel method of aTAKing cancer. J Cell Commun Signal. 2013;7:161–2.
127. Pal A, Huang W, Li X, Toy KA, Nikolovska-Coleska Z, Kleer CG. CCN6 modulates BMP signaling via the Smad-independent TAK1/p38 pathway, acting to suppress metastasis of breast cancer. Cancer Res. 2012;72:4818–28.
128. Pal A, Huang W, Toy KA, Kleer CG. CCN6 knockdown disrupts acinar organization of breast cells in three-dimensional cultures through up-regulation of type III TGF-beta receptor. Neoplasia. 2012;14:1067–74.

5

HDAC3 role in medication consumption in medication overuse headache patients

Claudia Pisanu[1], Stefano Caproni[2], Donatella Congiu[1], Letizia M. Cupini[3], Alessio Squassina[1], George P. Patrinos[4*], Ilenia Corbelli[2], Paolo Calabresi[2,5], Maria Del Zompo[1,6*] and Paola Sarchielli[2]

Abstract

Background: Medication overuse headache (MOH) is a common and debilitating disorder characterized by generation, perpetuation, and persistence of intense chronic migraine, caused by overuse of analgesics, triptans, or other acute headache compounds. It has been suggested that MOH could share some pathogenetic mechanisms with other kinds of drug addiction. In this regard, histone deacetylases 3 (HDAC3) seems to have a role in the memory processes involved in extinction of drug-seeking behavior in animal models. HDAC3 is inhibited by sodium valproate, a drug with proven efficacy in MOH. Recent evidence suggests an involvement of genetic factors in predisposition to medication overuse.

Results: In this association study, we sequenced all exons, intron/exon junctions, and 3′-5′UTR regions of *HDAC3* in 23 MOH patients to investigate its role in medication overuse. Associations between genotypes with continuous and dichotomous clinical characteristics were tested by multivariate analysis and Fisher's exact test, respectively. Sequencing of *HDAC3* revealed six single-nucleotide polymorphisms. The G allele of rs2530223 was significantly associated with the number of acute medications/month used and with the number of days/month in which medications were used ($p = 0.006$ and $p = 0.007$, respectively), but neither with headache frequency or intensity. None of the single-nucleotide polymorphisms (SNPs) was associated with clinical characteristics or response to sodium valproate.

Conclusions: *HDAC3* could be implicated in excessive medication consumption in MOH patients. Our preliminary findings provide support for the need of further investigation on larger independent samples to confirm and extend the role of *HDAC3* in medication overuse headache.

Keywords: Medication overuse headache, HDAC3, Sequencing, Sodium valproate

Background

Medication overuse headache (MOH) is a common and debilitating disorder characterized by generation, perpetuation, and persistence of intense chronic migraine, caused by overuse of analgesics, triptans, or other acute headache compounds [1]. Epidemiological studies show that MOH has become the third most frequent type of headache, with a prevalence of 1–2 % of the general population [2].

An increased risk of developing MOH has been shown in subjects with a family history of medication, drug, or alcohol abuse, suggesting a genetic predisposition to medication overuse [3]. Moreover, genetic variants have been suggested to have a role in migraine transformation into MOH [4], success of detoxification therapy [5], and relapse during the first year of follow-up [6].

The use of acute medication with psychotropic effects (barbiturates and opioids) has been associated with increased risk of migraine chronification [7]. MOH

* Correspondence: gpatrinos@upatras.gr; delzompo@unica.it
[4]Department of Pharmacy, University of Patras, School of Health Sciences, Patras, Greece
[1]Section of Neurosciences and Clinical Pharmacology, Department of Biomedical Sciences, University of Cagliari, SP8 Km. 0,700, 09042 Monserrato (CA), Italy
Full list of author information is available at the end of the article

patients show symptoms of withdrawal [3], a high rate of relapses [8], and decision-making deficits [9].

A neuroimaging study with 18F-fluorodeoxyglucose positron-emission tomography in MOH patients showed that a number of dysmetabolic brain areas involved in pain-processing recovered after withdrawal of medication, while long-lasting dysfunction was observed in orbitofrontal cortex [10], an area suggested to be involved in drug dependence and addiction [11]. A recent study has also identified persistent dysfunctions in the mesocorticolimbic dopamine circuit in MOH patients [12]. On the basis of this evidence, it has been speculated that MOH shares some pathogenetic mechanisms with other kinds of drug addiction [13, 14].

Histone deacetylases 3 (HDAC3) is a protein expressed in almost all tissues, including brain [15], responsible for the deacetylation of lysine residues of the core histones. Among other functions, HDAC3 has been shown to be involved in negative regulation of long-term memory formation [16]. It has been suggested that molecular mechanisms underlying drug overuse are similar to those regulating long-term associative memory [17]. HDAC3 inhibition has been found to increase the memory processes involved in the extinction of drug-seeking behavior in animal models [18]. Moreover, HDAC3 expression has recently been found to be increased in rat dorsal striatal neurons which were activated during drug-seeking tests after prolonged methamphetamine withdrawal compared to nonactivated Fos-negative neurons [19].

Interestingly, this enzyme is inhibited by sodium valproate (VPA), an anticonvulsant and mood stabilizer approved by FDA for migraine prevention and shown to be effective in the treatment of chronic daily headache [20, 21]. Although VPA has been proven to be efficacious in the treatment of MOH with a history of migraine without aura, the exact mechanism of action of this drug in MOH is not known, and a large percentage of treated patients do not respond [22].

In this study, we carried out an explorative investigation on the role of *HDAC3* genetic variants in medication overuse and response to VPA treatment in a sample of patients with MOH by sequencing of the functional regions of the gene.

Results

Sequencing of the *HDAC3* gene revealed five intronic single-nucleotide polymorphisms (SNP) (rs1421896, rs32954, rs2547547, rs149330805, and rs41290601) and the synonym variant located in exon 3, rs2530223 (Fig. 1). Percentages of successfully genotyped samples were 90 % for rs1421896 and rs32954, and 100 % for all the others SNPs. Genotyping was successful in all individuals. Rs32954 had a minor allele frequency (MAF) lower than 0.01 and was excluded from the analyses. All SNPs were already present in public databases (UCSC Genome Bioinformatics; NCBI), and no new variants were identified in our patients. All SNPs were in Hardy-Weinberg equilibrium (HWE) in our sample.

Multivariate analysis showed that rs2530223 was significantly associated with the number of acute medications/month used and days/month in which acute medications were used ($p = 0.02$ and eta squared = 0.32 for both variables), but not with frequency or intensity of headache. Specifically, GA and GG carriers showed a higher medication abuse compared to AA carriers. Since the means of the associated variables were similar for GA and GG carriers, we hypothesized a recessive model for the effect of the A allele on medication consumption, and we used this model for subsequent analysis. When we grouped G allele carriers, we found higher significance for number of drugs/month abused and days/month of drug abuse for both variables ($p = 0.006$, eta squared = 0.31; $p = 0.007$, eta squared = 0.31, respectively; Table 1). G carriers were not different from other subjects in regard to age or MOH duration (Table 1). Although not significant, there was a sex difference in our groups (in G carriers female

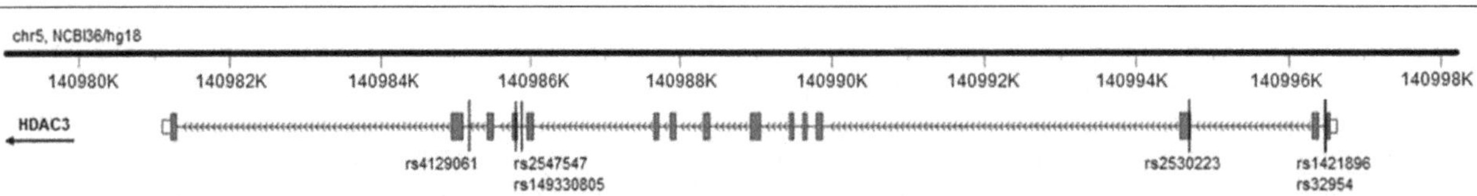

SNP	Alleles	MA	MAF SAMOHA	MAF European population
rs1421896	G/T	T	38%	40%
rs32954	A/G	A	0%	0%
rs2530223	G/A	A	41%	41%
rs2547547	A/G	G	7%	10%
rs149330805	C/T	C	2%	0.2%
rs41290601	C/T	C	2%	-

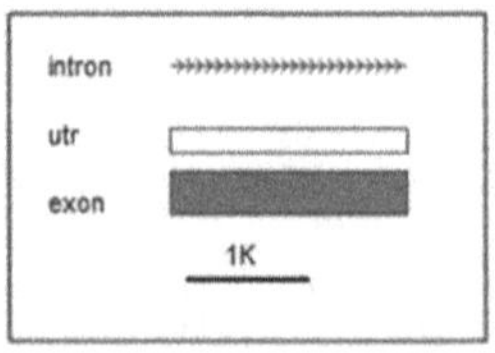

Fig. 1 Gene diagram of *HDAC3* gene including SNPs identified in our sample. Abbreviations: *SNP* single-nucleotide polymorphism, *MA* minor allele, *MAF* minor allele frequency. Allele frequencies for European population are reported accordingly to 1000 Genome Project [29]; data obtained through VarioWatch [23]. The diagram was created with FancyGene [31]

Table 1 Association between clinical characteristics and genotypes of rs2530223

	AA	GA/GG	Statistics	*p* value	Eta squared
Women/men	5/0	12/6		0.27	
Age (years)	42.2 ± 10.9	43.1 ± 9.5	0.18	0.5	
MOH duration	3.9 ± 3.8	5.4 ± 3.6	0.81	0.37	
Number of headache days/month	18.6 ± 1.8	21.9 ± 4.1	3.04	0.09	0.12
Headache intensity	2.0 ± 0.7	2.2 ± 0.6	0.44	0.51	0.02
Number of drugs/month abused	14.2 ± 4.1	23.8 ± 6.7	9.47	**0.006**	0.30
Days/month of drug abuse	11.4 ± 2.6	19.0 ± 5.3	9.06	**0.007**	0.31
VPA responders/nonresponders	4/1	9/9	–	0.33	

Continuous data are expressed in mean ± standard deviation; dichotomous data are expressed as frequencies
Headache intensity was measured with a 4-point scale with 0 = no pain, 1 = mild headache, 2 = moderate headache, 3 = severe headache. Headache attacks and drugs used during the baseline period were collected using a headache diary. Additional information on how these variables were collected is available in Sarchielli et al., 2014 [22]. Significant variables are indicated in bold
MOH medication overuse headache, *VPA* sodium valproate

prevalence was 66 %, while it was 100 % among G noncarriers). For the numbers of drug/month abused, sex did not give a significant contribution to the model when tested as a covariate ($p = 0.7$). For the number of days/month in which medications were used, sex was significant as a covariate ($p = 0.042$), and the model including sex and rs2530223 was significantly associated with numbers of days/month of abuse (model: $p = 0.003$; rs2530223: $p = 0.022$; sex: $p = 0.042$). When correcting for headache frequency, the impact of rs2530223 on number of medications used and days of abuse remained significant ($p = 0.03$ for both variables).

No *HDAC3* SNP was associated with response to VPA in our sample (data not shown). If used as a covariate in the linear model including rs2530223 and numbers of days/month of abuse, VPA response gave a nonsignificant contribution ($p = 0.8$), while the contribution of the SNP was still significant ($p = 0.01$). Thus, a different response to VPA does not seem to be influencing the hypothesized association between rs2530223 and medication consumption.

The analysis conducted with VarioWatch [23] showed that rs2530223 was predicted to have a "high" functional impact on *HDAC3*. VarioWatch assigns high functional impact to variants falling into an exonic splicing enhancer (ESE) site and into the protein domain. F-SNP database [24] showed that two out of four tools (ESRSearch and PESX) predicted an effect of rs2530223 on splicing regulation.

Discussion

Our exploratory study investigated for the first time the association between *HDAC3* variants, medication overuse, and other clinical variables in a sample of 23 MOH patients. To this purpose, we sequenced exons, intron/exon junctions, and 3′-5′UTR regions of the gene, and we identified six SNPs, all of which resulted cataloged in public databases. Our analyses showed a significant association of the G allele of rs2530223 with higher medication consumption, but not with attack frequency or intensity of headache. A recent study conducted in a small sample of MOH patients showed that the amount of acute medications taken for month was able to predict the prognosis at a 1-year follow-up [25]. This observation was confirmed by a recent prospective study conducted in a larger sample of MOH patients showing that overuse severity was associated with negative outcome at a 3-year follow-up [26]. Thus, understanding the basis of medication consumption in MOH patients appears to be of great relevance.

Our preliminary results suggest that rs2530223 could be implicated in excessive medication consumption independently of the necessity of acute medication for pain relief. The GG genotype of the same SNP has been associated with cigarette smoking in a Korean population of schizophrenia patients [$p = 0.0054$; odds ratio (95 % confidence interval) = 4.33 (1.41-13.25)] [27]. Prevalence of smoking in schizophrenia patients is three times higher compared to general population, but carriers of the rs2530223 GG genotype seem particularly predisposed to develop this habit [27].

Although rs2530223 is a synonym variant, it could be in strong linkage disequilibrium with rare functional variants that our study was not powered enough to detect. Moreover, VarioWatch predicted a high risk of functional impact of this SNP on *HDAC3*. Our results support previous evidence suggesting an involvement of genetic factors in predisposition to medication overuse in MOH patients [28].

Allele frequencies of rs2530223 are population specific, as the MAF in subjects with European, West African, or East Asian ancestry is 0.4, 0.16, and 0.63, respectively, accordingly to data from the 1000 Genome Project [29] obtained through VarioWatch [23]. Further studies in other ethnic groups are needed to assess the potential association of this SNP with medication consumption in other populations.

In our sample, subjects with the rs2530223 AA genotype were characterized by a lower headache frequency ($p = 0.09$). Thus, an alternative explanation for our results would be that subjects with this genotype show lower medication consumption due to a lower number of days/ month with headache. After correcting for headache frequency, the association between rs2530223 genotype and medication consumption was still significant ($p = 0.03$). While these results support our hypothesis that the SNP could play a role in medication overuse in these patients, the small sample size does not allow us to completely rule out a major contribution of headache frequency in driving significance. Findings from our study should be interpreted in light of the pilot nature of this investigation. The small sample size implemented could increase the risk for type 1 error and did not allow testing the effect of potentially relevant modifying factors in our model. Another limitation of the study is the small number of "AA" carriers in analysis under the recessive model. Strengths of our study include the prospective design and the choice to sequence *HDAC3* instead of target genotyping.

In conclusion, our pilot study suggests the involvement of *HDAC3* in excessive medication consumption in MOH patients. Our findings should be interpreted cautiously due to the limited sample size and might represent a first step of future extensive research aiming to clarify the role of *HDAC3* in medication overuse.

Conclusions

HDAC3 could be implicated in excessive medication consumption in MOH patients. These findings will serve as proof of concept for further investigations that will have to be performed on larger independent samples to confirm and extend our preliminary findings.

Methods

Subjects

This is an ancillary study from the sodium valproate in the treatment of medication overuse headache (SAMOHA) multicenter, randomized, double-blind, placebo-controlled study that enrolled 88 MOH patients for a 3-month treatment period with VPA (800 mg/day) or placebo after a 6-day outpatient detoxification regimen, followed by a 3-month follow-up. The 3-month responder rate (the proportion of patients achieving ≥50 % reduction in the number of days with headache per month) was higher in the VPA (45.0 %) than in the placebo arm (23.8 %) with an absolute difference of about 20 % ($p = 0.043$). VPA had safety and tolerability profiles comparable to placebo [22]. Informed written consent for the molecular study was obtained from 23 subjects included in the present work. All subjects undertook a venous blood draw before starting detoxification regimen and VPA therapy. The study was approved by the local Review Board. Table 1 shows the characteristics of the sample.

Laboratory procedures

Genomic DNA was extracted from peripheral blood leukocytes according to classical salting-out protocol. The human *HDAC3* gene is located on chromosome 5q31 and comprises 15 exons, for a length of 16 kb. The sequenced regions included all exons, intron/exon junctions, and 3′-5′UTR regions.

Sequencing was carried out using the Big Dye Terminator sequencing kit on an ABI-PRISM 3130XL Genetic Analyzer (Applied Biosystems) according to the manufacturer's protocol.

Statistical analysis

Sequences were analyzed with Sequence Scanner software v1.0 and aligned to the reference sequence of *HDAC3* (UCSC Genome Bioinformatics) using BioEdit, version 7.2.5. Deviation from the HWE was tested with chi-square test. Polymorphisms with a MAF <0.01 were excluded from the analyses. Association between genotypes with continuous clinical characteristics and response to VPA was tested by multivariate analysis and Fisher's exact test, respectively. Sex, headache frequency, and response to VPA were tested in the model as covariates. All the analyses were carried out with Haploview version 4.2 [30] and SPSS version 20 (IBM Statistics). A *P* value <0.05 was considered as statistically significant. Functional impact of associated variants was calculated with VarioWatch [23], a tool that assigns genomic variants a risk level on functional impact from "very low" to "very high". Analysis was conducted using standard parameters (selected region: 50 kbp upstream and 50 kbp downstream of SNP position). Effect of associated variants on splicing regulation was assessed with F-SNP [24], a database that predicts SNPs effect on splicing regulation by integrating information of four different tools: ESEfinder, RescueESE, ESRSearch, and PESX.

Abbreviations

ESE: exonic splicing enhancer; HDAC3: histone deacetylases 3; HWE: Hardy-Weinberg equilibrium; MAF: minor allele frequency; MOH: medication overuse headache; SAMOHA: sodium valproate in the treatment of medication overuse headache; SNP: single-nucleotide polymorphisms; VPA: sodium valproate.

Competing interests

No competing interests.

Authors' contributions

CP contributed in the study concept and design, analysis of data, and writing of the first draft of the manuscript. SC contributed in the acquisition, analysis, and interpretation of clinical data. DC performed the experiments and contributed in writing of the first draft of the manuscript. LMC contributed in selecting and collecting patients and biological samples from her Unit. AS contributed in data analysis and interpretation and revised the manuscript. GP contributed supervising the final version of the manuscript. IC contributed in selecting and collecting patients and biological samples from her Unit and in acquisition, analysis, and interpretation of clinical data. PC contributed in coordinating the clinical and molecular studies. MDZ coordinated the molecular study and contributed to study design and revising of the manuscript. PS coordinated the clinical study and contributed to study design and revising of the manuscript. All authors read and approved the final manuscript.

Financial support
This research was partly funded by "Agenzia Italiana del Farmaco" (AIFA) in the context of the project "AREA: Pharmacoepidemiological studies aimed at defining the benefit-risk profile of treatments and the impact of strategies for improving the appropriateness of drug use; TOPIC: Studies on pharmacological treatments of chronic headache" (announcement year 2006).

Author details
[1]Section of Neurosciences and Clinical Pharmacology, Department of Biomedical Sciences, University of Cagliari, SP8 Km. 0,700, 09042 Monserrato (CA), Italy. [2]Neurologic Clinic, University of Perugia, Perugia, Italy. [3]Headache and Cerebrovascular Diseases Center, Ospedale S. Eugenio, Rome, Italy. [4]Department of Pharmacy, University of Patras, School of Health Sciences, Patras, Greece. [5]IRCCS Fondazione "S. Lucia", Rome, Italy. [6]Institute of Neuroscience, CNR, Cagliari, Italy.

References

1. Terrazzino S, Tassorelli C, Sances G, Allena M, Viana M, Monaco F, et al. Association of haplotype combination of serotonin transporter gene polymorphisms with monthly headache days in MOH patients. Eur J Neurol. 2012;19:69–75.
2. Russell MB, Lundqvist C. Prevention and management of medication overuse headache. Curr Opin Neurol. 2012;25:290–5.
3. Katsarava Z, Fritsche G, Muessig M, Diener HC, Limmroth V. Clinical features of withdrawal headache following overuse of triptans and other headache drugs. Neurology. 2001;57:1694–8.
4. Cargnin S, Pautasso C, Viana M, Sances G, Mittino D, Cantello R, et al. Association of RAMP1 rs7590387 with the risk of migraine transformation into medication overuse headache. Headache. 2015;55:658–68.
5. Cargnin S, Viana M, Sances G, Bianchi M, Ghiotto N, Tassorelli C, et al. Combined effect of common gene variants on response to drug withdrawal therapy in medication overuse headache. Eur J Clin Pharmacol. 2014;70:1195–202.
6. Cargnin S, Viana M, Ghiotto N, Bianchi M, Sances G, Tassorelli C, et al. Functional polymorphisms in COMT and SLC6A4 genes influence the prognosis of patients with medication overuse headache after withdrawal therapy. Eur J Neurol. 2014;21:989–95.
7. Bigal ME, Serrano D, Buse D, Scher A, Stewart WF, Lipton RB. Acute migraine medications and evolution from episodic to chronic migraine: a longitudinal population-based study. Headache. 2008;48:1157–68.
8. Tassorelli C, Jensen R, Allena M, De Icco R, Sances G, Katsarava Z, et al. A consensus protocol for the management of medication-overuse headache: evaluation in a multicentric, multinational study. Cephalalgia. 2014;34:645–55.
9. Biagianti B, Grazzi L, Gambini O, Usai S, Muffatti R, Scarone S, et al. Decision-making deficit in chronic migraine patients with medication overuse. Neurol Sci. 2012;33:S151–5.
10. Fumal A, Laureys S, Di Clemente L, Boly M, Bohotin V, Vandenheede M, et al. Orbitofrontal cortex involvement in chronic analgesic-overuse headache evolving from episodic migraine. Brain. 2006;129:543–50.
11. London ED, Ernst M, Grant S, Bonson K, Weinstein A. Orbitofrontal cortex and human drug abuse: functional imaging. Cereb Cortex. 2000;10:334–42.
12. Ferraro S, Grazzi L, Muffatti R, Nava S, Ghielmetti F, Bertolino N, et al. In medication-overuse headache, fMRI shows long-lasting dysfunction in midbrain areas. Headache. 2012;52:1520–34.
13. Calabresi P, Cupini LM. Medication-overuse headache: similarities with drug addiction. Trends Pharmacol Sci. 2005;26:62–8.
14. Fuh JL, Wang SJ. Dependent behavior in patients with medication-overuse headache. Curr Pain Headache Rep. 2012;16:73–9.
15. de Ruijter AJ, van Gennip AH, Caron HN, Kemp S, van Kuilenburg AB. Histone deacetylases (HDACs): characterization of the classical HDAC family. Biochem J. 2003;370:737–49.
16. McQuown SC, Barrett RM, Matheos DP, Post RJ, Rogge GA, Alenghat T, et al. HDAC3 is a critical negative regulator of long-term memory formation. J Neurosci. 2011;31:764–74.
17. Robbins TW, Ersche KD, Everitt BJ. Drug addiction and the memory systems of the brain. Ann N Y Acad Sci. 2008;1141:1–21.
18. Malvaez M, McQuown SC, Rogge GA, Astarabadi M, Jacques V, Carreiro S, et al. HDAC3-selective inhibitor enhances extinction of cocaine-seeking behavior in a persistent manner. Proc Natl Acad Sci U S A. 2013;110:2647–52.
19. Li X, Rubio FJ, Zeric T, Bossert JM, Kambhampati S, Cates HM, et al. Incubation of methamphetamine craving is associated with selective increases in expression of BDNF and trkb, glutamate receptors, and epigenetic enzymes in cue-activated fos-expressing dorsal striatal neurons. J Neurosci. 2015;35:8232–44.
20. Yurekli VA, Akhan G, Kutluhan S, Uzar E, Koyuncuoglu HR, Gultekin F. The effect of sodium valproate on chronic daily headache and its subgroups. J Headache Pain. 2008;9:37–41.
21. Blumenfeld AM, Schim JD, Chippendale TJ. Botulinum toxin type A and divalproex sodium for prophylactic treatment of episodic or chronic migraine. Headache. 2008;48:210–20.
22. Sarchielli P, Messina P, Cupini LM, Tedeschi G, Di Piero V, Livrea P, et al. Sodium valproate in migraine without aura and medication overuse headache: a randomized controlled trial. Eur Neuropsychopharmacol. 2014;24:1289–97.
23. Cheng YC, Hsiao FC, Yeh EC, Lin WJ, Tang CY, Tseng HC, et al. VarioWatch: providing large-scale and comprehensive annotations on human genomic variants in the next generation sequencing era. Nucleic Acids Res. 2012;40:W76–81.
24. Lee PH, Shatkay H. F-SNP: computationally predicted functional SNPs for disease association studies. Nucleic Acids Res. 2008;36:D820–4.
25. Radat F, Chanraud S, Di Scala G, Dousset V, Allard M. Psychological and neuropsychological correlates of dependence-related behaviour in medication overuse headaches: a one year follow-up study. J Headache Pain. 2013;14:59.
26. Sances G, Galli F, Ghiotto N, Allena M, Guaschino E, Frustaci A, et al. Factors associated with a negative outcome of medication-overuse headache: a 3-year follow-up (the 'CARE' protocol). Cephalalgia. 2013;33:431–43.
27. Kim T, Park JK, Kim HJ, Chung JH, Kim JW. Association of histone deacetylase genes with schizophrenia in Korean population. Psychiatry Res. 2010;178:266–9.
28. Di Lorenzo C, Di Lorenzo G, Sances G, Ghiotto N, Guaschino E, Grieco GS, et al. Drug consumption in medication overuse headache is influenced by brain-derived neurotrophic factor Val66Met polymorphism. J Headache Pain. 2009;10:349–55.
29. 1000 Genomes Project Consortium. A map of human genome variation from population-scale sequencing. Nature. 2010;467:1061–73.
30. Barrett JC, Fry B, Maller J, Daly MJ. Haploview: analysis and visualization of LD and haplotype maps. Bioinformatics. 2005;21:263–5.
31. Rambaldi D, Ciccarelli FD. FancyGene: dynamic visualization of gene structures and protein domain architectures on genomic loci. Bioinformatics. 2009;25:2281–2.

6

Next-generation sequencing using a pre-designed gene panel for the molecular diagnosis of congenital disorders in pediatric patients

Eileen C. P. Lim[1], Maggie Brett[1], Angeline H. M. Lai[2,3], Siew-Peng Lee[1], Ee-Shien Tan[2,3], Saumya S. Jamuar[2,3], Ivy S. L. Ng[2,3] and Ene-Choo Tan[1,3*]

Abstract

Background: Next-generation sequencing (NGS) has revolutionized genetic research and offers enormous potential for clinical application. Sequencing the exome has the advantage of casting the net wide for all known coding regions while targeted gene panel sequencing provides enhanced sequencing depths and can be designed to avoid incidental findings in adult-onset conditions. A HaloPlex panel consisting of 180 genes within commonly altered chromosomal regions is available for use on both the Ion Personal Genome Machine® (PGM™) and MiSeq platforms to screen for causative mutations in these genes.

Methods: We used this Haloplex ICCG panel for targeted sequencing of 15 patients with clinical presentations indicative of an abnormality in one of the 180 genes. Sequencing runs were done using the Ion 318 Chips on the Ion Torrent PGM. Variants were filtered for known polymorphisms and analysis was done to identify possible disease-causing variants before validation by Sanger sequencing. When possible, segregation of variants with phenotype in family members was performed to ascertain the pathogenicity of the variant.

Results: More than 97 % of the target bases were covered at >20×. There was an average of 9.6 novel variants per patient. Pathogenic mutations were identified in five genes for six patients, with two novel variants. There were another five likely pathogenic variants, some of which were unreported novel variants.

Conclusions: In a cohort of 15 patients, we were able to identify a likely genetic etiology in six patients (40 %). Another five patients had candidate variants for which further evaluation and segregation analysis are ongoing. Our results indicate that the HaloPlex ICCG panel is useful as a rapid, high-throughput and cost-effective screening tool for 170 of the 180 genes. There is low coverage for some regions in several genes which might have to be supplemented by Sanger sequencing. However, comparing the cost, ease of analysis, and shorter turnaround time, it is a good alternative to exome sequencing for patients whose features are suggestive of a genetic etiology involving one of the genes in the panel.

Keywords: Congenital disorders, Gene panel, ICCG, Mutation screening, Next-generation sequencing

* Correspondence: tanec@bigfoot.com
[1]KK Research Centre, KK Women's and Children's Hospital, 100 Bukit Timah Road, Singapore 229899, Singapore
[3]Paediatrics Academic Clinical Programme, SingHealth Duke-NUS Graduate Medical School, Singapore 169857, Singapore
Full list of author information is available at the end of the article

Background

Congenital disorders comprise conditions present at birth or those that developed during infancy or early childhood. Presentations include structural abnormalities, neuromuscular disorders, developmental delay, and intellectual disability which collectively affect more than 10 % of children. The European Surveillance of Congenital Anomalies (EUROCAT) reported the prevalence of major congenital anomalies to be about 2.4 % of live births [1], while the Center for Disease Control and Prevention (CDC) reported 3.3 % for birth defects [2]. The prevalence of developmental disabilities is reported to be 13.9 % in the USA [3].

Less than half of these disorders have an identifiable cause such as aneuploidy, metabolic disorder, maternal infection, parental exposure to teratogenic agents, or intrapartum events. The remaining cases are thought to have a genetic etiology such as submiscroscopic chromosomal abnormalities or rare single/multiple nucleotide changes. The former can be detected by using chromosomal microarray analysis (CMA) which is now the recommended first-tier test for children with dysmorphism, multiple congenital anomalies, developmental delay/ intellectual disability, and/or autism spectrum disorder [4]. Although CMA is more sensitive than conventional karyotyping, the diagnostic yield for this group of disorders is still only about 20 % in multiple studies [5–7]. Genetic causes for the rest are likely due to small deletions and insertions, balanced translocations involving gene disruptions, and point mutations which cannot be detected by commonly used CMA platforms.

With massively parallel sequencing, many regions and even the entire genome can be interrogated simultaneously to identify such mutations. Although the cost of whole genome sequencing has become progressively lower in the last few years, data analysis and interpretation remain challenging. Due to the large number of short-reads, the sequence data has to be mapped back to the reference genome and filtered through known databases to identify variants for each individual, leading to long turnaround time from clinic testing to reporting. There is also the issue of incidental findings unrelated to the indication for testing and the American College of Medical Genetics and Genomics (ACMG) have recommended the reporting of pathogenic variants for 56 genes [8]. Subsequently, the ACMG recommended that patients be given the choice of opting out of receiving such information [9]. For these reasons, many laboratories still use Sanger sequencing of single or a few genes when there are known causal genes for the suspected disorders.

Exome sequencing can partly overcome the issue of data throughput but not the possibility of incidental findings. Targeted gene panels can address both by focusing on a set of relevant candidate genes with known diagnostic yield, while providing cost-related advantage as well as easier data analysis without the need for specialized computing infrastructure and expertise. The American Society of Human Genetics (ASHG) also recommends that gene testing should be limited to single genes or targeted gene panels based on the clinical presentations of the patient [10]. Compared to Sanger sequencing of single genes, targeted gene panel sequencing has much higher throughput, but each design needs to be evaluated for coverage and sensitivity before being put to routine clinical diagnostic use.

Among several pre-designed catalog panels for pediatric congenital disorders, there is one comprising 180 genes located within chromosomal regions with a high frequency of cytogenetic abnormalities in constitutional disorders [11] according to publicly available data from the International Collaboration for Clinical Genomics (ICCG—previously known as International Standards for Cytogenomic Arrays or ISCA) [12, 13]. To assess the coverage and sensitivity of this ICCG gene panel for high-throughput next-generation sequencing in congenital disorders, we used the Ion Torrent PGM platform to perform mutation screening of 15 pediatric patients with suspected genetic disorders.

Materials and methods

Ethics statement

The patients were previously recruited under two separate projects (CIRB Ref: 2007/831/F and 2010/238/F). Approval to conduct this sequencing study was provided by the SingHealth Central Institutional Review Board (CIRB Ref: 2013/798/F). All the subjects were minors, and written informed consent had been obtained from the parents.

Study samples

The 15 patients were previously recruited from the hospital's Genetics Clinics for testing of chromosomal imbalance using human 400 K CGH arrays (Agilent Technologies Inc., Santa Clara, USA). No significant pathogenic copy number changes were identified in all 15. Inclusion criteria include developmental delay/intellectual disability and multiple congenital anomalies. Each patient had been followed up and examined by a clinical geneticist. All of them have clinical features suggestive of a disorder associated with one of the 180 genes, although the features may not have been typical or completely fulfilled the clinical criteria of a specific syndrome at the time of recruitment.

DNA extraction

Genomic DNA was manually extracted from peripheral blood collected in EDTA tubes using the Gentra Puregene Blood Kit (Qiagen Inc., Valencia, USA) according to the manufacturer's instructions. DNA quality and quantity were measured on a Nanodrop Spectrophotometer (Thermo Scientific, Wilmington, USA).

Table 1 Summary of sequencing output and quality for each sample

Sample	Reads				Bases			
	Total	Mapped	On target	Mean depth	Aligned	≥Q20	On target	Uniformity[a]
1	1,348,756	1,322,761	91.29 %	203.4	98.59 %	87.61 %	55.36 %	92.47 %
2	1,389,395	1,361,138	91.29 %	209.9	98.58 %	87.80 %	54.95 %	92.55 %
3	1,552,042	1,522,728	91.16 %	234.3	98.63 %	87.82 %	55.29 %	92.37 %
4	1,494,165	1,470,215	91.90 %	226.8	98.71 %	87.87 %	55.06 %	92.76 %
5	1,369,435	1,346,412	91.91 %	210.2	98.78 %	88.89 %	54.65 %	92.90 %
6	1,663,702	1,633,814	91.20 %	252.4	98.72 %	88.33 %	55.03 %	92.43 %
7	1,602,753	1,569,980	91.01 %	242.7	98.67 %	88.75 %	55.14 %	92.36 %
8	1,694,348	1,662,379	91.25 %	256.8	98.69 %	88.80 %	54.90 %	92.36 %
9	1,431,017	1,398,943	90.08 %	211.7	98.30 %	88.04 %	54.83 %	92.52 %
10	1,717,174	1,677,112	90.16 %	253.2	98.24 %	87.83 %	55.57 %	92.12 %
11	1,408,352	1,373,789	89.67 %	205.5	98.12 %	87.42 %	55.28 %	92.56 %
12	1,511,078	1,484,377	90.97 %	227.3	98.42 %	88.06 %	54.93 %	92.51 %
13	1,554,866	1,521,948	90.96 %	235.1	98.44 %	89.17 %	55.07 %	92.11 %
14	1,578,886	1,547,559	91.48 %	239.6	98.54 %	89.31 %	55.09 %	92.54 %
15	1,558,185	1,525,061	90.91 %	234.0	98.50 %	88.91 %	55.03 %	92.40 %

[a]Percentage of target bases covered by at least 0.2x the average base read length

Library construction, sequencing, and data analysis

Genomic DNA (225 ng gDNA) was digested with 16 different restriction enzymes at 37 °C for 30 min to create a library of gDNA restriction fragments. Both ends of the targeted fragments were selectively hybridized to biotinylated probes from the HaloPlex ICCG panel (Agilent Technologies Inc., Santa Clara, CA, USA), which resulted in direct fragment circularization. During the 16-h hybridization process, HaloPlex ION Barcodes and Ion Torrent sequencing motifs were incorporated into the

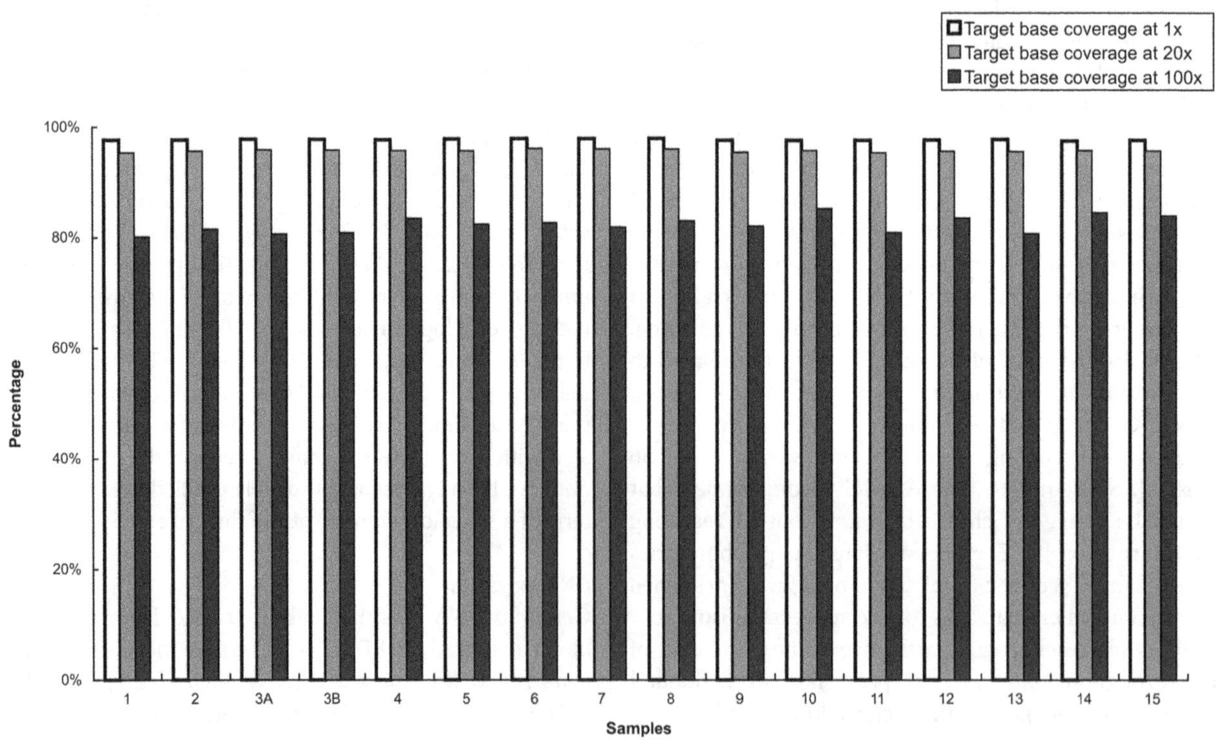

Fig. 1 Percentage of bases at the different read depths

Table 2 Mean coverage with highest and lowest number of reads for target regions for each gene

	Gene	Mean	Lowest	Highest
1	*ABCC8*	338.07	81.92	786.09
2	*ABCD1*	169.66	12.56	411.39
3	*ACSL4*[a]	164.77	21.30	492.11
4	*AFF2*	214.46	36.76	580.05
5	*ALX4*	222.07	84.73	558.92
6	*AP1S2*[a]	135.94	38.59	325.08
7	*APC*[a]	179.90	3.73	406.62
8	*AR*	223.99	43.85	529.40
9	*ATP7A*[a]	178.46	15.96	431.28
10	*ATRX*	158.16	10.57	441.01
11	*AVPR2*	212.24	91.24	401.30
12	*BMP4*[a]	277.08	184.26	355.73
13	*BMPR1A*[a]	249.32	92.33	500.82
14	*BMPR2*	221.72	39.06	545.08
15	*BRCA2*[a]	226.44	69.62	659.97
16	*BRWD3*	158.01	1.94	403.65
17	*BSND*	281.21	166.64	426.50
18	*BTK*[a]	248.63	71.65	522.36
19	*CACNA1C*	313.63	70.18	681.23
20	*CASK*	174.65	3.07	469.39
21	*CDKN1C*[a]	61.17	21.98	111.66
22	*CFC1*	0.00	0.00	0.06
23	*CHD7*[a]	238.95	6.00	491.12
24	*CHD8*[a]	241.14	3.17	571.36
25	*CHM*	138.15	0.00	424.06
26	*CHRNA7*	133.17	0.00	649.69
27	*CLCNKA*[a]	207.37	41.54	632.50
28	*CLCNKB*[a]	227.42	19.10	558.00
29	*CNTN4*[a]	258.10	74.48	742.09
30	*COL2A1*	311.23	28.83	762.32
31	*COL4A5*	145.99	6.30	492.06
32	*CREBBP*	307.73	66.01	682.75
33	*CUL4B*[a]	148.17	35.09	399.12
34	*CYP21A2*	42.13	0.00	317.76
35	*DCX*	191.11	31.11	424.96
36	*DHCR7*[a]	356.18	73.73	715.42
37	*DMRT1*	317.71	99.58	526.08
38	*DYM*[a]	199.54	35.51	538.64
39	*DYRK1A*	238.22	56.46	539.50
40	*EDNRB*[a]	244.22	108.94	440.60
41	*EHMT1*	322.86	0.00	914.42
42	*EMX2*	191.49	89.92	367.85
43	*EXT1*	255.03	122.82	531.24

Table 2 Mean coverage with highest and lowest number of reads for target regions for each gene *(Continued)*

44	*EXT2*	268.11	55.88	603.23
45	*EYA1*	259.46	9.39	471.54
46	*F8*	208.53	0.00	590.76
47	*F9*	194.99	29.24	362.11
48	*FANCA*	305.66	17.51	898.72
49	*FANCB*[a]	115.90	28.51	270.95
50	*FBN1*[a]	275.76	42.56	611.18
51	*FGD1*	232.34	56.74	586.70
52	*FGFR1*[a]	313.99	118.45	666.21
53	*FLNA*[a]	243.40	56.48	688.98
54	*FMR1*	156.86	48.89	329.36
55	*FOXC1*	93.65	76.19	114.03
56	*FOXG1*	96.79	77.95	125.85
57	*FOXL2*	93.73	75.81	114.31
58	*FZD4*	211.12	93.71	360.16
59	*GATA3*[a]	324.33	155.81	637.81
60	*GATA4*[a]	295.62	50.09	587.59
61	*GDF5*	155.05	113.49	212.75
62	*GJB2*[a]	249.56	200.76	298.70
63	*GLA*	214.53	82.27	473.23
64	*GLI2*	312.00	149.69	577.16
65	*GLI3*[a]	286.99	108.72	560.08
66	*GPC3*	216.44	42.47	424.44
67	*GPC6*	251.39	134.79	392.07
68	*GPR56*[a]	294.55	71.00	606.66
69	*GRIA3*	204.51	69.61	433.75
70	*HBA1*	50.15	0.00	182.69
71	*HBA2*	10.42	0.00	40.79
72	*HCCS*[a]	177.03	62.86	347.20
73	*HNF1B*	321.62	59.22	722.67
74	*HOXD13*	278.61	105.47	524.08
75	*HPRT1*	151.03	46.04	318.21
76	*IDS*	183.74	4.69	498.62
77	*IKBKG*	51.43	0.00	348.87
78	*IRF6*[a]	265.75	126.04	468.45
79	*JAG1*	308.99	57.19	644.27
80	*KAL1*	196.43	33.50	435.56
81	*KCNJ1*	341.18	200.92	557.14
82	*KCNQ1*	321.89	62.66	842.39
83	*L1CAM*[a]	238.10	33.83	531.65
84	*LAMP2*	161.71	16.59	374.76
85	*LEMD3*	162.74	55.42	325.70
86	*LHX4*	340.77	146.93	643.51
87	*LMX1B*	165.54	66.47	408.35

Table 2 Mean coverage with highest and lowest number of reads for target regions for each gene *(Continued)*

88	*MECP2*	116.40	21.60	224.22
89	*MID1*[a]	188.60	44.28	383.24
90	*MITF*	303.77	97.21	559.04
91	*MSX1*	148.47	85.95	232.61
92	*MSX2*	147.01	93.77	230.81
93	*MTM1*[a]	197.51	54.42	517.75
94	*MYCN*[a]	228.84	96.40	407.08
95	*NDP*[a]	237.17	92.91	444.75
96	*NDUFV1*	299.67	104.88	555.45
97	*NF2*	368.03	144.63	794.05
98	*NHS*	189.40	24.18	373.29
99	*NIPBL*[a]	172.28	15.79	382.14
100	*NLGN4X*[a]	251.27	119.13	470.66
101	*NOTCH2*	281.99	0.00	642.59
102	*NR5A1*[a]	222.01	116.84	407.74
103	*NRXN1*[a]	225.80	21.56	577.97
104	*NSD1*[a]	261.44	86.24	500.38
105	*OCA2*[a]	321.02	106.42	685.92
106	*OCRL*	178.97	13.16	440.97
107	*OFD1*	171.17	58.00	394.13
108	*OTC*	190.78	1.46	562.10
109	*OTX2*	311.41	198.51	476.69
110	*PAFAH1B1*[a]	234.58	15.99	516.41
111	*PAK3*	181.03	47.33	405.32
112	*PAX3*	235.81	80.62	569.70
113	*PAX6*[a]	242.37	25.79	599.28
114	*PAX9*[a]	258.47	7.00	540.15
115	*PGK1*	252.23	95.17	614.74
116	*PHEX*	200.00	48.82	439.78
117	*PHF6*[a]	165.22	63.07	315.44
118	*PIGB*	205.86	19.26	539.76
119	*PITX2*[a]	283.28	122.96	548.91
120	*PKD1*	99.18	0.00	512.88
121	*PKD2*	225.02	47.45	475.99
122	*PLP1*	247.34	9.76	525.11
123	*PREPL*[a]	215.09	36.12	484.89
124	*PRPS1*	247.30	102.55	418.52
125	*PTCH1*	270.35	12.72	733.37
126	*PTEN*	150.42	22.31	371.28
127	*PTPN11*	267.28	7.24	610.72
128	*RAI1*[a]	343.75	101.17	648.66
129	*RB1*	131.02	14.38	388.44
130	*RET*	271.31	71.71	635.08
131	*RPS19*[a]	321.73	108.91	519.38

Table 2 Mean coverage with highest and lowest number of reads for target regions for each gene *(Continued)*

132	*RS1*	222.95	115.25	327.74
133	*RUNX2*[a]	273.57	111.60	506.80
134	*SALL1*[a]	358.75	261.01	497.61
135	*SALL4*	275.10	113.08	406.79
136	*SATB2*[a]	308.41	180.72	485.31
137	*SCN1A*	184.22	17.84	385.17
138	*SGCE*	176.87	0.23	424.34
139	*SH2D1A*	221.35	64.88	432.85
140	*SHANK3*	244.90	12.74	621.93
141	*SHH*	161.98	64.47	259.27
142	*SIX3*	122.83	85.98	168.90
143	*SLC12A1*[a]	258.77	62.97	558.39
144	*SLC12A3*	280.89	56.97	814.03
145	*SLC16A2*	265.88	60.08	534.50
146	*SLC3A1*	226.04	90.48	481.54
147	*SLC6A8*	115.64	2.00	346.38
148	*SLC9A6*	140.59	40.48	373.83
149	*SMAD4*[a]	290.53	109.10	607.62
150	*SOX2*	195.01	156.36	240.25
151	*SPINK1*[a]	194.39	57.54	401.97
152	*SRY*	65.35	0.00	189.58
153	*SYN1*	211.18	33.53	488.47
154	*SYNGAP1*	209.23	41.07	495.34
155	*TBCE*[a]	274.69	89.15	774.41
156	*TBX1*[a]	281.13	28.78	628.34
157	*TBX3*	229.37	102.59	459.90
158	*TBX5*[a]	267.57	94.82	473.34
159	*TCF4*[a]	277.43	72.17	568.07
160	*TCOF1*	335.67	175.06	602.11
161	*TGFBR1*	211.80	1.52	479.34
162	*TGFBR2*	303.18	84.26	614.98
163	*TGIF1*	302.73	169.50	481.36
164	*TIMM8A*	166.52	37.46	370.74
165	*TRPS1*[a]	267.79	112.32	411.15
166	*TSC1*[a]	293.98	45.37	607.17
167	*TSC2*[a]	286.10	0.00	776.60
168	*TWIST1*	96.89	76.02	120.38
169	*UPF3B*	200.15	53.63	424.96
170	*USH1C*	283.03	38.50	767.39
171	*VHL*	130.75	57.24	269.80
172	*WT1*	335.43	112.21	654.89
173	*XIAP*[a]	132.08	31.85	278.12
174	*ZDHHC9*[a]	223.57	61.28	554.63
175	*ZEB2*[a]	261.68	97.71	474.05

Table 2 Mean coverage with highest and lowest number of reads for target regions for each gene *(Continued)*

176	*ZFPM2*	211.09	6.00	393.25
177	*ZIC1*	228.52	127.92	369.74
178	*ZIC2*	128.92	29.81	320.70
179	*ZIC3*	202.01	120.08	320.90
180	*ZIC4*	291.25	127.92	616.00

[a]Target regions do not include non-coding first exons

targeted fragments. Circularized target DNA-HaloPlex probe hybrids containing biotin were then captured by HaloPlex Magnetic Beads on the Agencourt SPRIPlate Super magnet magnetic plate. DNA ligase was added to close the nicks in the hybrids, and freshly-prepared NaOH was used to elute the captured target libraries. The target libraries were then amplified with 18 PCR cycles and purified using AMPure XP beads. Amplicons ranging from 150 to 550 bp were then quantified using an Agilent BioAnalyzer High Sensitivity DNA Assay kit on the 2100 Bioanalyzer to validate the enrichment of the libraries. Library preparation took approximately 1½ days.

Equimolar amounts of four multiplexed bar-coded libraries were pooled and clonally amplified by emulsion PCR, using the Ion PGM Template OT2 200 Kit 9 (Life Technologies, Carlsbad, CA, USA). The template-positive Ion Sphere Particles (ISPs) were then enriched with the Ion OneTouch™ ES and loaded on an Ion 318™ Chip v1. Four separate runs were performed for the 15 samples, with one sample sequenced twice on two different chips. Sequencing was carried out in the Ion PGM™ System using the Ion PGM™ Sequencing 200 Kit v2 according to the manufacturer's instructions with 500 flow runs.

The data from the sequencing runs were analyzed using the Torrent Suite v4.0.2 analysis pipeline, which includes raw sequencing data processing (DAT processing), splitting of the reads according to the barcode for the individual sample output sequence, classification, signal processing, base calling, read filtering, adapter trimming, and alignment QC. Single-nucleotide polymorphisms (SNP), multi-nucleotide polymorphisms (MNPs), insertions, and deletions were identified across the targeted subset of the reference using a plug-in Torrent Variant Caller (v4.0-r76860), with the parameter settings optimized for germ-line high frequency variants and minimal false positive calls. The output variant call format (VCF) file was then annotated through the web-based user-interfaced GeneTalk (GeneTalk GmbH, Berlin, Germany) and Ensembl Variant Effect Predictor [14].

Sequence variants were compared with data in dbSNP, 1000 Genomes and Human Genome Mutation Database. Variants not previously reported in healthy controls or previously classified as pathogenic were evaluated for coverage depth and also visually inspected using the Integrative Genomics Viewer before validation by dideoxy sequencing using standard protocol for BigDye® Terminator v3.1 Cycle Sequencing Kit (Life Technologies, Carlsbad, CA, USA). Segregation analysis was performed when DNA from family members was available. Sequencing was carried out on the Applied Biosystems® 3130 Genetic Analyzer (Life Technologies, Carlsbad, CA, USA). In addition, SIFT (sift.bii.a-star.edu.sg) and Polyphen2 (genetics.bwh.harvard.edu/pph2) were used to check the likely functional significance of missense variants for clinical interpretation.

Results

An average of 790 Mb was generated per chip (range 748–828 Mb). Loading densities of the targeted sequencing of four libraries (four samples were multiplexed in each library) ranged from 75 to 81 %. The total number of reads (usable sequence) ranged from 5.8 to 6.4 M, and average read length ranged from 124 to 131 bp. After filtering out polyclonal, low quality, and primer dimers, the percentage of usable reads ranged from 69 to 73 %. On average, each sample yielded 196 M bases from 1.5 M reads (Table 1 and Fig. 1) from 58,670 amplicons with a mean read length of 128 bp. One sample was sequenced twice, with near identical output obtained for both runs. The numbers of reads were 1,552,042 and 1,556,202 for total reads and 1,522,728 and 1,524,576 for mapped reads, and total numbers of bases sequenced were 199,024,281 and 200,813,003.

Approximately 97.4 % of the reads were aligned to the reference genome (hg19) and 91 % mapped to the target regions, with average base coverage ranging from 203× to 256× for individual samples. 97.7 % of the targets had minimum read depth of 20×, 95.6 % at >50× and 88.2 % at >100×. Full coverage was achieved for more than 95 % of targets in all 15 samples, and most (approximately 89.9 %) target bases did not show any bias toward forward or reverse strand read alignment. The average total coverage of all targeted bases was 95.7 % at 20× and 82.38 % at 100×. Coverage was also uniform across all samples. More than 88 % of called bases had a quality score of ≥Q20 (Table 1).

At the gene level, 137 of the 180 genes had mean coverage of at least 20×, of which 99 had a mean of >50× and 40 had a mean of >100× (Table 2). Despite the high target region coverage, amplification failed for at least 26 exons across the 180 genes. Thirteen genes (*CFC1, CHRNA7, CYP21A2, EHMT1, F8, HBA1, HBA2, IKBKG, NOTCH2, PKD1, SGCE, SRY, TSC2*) had at least one region that was not amplified and therefore not sequenced (lowest number of reads "0" in Table 2). The sequencing coverage of *CFC1, IKBKG, HBA1*, and *HBA2* was low with >50 % of these genes sequenced at >20× (Table 3). The gene with the highest mean coverage was *SALL1* (358×). The poorest coverage was for *CFC1*. Mean read depth for individual exons for three different genes were shown in Figs. 2, 3, and 4.

Overall, 2326 single-nucleotide variants (SNVs) and 25 indels were identified in the 15 patients. These variants identified from the Ion Reporter had an average coverage of 595× and an average Qscore of 38. Variant annotation indicated that 2203 were common variants present in dbSNP and 1000 Genome Project databases. The number of variants ranged from 154 to 175 per patient, with an average of 9.6 novel variants each. Synonymous variants were the most common.

Variants were prioritized for Sanger confirmation based on the individual's clinical presentations. Pathogenic variants were confirmed in six patients. The identified *CHD7* (two patients), *SHH*, *TCF4*, *TSC2*, and *MECP2* variants and the clinical features of these six patients are listed in Table 4. Another five patients had candidate variants

Table 3 Percentage of coverage for each gene at 20×

ABCC8	100.00 %	*DMRT1*	100.00 %	*HNF1B*	100.00 %	*OTX2*	100.00 %	*SLC16A2*	100.00 %
ABCD1	100.00 %	*DYM*	100.00 %	*HOXD13*	100.00 %	*PAFAH1B1*	100.00 %	*SLC3A1*	100.00 %
ACSL4	100.00 %	*DYRK1A*	100.00 %	*HPRT1*	100.00 %	*PAK3*	100.00 %	*SLC6A8*	94.71 %
AFF2	100.00 %	*EDNRB*	100.00 %	*IDS*	89.40 %	*PAX3*	100.00 %	*SLC9A6*	100.00 %
ALX4	100.00 %	*EHMT1*	99.47 %	*IKBKG*	26.71 %	*PAX6*	100.00 %	*SMAD4*	100.00 %
AP1S2	100.00 %	*EMX2*	100.00 %	*IRF6*	100.00 %	*PAX9*	99.61 %	*SOX2*	100.00 %
APC	98.72 %	*EXT1*	100.00 %	*JAG1*	100.00 %	*PGK1*	100.00 %	*SPINK1*	100.00 %
AR	100.00 %	*EXT2*	100.00 %	*KAL1*	100.00 %	*PHEX*	100.00 %	*SRY*	100.00 %
ATP7A	100.00 %	*EYA1*	100.00 %	*KCNJ1*	100.00 %	*PHF6*	100.00 %	*SYN1*	100.00 %
ATRX	99.29 %	*F8*	99.66 %	*KCNQ1*	100.00 %	*PIGB*	100.00 %	*SYNGAP1*	100.00 %
AVPR2	100.00 %	*F9*	100.00 %	*L1CAM*	100.00 %	*PITX2*	100.00 %	*TBCE*	100.00 %
BMP4	100.00 %	*FANCA*	100.00 %	*LAMP2*	100.00 %	*PKD1*	86.06 %	*TBX1*	100.00 %
BMPR1A	100.00 %	*FANCB*	100.00 %	*LEMD3*	100.00 %	*PKD2*	100.00 %	*TBX3*	100.00 %
BMPR2	100.00 %	*FBN1*	100.00 %	*LHX4*	100.00 %	*PLP1*	79.74 %	*TBX5*	100.00 %
BRCA2	100.00 %	*FGD1*	100.00 %	*LMX1B*	100.00 %	*PREPL*	100.00 %	*TCF4*	100.00 %
BRWD3	99.43 %	*FGFR1*	100.00 %	*MECP2*	100.00 %	*PRPS1*	100.00 %	*TCOF1*	100.00 %
BSND	100.00 %	*FLNA*	100.00 %	*MID1*	100.00 %	*PTCH1*	97.80 %	*TGFBR1*	93.58 %
BTK	100.00 %	*FMR1*	100.00 %	*MITF*	100.00 %	*PTEN*	100.00 %	*TGFBR2*	100.00 %
CACNA1C	100.00 %	*FOXC1*	100.00 %	*MSX1*	100.00 %	*PTPN11*	89.17 %	*TGIF1*	100.00 %
CASK	94.17 %	*FOXG1*	100.00 %	*MSX2*	100.00 %	*RAI1*	100.00 %	*TIMM8A*	100.00 %
CDKN1C	100.00 %	*FOXL2*	100.00 %	*MTM1*	100.00 %	*RB1*	100.00 %	*TRPS1*	100.00 %
CFC1	0.00 %	*FZD4*	100.00 %	*MYCN*	100.00 %	*RET*	100.00 %	*TSC1*	100.00 %
CHD7	100.00 %	*GATA3*	100.00 %	*NDP*	100.00 %	*RPS19*	100.00 %	*TSC2*	98.30 %
CHD8	99.11 %	*GATA4*	100.00 %	*NDUFV1*	100.00 %	*RS1*	100.00 %	*TWIST1*	100.00 %
CHM	95.10 %	*GDF5*	100.00 %	*NF2*	100.00 %	*RUNX2*	100.00 %	*UPF3B*	100.00 %
CHRNA7	84.46 %	*GJB2*	100.00 %	*NHS*	100.00 %	*SALL1*	100.00 %	*USH1C*	100.00 %
CLCNKA	100.00 %	*GLA*	100.00 %	*NIPBL*	100.00 %	*SALL4*	100.00 %	*VHL*	100.00 %
CLCNKB	100.00 %	*GLI2*	100.00 %	*NLGN4X*	100.00 %	*SATB2*	100.00 %	*WT1*	100.00 %
CNTN4	100.00 %	*GLI3*	100.00 %	*NOTCH2*	95.39 %	*SCN1A*	100.00 %	*XIAP*	100.00 %
COL2A1	100.00 %	*GPC3*	100.00 %	*NR5A1*	100.00 %	*SGCE*	94.86 %	*ZDHHC9*	100.00 %
COL4A5	98.76 %	*GPC6*	100.00 %	*NRXN1*	100.00 %	*SH2D1A*	100.00 %	*ZEB2*	100.00 %
CREBBP	100.00 %	*GPR56*	100.00 %	*NSD1*	100.00 %	*SHANK3*	96.32 %	*ZFPM2*	98.84 %
CUL4B	100.00 %	*GRIA3*	100.00 %	*OCA2*	100.00 %	*SHH*	100.00 %	*ZIC1*	100.00 %
CYP21A2	67.67 %	*HBA1*	30.07 %	*OCRL*	100.00 %	*SIX3*	100.00 %	*ZIC2*	100.00 %
DCX	100.00 %	*HBA2*	30.07 %	*OFD1*	100.00 %	*SLC12A1*	100.00 %	*ZIC3*	100.00 %
DHCR7	100.00 %	*HCCS*	100.00 %	*OTC*	91.74 %	*SLC12A3*	100.00 %	*ZIC4*	100.00 %

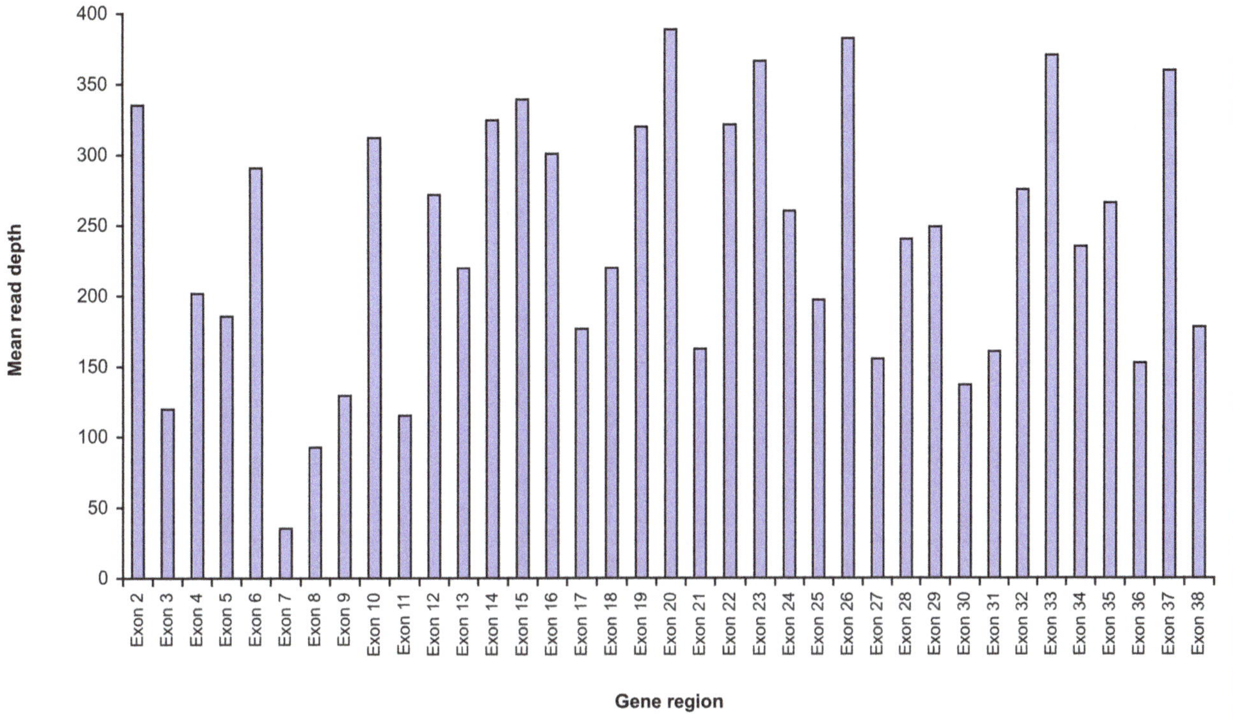

Fig. 2 Average target base read depth for exons 2–38 of *CHD7*

for which further evaluation and segregation analysis are ongoing.

Discussion

The HaloPlex ICCG panel is a pre-designed made-to-order panel targeting 180 genes. It follows the ICCG recommendations for design and resolution and is available through SureDesign from Agilent Technologies. The targeted panel includes genes in the most commonly altered chromosomal regions according to the ISCA/ICCG database. The 180 genes are covered by 2509 target regions which range in size from 2 to 6575 nucleotides. Depending on its size, a region is covered by between 1 and 547 amplicons.

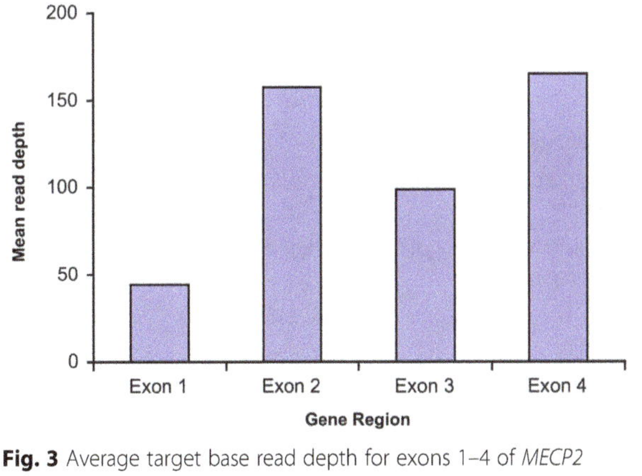

Fig. 3 Average target base read depth for exons 1–4 of *MECP2*

The recommended minimum read depth for clinical diagnostic sequencing is 20× [15, 16], which was achieved for over 90 % of the target for 170 genes. For *CHD7*, even the exon with the poorest coverage had a mean of 36 (Fig. 2). Of the remaining ten, four genes had 80–90 % coverage, and the other six (*CFC1*, *CYP21A*, *HBA1*, *HBA2*, *IKBKG*, *NOTCH2*, *PLP1*) had <80 %. More than half of the targets in these individual genes are within GC-rich regions. Less efficient PCR for these templates might have resulted in sequencing failure during library preparation, or insufficient sequence data were produced [17]. In addition, the HaloPlex protocol uses restriction enzymes which are sequence-dependent and nonrandom, this method might have contributed further to uneven coverage and also gaps in coverage [18]. For *IKBKG*, the presence of a pseudogene might have caused non-specific alignment and contributed to the low capture of target sequences [19]. Nijman et al. have almost no mapped reads in *IKBKG* in their targeted sequencing, and generally poor coverage of *CFC1* and *IKBKG* had been reported in multiple studies [20–22]. For the gene with the poorest coverage *CFC1*, all six exons had no reads across all 15 samples. This gene is associated with the generation of left-right asymmetry via the TGF pathway. There were 23 mutations in HGMD, 13 of which were found in patients with congenital

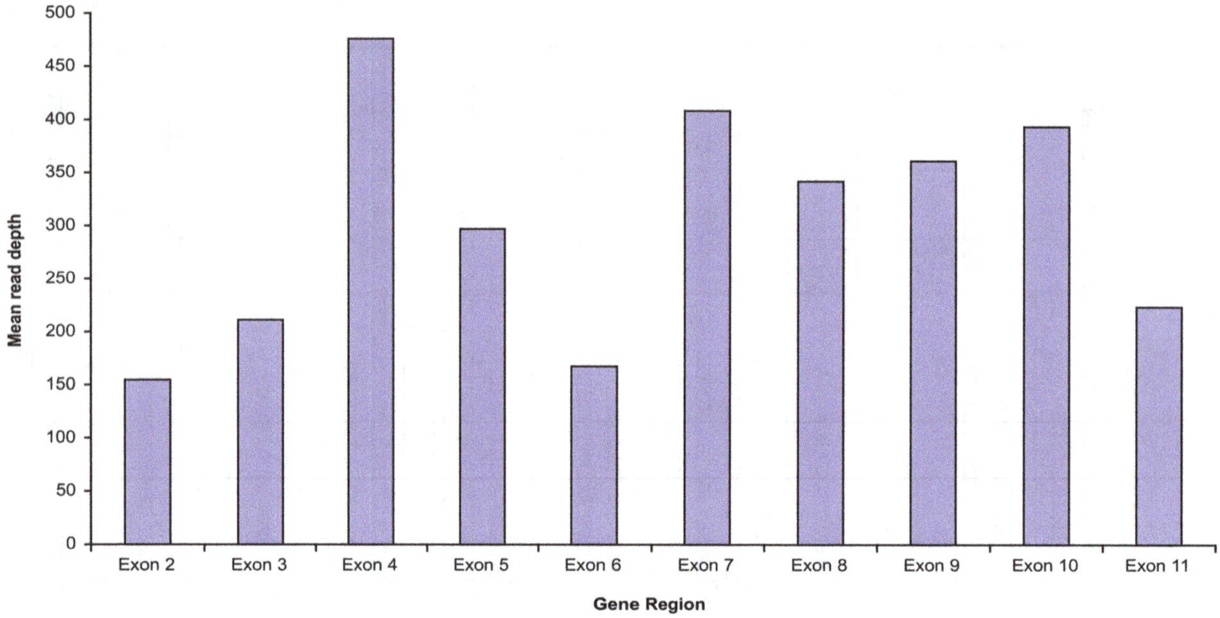

Fig. 4 Average target base read depth for exons 2–11 of *SATB2*

heart disease [23]. This panel would not be useful for patients with clinical suspicion of *CFC1* gene mutations.

The first exon of 64 genes was not included in the design (indicated with "*" in Table 2). All the 64 genes have one or more non-coding exon. The entire exon 1 of these genes (and additional exons for some others) contains only untranslated regions. In general, amplification of exon 1 of some genes was problematic because of the generally higher GC content and sequence complexity [24–26]. Our results showed that *MECP2* had an average target base read depth of 118×. The coverage for exon 1 is the lowest among all, but it is still two times that of the minimum of 20× recommended for clinical diagnostics (Fig. 3). *SATB2* had an average target base read depth of 300×, but exon 1 was not covered in the design (Fig. 4). Nevertheless, including non-coding exons in the design might improve the yield of NGS as variants affecting splicing of non-coding exons have been reported to be disease-causing [27].

Many congenital disorders do not have unique and exclusive features, and the presentations may be non-specific. Even for syndromic disorders, there are overlapping features, and the phenotypic features in some patients may be atypical, making it challenging for the clinical geneticists to come to a diagnosis based on clinical history and examination. All the 15 patients in this study have constitutional disorders and suspicion of chromosomal disorders, but CMA did not find any pathogenic copy number abnormality. With this targeted panel,

Table 4 Pathogenic variants identified and the respective patients' associated clinical features

Patient	Gender	Age[a]	Gene	Nucleotide change	Amino acid change	Clinical features
1	M	1d	CHD7	NM_017780.3:c.7891C > T	p.R2631X	Hypoplastic left heart, choanal atresia, oesophageal atresia
2	F	1y4m	CHD7	NM_017780.3c.601C > T	p.Q201X	PDA, aortic stenosis, coloboma, hypotonia
3	F	3y9m	MECP2	NM_004992.3:c.763C > T	p.R255X	Developmental delay, hypotonia, neurodevelopmental regression, epilepsy
4	F	2w	SHH	NM_000193.3:c.413C > A	p.S138Y	Alobar HPE, PDA, hypotelorism, single nostril, choanal atresia, overlapping fingers
5	M	5y11m	TCF4	NM_001083962.1:c.1739G > A	p.R580Q	GDD, microcephaly, epicanthic folds, hypertelorism, drooling, no speech
6	F	5y8m	TSC2	NM_000548.3:c.3364delC	p.R1121Vfs*69	Bilateral large renal cysts, ballotable left kidney, cardiac rhabdomyoma, iris pigmentation & hamartomas, epilepsy

GDD global developmental delay, *HPE* holoprosencephaly, *PDA* patent ductus arterio
[a]Age at enrollment (d = day, y = year, m = month)

we were able to reach a molecular diagnosis for six patients after reviewing the results with their primary physicians (Table 4). Pathogenic *CHD7* variants were detected in two patients with clinical features consistent with CHARGE syndrome. Both *CHD7* variants identified (p.R2613X and p.Q201X) have been previously reported in other CHARGE patients [28]. A pathogenic p.R255X *MECP2* variant was detected in a patient with clinical features of Rett syndrome. This variant has also been reported previously [29]. The patients with the truncating *TSC2* variant and the missense *SHH* variant also showed clinical features consistent with the respective causative genes. These two variants are novel and the missense variant is predicted to be pathogenic according to both SIFT and Polyphen. Similarly, the clinical features of the patient with the *TCF4* variant are found to be consistent with Pitt-Hopkins syndrome upon retrospective review of the patient's progressive features by the attending physician. This p.R580Q *TCF4* variant has been reported as pathogenic in patients with Pitt-Hopkins syndrome [30].

The identification of a patient's causative mutation has the translational benefit of providing the parents with an answer for their child's condition. In addition, it provides a guide to the attending clinician on the management and prognosis of the patient. A molecular diagnosis would also facilitate access to clinical trials and programs for special needs children. The use of appropriate gene panels obviates the need for subjective clinical decision on which gene(s) to test in each patient, and may lead to a standard testing workflow for each group of disorders. Generally for those whose diagnosis can be narrowed down to a few suspected genetic syndromes, targeted gene panels would be superior to exome sequencing which has more limitations in the diagnostic setting due to coverage deficiencies in some genes and longer turnaround time. Higher-average read depth could be attained at a lower cost, making it superior to exome sequencing in terms of cost, sensitivity, and expected diagnostic yield [31, 32].

Conclusions

The Haloplex ICCG panel had good coverage except for ten of the target genes. Consideration would have to be made for the low coverage for some regions in several genes which might have to be supplemented by Sanger sequencing. However, comparing the cost, ease of analysis, and shorter turnaround time, it is a good alternative to exome sequencing for patients whose features are suggestive of a genetic etiology involving one of the genes in the panel.

Competing interests

All authors declare that they have no competing interests.

Authors' contributions

ECT designed the study and obtained the funding. EL and SPL carried out the sequencing experiments. EL, MB, and SJ performed the analysis and interpretation of the sequencing data. MB, AL, EST, and IN carried out the selection of patients, clinical assessment, and phenotype correlation. EL and ECT prepared the manuscript. All authors read and approved the manuscript.

Acknowledgements

This work is supported by NMRC/CG/006/2013 and NMRC/PPG/KKH12010-Theme3 from the National Medical Research Council, Ministry of Health, Republic of Singapore. We thank K Chang and CH Kuick for the use of the Ion Torrent PGM.

Author details

[1]KK Research Centre, KK Women's and Children's Hospital, 100 Bukit Timah Road, Singapore 229899, Singapore. [2]Genetics Service, Department of Paediatrics, KK Women's and Children's Hospital, Singapore 229899, Singapore. [3]Paediatrics Academic Clinical Programme, SingHealth Duke-NUS Graduate Medical School, Singapore 169857, Singapore.

References

1. Dolk H, Loane M, Garne E. The prevalence of congenital anomalies in Europe. Adv Exp Med Biol. 2010;686:349–64.
2. Birth defects [http://www.cdc.gov/ncbddd/birthdefects/index.html]. Accessed 4 Aug 2015.
3. Boyle CA, Boulet S, Schieve LA, Cohen RA, Blumberg SJ, Yeargin-Allsopp M, et al. Trends in the prevalence of developmental disabilities in US children, 1997–2008. Pediatrics. 2011;127:1034–42.
4. Miller DT, Adam MP, Aradhya S, Biesecker LG, Brothman AR, Carter NP, et al. Consensus statement: chromosomal microarray is a first-tier clinical diagnostic test for individuals with developmental disabilities or congenital anomalies. Am J Hum Genet. 2010;86:749–64.
5. Bartnik M, Wisniowiecka-Kowalnik B, Nowakowska B, Smyk M, Kedzior M, Sobecka K, et al. The usefulness of array comparative genomic hybridization in clinical diagnostics of intellectual disability in children. Dev Period Med. 2014;18:307–17.
6. Battaglia A, Doccini V, Bernardini L, Novelli A, Loddo S, Capalbo A, et al. Confirmation of chromosomal microarray as a first-tier clinical diagnostic test for individuals with developmental delay, intellectual disability, autism spectrum disorders and dysmorphic features. Eur J Paediatr Neurol. 2013;17:589–99.
7. Chong WW, Lo IF, Lam ST, Wang CC, Luk HM, Leung TY, et al. Performance of chromosomal microarray for patients with intellectual disabilities/developmental delay, autism, and multiple congenital anomalies in a Chinese cohort. Mol Cytogenet. 2014;7:34.
8. Green RC, Berg JS, Grody WW, Kalia SS, Korf BR, Martin CL, et al. ACMG recommendations for reporting of incidental findings in clinical exome and genome sequencing. Genet Med. 2013;15:565–74.
9. ACMG Board of Directors. ACMG policy statement: updated recommendations regarding analysis and reporting of secondary findings in clinical genome-scale sequencing. Genet Med. 2015;17:68–9.
10. Botkin JR, Belmont JW, Berg JS, Berkman BE, Bombard Y, Holm IA, et al. Points to consider: ethical, legal, and psychosocial implications of genetic testing in children and adolescents. Am J Hum Genet. 2015;97:6–21.
11. Haloplex disease research panels [http://www.chem.agilent.com/Library/datasheets/Public/HaloPlexDiseaseResearchPanels5991-2526ENa.pdf]. Accessed 4 Aug 2015.
12. Kaminsky EB, Kaul V, Paschall J, Church DM, Bunke B, Kunig D, et al. An evidence-based approach to establish the functional and clinical significance of copy number variants in intellectual and developmental disabilities. Genet Med. 2011;13:777–84.
13. Moreno-De-Luca D, Sanders SJ, Willsey AJ, Mulle JG, Lowe JK, Geschwind DH, et al. Using large clinical data sets to infer pathogenicity for rare copy number variants in autism cohorts. Mol Psychiatry. 2013;18:1090–5.
14. Yourshaw M, Taylor SP, Rao AR, Martin MG, Nelson SF. Rich annotation of DNA sequencing variants by leveraging the Ensembl Variant Effect Predictor with plugins. Brief Bioinform. 2014;16:255–64.

15. Rehm HL, Bale SJ, Bayrak-Toydemir P, Berg JS, Brown KK, Deignan JL, et al. ACMG clinical laboratory standards for next-generation sequencing. Genet Med. 2013;15:733–47.
16. Yohe S, Hauge A, Bunjer K, Kemmer T, Bower M, Schomaker M, et al. Clinical validation of targeted next-generation sequencing for inherited disorders. Arch Pathol Lab Med. 2015;139:204–10.
17. Bragg LM, Stone G, Butler MK, Hugenholtz P, Tyson GW. Shining a light on dark sequencing: characterising errors in Ion Torrent PGM data. PLoS Comput Biol. 2013;9:e1003031.
18. Coonrod EM, Durtschi JD, VanSant WC, Voelkerding KV, Kumanovics A. Next-generation sequencing of custom amplicons to improve coverage of HaloPlex multigene panels. Biotechniques. 2014;57:204–7.
19. Aksyonov SA, Bittner M, Bloom LB, Reha-Krantz LJ, Gould IR, Hayes MA, et al. Multiplexed DNA sequencing-by-synthesis. Anal Biochem. 2006;348:127–38.
20. Brett M, McPherson J, Zang ZJ, Lai A, Tan ES, Ng I, et al. Massively parallel sequencing of patients with intellectual disability, congenital anomalies and/or autism spectrum disorders with a targeted gene panel. PLoS One. 2014;9:e93409.
21. Nijman IJ, van Montfrans JM, Hoogstraat M, Boes ML, van de Corput L, Renner ED, et al. Targeted next-generation sequencing: a novel diagnostic tool for primary immunodeficiencies. J Allergy Clin Immunol. 2014;133:529–34.
22. Kammermeier J, Drury S, James CT, Dziubak R, Ocaka L, Elawad M, et al. Targeted gene panel sequencing in children with very early onset inflammatory bowel disease—evaluation and prospective analysis. J Med Genet. 2014;51:748–55.
23. Human gene mutation database [https://portal.biobase-international.com/hgmd/pro/gene.php?gene=CFC1]. Accessed 2 Sep 2015.
24. Gnirke A, Melnikov A, Maguire J, Rogov P, LeProust EM, Brockman W, et al. Solution hybrid selection with ultra-long oligonucleotides for massively parallel targeted sequencing. Nat Biotechnol. 2009;27:182–9.
25. Hu H, Wrogemann K, Kalscheuer V, Tzschach A, Richard H, Haas SA, et al. Mutation screening in 86 known X-linked mental retardation genes by droplet-based multiplex PCR and massive parallel sequencing. Hugo J. 2009;3:41–9.
26. Porreca GJ, Zhang K, Li JB, Xie B, Austin D, Vassallo SL, et al. Multiplex amplification of large sets of human exons. Nat Methods. 2007;4:931–6.
27. Eisenberger T, Neuhaus C, Khan AO, Decker C, Preising MN, Friedburg C, et al. Increasing the yield in targeted next-generation sequencing by implicating CNV analysis, non-coding exons and the overall variant load: the example of retinal dystrophies. PLoS One. 2013;8:e78496.
28. Bartels CF, Scacheri C, White L, Scacheri PC, Bale S. Mutations in the CHD7 gene: the experience of a commercial laboratory. Genet Test Mol Biomarkers. 2010;14:881–91.
29. Amir RE, Van den Veyver IB, Wan M, Tran CQ, Francke U, Zoghbi HY. Rett syndrome is caused by mutations in X-linked MECP2, encoding methyl-CpG-binding protein 2. Nat Genet. 1999;23:185–8.
30. Amiel J, Rio M, de Pontual L, Redon R, Malan V, Boddaert N, et al. Mutations in TCF4, encoding a class I basic helix-loop-helix transcription factor, are responsible for Pitt-Hopkins syndrome, a severe epileptic encephalopathy associated with autonomic dysfunction. Am J Hum Genet. 2007;80:988–93.
31. Ankala A, da Silva C, Gualandi F, Ferlini A, Bean LJ, Collins C, et al. A comprehensive genomic approach for neuromuscular diseases gives a high diagnostic yield. Ann Neurol. 2015;77:206–14.
32. Consugar MB, Navarro-Gomez D, Place EM, Bujakowska KM, Sousa ME, Fonseca-Kelly ZD, et al. Panel-based genetic diagnostic testing for inherited eye diseases is highly accurate and reproducible, and more sensitive for variant detection, than exome sequencing. Genet Med. 2015;17:253–61.

7

Exploring the interaction among EPHX1, GSTP1, SERPINE2, and TGFB1 contributing to the quantitative traits of chronic obstructive pulmonary disease in Chinese Han population

Li An[1], Yingxiang Lin[1], Ting Yang[2] and Lin Hua[3,4*]

Abstract

Background: Currently, the majority of genetic association studies on chronic obstructive pulmonary disease (COPD) risk focused on identifying the individual effects of single nucleotide polymorphisms (SNPs) as well as their interaction effects on the disease. However, conventional genetic studies often use binary disease status as the primary phenotype, but for COPD, many quantitative traits have the potential correlation with the disease status and closely reflect pathological changes.

Method: Here, we genotyped 44 SNPs from four genes (EPHX1, GSTP1, SERPINE2, and TGFB1) in 310 patients and 203 controls which belonged to the Chinese Han population to test the two-way and three-way genetic interactions with COPD-related quantitative traits using recently developed generalized multifactor dimensionality reduction (GMDR) and quantitative multifactor dimensionality reduction (QMDR) algorithms.

Results: Based on the 310 patients and the whole samples of 513 subjects, the best gene-gene interactions models were detected for four lung-function-related quantitative traits. For the forced expiratory volume in 1 s (FEV1), the best interaction was seen from EPHX1, SERPINE2, and GSTP1. For FEV_1%pre, the forced vital capacity (FVC), and FEV_1/FVC, the best interactions were seen from SERPINE2 and TGFB1.

Conclusion: The results of this study provide further evidence for the genotype combinations at risk of developing COPD in Chinese Han population and improve the understanding on the genetic etiology of COPD and COPD-related quantitative traits.

Keywords: COPD, SNP, Interaction, Quantitative traits, MDR

Background

Chronic obstructive pulmonary disease (COPD) is defined as airflow limitation that is not fully reversible [1]. Cigarette smoking is the major risk factor for COPD, but smokers show considerable variation in their risk of developing airflow obstruction [2]. Although a series of studies have found the genetics contributions from some genes by analyzing individual effects of single nucleotide polymorphisms (SNPs) [3], but in most cases with a large proportion of the genetic component left unexplained, the genetic risk factors for COPD are still largely unknown. Recent studies have approved that complex traits cannot be explained by any single SNP variant, and the characterization of gene-gene interactions and gene-environment interactions may be the key to understand the underlying pathogenesis of complex diseases [4]. It is therefore suggested that identifying the possible jointed effects of gene-gene interaction will help discover the potential susceptibility factors of COPD risk.

* Correspondence: hualin7750@ccmu.edu.cn
[3]School of Biomedical Engineering, Capital Medical University, Beijing 100069, China
[4]Beijing Key Laboratory of Fundamental Research on Biomechanics in Clinical Application, School of Biomedical Engineering, Capital Medical University, Beijing 100069, China
Full list of author information is available at the end of the article

Recent advances in genetic studies have implicated that COPD represents a complex disease with genetics contributions from multiple genes. For example, although many studies did not find the association between EPHX1 and the susceptibility to COPD or disease severity [5, 6], Vibhuti et al. [7] approved that and the combination of 113H/139H alleles of mEPHX and 105V/114V alleles of GSTP1 genotypes with same alleles is associated with imbalanced oxidative stress and lung function in COPD patients. In addition, Artigas et al. [8] investigated the combined effect of the risk alleles at six loci (TNS1, GSTCD, HTR4, AGER, THSD4, and HHIP) and found their joint effects on lung function and COPD risk. Therefore, as a complex polygenic disease, COPD is likely affected by the operation of multiple genes and the coincident actions of several genetic events. However, most conventional genetic studies often use binary disease status as the primary phenotype, but for COPD, many quantitative traits have been shown to correlate with the disease status and to have greater sensitivity in detecting early pathological changes. For example, a ratio between forced expiratory volume in 1 s (FEV_1) and forced vital capacity (FVC) has emphasized the importance of the functional assessment of usually progressive, non-fully reversible airflow limitation [9]. The BODE index, a multidimensional parameter including the body-mass index (B), the degree of airflow obstruction (O), functional dyspnea (D), and exercise capacity (E), was reported to be superior to FEV_1 in reflecting the severity of COPD and effective in predicting the mortality in patients with COPD [10]. Therefore, it is suggested that important insight can be garnered from investigating genotype combinations contributing to the COPD-related quantitative traits, which will help improve the understanding of the genetic etiology of COPD.

Recently, some extension algorithms for detecting and characterizing epistatic interactions in the context of quantitative outcomes named as generalized multifactor dimensionality reduction (GMDR) [11] and quantitative multifactor dimensionality reduction (QMDR) were developed [12], and these algorithms allow researchers to build more accurate models that involve multiple genotype combinations contributing to disease-related quantitative traits. By summarizing a group/body of evidence, we found four genes: EPHX1, GSTP1, SERPINE2, and TGFB1, that are reported to be associated with COPD, and these associations have been confirmed by replication and meta-analysis [13]. Therefore, in the present study, we genotyped 44 SNPs (Additional file 1) involved in these four genes in 310 COPD patients and 203 controls which belonged to the Chinese Han population to explore the joint gene-gene interactions contributing to COPD-related quantitative traits based on the GMDR and QMDR algorithms. We also used a web-based tool GeneMANIA [14] to find genes that interact in any way (physically, genetically, etc.) with our studied four genes in this paper. Our study provides further evidences to identify genotype combinations at risk of developing COPD in Chinese Han population and improve the understanding of the genetic etiology of COPD.

Results

General characteristics of COPD-related quantitative traits for patients

The general characteristics of COPD-related quantitative traits for patients are shown in Additional file 2. Especially, the distribution of the modified Medical Research Council dyspnea scale (MMRC) is as follows: 52 patients (16.8 %) MMRC 0, 144 (46.5 %) MMRC 1, 84 (27.1 %) MMRC 2, 11 (3.5 %) MMRC 3, and 19 (6.1 %) MMRC 4, with a median of 1 (P_5–P_{95}, 0–4). This MMRC distribution indicates that the degrees of various physical activities that precipitate dyspnea of the COPD patients in our study are mild. The distribution of BODE index is as follows: 9 patients (2.9 %) BODE 0, 56 (18.1 %) BODE 1, 93 (30.0 %) BODE 2, 71 (22.9 %) BODE 3, 36 (11.6 %) BODE 4, 26 (8.4 %) BODE 5, 11 (3.5 %) BODE 6, 4 (1.3 %) BODE 7, 3 (1.0 %) BODE 9, and 1 (0.3 %) BODE 10, with a median of 2 (P_5–P_{95}, 1–6). The BODE distribution also indicates that the severity of our COPD patients is mild. In addition, in terms of the effect of a single SNP, except rs41266229 (EPHX1) and rs729631 (SERPINE2) which display the significant difference between the COPD patients and normal controls after passing the multiple testing corrections [13], no significant differences were seen from other single SNP (Additional file 1).

Single marker analysis for COPD-related quantitative traits based on patients

In the current study, we performed the analysis of single marker effect for seven COPD-related quantitative traits. We included covariates age, sex, and pack-years of smoking in the model. For the seven COPD-related quantitative traits, except rs729631 (SERPINE2) which showed a strong association with FVC, no single marker effects showed a significant association after being corrected by Bonferroni procedure (Table 1). It appears that most of these candidate SNPs do not show independent associations with COPD-related quantitative traits.

The best two-way gene-gene interaction models for COPD-related quantitative traits using GMDR, QMDR, and traditional quantitative trait locus (QTL)

In Table 2, we listed the best interaction models identified by QMDR from tenfold cross-validation for COPD-related quantitative traits after being adjusted by covariates age, sex, and pack-years of smoking based on 310 patients. For FEV_1, the best model is the interaction between EPHX1

Table 1 Single marker effects for six[a] COPD-related quantitative traits ($n = 310$ patients)

Six COPD-related quantitative traits																	
FEV_1			FEV_1%pre			FVC			FEV_1/FVC (%)			BODE			6MWT		
Main effects	p^*	p^{**}	Main effects	p^*	p^{**}	Main effects	p^*	p^{**}	Main effects	p^*	p^*	Main effects	p^*	p^{**}	Main effects	p^*	p^{**}
SERPINE2 (rs729631)	0.004	0.176	EPHX1 (rs868966)	0.048	1.000	EPHX1 (rs868966)	0.010	0.440	EPHX1 (rs3738040)	0.005	0.220	SERPINE2 (rs4674841)	0.008	0.352	EPHX1 (rs3766934)	0.027	1.000
SERPINE2 (rs975278)	0.016	0.704				EPHX1 (rs2854450)	0.022	0.968	EPHX1 (rs1877724)	0.007	0.308	EPHX1 (rs2234922)	0.019	0.836	SERPINE2 (rs4674841)	0.045	1.000
SERPINE2 (rs4674841)	0.037	1.000				EPHX1 (rs3738040)	0.023	1.000	EPHX1 (rs2292558)	0.015	0.660	GSTP1 (rs1138272)	0.020	0.880	SERPINE2 (rs6734100)	0.046	1.000
SERPINE2 (rs17196253)	0.013	0.572				EPHX1 (rs1877724)	0.045	1.000	GSTP1 (rs1138272)	0.028	1.000	SERPINE2 (rs13392495)	0.025	1.000			
SERPINE2 (rs3820766)	0.029	1.000				SERPINE2 (rs729631)	2.27E-05	0.001	SERPINE2 (rs729631)	0.002	0.088	SERPINE2 (rs2118409)	0.032	1.000			
									SERPINE2 (rs975278)	0.035	1.000	GSTP1 (rs36211088)	0.032	1.000			

[a]There was no significant main effect for MMRC before being corrected by Bonferroni procedure

$^*p < 0.05$ before corrected by Bonferroni procedure; $^{**}p$ after corrected by Bonferroni procedure

Table 2 The best models identified by QMDR for COPD-related quantitative traits in Chinese Han population ($n = 310$ patients)

COPD-related quantitative traits	The best two-way interaction models	T-CV score	CV consistency	Permutated *P* value
FEV_1	EPHX1(rs2292568)*GSTP1(rs4147581)	2.6390	7/10	0.019*
FEV_1%pre	EPHX1(rs1051741)*TGFB1(rs6957)	1.9234	7/10	0.042*
FVC	SERPINE2(rs7583463)*TGFB1(rs2241713)	2.2735	8/10	0.028*
FEV_1/FVC (%)	SERPINE2(rs17196253)*SERPINE2(rs6748795)	0.3566	3/10	NS
BODE	SERPINE2(rs4674841)*SERPINE2 (rs6748795)	−0.3295	4/10	NS
MMRC	SERPINE2(rs2118409)*SERPINE2 (rs6712954)	1.467	2/10	NS
6MWT	SERPINE2(rs7583463)*SERPINE2 (rs2118409)	1.229	7/10	NS

CV cross-validation, *NS* not significant
**P* value obtained from the 1000 permutation testing

(rs2292568) and GSTP1 (rs4147581). The 1000 permutation testing revealed a significant *P* value of 0.019. The average maximum of FEV_1 (1.82) was seen from rs2292568 (CC)*rs4147581 (GG), whereas the average minimum of FEV_1 (1.08) was seen from rs2292568 (CT)*rs4147581 (GG) (Fig. 1a). This indicated that having two minor alleles for the EPHX1 gene corresponded to an average maximum value of FEV_1. For FEV_1%pre, the best interaction was detected between rs1051741 (EPHX1) and rs6957 (TGFB1). The 1000 permutation testing also revealed a significant *P* value of 0.042. The average maximum of FEV_1%pre (59.92) was seen from rs1051741 (CT)*rs6957 (AA), whereas the average minimum of FEV_1%pre (35.57) was seen from rs1051741 (CT)*rs6957 (AG) (Fig. 1b). For FVC, the best model is the interaction between SERPINE2 (rs7583463) and TGFB1 (rs2241713) which shows a significant *P* value of 0.028 based on the 1000 permutation testing. The average maximum of FVC (3.18) was seen from rs7583463 (AA)*rs2241713 (CG), whereas the average minimum of FVC (2.40) was seen from rs7583463 (CC)*rs2241713 (GG) (Fig. 1c). However, for the other four COPD-related quantitative traits, the best interaction models were found within the gene itself but not found between genes, and the 1000 permutation testing did not find their significance ($P > 0.05$). For FEV_1/FVC, 6-min walk test (6MWT), BODE, and MMRC, the best interactions are rs17196253 (SERPINE2) and rs6748795 (SERPINE2) (Fig. 1d), rs7583463 (SERPINE2) and rs2118409 (SERPINE2) (Fig. 1e), rs4674841 (SERPINE2) and rs6748795 (SERPINE2) (Fig. 1f), and rs2118409 (SERPINE2) and rs6712954 (SERPINE2) (Fig. 1g), respectively. The description and comparison among multiple genotype combinations contributing to seven COPD-related quantitative traits are shown in Additional file 3. For the 310 patients, after being adjusted by covariates, the most significant gene-gene interactions identified by traditional QTL were consistent with those interactions obtained from QMDR in five quantitative traits: FEV_1, FEV_1%pre, FVC, FEV_1/FVC, and BODE (Additional files 4 and 5). For MMRC and 6MWT, there were some discrepancies between QMDR and traditional QTL. We know that QTL is less sensitive in detecting the local effects, whereas QMDR can find the genotype combinations that distinguish the high- and low-level groups optimally. Therefore, when there is good discrimination between the low- and high-level groups in terms of traits, these two methods can both detect the interactions with good power.

In addition, for lung-function-related quantitative traits (FEV_1, FEV_1%pre, FVC, and FEV_1/FVC), we further detected the two-way gene-gene interaction using GMDR, QMDR, and traditional QTL based on the whole samples (310 patients and 203 controls). GMDR, QMDR, and traditional QTL all found that the best interaction model was EPHX1 and GSTP1 for FEV_1, SERPINE2 and TGFB1 for FVC, and FEV_1/FVC (Table 3 and Additional file 4).

The best three-way gene-gene interactions models for COPD-related quantitative traits using GMDR and QMDR

In Table 4, we listed the best three-way gene-gene interaction models identified by QMDR from tenfold cross-validation for COPD-related quantitative traits after being adjusted by covariates age, sex, and pack-years of smoking based on 310 patients. For FEV_1, the best model was seen from GSTP1, EPHX1, and SERPINE2. For FEV_1%pre, FVC, and FEV_1/FVC, the best models were seen from SERPINE2 and TGFB1. For BODE, EPHX1 and SERPINE2 were found to be the best interaction. For MMRC, interaction between GSTP1, TGFB1, and SERPINE2 was the best model with a significant permutated *P* value of 0.022. For 6MWT, the best model was SERPINE2 and GSTP1.

In addition, for four lung-function-related quantitative traits, we also detected the three-way gene-gene interactions using GMDR and QMDR based on the whole samples. GMDR and QMDR all found that the best interaction model was EPHX1, GSTP1, and SERPINE2 for FEV_1 and SERPINE2 and TGFB1 for FVC (Table 5).

Gene-gene interactions in the network

To extend/explore the potential joint genetic effects of these four genes (EPHX1, GSTP1, SERPINE2, and TGFB1), we also used a web-based tool GeneMANIA

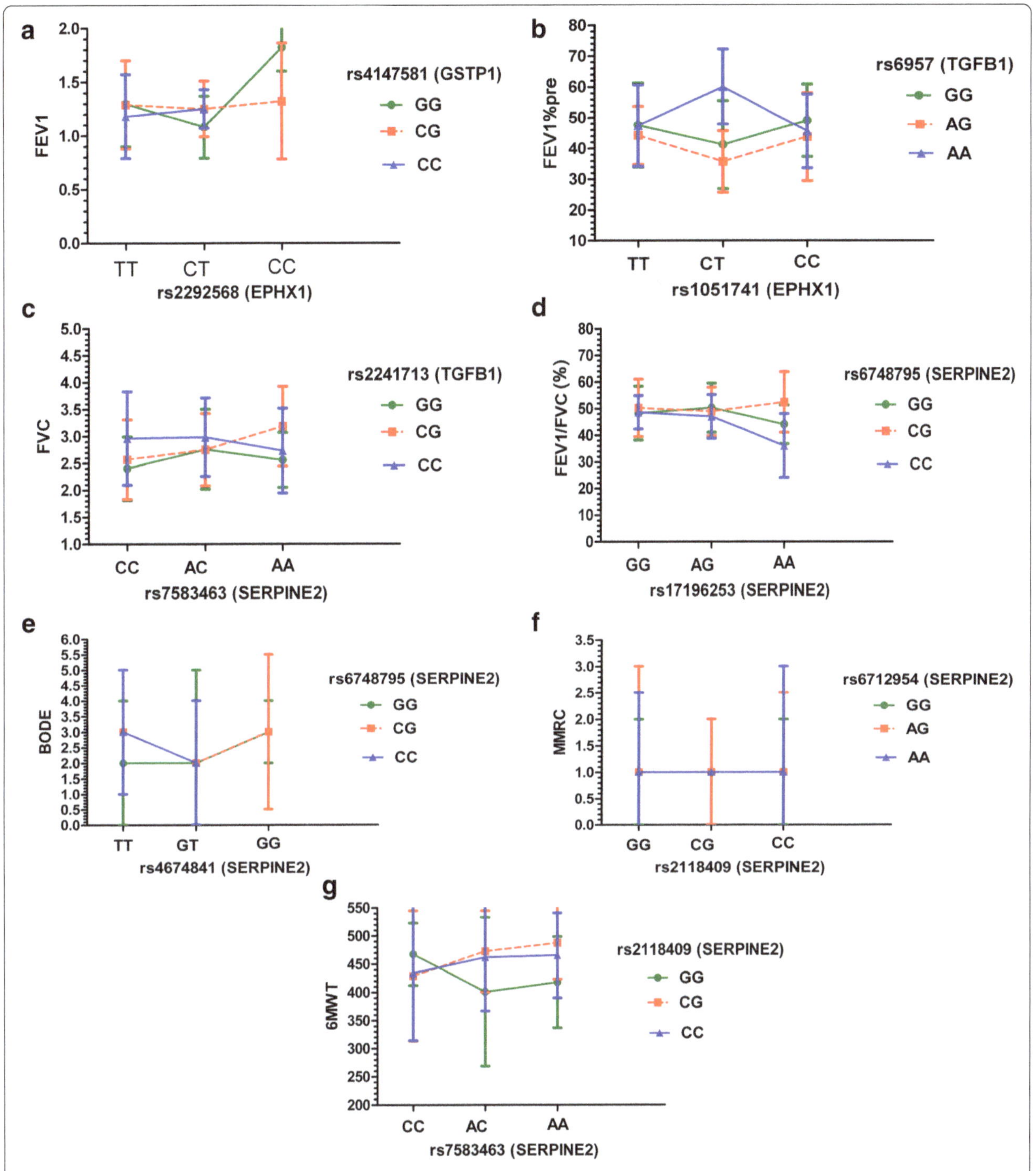

Fig. 1 The best gene-gene interaction models for COPD-related quantitative traits using QMDR method. **a** FEV_1. **b** FEV_1%pre. **c** FVC. **d** FEV_1/FVC (%). **e** BODE. **f** MMRC. **g** 6MWT. For FEV_1, FEV_1%pre, FVC, FEV_1/FVC, and 6MWT, the *y-axis* represents the mean of the trait and the *error bar* represents the standard deviation. For BODE and MMRC, the *y-axis* represents the median of the trait and the *error bar* represents the quartile interval

[14] to find their interactions in any way (physically, genetically, etc.) in the network. We found that except EPHX1 which interacted with GSTP1 directly in the network, these four genes interacted with each other indirectly by passing a transcription factor named FOS (Fig. 2). Previous study confirmed the altered expression of gene encode for FOS in the lung tissues from COPD by using real-time quantitative

Table 3 The best two-way models identified by QMDR and GMDR for four lung-function-related quantitative traits in Chinese Han population ($n = 310$ patients + 203 controls)

COPD-related quantitative traits	The best two-way interaction models based on QMDR			The best two-way interaction models based on GMDR		
	Gene-gene interaction	CV consistency	Permutated *P* value	Gene-gene interaction	CV consistency	Permutated *P* value
FEV_1	rs2260863(EPHX1)*rs4147581(GSTP1)	5/10	0.031*	rs3766934(EPHX1)*rs947895(GSTP1)	3/10	NS
FEV_1%pre	rs10151740(EPHX1)*rs1800469(TGFB1)	2/10	NS	rs2260863(EPHX1)*rs861442(SERPINE2)	3/10	NS
FVC	rs7583463(SERPINE2)*rs2241713(TGFB1)	5/10	NS	rs6748795(SERPINE2)*rs2241713(TGFB1)	4/10	0.036*
FEV_1/FVC (%)	rs17196253(SERPINE2)*rs2241713(TGFB1)	8/10	0.027*	rs729631(SERPINE2)*rs2241713(TGFB1)	2/10	NS

***CV* cross-validation, *NS* not significant**
***P* value obtained from the 1000 permutation testing**

Table 4 The best three-way models identified by QMDR for COPD-related quantitative traits in Chinese Han population ($n = 310$ patients)

COPD-related quantitative traits	The best three-way interaction models	T-CV score	CV consistency	Permutated P value
FEV_1	rs4147581(GSTP1)*rs2292568(EPHX1)*rs4674843(SERPINE2)	0.9948	3/10	NS
FEV_1%pre	rs282254(SERPINE2)*rs6738983(SERPINE2)*rs2241713(TGFB1)	0.4451	3/10	NS
FVC	rs2241715(TGFB1)*rs282254(SERPINE2)*rs6738983(SERPINE2)	−0.2469	2/10	NS
FEV_1/FVC (%)	rs10191694(SERPINE2)*rs282254(SERPINE2)*rs2241713(TGFB1)	0.0393	4/10	NS
BODE	rs13392495(SERPINE2)*rs2118409(SERPINE2)*rs2234922(EPHX1)	−0.1974	2/10	NS
MMRC	rs4147581(GSTP1)*rs2241718(TGFB1)*rs2118409(SERPINE2)	−2.3572	2/10	0.022*
6MWT	rs4674841(SERPINE2)*rs7583463(SERPINE2)*rs947895(GSTP1)	0.9901	2/10	NS

CV cross-validation, *NS* not significant
**P* value obtained from the 1000 permutation testing

RT-PCR [15]. However, Demoly et al. found that FOS was rarely expressed in the normal and pathological chronic bronchitis and lung cancer proliferative compartment of the human bronchi, suggesting its low role in cell proliferation of the large airways [16]. Considering that FOS is the center of the interaction network involved in these four genes, it should be focused on in further studies.

Discussion

Up to now, although there are many different candidate genes which have been investigated for their potential roles in lung function impairment in smokers [17, 18], few works were interested to study the combinations of polymorphisms in COPD quantitative traits. In this paper, our study tested for the association of genetic interaction with seven COPD-related quantitative traits using recently developed GMDR and QMDR algorithms. We got the support for the lack of single marker associations between these SNPs and COPD-related quantitative traits; however, our quantitative trait interaction analysis yielded several interesting candidate gene-gene interactions. For FEV_1, the best interaction was seen from EPHX1, SERPINE2, and GSTP1. For FEV_1%pre, FVC, and FEV_1/FVC, the best interaction models were seen from SERPINE2 and TGFB1. Interestingly, we found EPHX1 interact with GSTP1 directly for FEV_1 trait for COPD patients, which is consistent with the interaction identified by GeneMANIA. In previous studies, Lakhdara et al. have suggested that combined EPHX1, GSTP1, GSTM1 and GSTT1 genetic polymorphisms may play a significant role in the development of COPD, emphysema and decline of the lung function based on the analysis for Tunisian population [18]. Salam et al. found that EPHX1 and GSTP1 variants contribute to the occurrence of childhood asthma and increase asthma susceptibility to exposures from major roads based on the analysis for white children in Southern California [19]. Su et al. performed two-way and three-way gene-gene interactions to find the combining effect of GSTP1, INSIG2, and IL4Ra to lifetime asthma based on the Taiwan seventh-grade children [20]. Therefore, our results provide new evidences that COPD candidate genes may show interactive effects with lung-function-related traits. However, for 6MWT, MMRC, and BODE, the best interaction models only existed in SERPINE2 itself. Because COPD is a complex disease which is caused by the genetics contributions from multiple genes, therefore, genes derived from multiple gene-gene interactions may help reveal their cumulative effect effectively. SERPINE2 occurring in multiple gene-gene interactions has been approved for its association with COPD. In fact, many previous findings have confirmed that SERPINE2 gene polymorphisms are associated to COPD and may be involved particularly in the development of panlobular emphysema [21].

In addition, we know that the advantage of MDR is not only that it can deal with sparse and high-dimension data and therefore might uncover non-linear SNP-SNP interactions that are missed by QTL but also it can detect high-order interactions between genes which cannot be performed by QTL as the model complexity increases with the order of interactions. In the present study, we used GMDR and QMDR to detect the three-way interactions between genes and found that the best interactions were seen from some of these four genes. Furthermore, we have determined that the genes more frequently detected by GMDR, QMDR, and QTL were more likely to be functional, such as SERPINE2 [22]. This suggests that our results do not occur only by chance but might reveal some real biological links between genes. Especially, the interaction between EPHX1 and GSTP1 were approved by GeneMANIA web-based tool. The interactions detected by GMDR and QMDR seem more diverse and less influenced by the SNP main effects.

Moreover, we know that the most common variable selection strategy for interaction studies often select SNPs with main effects to test for the interactions. However, such an approach might cause the miss of some of the true interactions between genes. It has been reported

Table 5 The best three-way models identified by QMDR and GMDR for four lung-function-related quantitative traits in Chinese Han population ($n = 310$ patients + 203 controls)

COPD-related quantitative traits	The best three-way interaction models based on QMDR			The best three-way interaction models based on GMDR		
	Gene-gene interactions	CV consistency	Permutated *P* value	Gene-gene interactions	CV consistency	Permutated *P* value
FEV_1	rs4147581(GSTP1)*rs2260863(EPHX1)*rs6736436(SERPINE2)	4/10	NS	rs868966(EPHX1)*rs7583463(SERPINE2)*rs947895(GSTP1)	4/10	NS
FEV_1%pre	rs282254(SERPINE2)*rs6738983(SERPINE2)*rs2241713(TGFB1)	4/10	0.041*	rs282254(SERPINE2)*rs729631(SERPINE2)*rs1051740(EPHX1)	2/10	NS
FVC	rs2241715(TGFB1)*rs282254(SERPINE2)*rs6738983(SERPINE2)	2/10	NS	rs2241713(TGFB1)*rs6748795(SERPINE2)*rs7579646(SERPINE2)	4/10	0.035*
FEV_1/FVC (%)	rs10191694(SERPINE2)*rs868966(EPHX1)*rs2241713(TGFB1)	4/10	NS	rs4674843(SERPINE2)*rs282254(SERPINE2)*rs2241713(TGFB1)	5/10	0.039*

CV cross-validation, *NS* not significant
*P value obtained from the 1000 permutation testing

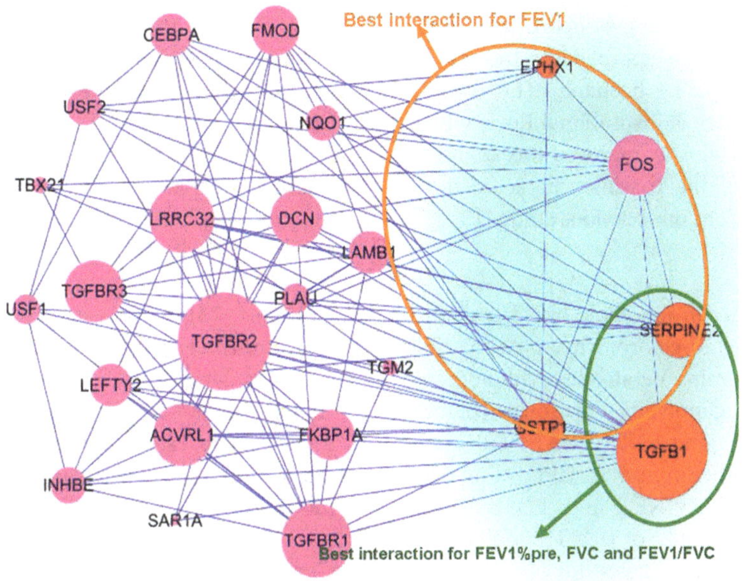

Fig. 2 The interaction of four genes in the network using GeneMANIA web tool. The *red circles* indicate the four genes studied in this paper, and other *pink circles* indicate the interacted genes in the network acquired from GeneMANIA web tool. The *larger size circles* indicate the genes with the greater degree in the network

that the false positive report probability (FPRP) [23] depends on prior probability that the association is real and the statistical power of the test, therefore selecting genes based on their functions can clearly reduce the FPRP [24]. In the present study, we select four genes: EPHX1, GSTP1, SERPINE2, and TGFB1 to explore their interaction effects contributing to COPD-related quantitative traits. In fact, our selected genes are based on the priori evidences that they are functionally important in the COPD development [13]. This selection may help reduce the FPRP. In the future, the further validation of the gene-gene interactions found in this study using other independent datasets will strengthen to confirm our results and provide further insight into the role of interacting genes in COPD etiology.

Furthermore, we must point out the limitations of the present study. Firstly, we limited our studies to interactions within four COPD-related genes, but interactions between genes based on the other priori biology evidences or on pathways may be related to disease risk as well and warrant further exploration. Secondly, a newly developed multivariate quantitative multifactor dimensionality reduction (Multi-QMDR) algorithm is approved to have better performance than QMDR and GMDR when multiple quantitative phenotypes are available [25]. This method summarized the multivariate phenotypes into a univariate score by dimensional reduction analysis, and then classify the samples accordingly into high-risk and low-risk groups. Although GMDR and QMDR are appropriate for analyzing the interactions of smaller number of biomarkers, Multi-QMDR will outperform these two methods when detecting the interactions between a greater number of biomarkers [25]. In our future work, Multi-QMDR will be used for exploring interaction effects between large numbers of variables including genetic and environment factors. Finally, a relatively small population was recruited and the relative small sample size might affect the results. After the patients were classified according to the genotype combinations, the size of the subgroups became small and this may also affect the statistical power [26]. Indeed, we can see that some best interactions were not significant after being adjusted by the permutation tests. Maybe added sample size can change this case. Therefore, our findings should be considered with caution. In the future, we will use a larger population and study more candidate genes taking into account the gene-gene or gene-environment interactions contributing to COPD phenotype or quantitative traits to elucidate the genetic pathogenesis of COPD.

Methods

Study population

We recruited 310 unrelated COPD patients aged 40–75 years from respiratory outpatient clinics at 12 hospitals in Beijing from October 2007 to March 2009. The cases are physician-diagnosed COPD; the pulmonary function test shows FEV_1/FVC of less than 0.7 and $FEV_1\%pre$ of less than 0.8 predicted and no evidence of primary asthma or other respiratory diseases. The control group comprised of 203 subjects with the same age range as the case group. They have no history of respiratory symptoms and exhibit normal pulmonary function of FEV_1/FVC of more than 0.7

and FEV_1%pre of more than 0.8 predicted. Written informed consent was obtained from every participating subject, and the study protocol was approved by the research ethics boards of all participating hospitals. The complete name of the ethics committee is Institutional Review Board of Beijing Chaoyang Hospital who approved this study. The detailed entry criteria and the baseline characteristics of study subjects were seen from our previous study [13, 27].

Genotyping of SNPs

Genomic DNA was isolated from whole blood leukocytes by the conventional phenol-chloroform method. SNPs were genotyped using Illumina VeraCode technology performed on BeadXpress genotyping platform (Illumina Inc., USA). Forty-four tagging SNPs (MAF > 0.05) were genotyped to capture the common variants of the four genes (EPHX1, GSTP1, SERPINE2, and TGFB1) under pairwise mode with r^2 threshold of 0.8. The detailed description was seen from our previous study [13, 27].

COPD-related quantitative traits

In the present study, for COPD patients, we focused on seven COPD-related quantitative traits to perform our analysis. These traits were described simply as follows:

FEV_1 and FEV_1%pre: FEV_1 is called the forced expiratory volume in one second, indicating the volume in a 1-s forced exhalation. It is then converted to a percentage of predicted based on your height, weight, and race normal named as *FEV_1%pre*. FEV_1%pre is a key value to be known by smokers and COPD patients in order to assess the severity of the disease [28]. In the present study, the FEV_1%pre of COPD patients is less than 0.8.

FVC is called the forced vital capacity, indicating the amount of air exhaled forcefully and quickly after maximum inspiration [29].

FEV_1/FVC is a calculated ratio used in the diagnosis of obstructive and restrictive lung disease. It represents the proportion of a person's vital capacity that they are able to expire in the first second of expiration [30]. In the present study, the FEV_1/FVC of COPD cases is less than 70 %.

6MWT is the 6-min walk test which is the most commonly used exercise test in pulmonary rehabilitation. In the current study, the 6MWT was carried out according to the ATS guidelines [31]. Each patient was ordered to walk in a solid and flat corridor for 6 min as soon as possible. The test was repeated twice with an interval of at least 30 min. The best walking distances for two 6MWTs for each patient were recorded as the 6-min walking distance (6MWD).

MMRC is the modified Medical Research Council dyspnea scale which uses a simple grading system to assess a patient's level of dyspnea. The MMRC dyspnea scale classified the breathless into six grades (0 to 5) according to self-perceived breathlessness during daily activities [32]. Grade 5 represents the most severe category.

BODE index is a multidimensional index comprising the BMI, degree of airway obstruction (FEV_1%pre), functional dyspnea (MMRC dyspnea scale), and exercise capacity (6MWT). For the calculation of the BODE index, we used an empirical model as previously described [33]. For the first parameter, the value was 0 or 1. For the last three parameters, the patient received points ranging from 0 (lowest value) to 3 (highest value). The BODE index was the sum of points for each variable, ranging from 0 to 10. A higher BODE index score indicates a greater probability of patient mortality [34].

Considering that 6MWT, BODE, and MMRC are measure indexes only appropriate for COPD patients, therefore the quantitative traits measured for normal controls are four lung-function-related traits: FEV_1, FEV_1%pre, FVC, and FEV_1/FVC, which were subjected to our further analysis.

Statistical analysis

General characteristics of COPD-related quantitative traits for COPD patients

The general characteristics of COPD-related traits for patients are described, and the comparison among multiple genotype combination is performed using the analysis of variance (ANOVA) or Kruskal-Wallis test. A *P* value of <0.05 is considered statistically significant. All statistical analysis was completed using SPSS version 19.0 (SPSS Inc., Chicago, IL).

Single marker analysis for COPD-related quantitative traits based on patients

For seven COPD-related quantitative traits for patients, we used the QTL method (general linear model) to perform single marker analysis using the PLINK software (http://pngu.mgh.harvard.edu/~purcell/plink/), and we used an additive model for gene effects. We included covariates age, sex, and pack-years of smoking in the model. A correction for multiple comparisons was performed using the Bonferroni procedure [35].

Gene-gene interaction analysis for COPD-related quantitative traits

In the present study, we used recently developed GMDR and QMDR algorithms to test for the two-way and three-way gene-gene interactions with COPD-related quantitative traits based on the COPD patients and the whole samples, respectively. GMDR uses score-related statistics derived from a generalized linear regression model and allows covariates to be adjusted [11]. QMDR extends the MDR algorithm and works with quantitative or continuous phenotypes. Instead of comparing the case-control ratio of each multi-locus genotype to a fixed threshold, QMDR compares the mean value of each multi-locus genotype to the overall mean. The outcome between high- and low-level groups defined by the QMDR attribute is compared using a *T* test and then he *T* statistic is used as a training score to choose the best model [12]. In addition, we also used the QTL method (general linear model) to identify the two-way gene-gene interactions, and gene-gene pairs were considered significant if *P* value is smaller than 0.05. Those interactions with most significant *P* values were considered as the best two-way interaction models. The QTL was performed with the PLINK software (http://pngu.mgh.harvard.edu/~purcell/plink/). Considering that the covariates like age, sex, and smoking status might have a strong main effect and may potentially interfere with the ability of MDR and QTL to achieve their goal [35], we therefore included age, sex, and pack-years of smoking in these methods, respectively.

Gene-gene interactions in the network

To extend/explore the potential joint genetic effects of these four genes (EPHX1, GSTP1, SERPINE2, and TGFB1) with other genes, we also used a web-based tool GeneMANIA [14] to find their interaction in any way (physically, genetically, etc.) in the network. Because GeneMANIA does not support pseudogenes, we thus manually queried the four genes: EPHX1, GSTP1, SERPINE2, and TGFB1, and used the automatic weighting for the network. For the network creation, we used only physical interactions, predicted interaction, pathways, and co-expression. GeneMANIA was accessed on 31 May 2013.

Conclusion

In conclusion, our study suggests the potential interactions between EPHX1, SERPINE2, GSTP1, and TGFB1 contributing to COPD-related quantitative traits, such as FEV_1, FEV_1%pre and FVC. The MDR approaches used in this paper that have the potential in the identification of complex biological links contribute to COPD development processes. Our study provides further evidence for the genotype combinations at risk of developing COPD in Chinese Han population and improves understanding on the genetic etiology of COPD.

Additional files

Additional file 1: Forty-four captured tagging SNPs involved in four genes (EPHX1, SERPINE2, GSTP1, and TGFB1) and their association with COPD phenotype using genotype-based chi-square tests. (DOC 103 kb)

Additional file 2: The general characteristics of COPD-related quantitative traits for COPD patients ($n = 310$).

Additional file 3: The description and comparison among multiple genotype combination contributing to seven COPD-related quantitative traits based on QMDR ($n = 310$ patients).

Additional file 4: The best models identified by traditional QTL for COPD-related quantitative traits in Chinese Han population.

Additional file 5: Gene-gene interaction models for COPD-related quantitative traits using traditional QTL method based on 310 patients.

Competing interests
The authors declare that they have no competing interests.

Authors' contributions
LA gave the initial instructions for the work. LA, YL, and TY collected the data. LH analyzed the data. LA and LH wrote and edited the manuscript. All authors read and approved the final version of the manuscript.

Acknowledgements
This work is supported by the Beijing Natural Science Foundation (Grant Nos. 7142015) and the National Science Foundation of China (Grant Nos. 31100905). This study is also supported by the foundation-clinical cooperation project of the Capital Medical University (14JL43).

Author details
[1]Beijing Key Laboratory of Respiratory and Pulmonary Circulation Disorders, Beijing Institute of Respiratory Medicine, Department of Respiratory and Critical Care Medicine, Beijing Chao-Yang Hospital, Capital Medical University, Beijing 100020, China. [2]Department of Respiratory and Critical Care Medicine, China-Japan Friendship Hospital, Beijing 100029, China. [3]School of Biomedical Engineering, Capital Medical University, Beijing 100069, China. [4]Beijing Key Laboratory of Fundamental Research on Biomechanics in Clinical Application, School of Biomedical Engineering, Capital Medical University, Beijing 100069, China.

References

1. Vestbo J, Hurd SS, Agustí AG, et al. Global strategy for the diagnosis, management, and prevention of chronic obstructive pulmonary disease: GOLD executive summary. Am J Respir Crit Care Med. 2013;187(4):347–65.
2. Pillai SG, Ge D, Zhu G, et al. A genome-wide association study in chronic obstructive pulmonary disease (COPD): identification of two major susceptibility loci. PLoS Genet. 2009;5(3):e1000421.
3. Smolonska J, Wijmenga C, Postma DS, Boezen HM. Meta-analyses on suspected chronic obstructive pulmonary disease genes. Am J Respir Crit Care Med. 2009;180:618–31.
4. Yang P, Ho JW, Yang YH, Zhou BB. Gene-gene interaction filtering with ensemble of filters. BMC Bioinformatics. 2011;12 Suppl 1:S10.
5. Chappell S, Daly L, Morgan K, et al. Genetic variants of microsomal epoxide hydrolase and glutamate-cysteine ligase in COPD. Eur Respir J. 2008;32:931–7.
6. Siedlinski M, Postma DS, Smit HA, Boezen HM. No effects of EPHX1 polymorphisms on the level or change of FEV1 in the general population. Eur Respir J. 2009;33(2):446–9.
7. Vibhuti A, Arif E, Deepak D, Singh B, Pasha MAQ. Genetic polymorphisms of GSTP1 and mEPHX correlate with oxidative stress markers and lung function in COPD. Biochem Biophys Res Commun. 2007;359(1):136–42.
8. Artigas MS, Wain LV, Repapi E, et al. Effect of five genetic variants associated with lung function on the risk of chronic obstructive lung disease, and their joint effects on lung function. Am J Respir Crit Care Med. 2011;184:786–95.

9. Guerra S. Asthma and chronic obstructive pulmonary disease: natural history, phenotypes, and biomarkers. Curr Opin Allergy Clin Immunol. 2009; 9(5):409–16.
10. Liu S-F, Tseng C-W, Tu M-L, et al. The clinical COPD questionnaire correlated with BODE index—a cross-sectional study. The ScientificWorld Journal. 2012; 2012:Article ID 361535.
11. Lou X-Y, Chen G-B, Yan L, Elston RC, Li MD, et al. A generalized combinatorial approach for detecting gene-by-gene and gene-by-environment interactions with application to nicotine dependence. Am J Hum Genet. 2007;80:1125–37.
12. Gui J, Moore JH, Williams SM, et al. A simple and computationally efficient approach to multifactor dimensionality reduction analysis of gene-gene interactions for quantitative traits. PLoS One. 2013;8(6):e66545.
13. Hua L, An L, Li L, Zhang Y, Wang C. A bioinformatics strategy for detecting the complexity of chronic obstructive pulmonary disease in northern Chinese Han population. Genes Genet Syst. 2012;87:197–209.
14. Mostafavi S, Ray D, Warde-Farley D, Grouios C, Morris Q. GeneMANIA: a real-time multiple association network integration algorithm for predicting gene function. Genome Biol. 2008;9 Suppl 1:S4.
15. Ning W, Li C-J, Kaminski N, et al. Comprehensive gene expression profiles reveal pathways related to the pathogenesis of chronic obstructive pulmonary disease. PNAS. 2004;101(41):14895–900.
16. Demoly P, Chanez P, Pujol J-L, et al. Fos immunoreactivity assessment on human normal and pathological bronchial biopsies. Respir Med. 1995;89(5): 329–35.
17. Joos L, He J-Q, Shepherdson MB, et al. The role of matrix metalloproteinase polymorphisms in the rate of decline in lung function. Hum Mol Genet. 2002;11(5):569–76.
18. Lakhdara R, Dendena S, Knanib J, et al. Combined analysis of EPHX1, GSTP1, GSTM1 and GSTT1 gene polymorphisms in relation to chronic obstructive pulmonary disease risk and lung function impairment. Dis Markers. 2011;20: 253–63.
19. Salam MT, Lin PC, Avol EL, Gauderman WJ, Gilliland FD. Microsomal epoxide hydrolase, glutathione S-transferase P1, traffic and childhood asthma. Thorax. 2007;62(12):1050–7.
20. Su M-W, Tung K-Y, Liang P-H, et al. Gene-gene and gene-environmental interactions of childhood asthma: a multifactor dimension reduction approach. PLoS One. 2012;7(2):e30694.
21. Kukkonen MK, Tiili E, Vehmas T, Oksa P, Piirilä P, Hirvonen A. Association of genes of protease-antiprotease balance pathway to lung function and emphysema subtypes. BMC Pulm Med. 2013;13:36.
22. Fujimoto K, Ikeda S, Arai T, et al. Polymorphism of SERPINE2 gene is associated with pulmonary emphysema in consecutive autopsy cases. BMC Med Genet. 2010;11:159.
23. Wacholder S, Chanock S, Garcia-Closas M, Ghormli LE, Rothman N. Assessing the probability that a positive report is false: an approach for molecular epidemiology studies. J Natl Cancer Inst. 2004;96(6):434–42.
24. Briollais L, Wang Y, Rajendram I, Onay V, Shi E, Knight J, Ozcelik H. Methodological issues in detecting gene-gene interactions in breast cancer susceptibility: a population-based study in Ontario. BMC Med. 2007;5:22.
25. Yu W, MS Kwon MS, Park T. Multivariate quantitative multifactor dimensionality reduction for detecting gene-gene interactions. Hum Hered. 2015;79:168–81.
26. Koran MEI, Hohman TJ, Meda SA, Thornton-Wells TA, Initiative ADN. Genetic interactions within inositol-related pathways are associated with longitudinal changes in ventricle size. J Alzheimers Dis. 2014;38(1):145–54.
27. An L, Yang T, Zhang Y, Lin Y, Zhang H, Jiao X, Hua L, Dai H, Wang C. Association of SERPINE2 gene with the risk of chronic obstructive pulmonary disease and spirometric phenotypes in northern Han Chinese population. Mol Biol Rep. 2011;39(2):1427–33.
28. Tashkin DP, Celli BR, Decramer M, Lystig T, Liu D, Kesten S. Efficacy of tiotropium in COPD patients with FEV1 ≥ 60 % participating in the UPLIFT® trial. COPD. 2012;9(3):289–96.
29. Yuan W, He X, Xu Q-F, Wang H-Y, Casaburi R. Increased difference between slow and forced vital capacity is associated with reduced exercise tolerance in COPD patients. BMC Pulm Med. 2014;14:16.
30. Swanney MP, Ruppel G, Enright PL, et al. Using the lower limit of normal for the FEV1/FVC ratio reduces the misclassification of airway obstruction. Thorax. 2008;63:1046–51.
31. Laboratories ATSCoPSfCPF. ATS statement: guidelines for the six-minute walk test. Am J Respir Crit Care Med. 2002;166:111–7.
32. Bestall JC, Paul EA, Garrod R, Garnham R, Jones PW, Wedzicha JA. Usefulness of the Medical Research Council (MRC) dyspnoea scale as a measure of disability in patients with chronic obstructive pulmonary disease. Thorax. 1999;54:581–6.
33. Celli BR, Cote CG, Marin JM, et al. The body-mass index, airflow obstruction, dyspnea, and exercise capacity index in chronic obstructive pulmonary disease. N Engl J Med. 2004;350:1005–12.
34. Regueiro EMG, Lorenzo VAPD, Basso RP, Pessoa BV, Jamami M, Costal D. Relationship of bode index to functional tests in chronic obstructive pulmonary disease. Clinics (Sao Paulo). 2009;64(10):983–8.
35. Gui J, Andrew AS, Andrews P, Nelson HM, Kelsey KT, Karagas MR, Moore JH. A simple and computationally efficient sampling approach to covariate adjustment for multifactor dimensionality reduction analysis of epistasis. Hum Hered. 2010;70:219–25.

8

Transcriptome analysis reveals manifold mechanisms of cyst development in ADPKD

Rita M. C. de Almeida[1,2], Sherry G. Clendenon[3], William G. Richards[4], Michael Boedigheimer[4], Michael Damore[4], Sandro Rossetti[5], Peter C. Harris[5], Britney-Shea Herbert[6], Wei Min Xu[7], Angela Wandinger-Ness[8], Heather H. Ward[9], James A. Glazier[3] and Robert L. Bacallao[7*]

Abstract

Background: Autosomal dominant polycystic kidney disease (ADPKD) causes progressive loss of renal function in adults as a consequence of the accumulation of cysts. ADPKD is the most common genetic cause of end-stage renal disease. Mutations in polycystin-1 occur in 87% of cases of ADPKD and mutations in polycystin-2 are found in 12% of ADPKD patients. The complexity of ADPKD has hampered efforts to identify the mechanisms underlying its pathogenesis. No current FDA (Federal Drug Administration)-approved therapies ameliorate ADPKD progression.

Results: We used the de Almeida laboratory's sensitive new transcriptogram method for whole-genome gene expression data analysis to analyze microarray data from cell lines developed from cell isolates of normal kidney and of both non-cystic nephrons and cysts from the kidney of a patient with ADPKD. We compared results obtained using standard Ingenuity Volcano plot analysis, Gene Set Enrichment Analysis (GSEA) and transcriptogram analysis. Transcriptogram analysis confirmed the findings of Ingenuity, GSEA, and published analysis of ADPKD kidney data and also identified multiple new expression changes in KEGG (Kyoto Encyclopedia of Genes and Genomes) pathways related to cell growth, cell death, genetic information processing, nucleotide metabolism, signal transduction, immune response, response to stimulus, cellular processes, ion homeostasis and transport and cofactors, vitamins, amino acids, energy, carbohydrates, drugs, lipids, and glycans. Transcriptogram analysis also provides significance metrics which allow us to prioritize further study of these pathways.

Conclusions: Transcriptogram analysis identifies novel pathways altered in ADPKD, providing new avenues to identify both ADPKD's mechanisms of pathogenesis and pharmaceutical targets to ameliorate the progression of the disease.

Keywords: Kidney, Transcriptogram, Cystic kidney disease, Autosomal dominant polycystic kidney disease, Bioinformatics, Pathway identification

Background

Autosomal dominant polycystic kidney disease (ADPKD) is a monogenic disorder associated with cystic renal disease, liver cysts, cardiac valve abnormalities, and berry aneurysms [1]. Progressive accumulation of renal cysts in ADPKD culminates in kidney failure, usually during the fifth or sixth decades of life. With a disease incidence of 1 in 800, ADPKD is one of the most common human genetic disorders. Despite extensive research, no Federal Drug Administration (FDA)-approved treatments prevent or delay disease progression, limiting patient treatment options to dialysis or kidney transplantation [2].

Two gene loci are responsible for ADPKD; HmPKD1 (human polycystic kidney disease gene 1) and HmPKD2 (human polycystic kidney disease gene 2) located on chromosomes 16 and 4, respectively. The gene products of these loci are polycystin-1 (PC-1) and polycystin-2 (PC-2), proteins that form a heteromeric complex in

* Correspondence: rbacalla@iupui.edu
[7]Division of Nephrology, Department of Medicine, Richard Roudebush VAMC and Indiana University School of Medicine, Indianapolis, IN 46202, USA
Full list of author information is available at the end of the article

primary cilium of renal cells [3–5]. Primary cilia are mechanically sensitive and serve as a flow sensor in renal tubular epithelia [6]. Due to the subcellular localization of polycystins, and the pleiotropic phenotypes associated with their mutations, Hildebrandt et al. called ADPKD the grandfather of ciliopathies [7].

Since ADPKD perturbs the Jnk/Stat (cJun N-terminal kinases/signal transducer and activator of transcription 1), MAPK (mitogen-activated protein kinase), mTOR (mammalian target of rapamycin), Wnt/Wgless (Wingless-related integration site/Wingless)and Erk (extracellular signal regulated kinase) kinase pathways [8], somatostatin analogues, vasopressin receptor antagonists, mTOR inhibitors, and statins have been tested for their ability to ameliorate the course of ADPKD. While mTOR inhibitors reduced cyst growth in murine polycystic kidney disease (PKD) models, they did not slow progression of renal impairment in human trials [9–11]. The FDA did not approve a recent vasopressin receptor antagonist, which inhibited cyst growth in several animal models of polycystic kidney disease, and slowed increases in total kidney volume and decreased estimated creatinine clearance in humans [12–14]. Because cyst formation in ADPKD begins in utero, drugs that can prevent initial cyst formation are not likely to be acceptable in a clinical setting [15, 16]. However, it is possible that the signaling pathways that initially drive cyst emergence are the unique entry points for treatment. We therefore concentrate on identifying the properties of ADPKD cells derived from normal nephrons and cysts from the same kidney to compare to kidney cells derived from an end-stage cystic kidney and normal human renal cortex. Our eventual goal would be to identify signaling pathways that provide a unique opening for targeted therapy in ADPKD.

The paucity of ADPKD drug candidates partially results from the difficulty in identifying pathways that promote cyst growth in renal cells but are not essential in other adult cell types. Standard gene-chip analysis of expressed mRNA shows that ADPKD perturbs Wnt/Wgless and Notch signaling [17, 18]. Decreased Notch signaling and mutated components in the Wnt pathway can cause renal cystic disease [18–20]. However, the Wnt/Wgless and Notch signaling pathways are essential to cell fate transitions and assignments in most cell types [21], so targeting these pathways would likely result in widespread and damaging bystander effects. Similarly, renal epithelial cells with an HmPKD1 mutation express many markers of immature cell differentiation, including increased proliferation rates, altered cell-ECM (extracellular matrix) adhesion, and increased apoptosis. However, most of these pathways are ubiquitous and thus not promising drug targets. To identify promising therapeutic targets, we need to compare expression patterns in cells from normal human renal cortex, normal nephrons in ADPKD patents, and in cysts from the same patients to identify pathways uniquely active in cystogenesis and not essential in other adult tissues. Identifying optimal drug targets also requires a coherent biological context that connects clusters of gene perturbations to the mechanisms of cyst formation, not just identification of individual perturbed genes in cystic ADPKD cells.

The de Almeida laboratory developed transcriptogram whole-genome gene expression data analysis to identify perturbed molecular networks and pathways more sensitively than conventional gene-chip analysis methods [22–24]. Transcriptogram analysis orders genes into a list using a Monte Carlo simulation that minimizes the distance within the list between associated gene products, so proximity in the list correlates with the degree of co-participation in biological processes. Calculating the average transcription level for genes within a moving window produces a transcriptogram profile which reveals any differentially expressed pathways. This robust statistical approach couples enhanced significance assessment with assessment of false discovery rates (FDRs). Transcriptogram analysis identifies rich sets of biological signaling interactions for later integrated hypothesis testing.

Results and discussion

We generated three different telomerase-immortalized cell lines, derived from isolates of (i) a normal kidney of a 57-year-old male (designated as normal cells, NK), (ii) non-cystic tissue from the kidney of a 36-year-old male (designated as non-cystic ADPKD cells, NC-ADPKD), and (iii) cystic tissue from the same donor (designated as cystic ADPKD cells, C-ADPKD). The additional ADPKD cell line in this paper is a previously characterized telomerase immortalized cell line isolated from an end-stage polycystic kidney [25]. We refer to the expression patterns of the NK cells as normal. We refer to expression of a gene or pathway in ADPKD, NC-ADPKD, or C-ADPKD cells as higher-than-normal if the expression level in those cells is significantly greater than in NK cells. Conversely, we refer to expression of a gene or pathway in ADPKD, NC-ADPKD, or C-ADPKD cells as lower-than-normal if the expression level in those cells is significantly lower than in NK cells. Differences between the NC-ADPKD and NK cells are particularly significant because they may identify early changes permissive for cyst formation in morphologically normal kidney tissue. We obtained microarray data for genome-wide gene expression for all cell lines in triplicate. We then analyzed the resulting data using three different, complementary methods: single gene expression analysis using QIAGEN's Ingenuity Pathway Analysis (IPA QIAGEN Redwood City), Gene Set Enrichment Analysis (GSEA) [26], and the transcriptogram method [22, 23, 27].

Mouse and human renal cells with aberrant polycystin-1 have impaired ciliary mechanosensation, and this impairment has been proposed as a cellular mechanism that promotes cystogenesis [28]. However, most cyst epithelia of human ADPKD kidneys express full-length polycystin-1 (PC-1) and polycystin-2 (PC-2) at normal or increased abundance [29–31]. Our PC-1 microarray data agrees with these observations (Fig. 1). Our microarray data show equal expression of PC-2 in NC-ADPKD and NK cells and reduced expression in C-ADPKD cells, a finding of uncertain significance.

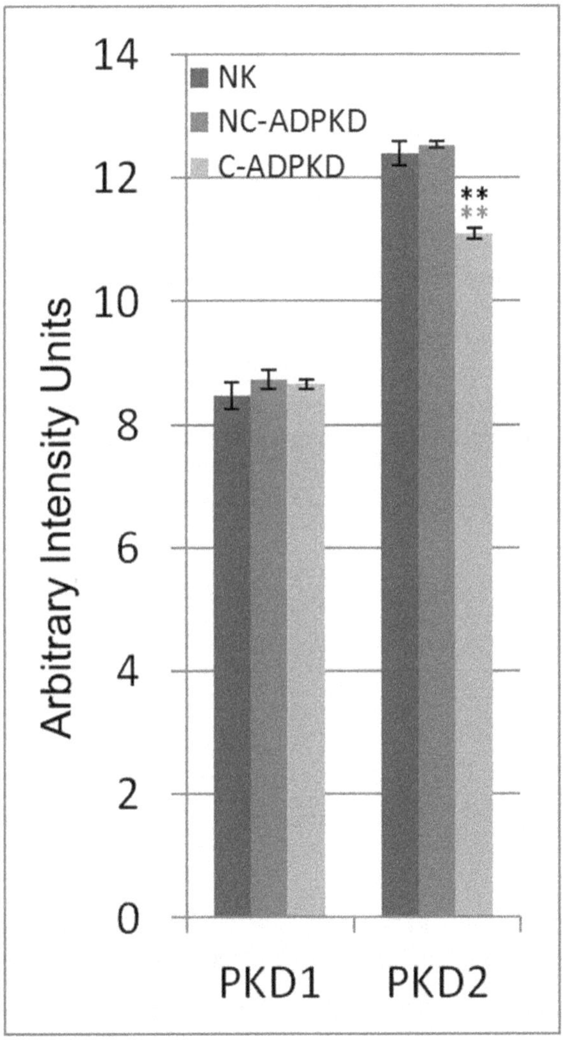

Fig. 1 PKD1 and PKD2 gene expression in the NK, NC-ADPKD, and C-ADPKD cells. PKD1 expression is not different from normal in the NC-ADPKD and C-ADPKD cells. PKD2 expression is normal in the NC-ADPKD cells but significantly lower than normal in C-ADPKD cells. Bars show mean ± s.e., $**p < 0.01$, $*p < 0.05$ (*black asterisk* is in comparison to NK, *gray asterisk* is in comparison to NC-ADPKD)

Volcano plots: single-gene analyses

Ingenuity pathway analysis scores each gene independently to create a list of all genes which change significantly in expression between two states. We averaged gene expression levels over the replicates for each cell line after normalization and compared cell lines by calculating the fold change (FC) as the ratio between the averages. We also obtained P values for each gene expressed. We present the results as Volcano plots (Fig. 2). Setting a significance threshold of FC > 2 and $P < 0.01$, we found 80 genes with significantly altered expression levels between the NK and NC-ADPKD cells, 968 genes with significantly altered expression levels between the NK and C-ADPKD cells, and 1182 genes with significantly altered expression levels between the C-ADPKD and NC-ADPKD cells (Additional file 1). These long lists of differentially expressed genes, by themselves, do not provide immediate insights into the biological mechanisms of ADPKD.

GSEA: Gene Set Enrichment Analyses

GSEA determines whether an a priori defined set of genes shows statistically significant, concordant differences between two biological states [26, 32, 33]. GSEA evaluates genome-wide expression profiles from cells belonging to two classes. We performed GSEA on the three pairs: NK versus NC-ADPKD cells, NK versus C-ADPKD cells, and NC-ADPKD versus C-ADPKD cells to identify differential expression in Kyoto Encyclopedia of Genes and Genomes (KEGG) pathways and in Gene Ontology: Biological Process (GO) terms. We set a significance threshold for the gene set permutation FDR <0.05. Table 1 summarizes the GSEA results and Table **2** lists all significantly altered KEGG pathway and GO term gene sets.

All GSEA-detected pathway differences between NK and NC-ADPKD cells related to 'metabolism' (We will use single '' to identify terms from GO and KEGG). GSEA-detected pathway differences between NK and C-ADPKD cells relate to 'chemokine signaling,' 'cell migration,' and 'cell-cell adhesion,' but not 'metabolism'. GSEA-detected pathway differences between NC-ADPKD and C-ADPKD cells relate to 'chemokine signaling,' 'cell migration,' and 'cell-cell adhesion' but not 'metabolism'. However, transcriptogram analyses (see below) show that expression of metabolome genes differs between these pairs as well, but too weakly for GSEA to detect, likely due to the competitive character of GSEA analysis [33].

Transcriptograms: genome-wide landscapes of gene expression

Transcriptograms project expression profiles onto a gene list that is ordered with genes belonging to the same KEGG pathway or GO term clustered in the list. We built an ordered list of 9684 genes (Additional file 2)

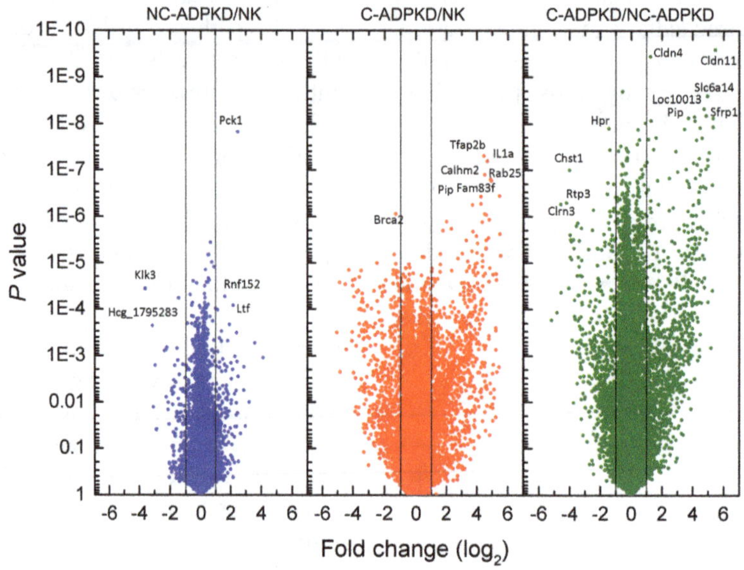

Fig. 2 Volcano plot of single gene analysis. Plots of log *P* value versus $\log_2$ fold change for NC-ADPKD/NK, C-ADPKD/NK, and NC-ADPKD/C-ADPKD cells. The two *vertical lines* in each panel mark twofold change. *Labels* indicate representative genes with highly significant fold changes. See Additional file 1 for full lists of significantly changed genes

using a Monte Carlo Simulation that minimizes distances between associated gene products. Specifically, proximity in the list correlates with co-participation in biological processes, based on protein-protein association information available from the STRING database [34, 35]. Transcriptogram values then correspond to the average expression level of the genes located in a window of radius $r = 30$ (window size $2r + 1 = 61$) along the ordered list. Overlay of selected GO terms and KEGG pathways onto the ordered list then serves as a key to the biological correlates of expression differences and thus aids interpretation of transcriptograms of experimental

Table 1 GSEA analysis summary

GSEA summary for NC-ADPKD/NK						
Upregulated in		# gene sets	FDR < 0.25	FDR < 0.05	$P < 0.05$	$P < 0.01$
NK	KEGG	162	15	**5**	11	7
	GOBP	467	0	0	6	1
NC-ADPKD	KEGG	162	0	0	20	3
	GOBP	467	10	0	41	18
GSEA summary for C-ADPKD/NK						
Upregulated in		# gene sets	FDR < 0.25	FDR < 0.05	$P < 0.05$	$P < 0.01$
NK	KEGG	162	2	0	8	0
	GOBP	467	0	0	11	2
C-ADPKD	KEGG	162	15	**3**	17	12
	GOBP	467	1	**1**	46	13
GSEA summary for NC-ADPKD/C-ADPKD						
Upregulated in		# gene sets	FDR < 0.25	FDR < 0.05	$P < 0.05$	$P < 0.01$
NC-ADPKD	KEGG	162	11	0	10	4
	GOBP	467	17	0	24	13
C-ADPKD	KEGG	162	11	**4**	18	10
	GOBP	467	3	**1**	42	15

Numbers of gene sets that reach significance in comparisons of two GSEA classes, FDR < 0.05, are bold. *FDR* false discovery rate, *P* nominal *P* value, as described by Subramanian et al. 2005 [26]. GSEA expresses all differences as upregulation to minimize class bias due to the intrinsic asymmetry of the method

Table 2 KEGG pathways and GO terms identified as differentially expressed by GSEA analysis

	Size	ES	NES	Normal *P* value	FDR	FWER *P* value
NC-ADPKD/NK, upregulated in NK						
KEGG_drug_metabolism_cytochrome_p450	42	0.8	2.17	0	0	0
KEGG_metabolism_of xenobiotics_by_cytochrome p450	42	0.7	2.06	0	0	0.001
KEGG_histidine_metabolism	22	0.8	1.94	0	0.006	0.019
KEGG_glutathione_metabolism	38	0.7	1.86	0	0.013	0.049
KEGG_fatty_acid_metabolism	32	0.6	1.73	0.004	0.048	0.209
C-ADPKD/NK, upregulated in C-ADPKD						
KEGG_chemokine_signaling_pathway	144	−1	−1.73	0	0.01	0.011
KEGG_axon_guidance	99	−1	−1.68	0	0.03	0.066
KEGG_leukocyte_transendothelial_migration	86	−1	−1.66	0.001	0.028	0.092
GOBP_cell_cell_adhesion	48	0.8	1.8	0	0.001	0.001
NC-ADPKD/C-ADPKD, upregulated in C-ADPKD						
KEGG_leukocyte_transendothelial_migration	86	−1	−1.82	0	0	0
KEGG_chemokine_signaling_pathway	144	−1	−1.74	0	0.024	0.05
KEGG_tight_junction	101	−1	−1.73	0	0.02	0.063
KEGG_axon_guidance	99	−1	−1.73	0	0.016	0.066
GOBP_cell_cell_adhesion	48	0.8	1.8	0	0.007	0.008

Listing of KEGG pathways and GO terms with FDR < 5 %. GSEA expresses all differences as upregulation to minimize class bias due to the intrinsic asymmetry of the method

gene expression data (Fig. 3). The x-axis corresponds to the ordered gene list. Peaks represent regions of the list enriched with genes belonging to specific pathways or terms. We normalize the density profiles of term enrichment so that when all genes within a window participate in that pathway or term, the center point of that interval has a value of one. This paper presents transcriptograms as three-part panels, with the transcriptogram itself in the upper third of the panel, the P values for the transcriptogram in the middle third of the panel (with horizontal

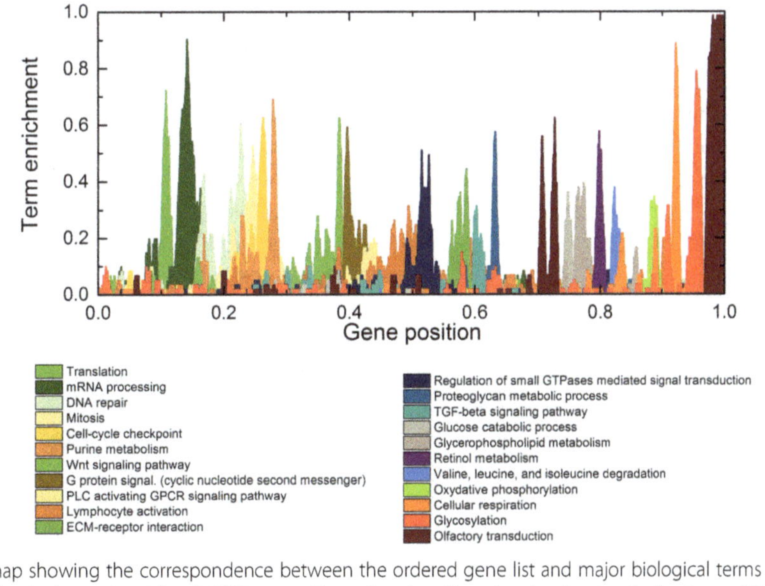

Fig. 3 Term enrichment map showing the correspondence between the ordered gene list and major biological terms and pathways. The x-axis indicates the relative position in the ordered list of 9684 genes. The colored profiles give the density distributions within the list of specific GO terms or KEGG pathways. A term enrichment value of 1 on the y-axis indicates that all genes in an interval of radius $r = 30$ participate in a given GO term or KEGG pathway. *Peaks* mark regions enriched with genes related to the term or pathway indicated in the legend. The legend orders the terms/pathways from left to right

lines indicating $p = 0.05$ and 0.01), and plots of peaks from the term enrichment density profile that correspond to significant peaks in the transcriptogram in the lower third of the panel. We calculated FDR values for all comparisons (Table 3).

Using transcriptogram analysis, we first compared the expression profiles of NK and NC-ADPKD samples (Fig. 4). Across most of the ordered list, the standard errors of the expression levels of genes for the NK and NC-ADPKD cells overlap, showing that gene expression levels of these genes in NC-ADPKD cells do not differ significantly from normal. However, gene positions between 0.22 and 0.26 and the intervals centered at positions 0.46 and 0.88 show significant differences ($P < 0.01$ and FDR < 0.12). The term enrichment profile shows that these significant peaks correspond to 'cell cycle,' 'locomotory behavior,' 'NOD (nucleotide-binding oligomerization domain)-like receptor signaling,' and 'Potassium ion transport' (Fig. 4). When we analyzed the gene lists from each interval of differential expression to identify additional pathways and terms, we found additional differentially expressed gene sets related to 'cell cycle,' 'nucleotide metabolism,' 'genetic information processing,' 'immune response,' and 'ion transport' (Figs. 7, 8, 9, 11, 13). We examined individual gene expression profiles from two of these pathways, 'NOD-like receptors' and 'potassium ion transport'. Genes differentially expressed at significant levels (Figs. 12a, 11b) may be potential targets for drug interventions to prevent or ameliorate very early stages of cyst growth.

Transcriptogram analysis comparing the NK and C-ADPKD samples (Fig. 5) detected additional regions of significant difference (where $P < 0.01$ and FDR < 0.12). The term enrichment profile shows that these significant peaks correspond to alterations in 'RNA processing,' 'cell cycle,' 'nucleic acid processing and metabolism,' 'G-protein signaling,' 'immune response,' and 'cell fate' related pathways including 'Calcium signaling' and 'JAK-STAT' pathways, 'wound healing,' 'extracellular matrix,' 'cell adhesion and tight junctions,' as well as energy-related gene sets for 'oxidative phosphorylation' and the 'TCA (tricarboxylic acid cycle) cycle,' and the 'drug-metabolism related cytochrome P450'. Analysis of the gene lists from each interval of differential expression identified additional related pathways and terms (Figs. 7, 8, 9, 10, 11, 12, 13, and 14). Overall, C-ADPKD cells have lower-than-normal metabolic rates and lower-than-normal expression levels of genes associated with 'cell proliferation,' 'RNA (ribonucleic acid) metabolism,' and 'sugar, lipid and energy metabolism'. Additionally, their interaction with the extracellular environment is strongly altered as indicated by enhanced expression of 'cell adhesion,' 'tight junction,' and 'cell surface signaling' pathways. Thus, C-ADPKD cells have abnormal interactions with their extracellular environment.

Table 3 False discovery rates

False discovery rates			
P value	NC-ADPKD/NK	C-ADPKD/NK	C-ADPKD/NC-ADPKD
0.1	0.131545	0.140392	0.0970966
0.05	0.137393	0.120033	0.0869387
0.01	0.100738	0.112763	0.0809876
0.005	0.100182	0.1156	0.0804989
0.001	0	0.106	0.0800862
0.0005	0	0	0.0800589
0.0001	0	0	0.08
5.00E−05	0	0	0.08

False discovery rates (FDR) for relative transcriptograms obtained using 500 sample-label permutations

Although cell cycle regulation is abnormal in both NC-ADPKD and C-ADPKD cells, expression of cell-cycle-related genes is higher-than-normal in NC-ADPKD samples and lower-than-normal in C-ADPKD samples. Additional pathways and terms identified from gene lists of the cell cycle or RNA metabolism-associated intervals (Figs. 7, 8, and 9) present a consistent pattern: expression in the NC-ADPKD sample is higher than normal and expression in C-ADPKD sample is lower than normal. This pattern of cell-cycle regulation disruption deserves future investigation since the genes included in this gene set initiate and regulate cell cycle progression making it difficult to predict the net effect on cell proliferation.

We then used transcriptogram analysis to compare NC-ADPKD and C-ADPKD samples (Fig. 6). Because NC-ADPKD and NK samples have very similar expression profiles (Fig. 4), the transcriptogram comparison of NC-ADPKD to C-ADPKD samples is similar to the transcriptogram comparison of NK to C-ADPKD samples. However, because NC-ADPKD and C-ADPKD samples derive from cystic and non-cystic tissues from the same kidney, standard errors and consequently, *P* values for this comparison are very small. However, the location of the most significant peaks and valleys are nearly identical in both comparisons. Many of the pathways and terms differentially expressed between NC-ADPKD and C-ADPKD samples (Figs. 6, 7, 8, 9, and 10) are also differentially expressed between NK and C-ADPKD samples.

Gene sets associated with significantly altered transcriptogram intervals

Transcriptogram values indicating significant differential expression do not directly refer to pathways or terms, but rather to intervals of the ordered list enriched with genes for specific pathways and terms. Therefore, subsequent to transcriptogram analysis (Figs. 3, 4, and 5), we fed the gene lists from each identified interval of differential expression into the publicly available David functional

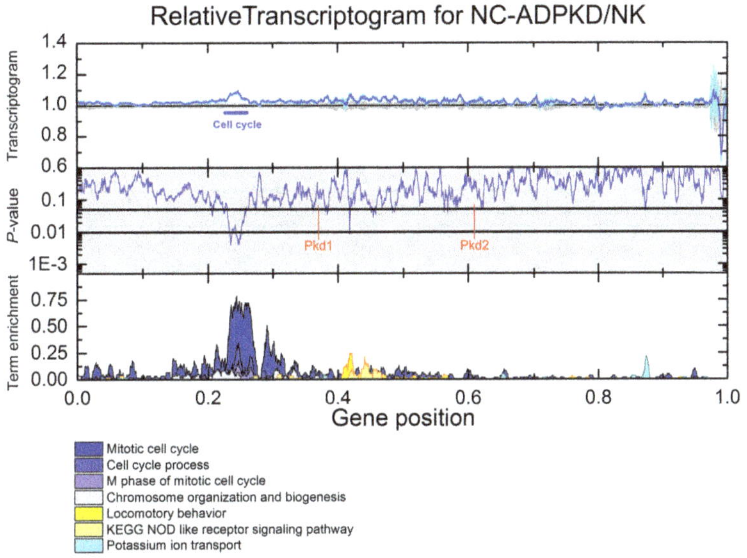

Fig. 4 Relative transcriptogram for NC-ADPKD/NK. The *x*-axis indicates the relative positon in the ordered list of 9684 genes. *Upper panel* the relative transcriptograms are presented as means ± s.e.m. with NC-ADPKD (*blue line* ± *cyan region*) and NK (*black line* ± *gray region*) given relative to NK. *Center panel* (*shaded gray*): *P* value from a two-tailed Weyl's *t* test is plotted for each point of the transcriptograms. *Horizontal lines* mark $P = 0.05$ and $P = 0.01$. Location in the ordered list of Pkd1 and Pkd2, the causative genes for ADPKD, is shown. *Lower panel* Term enrichment for transcriptogram regions with significantly changed expression. A term enrichment value of 1 on the *y*-axis indicates that all genes in an interval of radius $r = 30$ participate in a given GO term or KEGG pathway. As an example of how to read the relative transcriptogram figures, NC-ADPKD cells have higher-than-normal gene expression in the region of the peak labeled 'cell cycle' in the *upper panel* with a significance of $P < 0.01$ (*middle panel*). This region is enriched with genes associated with 'cell cycle' KEGG terms and GO pathways (marked with a *bar* and identified by referring to the *lower panel*, which shows term enrichment)

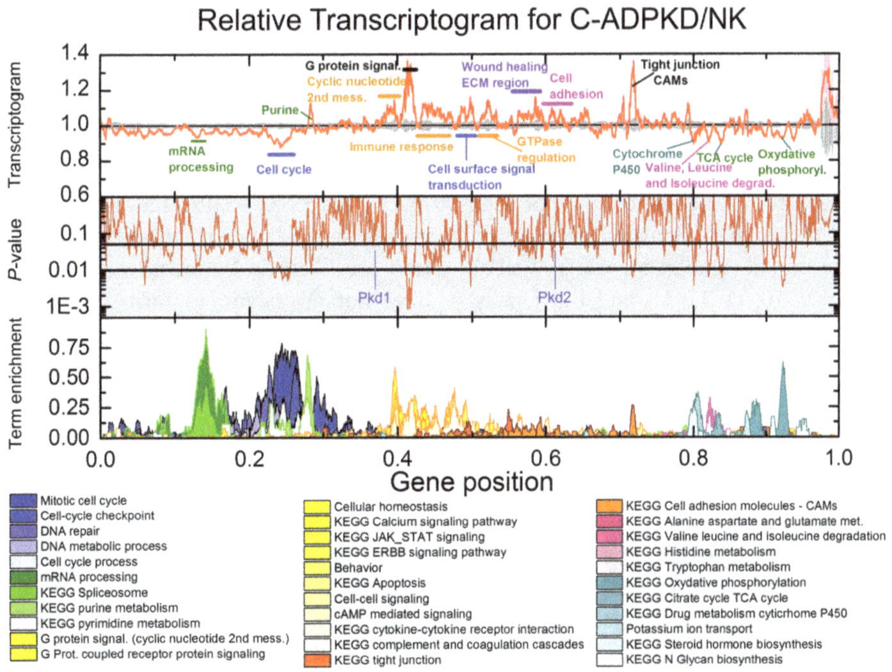

Fig. 5 Relative transcriptogram for C-ADPKD/NK. The *x*-axis indicates the relative position in the ordered list of 9684 genes. *Upper panel* We present the relative transcriptograms as means ± s.e.m. with C-ADPKD (*red line* ± *pink region*) and NK (*black line* ± *gray region*) given relative to NK. *Center panel* (*shaded gray*): *P* value from a two-tailed Weyl's *t* test for each point of the transcriptogram. *Horizontal lines* mark $P = 0.05$ and $P = 0.01$. We label the location in the ordered list of Pkd1 and Pkd2, the causative genes for ADPKD. *Lower panel* Term enrichment for transcriptogram regions with gene expression significantly different from normal. A term enrichment value of 1 on the y-axis indicates that all genes in an interval of radius $r = 30$ participate in a given GO term or KEGG pathway

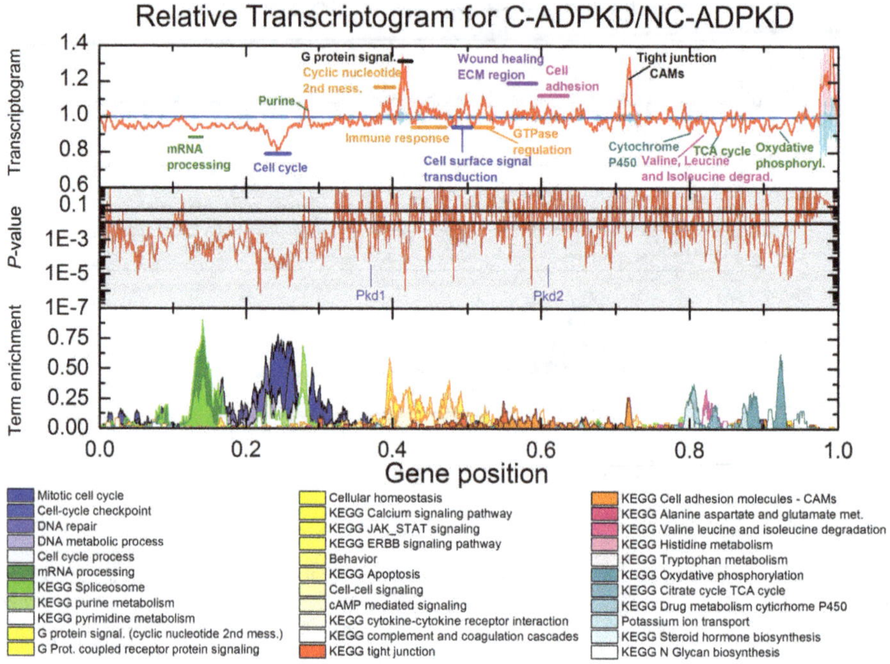

Fig. 6 Relative transcriptogram for C-ADPKD/NC-ADPKD. The *x*-axis indicates the relative positon in the ordered list of 9684 genes. *Upper panel* The relative transcriptograms are presented as means ± s.e.m. with C-ADPKD (red line ± pink region) and NC-ADPKD (blue line ± cyan region) relative to NC-ADPKD. Center panel (shaded gray): *P* value from a two tailed Weyl's *t* test for each point of the transcriptogram. Horizontal lines mark $P = 0.05$ and $P = 0.01$. We label the location in the ordered list of Pkd1 and Pkd2, the causative genes for ADPKD. Lower panel: Term enrichment for transcriptogram regions with gene expression significantly different from normal. A term enrichment value of 1 on the *y*-axis indicates that all genes in an interval of radius $r = 30$ participate in a given GO term or KEGG pathway. *P* values between C-ADPKD and NC-ADPKD cells are smaller than between either C-ADPKD or NC-ADPKD and NK cells (see Figs. 4 and 5) because C-ADPKD and NC-ADPKD cells were derived from the same individual, allowing us to discriminate additional differentially expressed regions

tools [36, 37] to identify additional KEGG pathways (pathways) and GO terms (terms) associated with those intervals. We then had to consider the differential expression of particular pathways and terms independently. For each of these pathways and terms, we calculated average expression levels and determined significance using Welch's two tail *t* test (Figs. 7, 8, 9, 10, 11, 12, 13, and 14). Finally, we categorized these pathways and terms according to the KEGG pathway map and GO term hierarchies, grouping together functionally overlapping pathways and terms from KEGG and GO.

Differentially regulated KEGG pathways and GO terms identified from gene set analyses

NC-ADPKD samples had higher-than-normal and C-ADPKD samples lower-than-normal expression of pathways and terms associated with 'cell proliferation' (Fig. 7). Both NC-ADPKD and C-ADPKD samples had higher-than-normal expression of 'cell-death-related' terms. These expanded results agree with the terms identified using the transcriptogram ordered gene list (Figs. 3, 4, and 5). Consistent with the changes seen in 'cell growth,' 'genetic information processing,' (Fig. 8) and 'amino acid metabolism' (Fig. 9), pathways and terms are higher than normal in NC-ADPKD samples and lower than normal in C-ADPKD samples. The one exception to this pattern, the KEGG 'ribosome pathway,' is higher than normal in both NC-ADPKD and C-ADPKD samples. These results suggest that treatments that target cell proliferation are likely to be effective in patients in which cysts have not yet begun to form and ineffective in patients with significant cyst formation. Pathways and terms with abnormal expression in NC-ADPKD samples pique our interest because changes that occur before cysts form have the greatest potential as targets for amelioration of cyst formation.

Conventional gene chip analysis has not identified pathways that explained the cell de-differentiation observed in cystic cells [38, 39]. Our analysis has revealed a group of signal transduction pathways and terms that are abnormal in ADPKD (Fig. 10). Both NC-ADPKD and C-ADPKD samples have higher-than-normal expression of most signal-transduction pathways. Elevated 'cyclic nucleotide related' pathways are not surprising, given cyclic AMP's role in promoting cyst expansion [40, 41]. Both NC-ADPKD and C-ADPKD samples have higher-than-normal expression of Wnt and Notch pathways, which enhance proliferation, increase resistance to apoptosis

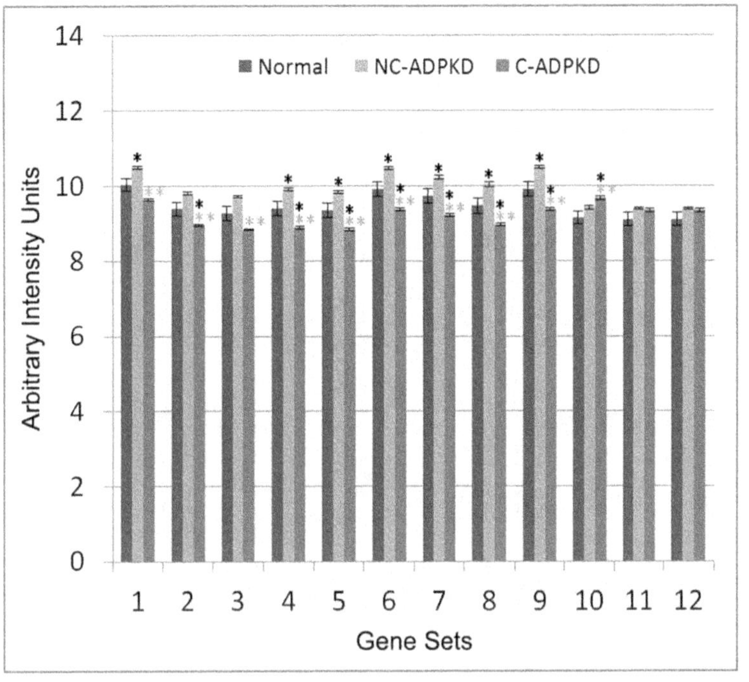

Fig. 7 Both cell growth and cell death are altered in ADPKD. NC-ADPKD cells have higher-than-normal expression and C-ADPKD cells have lower-than-normal expression of genes from 'cell growth' gene sets. Both NC-ADPKD and C-ADPKD cells have higher-than-normal expression of genes from 'cell death' gene sets. We present data as mean ± s.e.m., $^{**}P < 0.01$, $^{*}P < 0.05$ (*black asterisk* is in comparison to NK, *gray asterisk* is in comparison to NC-ADPKD). *Cell Growth Gene Sets:* (1) KEGG_CELL_CYCLE, (2) CELL_CYCLE, (3) CELL_CYCLE_CHECKPOINT, (4) CELL_CYCLE_PROCESS, (5) CELL_CYCLE_PHASE, (6) MITOTIC_M_PHASE, (7) MITOTIC_CELL_CYCLE, (8) M_PHASE, (9) MITOSIS. *Cell Death Gene Sets:* (10) KEGG_APOPTOSIS, (11) APOPTOTIC_PROCESS, (12) PROGRAMMED_CELL_DEATH

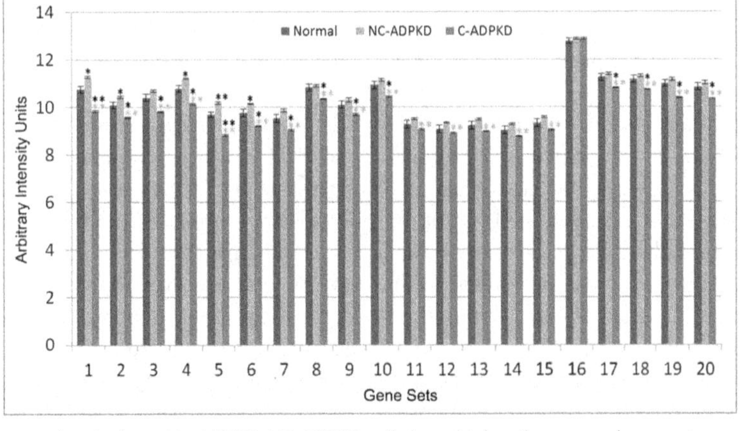

Fig. 8 Genetic information processing is altered in ADPKD. NC-ADPKD cells have higher-than-normal expression and C-ADPKD cells have lower-than-normal expression of genes from all 'Genetic information processing' gene sets except the KEGG ribosome gene set. We present data as mean ± s.e.m., $^{**}P < 0.01$, $^{*}P < 0.05$ (*black asterisk* is in comparison to NK, *gray asterisk* is in comparison to NC-ADPKD). *Genetic Information Processing Gene Sets:* (1) KEGG_DNA_REPLICATION, (2) KEGG_BASE_EXCISION_REPAIR, (3) KEGG_NUCLEOTIDE_EXCISION_REPAIR, (4) KEGG_MISMATCH_REPAIR, (5) KEGG_HOMOLOGOUS_RECOMBINATION, (6) DNA_REPLICATION, (7) DNA_REPAIR, (8) KEGG_RNA_POLYMERASE, (9) KEGG_BASAL_TRANSCRIPTION_FACTORS, (10) KEGG_SPLICEOSOME, (11) TRANSCRIPTION, (12) REGULATION_OF_TRANSCRIPTION, (13) TRANSCRIPTION_DNA_DEPENDENT, (14) REGULATION_OF_TRANSCRIPTION_DNA_DEPENDENT, (15) TRANSCRIPTION_FROM_RNA_POLYMERASE_II_PROMOTER, (16) KEGG_RIBOSOME, (17) RIBONUCLEOPROTEIN_COMPLEX_BIOGENESIS_AND_ASSEMBLY, (18) PROTEIN_RNA_COMPLEX_ASSEMBLY, (19) MRNA_PROCESSING_GO_0006397, (20) RNA_SPLICING_VIA_TRANSESTERIFICATION_REACTIONS

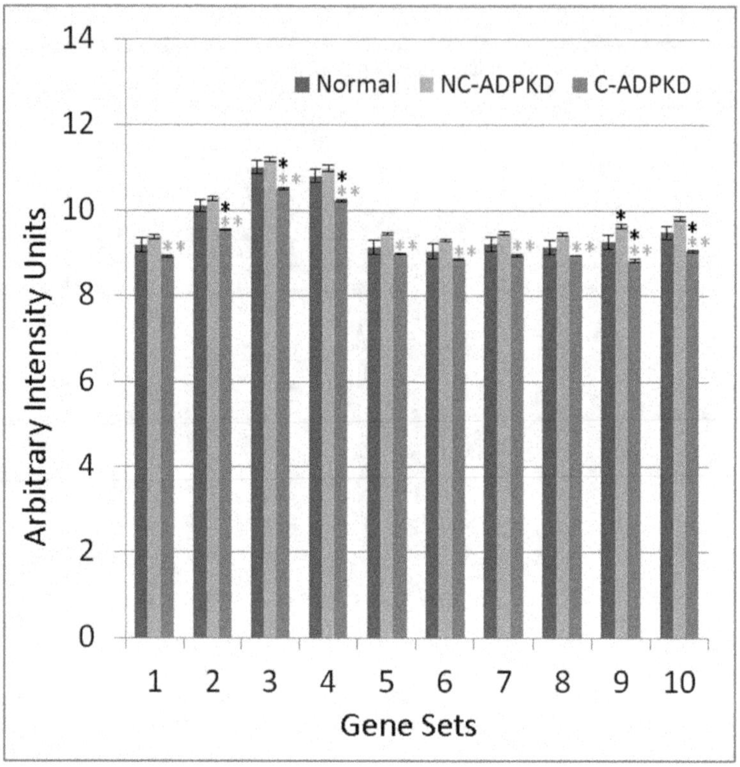

Fig. 9 Nucleotide metabolism is abnormal in ADPKD. NC-ADPKD cells have higher-than-normal expression and C-ADPKD cells have lower-than-normal expression of genes from all 'Nucleotide Metabolism' gene sets. We present data as mean ± s.e.m., $**P < 0.01$, $*P < 0.05$ (*black asterisk* is in comparison to NK, *gray asterisk* is in comparison to NC-ADPKD). *Nucleotide Metabolism Gene Sets:* (1) KEGG_PURINE_METABOLISM, (2) KEGG_PYRIMIDINE_METABOLISM, (3) RNA_SPLICING, (4) MRNA_METABOLIC_PROCESS, (5) NEGATIVE_REGULATION_OF_TRANSCRIPTION, (6) REGULATION OF NUCLEOBASE_NUCLEOSIDE_NUCLEOTIDE_AND_NUCLEIC_ACID_METABOLIC_PROCESS, (7) RNA_BIOSYNTHETIC_PROCESS, (8) NEGATIVE_REGULATION_OF NUCLEOBASE_NUCLEOSIDE_NUCLEOTIDE_AND_NUCLEIC_ACID_METABOLIC_PROCESS, (9) CHROMOSOME_ORGANIZATION_AND_BIOGENESIS, (10) DNA_METABOLIC_PROCESS

and inhibit differentiation of epithelial cells [42]. The excess expression is greater in NC-ADPKD than in C-ADPKD samples, again suggesting possible targets for prevention of cyst initiation.

Chronic non-resolving inflammation accompanies cyst accumulation in ADPKD [43]. Our analysis identified multiple 'immune response' pathways with abnormal expression (Fig. 11). All but one of the identified 'immune response' pathways had higher-than-normal expression in NC-ADPKD samples and further increased expression in C-ADPKD samples, consistent with increased inflammatory response as cysts accumulate. Notably, the morphologically normal NC-ADPKD-derived cells already showed higher-than-normal expression of 'immune response' pathways, suggesting that components of the immune response could provide targets to ameliorate the progression of ADPKD. An exception to this pattern was the lower-than-normal expression of the KEGG 'complement and coagulation' pathway in C-ADPKD samples.

'Response-to-stimulus' gene groups are overexpressed in kidney carcinoma [44]. Our analysis identifies multiple 'response-to-stimulus' terms with increased expression in ADPKD (Fig. 12), suggesting mechanistic similarities between PKD and kidney carcinoma [45]. All but one of the identified 'response-to-stimulus' terms had higher-than-normal expression in NC-ADPKD samples and further increased expression in C-ADPKD samples. In C-ADPKD samples, expression of 'response-to-endogenous-stimulus' genes was lower than normal and also lower than in NC-ADPKD samples.

Establishment and maintenance of epithelial cell polarity are prerequisites for normal function of all epithelial organs. Epithelia depend on cell adhesion molecules to adapt and respond to mechanical forces and cell density, while tight junctions control diffusion across the epithelial layer. Transcriptogram analysis shows that both NC-ADPKD and C-ADPKD cells have higher-than-normal expression of genes in the 'cell-adhesion-molecule' and 'tight-junction' KEGG pathways (Fig. 12). Nephron segments differentially express multiple tight-junction proteins which may determine segment specific paracellular permeability [46]. ADPKD cyst epithelia express claudin-7 in an abnormal distribution on the apical and basolateral membrane [47]. Decreased presence of strong E-cadherin

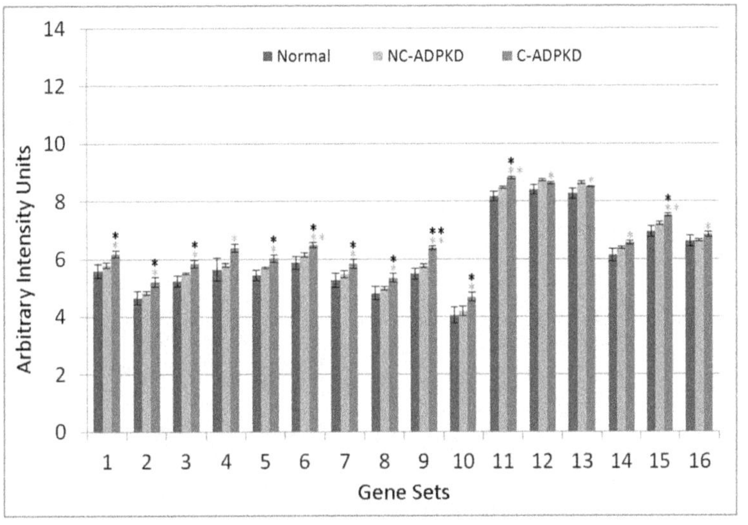

Fig. 10 ADPKD upregulates signal transduction. NC-ADPKD and C-ADPKD cells have higher-than-normal expression of genes from all signal transduction gene sets. Expression levels in NC-ADPKD cells are intermediate between those of NK and C-ADPKD cells, exception that expression levels of Wnt and Notch signaling pathways are higher in NC-ADPKD cells. These pathways are normally active primarily during embryonic development. We present data as mean ± s.e.m., $^{**}P < 0.01$, $^{*}P < 0.05$ (*black asterisk* is in comparison to NK, *gray asterisk* is in comparison to NC-ADPKD). *Signal Transduction Gene Sets:* (1) G_PROT._COUPLED_RECEPTOR_PROTEIN_SIGNALING, (2) G_PROT._SIGNALING_COUPLED_TO_CYCLIC_NUCLEOTIDE_2ND_MESS, (3) G_PROT._SIGNALING_COUPLED_TO_CAMP_NUCLEOTIDE_2ND_MESS, (4) G_PROT._SIGNALING_ADENYLATE_CYCLASE_ACTIVATING, (5) CAMP_MEDIATED_SIGNALING, (6) CELL_CELL_SIGNALING, (7) SYNAPTIC_TRANSMISSION, (8) CYCLIC_NUCLEOTIDE_MEDIATED_SIGNALING, (9) KEGG_CYTOKINE_CYTOKINE_RECEPTOR_INTERACTION, (10) KEGG_NEUROACTIVE_LIGAND_RECEPTOR_INTERACTION, (11) KEGG_ERBB_SIGNALING_PATHWAY, (12) KEGG_WNT_SIGNALING_PATHWAY, (13) KEGG_NOTCH_SIGNALING_PATHWAY, (14) KEGG_CALCIUM_SIGNALING_PATHWAY, (15) KEGG_JAK_STAT_SIGNALING_PATHWAY, (16) KEGG_ABC_TRANSPORTERS

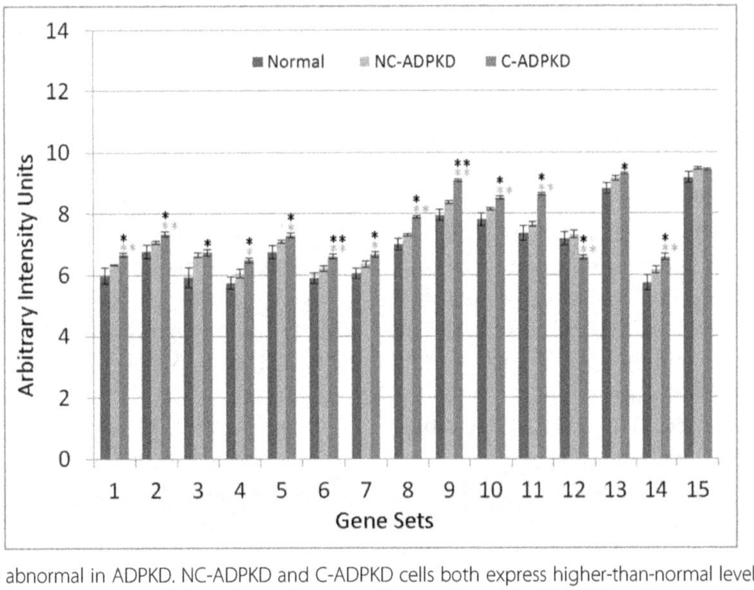

Fig. 11 Immune response is abnormal in ADPKD. NC-ADPKD and C-ADPKD cells both express higher-than-normal levels of genes from 'immune response' gene sets, exception that C-ADPKD cells have lower-than-normal expression of the KEGG 'Complement and Coagulation cascade' gene set (12). We present data as mean ± s.e.m., $^{**}P < 0.01$, $^{*}P < 0.05$ (*black asterisk* is in comparison to NK, *gray asterisk* is in comparison to NC-ADPKD). *Immune Response Gene Sets:* (1) INFLAMMATORY_RESPONSE, (2) IMMUNE_RESPONSE, (3) HUMORAL_IMMUNE_RESPONSE, (4) CELL_ACTIVATION, (5) IMMUNE_SYSTEM_PROCESS, (6) LEUKOCYTE_ACTIVATION, (7) LYMPHOCYTE_ACTIVATION, (8) KEGG_CHEMOKINE_SIGNALING_PATHWAY, (9) KEGG_NOD_LIKE_RECEPTOR_SIGNALING_PATHWAY, (10) KEGG_T_CELL_RECEPTOR_SIGNALING_PATHWAY, (11) KEGG_LEUKOCYTE_TRANSENDOTHELIAL_MIGRATION, (12) KEGG_COMPLEMENT_AND_COAGULATION_CASCADES, (13) KEGG_CYTOSOLIC_DNA_SENSING_PATHWAY, (14) KEGG_HEMATOPOIETIC_CELL_LINEAGE, (15) KEGG_FC_GAMMA_R_MEDIATED_PHAGOCYTOSIS

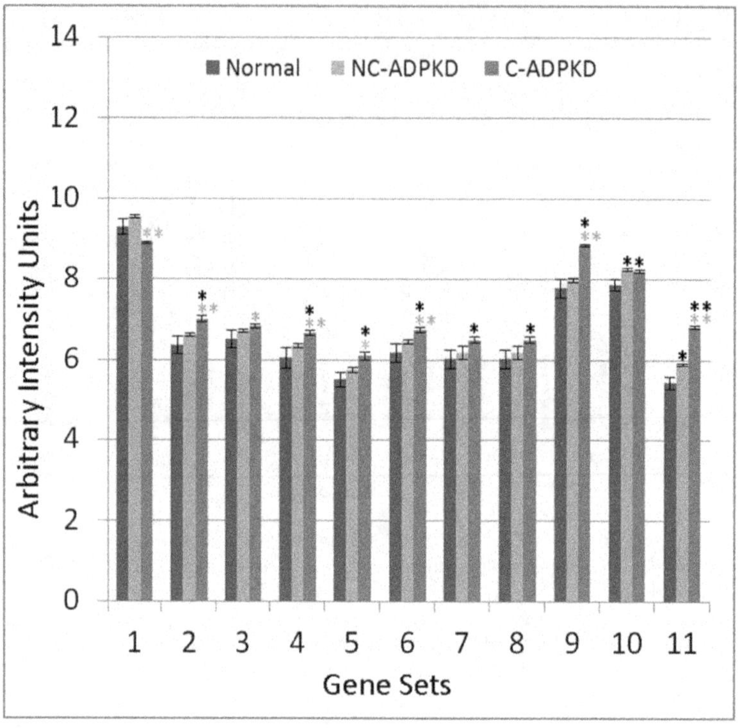

Fig. 12 Response to stimulus and cellular processes are abnormal in ADPKD. Both NC-ADPKD and C-ADPKD cells have higher-than-normal expression of genes in the 'response to stimulus' gene sets (1–8), except that C-ADPKD cells have lower-than-normal expression of genes in the 'response to endogenous stimulus' gene set. C-ADPKD cells have higher-than-normal expression of genes in the 'cellular processes' gene sets (9–11). Data are represented as mean ± s.e.m., $^{**}P < 0.01$, $^{*}P < 0.05$ (*black asterisk* is in comparison to NK, *gray asterisk* is in comparison to NC-ADPKD). *Response to Stimulus Gene Sets:* (1) RESPONSE_TO_ENDOGENOUS_STIMULUS, (2) RESPONSE_TO_EXTERNAL_STIMULUS, (3) REGULATION_OF_RESPONSE_TO_STIMULUS, (4) DEFENSE_RESPONSE, (5) CELLULAR_DEFENSE_RESPONSE, (6) RESPONSE_TO_WOUNDING, (7) COAGULATION, (8) BLOOD_COAGULATION. *Cellular Processes Gene Sets:* (9) KEGG_TIGHT_JUNCTION, (10) KEGG_GAP_JUNCTION, (11) LOCOMOTORY_BEHAVIOR

adhesion molecules on the tubule cell surface, accompanied by upregulation of weaker cell-cell adhesion by N-cadherin and cadherin-8 are also known components of ADPKD [48, 49]. This lower-than-normal cell-cell adhesion accompanies higher-than-normal expression of cell motility terms, both hallmarks of epithelial to mesenchymal transition and cellular de-differentiation.

Defects in urine concentration are a well-established component of ADPKD [50]. NC-ADPKD samples had slightly higher-than-normal and C-ADPKD samples had significantly lower-than-normal expression of 'vasopressin-regulated water reabsorption' [51] and 'proximal tubule bicarbonate reclamation' [52] pathways (Fig. 13).

ADPKD causes widespread disruptions of metabolism (Fig. 14). Of the metabolic pathways and terms identified, 'cofactor and vitamin metabolism' and 'amino acid and energy metabolism' were all decreased in C-ADPKD samples. 'Carbohydrate, drug, lipid and glycan metabolism' pathways were lower than normal in C-ADPKD samples with the exception of 'fructose and mannose,' 'galactose,' and 'amino sugar and nucleotide sugar metabolism'. 'Drug metabolism cytochrome P450' pathway expression levels were lower than normal in both NC-ADPKD and C-ADPKD samples. 'Lipid metabolism' pathway expression was significantly abnormal, but with mixed expression effects. 'Glycan metabolism' pathway expression was slightly higher than normal in NC-ADPKD samples and lower than normal in C-ADPKD samples.

The differential expression of pathways and terms (Figs. 7, 8, 9, 10, 11, 12, 13, and 14) in the gene sets associated with significantly altered transcriptogram intervals (Figs. 4, 5, and 6) provides strong evidence that:

1) 'Proliferation,' 'genetic information processing,' and 'nucleotide metabolism' pathways and terms are higher-than-normal in NC-ADPKD and lower-than-normal in C-ADPKD, while 'apoptosis' is higher-than-normal in both NC-ADPKD and C-ADPKD.
2) 'Immune response' pathways and terms overall are upregulated in both NC-ADPKD and C-ADPKD.
3) Changes in 'signal transduction' and 'cellular process' pathways are consistent with de-differentiation of epithelial cells in ADPKD.
4) 'Metabolism' pathways and terms overall are downregulated in ADPKD.

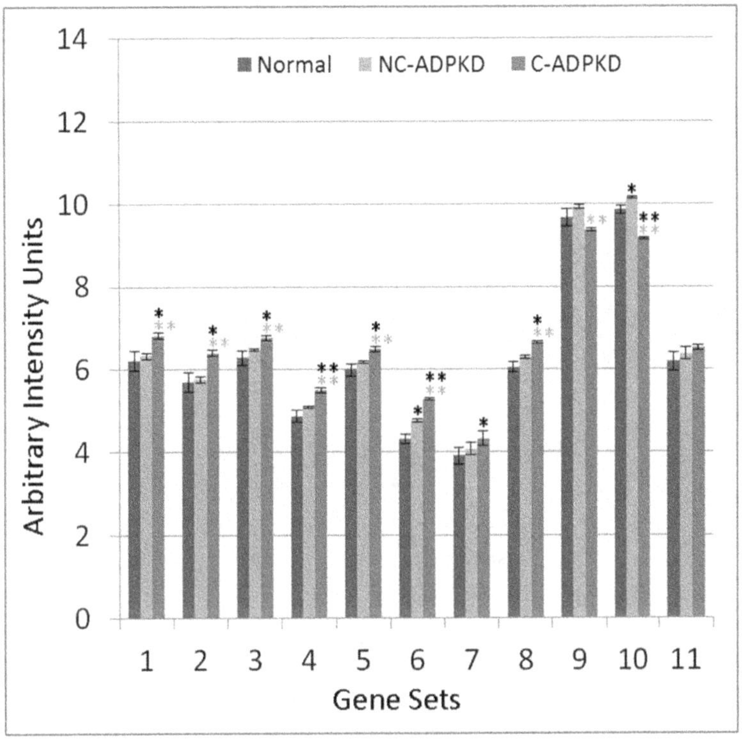

Fig. 13 Ion homeostasis and transport are abnormal in ADPKD. NC-ADPKD cells have higher-than-normal and C-ADPKD cells have much higher-than-normal expression of genes in 'ion homeostasis' gene sets (1–8). NC-ADPKD cells have higher-than-normal expression of genes in 'transport' gene sets (9–11). We represent data as mean ± s.e.m, $^{**}P < 0.01$, $^{*}P < 0.05$ (*black asterisk* is in comparison to NK, *gray asterisk* is in comparison to NC-ADPKD). *Ion Homeostasis Gene Sets:* (1) ION_HOMEOSTASIS, (2) CELLULAR_CATION_HOMEOSTASIS, (3) ION_TRANSPORT, (4) METAL_ION_TRANSPORT, (5) CATION_TRANSPORT, (6) POTASSIUM_ION_TRANSPORT, (7) CALCIUM_ION_TRANSPORT, (8) MONOVALENT_INORGANIC_CATION_TRANSPORT. *Transport Gene Sets:* (9) KEGG_VASOPRESSIN_REGULATED_WATER_REABSORPTION, (10) KEGG_PROXIMAL_TUBULE_BICARBONATE_RECLAMATION, (11) REGULATION_OF_BODY_FLUID_LEVELS

We therefore posit that genes from the pathways and terms that are uniquely altered in NC-ADPKD samples (e.g., before cysts have formed) have the greatest potential as drug targets for ameliorating cyst formation.

Finding individual candidate genes

We next examine the expression levels of the individual genes (Fig. 15) in selected pathways and terms which transcriptogram analysis identifies as differentially expressed at a significant level (Figs. 7, 8, 9, 10, 11, 12, 13 and 14). Selection of pathways and terms for further examination was based on significance level and relevance to the existing literature. These genes likely play key roles in development of ADPKD and are thus potential targets for drug therapies to prevent or delay ADPKD. Figure 15 shows the levels of expression of individual genes from three pathways and terms, 'Nod-like receptor signaling' a term from 'immune response,' 'potassium ion transport' a term from 'ion homeostasis,' and 'oxidative phosphorylation' a term from 'energy metabolism'. We then confirmed expression levels of individual genes in these pathways and terms using qRT-PCR (Additional file 3).

The intracellular NOD-like receptor (NLR) family plays a central role in regulation of the innate immune response. The NLRs NOD1 and NOD2 sense bacterial peptidoglycan fragments and respond by stimulating the activation of NF-κB (nuclear factor kappa beta) and MAPK, cytokine production, and apoptosis. The NLRs NALP1 (NLR-pyrin containing), NALP3 and Ipaf activate caspase-1 through inflammasomes, which generate pro-inflammatory cytokines. NOD-like receptor signaling contributes to multiple renal diseases with inflammatory components, including ureteric obstruction, ischemia reperfusion injury, glomerulonephritis, sepsis, hypoxia, glycerol-induced renal failure, and crystal nephropathy [53–55]. However, neither the Volcano plots nor GSEA analysis found abnormal activity of NOD-like receptor signaling in ADPKD cells. We examined expression of the 20 individual genes involved in the KEGG 'NOD-like receptor signaling' pathway (Fig. 15a) that were present in our microarrays. In NC-ADPKD cells, all but one of the 20 NOD-like receptor signaling genes had higher-than-normal expression (Fig. 15a), suggesting that that reducing NOD-like receptor signaling early in ADPKD might ameliorate the progression of the disease. C-ADPKD cells

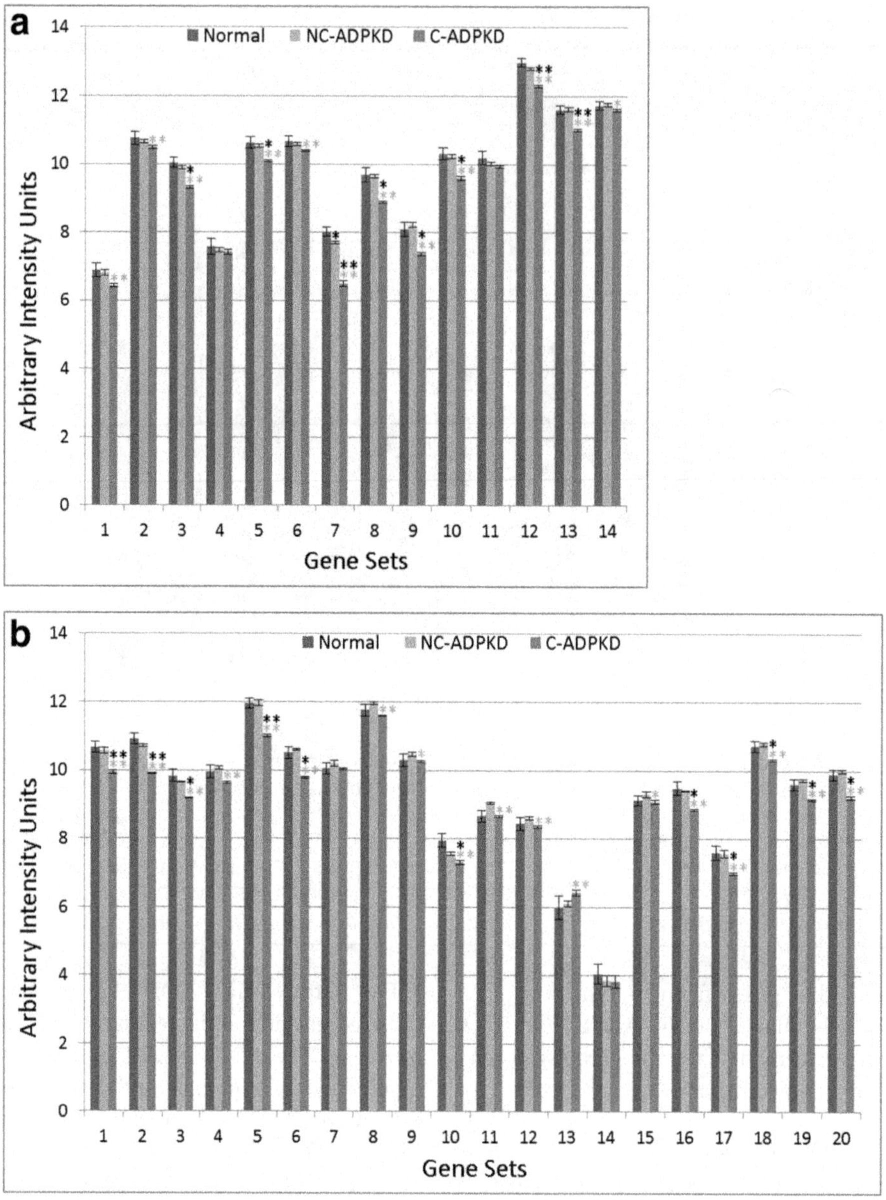

Fig. 14 (See legend on next page.)

(See figure on previous page.)
Fig. 14 ADPKD broadly perturbs metabolism. **a** Cofactor and vitamin, amino acid, and energy metabolism and **b** carbohydrate, drug, lipid, and glycan metabolism. C-ADPKD cells have lower-than-normal expression of genes in 'cofactor and vitamin' gene sets (A1-2) compared to both NK and NC-ADPKD cells. Both NC-ADPKD and C-ADPKD cells have lower-than-normal expression of genes in 'amino acid' gene sets (A3-11). C-ADPKD cells have lower-than-normal expression of genes in 'energy metabolism' gene sets (A12-14). C-ADPKD cells have lower-than-normal expression of genes in all 'carbohydrate metabolism' gene sets (B1-9) except for the KEGG 'histidine metabolism' gene set. C-ADPKD cells have lower-than-normal expression of genes in the 'drug metabolism' gene set (B10). C-ADPKD cells have lower-than-normal expression of genes in all 'lipid metabolism' (B11-18) gene sets except for the KEGG 'arachidonic acid metabolism' gene set (B13). C-ADPKD cells have lower-than-normal expression of genes in 'glycan metabolism' gene sets (B19-20). We present data as mean ± s.e.m., $^{**}P < 0.01$, $^{*}P < 0.05$ (*black asterisk* is in comparison to NK, *gray asterisk* is in comparison to NC-ADPKD). **a** Cofactor and vitamin, amino acid, and energy metabolism gene sets. *Cofactor and Vitamin Gene Sets:* (1) KEGG_RETINOL_METABOLISM, (2) KEGG_PORPHYRIN_AND_CHLOROPHYLL_METABOLISM. *Amino Acid Metabolism Gene Sets:* (3) KEGG_ALANINE_ASPARTATE_AND_GLUTAMATE_METABOLISM, (4) KEGG_GLYCINE_SERINE_AND_THREONINE_METABOLISM, (5) KEGG_VALINE_LEUCINE_AND_ISOLEUCINE_DEGRADATION, (6) KEGG_ARGININE_AND_PROLINE_METABOLISM, (7) KEGG_HISTIDINE_METABOLISM, (8) KEGG_TRYPTOPHAN_METABOLISM, (9) KEGG_BETA_ALANINE_METABOLISM, (10) KEGG_SELENOAMINO_ACID_METABOLISM, (11) KEGG_GLUTATHIONE_METABOLISM. *Energy Metabolism Gene Sets:* (12) KEGG_OXIDATIVE_PHOSPHORYLATION, (13) MITOCHONDRIAL_TRANSPORT, (14) MITOCHONDRION_ORGANIZATION_AND_BIOGENESIS. **b** Carbohydrate, drug, lipid and glycan metabolism gene sets. *Carbohydrate Metabolism Gene Sets:* (1) KEGG_GLYOXYLATE_AND_DICARBOXYLATE_METABOLISM, (2) KEGG_PROPANOATE_METABOLISM, (3) KEGG_BUTANOATE_METABOLISM (4) KEGG_GLYCOLYSIS_GLUCONEOGENESIS, (5) KEGG_CITRATE_CYCLE_TCA_CYCLE, (6) KEGG_PYRUVATE_METABOLISM, (7) KEGG_FRUCTOSE_AND_MANNOSE_METABOLISM, (8) KEGG_GALACTOSE_METABOLISM, (9) KEGG_AMINO_SUGAR_AND_NUCLEOTIDE_SUGAR_METABOLISM. *Drug Metabolism Gene Sets;* (10) KEGG_DRUG_METABOLISM_CYTOCHROME_P450. *Lipid Metabolism Gene Sets:* (11) KEGG_GLYCEROLIPID_METABOLISM, (12) KEGG_GLYCEROPHOSPHOLIPID_METABOLISM, (13) KEGG_ARACHIDONIC_ACID_METABOLISM, (14) KEGG_LINOLEIC_ACID_METABOLISM, (15) KEGG_SPHINGOLIPID_METABOLISM, (16) KEGG_FATTY_ACID_METABOLISM, (17) KEGG_STEROID_HORMONE_BIOSYNTHESIS, (18) PHOSPHOLIPID_BIOSYNTHETIC_PROCESS. *Glycan Metabolism Gene Sets:* (19) KEGG_N_GLYCAN_BIOSYNTHESIS, (20) KEGG_GLYCOSYLPHOSPHATIDYLINOSITOL_GPI_ANCHOR_BIOSYNTHESIS

also had higher-than-normal expression levels of several of these genes, including tumor necrosis factor (TNF). TNF blockers are an approved treatment for debilitating chronic inflammatory diseases, in particular rheumatoid arthritis (RA) so tumor necrosis factor (TNF) blockers specifically and NOD-like receptor signaling blockers in general may be worth testing for treatment of ADPKD. Even if they do not slow cyst progression, they may reduce the chronic pain associated with inflammatory diseases like ADPKD.

The kidney is the primary regulator of total body potassium content. Maintenance of proper levels and distribution of potassium across the cell membrane is critical for normal cell function [56]. Further, potassium channels are critical for cAMP-dependent chloride secretion and cyst growth in ADPKD [57]. We examined expression of the 11 individual genes in our microarrays with the GO 'potassium ion transport' label (Fig. 15c). Our analysis revealed changes of expression of 'potassium ion transport' as a category and of individual genes within that category, which neither Volcano plotting or GSEA analysis was able to identify.

$Pkd1^{-/-}$ cells and kidneys from cystic mice preferentially rely on aerobic glycolysis for their energy demands, a metabolic switch similar to the Warburg effect in cancer cells [58]. Our analysis revealed changes in pathways and terms related to 'energy metabolism' that conventional volcano and GSEA analysis missed. We examined expression of the 20 individual genes in the KEGG 'oxidative phosphorylation' pathway (Fig. 15b) that were present in our microarrays. Expression of all oxidative phosphorylation related genes was significantly lower than normal in both C-ADPKD and NC-ADPKD samples, with greater reduction in C-ADPKD samples. Volcano plotting also identified phosphoenolpyruvate carboxy-kinase 1 (Pck1) as significantly differentially expressed (Fig. 1); the Pck1 enzyme is a main control point for the regulation of gluconeogenesis. Pck1 expression in NC-ADPKD samples is 5.58 times higher than normal ($p = 1.54 \times 10^{-8}$) and is 0.58 times lower than normal (not significant) in C-ADPKD samples.

Discussion

In this communication, we compare gene expression profiles between a paired age and sex-matched pair of telomerase immortalized human cell lines (NK and PKD). A second grouped pair of immortalized human cell lines (NC-ADPKD and C-ADPKD) was derived from renal cysts and normal appearing nephrons from the same human male polycystic kidney. The choice to use immortalized cell lines as the source material to isolate RNA was based on our prior unsuccessful attempts to obtain good-quality RNA from polycystic kidneys. Due to their large size and the need to cross clamp the kidneys at the renal pedicle, we obtained poor-quality RNA isolated from the nephrectomy specimen likely because of prolonged warm ischemia time. While the use of cell lines allowed us to eliminate the issue of RNA degradation, it also brings forward the question as to how generalizable is the data presented in this communication. In our review, the group that solved the problem of obtaining high-quality RNA from polycystic kidney surgical specimens was Song et al. [17]. Our preliminary analysis of that data set using the transcriptogram approach shows a close concordance between our data and Song's data. This comparison will be the subject of a future communication.

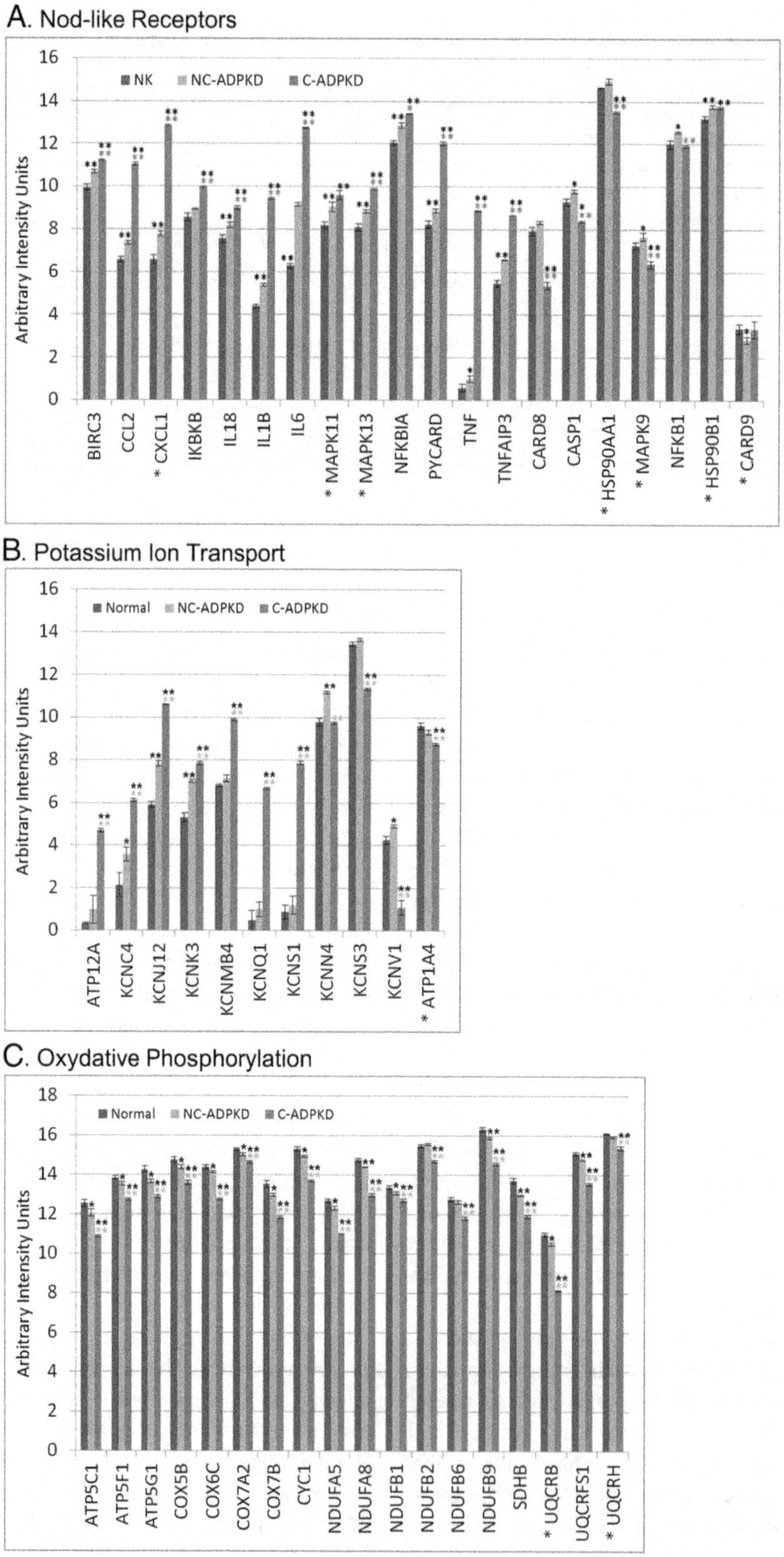

Fig. 15 (See legend on next page.)

(See figure on previous page.)
Fig. 15 Comparisons of individual gene expression levels for genes selected from differentially expressed gene sets. **a** NOD-like receptor signaling, **b** potassium ion transport, and **c** oxidative phosphorylation. To simplify presentation of these gene sets, where we used two or more probes in the microarray for a single gene, we give mean values and mark the gene names with an "asterisk". Within gene sets, we can discern changes in individual genes responsible for differential expression of the pathways. We present data as mean ± s.e.m., $^{**}P < 0.01$, $^{*}P < 0.05$ (*black asterisk* is in comparison to NK, *gray asterisk* is in comparison to NC-ADPKD). Additional file 4 provides additional information on each gene

Other evaluations of gene expression data have relied on murine cell lines or RNA isolated from newly formed cysts from conditional knockout models, and results from these studies identify similar themes for aberrant signaling such as immune defense, cell structure and motility, cellular proliferation, apoptosis, and metabolic control [59–62]. These are GSEA findings that are also observed in our study suggesting that a subset of findings observed in our cell lines are generalizable.

Current analyses of genome-wide gene expression measurements (microarrays or RNASeq, for example) such as single gene Volcano plots (Fig. 1) and GSEA gene set analysis (Tables 1 and 2) have failed to identify patterns of gene expression that define specific diseases or reveal the entirety of their molecular mechanisms of pathogenesis. Our ADPKD transcriptogram analysis (Figs. 4, 5, and 6) identified more significantly altered KEGG pathways and GO terms than either Volcano plots (Fig. 2) or GSEA analysis (Tables 1 and 2). Importantly, transcriptogram analysis identifies additional pathways and terms which are consistent with what we know about signaling, functional, and morphological changes that occur in ADPKD, clarifying the mechanisms by which PKD mutations drive cyst formation.

Comparing global gene expression profiles between NK, ADPKD, NC-ADPKD, and C-ADPKD shows that the NC-ADPKD gene profile is most similar to the NK line expression profile. The NK cell line profile is markedly different from both the C-ADPKD and end-stage ADPKD cell line gene expression profiles (Additional file 5: Figure S5). NC-ADPKD, C-ADPKD, and ADPKD cell lines all have truncation mutations in one allele of the PC-1 gene. However, when we sequenced the PC-1 genomic clones, we found no evidence for second somatic mutations in the PC-1 gene [25]. Additionally, there were no differences in total polycystin-1 and 2 protein expression in the ADPKD cell line [25]. The sole distinguishing feature between the NK and ADPKD cell lines was the absence of polycystin-1 in the cilia of the ADPKD cells [63]. Our transcriptogram analysis suggests that some other genetic event, i.e., a second hit, causes the dramatic shift in gene expression which transforms non-cystic ADPDK cells into cystic ADPKD cells [64]. The transition in expression profiles may have been determined during the early steps of cyst emergence that set the subsequent gene expression profile to reflect a fundamentally altered differentiation profile [17] [65]. Alternatively, a second somatic mutation that launched cyst emergence occurred in some other cystogenic gene site where we have incomplete information at present [66, 67]. Notably, in a murine conditional PKD1 knockout, cyst formation is most robust with PKD1 inactivation up to post-natal day 14 [68]. In other knock out models, cyst formation also requires a kidney injury and repair cycle to yield robust cystogenesis suggesting that there is a developmental window, recapitulated during cell repair that leads to a risk of cyst formation when polycystin-1 levels are abnormal [69].

Several of the many signaling pathways altered in cystic epithelia deserve special consideration [70]. Several potassium channel genes are overexpressed in our cystic cell lines. These potassium channel genes are KCNC4 (potassium voltage-gated channel subfamily C member 4), KCNJ12 (potassium voltage-gated channel subfamily J member 12), KCNK3 (potassium two pore domain channel subfamily K member 3), KCNMB4 (potassium calcium-activated channel subfamily M regulatory beta subunit 4), KCNQ1 (potassium voltage-gated family Q member 1), and KCNS1 (potassium voltage-gated channel modifier subfamily S member 1). NC-ADPKD cells have higher-than-normal and C-ADPKD cells have lower-than-normal expression of KCNN4 (potassium calcium-activated channel subfamily N member 4), KCNV1 (potassium voltage gated channel modifier subfamily V member 1), and KCNS3 (potassium voltage-gated channel subfamily A member 3). Notably, KCNN4 is responsible for calcium-dependent cyst fluid secretion and is thus a potential therapeutic target to inhibit cyst growth [57]. Many of these channels act to hyperpolarize the cell membrane, and voltage-sensitive K channel membrane depolarization induces nano-scale assembly of phosphatidyl serine, which in turn results in nano-scale clustering sites for K-ras, thereby promoting cell cycle progression via MAPK downstream signaling [71, 72]. Experimental studies have demonstrated that cyst expansion results in cell stretching [73]. Since some K channels are stretch activated, K channel activation of proliferation could lead to feedback, where cyst expansion driven by fluid secretion directly accelerates cell-cycle progression [73–76].

Our transcriptogram analysis found significantly higher-than-normal expression of downstream mediators of the 'inflammasome signaling' pathway in NC-ADPKD and C-ADPKD samples, which may accelerate disease pathogenesis [53, 77–80]. This signaling cascade includes nucleotide-binding oligomerization domain receptors or

NOD-like receptors, which have been implicated in renal diseases including ureteric obstruction, ischemia reperfusion injury, glomerulonephritis, sepsis, hypoxia, glycerol-induced renal failure, and crystal nephropathy [53–55, 81]. Our data show that NOD-like receptor signaling may also play an important role in ADPKD. NC-ADPKD and C-ADPKD samples had higher-than-normal ($p < 0.01$) expression of a number of other inflammasome signaling genes, including: interleukin (IL) 6, IL1β, NFκB1A, CCL2 (chemokine (C-C motif) ligand), BIRC3, TNFAIP3, IL18, PYCARD (also called ASC), and MAPK13.

Inflammasome signaling, a part of the innate immune system, includes membrane receptors that recognize conserved pathogen-associated molecular patterns (PAMPs) on invading pathogens or host-derived danger-associated molecular patterns (DAMPs) released in response to stress, reactive oxygen species generation, or cell death [78]. Both Toll-like receptors and C-type lectin pattern recognition receptors (PRRs) can initiate inflammasome signaling at the cell membrane [55]. Additional PRRs include the retinoic acid-inducible gene (RIG-1)-like receptors which recognize double-stranded RNAs (dsRNA) and NOD-like receptors which recognize microbe-associated molecular pattern signatures (MAMPS) and DAMPs. Other intracellular monitors of the system include HIN-200 receptors and RIG-1-like receptors [82–84]. Inflammasome signaling begins with a priming phase, initiated by receptors that signal through myeloid differentiation primary response (MyD88) pathways and other NFκB activating pathways such as IL-1R and the tumor necrosis factor receptor (TNFR) [55, 85]. Priming promotes IL1β, NRLP3, and IL18 transcription and protein synthesis and requires interleukin 1 receptor-associated kinase (IRAK1) activation [86]. K^{-+}efflux, adenosine tri-phosphate (ATP), reactive oxygen species (ROS), pore-forming toxins, or crystals [87–91] all lead to inflammasome activation. The purinergic receptor P2X7 [78, 89, 92, 93] is another inflammasome activator, which is more active under conditions of low fluid shear stress. ADPKD cells, lining cyst walls, are sheltered from fluid shear normally found in tubule lumens; hence, it is likely that in vivo P2X7 is more active [29]. Following inflammasome activation, NOD-like receptors such as NLRP3 form macromolecular complexes with ASC (apoptosis-associated speck-like protein, PYCARD), an adaptor with a caspase recruitment domain (CARD) that bridges NLRs and caspase-1 [94]. This macromolecular complex activates caspace-1, which enzymatically cleaves the pro-inflammatory cytokines IL-1β and IL-18 [95]. Inflammasome signaling has transcriptional effects mediated via MAPK to induce NFκB and the pro-inflammatory cytokines IL-1β and IL-18 [86].

The cystic epithelial cells in our study have higher-than-normal expression of the inflammasome adaptor PYCARD/ASC and the signal modulators BIRC3, preparing them to over-respond to inflammasome signals [80, 95]. The cystic epithelial cells also have higher-than-normal levels of the mRNAs encoding downstream effectors of inflammasome signaling, which likely increase expression of IL1β, IL-18, TNFα, monocyte chemotactic protein-1 (MCP-1), and IL-6 [96–98]. While many of these protein biomarkers correlate with disease severity in either animal models of renal cyst disease or urine from patients with ADPKD [99, 100], our analysis indicates that they may also drive cyst genesis and expansion.

Intense fibrosis and loss of functional parenchyma accompany kidney enlargement during ADPKD disease progression [101, 102]. Our transcriptome analysis suggest that cystic epithelial cells can excessively augment innate inflammatory responses that may accelerate fibrosis and stimulate a chronic inflammatory state by driving macrophage polarization and activation [103]. Since intracellular levels of calcium are low in ADPKD cells [70, 104, 105] and levels of P2X7 gene expression are lower than normal [25], reactive oxygen species are the most likely trigger of inflammasome assembly [88]. Even though P2X7 message levels are lower than normal in ADPKD cells, primary cultured cyst epithelial cells secrete high levels of ATP [29, 106], leading to maximal stimulation of any P2X7 receptors that are present. Since P2X7 activation co-stimulates formation of the NALP inflammasome, cystic epithelial cells may be the primary sources of the IL18 and IL1β identified in cyst fluid [100, 107].

Recent evidence suggests that other K channels can activate transport vesicle release in response to inflammasome activation, and the resultant vesicle cargo protein composition depends on the K channel responsible for membrane depolarization [92]. Thus, aberrant endogenous K-channel expression in cystic epithelia may impair auto regulatory responses to interleukin secretion.

We propose a scenario for the persistent inflammation seen in ADPKD kidneys based on our transcriptogram analysis. Our findings show higher-than-normal mRNA expression of MCP-1 in C-ADPKD cells, which would promote mononuclear cell infiltration into cystic kidney parenchyma. Within the parenchyma, IL1β, IL-18, and IL-6 can all activate infiltrated mononuclear cells. High levels of DAMPs released by apoptotic cells, and DAMPs such as hyaluronic acid and protein fragments resulting from proteolytic extracellular matrix fragments in ADPKD cystic kidneys would then further push mononuclear cells towards an M2 phenotype [99, 107–111]. These M2-like monocytes would continuously secrete transforming growth factor (TGF-β) and connective tissue growth factor (CTGF), which would convert cells in the interstitium to myofibroblasts [78, 102]. Other M2-like monocytes would stimulate epithelial cell proliferation thereby driving cyst expansion [103]. The same signals would stimulate Th1 cells to secrete IFN-γ, IL-13, and Th2 cells to secrete IL-4 and IL-5 and Treg cells to secrete IL-10 and TGF-β, exacerbating the dysregulated inflammatory cascade [86]. This pathogenic picture suggests that pharmacologic interventions which attenuate the inflammatory cascade should delay cyst expansion and fibrosis in ADPKD.

Conclusions

Our analysis of ADPKD provides a workflow which applies to the hierarchical analysis of any large-scale microarray study. We begin with transcriptogram analysis as a method of global triage to identify intervals of altered expression in the ordered gene list, then determine which genes in those intervals of KEGG pathways or GO terms that are differentially expressed (e.g.,'potassium ion transport' in Fig. 14), and finally explore the significance of altered expression profiles of single genes within those altered pathways and terms (Fig. 15). The transcriptograms provide crucial mechanistic context for understanding the significance of altered gene expression.

Methods

Cell lines and culture conditions

All cell lines derived from human kidneys under a protocol were approved by the Indiana University Institutional Review Board. We immortalized all cell lines with human telomerase as previously described and maintained them in continuous culture [25]. We grew cells with renal epithelial growth media supplemented with 5% fetal bovine serum (Lonza, Bazel, Switzerland and GE Healthcare HyClone, Little Chalfont, Buckinghamshire, UK) and maintained them at 37 °C, 5% CO_2 atmosphere. We passaged cells twice-weekly using trypsin-EDTA (Sigma-Aldrich, St. Louis, MO). We micro-dissected the source tissue for the NC-ADPKD and C-ADPKD cell lines from an early stage polycystic kidney from a 36-year-old male. We isolated NC-ADPKD cells from intact renal tubules and C-ADPKD cells from surface cysts. All cell lines expressed the proximal tubule markers ANPEP (alanyl aminopeptidase, membrane), FAH (fumarylacetoacetate hydrolase), SLC5A2 (sodium glucose transporter 5A2), LRP2 (LDL receptor related protein), and HNF1A (hepatocyte nuclear factor 1 homeobox A). They did not express proximal marker CUBN (cubulin). All lines expressed the cortical thick ascending limb marker UMOD (uromodulin). No lines expressed SLC12A1 (solute carrier family 12 member 1) or KCNJ1 (potassium voltage-gated channel subfamily J) . All cell lines expressed the distal convoluted tubule markers KLK1 (kallikrein-1) and KL (klotho). Only the NC-ADPKD cells expressed SLC12A3 (solute carrier family 12 member 3). The NK cell line expressed PVALB (parvalbumin). All cell lines expressed the collecting duct markers, AQP2 (aquaporin 2), and SCNN1G (sodium channel epithelial 1 subunit gamma), while no cell lines expressed FXYD2 (sodium/potassium-transporting ATPase gamma). The gene-expression profiles suggest that the cultured cells likely originate from proximal tubule segments. In contrast, the NK kidney cell line is a mixed cell population made from whole kidney collagenase digest. Herbert et al. have described the NK and ADPKD Q4004X cells [25]. We sequenced the HmPKD1 gene using a protocol of Herbert et al., revealing a heterozygous truncation mutation at amino acid 2556 (Q2556X) [25].

Chemicals and reagents

We purchased all buffers and inorganic chemicals from Sigma-Aldrich (Sigma-Aldrich, St. Louis, MO). We isolated total RNA from cells using TRIzol Reagent (Thermo Fischer Scientific, Waltham, MA) according to manufacturer's directions. We plated cells onto Costar membrane filter supports at a density of 50,000 cells/cm^2 and grew them for 5 days to ensure confluence [25].

We labeled 200 ng of purified total RNA using the Agilent QuickAmp labeling kit, 1-color (Agilent Technologies, Palo Alto, CA) and hybridized purified cRNA to a custom Agilent Human Whole Genome 4x180K array, which replicates the content of the v2 4x44k array at least four times (AMIDID 026822). After hybridization at 65 °C, 20 rpm for 17 h, we washed arrays in wash buffer 1 (6XSSC (saline sodium citrate), 0.005 % TritonX-102) for 5 min at room temperature and wash buffer 2 (0.06X SSC, 0.005 % Triton X-102) for 5 min at 37 °C. We scanned arrays on the Agilent High-Resolution Microarray B-series Scanner (G2505B) and quantified the images using Agilent Feature Extraction software (version 10.7).

Microarray data preprocessing and normalization

We processed extracted feature (reporter) intensities from each array separately by subtracting a constant to bring the minimum intensity to 1 and then taking the log, base 2. We mapped the transformed intensities using a non-linear function to ensure that the cumulative distribution profiles of the intensities were comparable between all arrays. We present the resulting comparable feature intensities in arbitrary units. We removed features with low intensity from the analysis if the 90th percentile was below the limit of detection (LoD), which we estimated as the mean of a set of negative controls plus 1.96 times the standard deviation of the negative controls. We also removed features with low range across all samples, which we defined as having a difference between the 95th percentile and 5th percentile of less than log 2 (1.5-fold). We summarized the replicate probes by averaging and constructed a mixed-effects linear model of expression using factors for tissue type (cysts or kidney), status (ADPKD or NK), and cell line (NK, C-ADPKD, NC-ADPKD, ADPKD), treating cell line as a random effect.

Volcano plotting

We averaged gene expression levels over the replicates for each cell line after normalization and compared the cell lines by calculating the FC. We defined FC as the ratio between the averages and we determined P values for each gene expressed. Volcano plots use FC as the x-axis and the P value as the y-axis (Fig. 2). We defined significantly changed genes as those with thresholds of FC > 2 and $P < 0.01$.

Gene Set Enrichment Analysis (GSEA)

We performed gene set enrichment analysis using the application available at the Broad Institute Gene Set Enrichment Analysis website [26, 33]. We estimated the signal-to-noise ratio and false discovery rates (FDR), from 1000 gene-set permutations, due to the low number of samples in each class ($n = 3$). We tested the Gene Ontology: Biological Process terms and KEGG pathways gene sets. Since we used gene permutations, we considered gene sets to be differentially expressed if FDR < 0.05. We calculated GSEA for NC-ADPKD versus NK, C-ADPKD versus NK, and C-ADPKD versus C-ADPKD.

Transcriptogram analysis

Ordering the gene list

Transcriptograms give an integrated visualization of genome-wide gene expression data by projecting expression levels onto a functionally ordered gene list to produce a genome-wide expression profile [23, 27, 34]. The gene list ordering is based on STRING database protein-protein interactions [34] with confidence scores over 0.800 drawn from all methods to infer associations, with the exception of text mining. The ordering process is performed using a Monte Carlo algorithm that minimizes a cost function:

$$F = \sum_{i=1}^{N-1} \sum_{j=i+1}^{N} d^{\,\alpha}_{i\,j} \left(|A_{i\,j} - A_{i+1\,j}| + |A_{i\,j} - A_{i-1\,j}| + |A_{i\,j} - A_{i\,j+1}| + |A_{i\,j} - A_{i\,j-1}| \right), \tag{1}$$

where N is the number of genes in the list and A is the association matrix. $A_{i\,j} = 1$ when the products of the genes at positions i and j in the list associate and $A_{i\,j} = 0$ otherwise. $d_{i\,j} = |i - j|$ measures the distance between the locations of genes i and j in the list. Minimizing F causes associated genes to cluster in the list. Minimization starts with a randomly ordered list of all genes whose products have at least one association. Each step chooses a pair of genes randomly, tentatively swaps their positions, and calculates the change in the cost function ΔF. The algorithm accepts the position swap whenever $\Delta F \leq 0$. If $\Delta F > 0$, the algorithm accepts the swap with probability $\exp{-\frac{\Delta F}{T}}$. T is a fluctuation amplitude that allows the configuration to escape from local minima of ΔF. One Monte-Carlo step (MCS) equals N attempted gene-pair exchanges. The simulated annealing algorithm starts with T large and decreases T by a small amount once every 100 MCS. The ordering algorithm produces a gene list (Additional file 2) where the probability that any two genes associate decays exponentially with their distance in the list.

Visualizing KEGG pathway and GO term profiles in the ordered list

Because STRING database interactions use KEGG pathway maps for benchmarking and calibration [112], genes in close proximity in the list are probably in the same KEGG pathway. Consequently, the ordered list groups genes by biological function. We used David's Annotational Tools [113] to obtain a list of the GO terms and KEGG pathways that associate to intervals of the ordered list. For each of these GO terms and KEGG pathways, we obtain a profile by creating an N-element vector, $\overrightarrow{h}$, and setting $h_i = 1$, if the gene at position i in the list participates in the specified GO term or KEGG pathway and $h_i = 0$, if the gene at position i in the list does not participate in the specified GO term or KEGG pathway [113, 114]. For each pathway or term, we obtained a profile for $r = 30$. A value of 1 indicates that all genes in an interval participate in a given GO term or KEGG pathway. We read the resulting profiles along the ordered list as indicative of the level of enrichment with genes of a given GO term or KEGG pathway. Interpretation of transcriptograms is then facilitated by comparing the enrichment profiles from regions with significant difference in their transcriptograms.

Transcriptogram calculation

We next map the microarray data onto the ordered list. We then smooth the raw profile to obtain a final *transcriptogram profile*, a new $N - 2r - 1$ element vector, $\overrightarrow{k}$ using a running average with a window of size $2r + 1$ ($r = 30$):

$$k_i = \frac{1}{2r+1} \sum_{j=-r}^{r} h_{i+j}, \tag{2}$$

where $i \in \{r + 1, N - r - 1\}$. The resulting profile is the transcriptogram for the expression data. Profile peaks in $\overrightarrow{k}$ can be interpreted by comparison with the KEGG pathways and GO terms enriched in that region of the ordered list.

Class comparison

We next compare transcriptograms between sample classes. First, we produce the transcriptograms. We next average the transcriptograms for all the samples of each class, producing a class-average transcriptogram profile, $\langle \overrightarrow{k} \rangle$ and corresponding standard error profile $\overrightarrow{\sigma}_k$. To compare a reference (R) and perturbed (P) expression pattern, we divide the perturbed by the normal value for each averaged transcriptogram profile element to obtain the relative transcriptogram $\overrightarrow{\Delta}_{P/R}$:

$$\Delta_i = \frac{k_i^P}{k_i^R}. \tag{3}$$

Regions in $\overrightarrow{\Delta}_{P,R}$ with $\Delta_i \gg 1$ or $\ll 1$ indicate specific perturbed gene expression. The upper panels in Figs. 4, 5, and 6 show the relative transcriptograms.

Significance evaluation

We estimate the significance of differences between two transcriptogram classes using a two-tailed Welch's t test on the class averages to obtain a P value for each list position and by creating 500 random permutations of the sample labels (phenotypes) to estimate the FDR. The middle panels in Figs. 4, 5, and 6 show the P value for each list position.

Additional files

Additional file 1: Lists of genes which Volcano plotting identifies as abnormally expressed.

Additional file 2: Ordered gene list.

Additional file 3: Microarray validation by qRT-PCR.

Additional file 4: Protein expression information on NOD-like receptor signaling, potassium ion transport, and oxidative phosphorylation gene sets from the human protein atlas.

Additional file 5: Relative transcriptogram for ADPKD cells.

Abbreviations

ADPKD: Autosomal dominant polycystic kidney disease; ANPEP: Alanyl aminopeptidase, membrane; ASC: Apoptosis-associated speck-like protein; ATP: Adenosine tri-phosphate; C-ADPKD: Cystic autosomal dominant polycystic kidney disease; CARD: Caspase recruitment domain; CCL2: Chemokine (C-C motif) ligand 2; CTGF: Connective tissue growth factor; CUBN: Cubulin; DAMPs: Damage-associated molecular patterns; DNA: Deoxyribonucleic acid; ECM: Extracellular matrix; Erk: Extracellular signal regulated kinase; FAH: Fumarylacetoacetate hydrolase; FC: Fold change; FDA: Federal Drug Administration; FDR: False discovery rate; FXYD: Sodium/potassium-transporting ATPase gamma; G PROT: G protein; GO: Gene ontology; GSEA: Gene Set Enrichment Analysis; HmPKD1: Human polycystic kidney disease gene 1; HmPKD2: Human polycystic kidney disease gene 2; HNF1A: Hepatocyte nuclear factor 1 homeobox A; IL: Interleukin; IRAK1: Interleukin 1 receptor associated kinase 1; Jnk: cJun N-Terminal kinase; KCNC4: Potassium voltage-gated channel subfamily C member 4; KCNJ1: Potassium voltage-gated channel subfamily J; KCNJ12: Potassium voltage-gated channel subfamily J member 12; KCNK3: Potassium two pore domain channel subfamily k member 3; KCNMB4: Potassium calcium-activated channel subfamily M regulatory beta subunit 4; KCNN4: Potassium calcium-activated channel subfamily N member 4; KCNQ1: Potassium voltage gated family Q member 1; KCNS1: Potassium voltage gated channel modifier subfamily S member 1; KCNS3: Potassium voltage gated channel subfamily A member 3; KCNV1: Potassium voltage gated channel modifier subfamily V member 1; KEGG: Kyoto Encyclopedia of Genes and Genomes; KL: Klotho; KLK1: Kallikrein-1; LRP: LDL receptor-related protein; MAPK: Mitogen-activated protein kinase; MCP: Monocyte chemotactic protein; mTOR: Mammalian target of rapamycin; MyD88: Myeloid differentiation primary response 88; NALP1: NLR pyrin containing; NC ADPKD: Non-cystic autosomal dominant polycystic kidney disease; NF-kB: Nuclear factor kappa beta; NK: Normal kidney; NLR: NOD-like receptor; NLRP3: NOD-like receptor protein; NOD: Nucleotide-binding oligomerization domain; P2X: Purinergic receptor; PAMPs: Pathogen associated molecular patterns; PC-1: Polycystin 1; PC-2: Polycystin 2; Pck1: Phosphoenolpyruvate carboxy-kinase 1; PKD: Polycystic kidney disease; PRRs: Pattern recognition receptors; PVALB: Parvalbumin; qRT-PCR: Quantitative reverse transcriptase polymerase chain reaction; RA: Rheumatoid arthritis; RIG-1: Retinoic acid inducible protein; RNA: Ribonucleic acid; ROS: Reactive oxygen species; SCNN1G: Sodium channel epithelial 1 subunit gamma; SLC12A1: Solute carrier family 12 member 1; SLC12A3: Solute carrier family 12 member 3; SLC5A2: Sodium glucose transporter 5A2; Stat: Signal transducer and activator of transcription 1; TCA: Tricarboxylic acid; TGF: Transforming growth factor; TNF: Tumor necrosis factor; Treg: Regulatory T cell; UMOD: Uromodulin; Wgless: Wingless; Wnt: Wingless-related integration site

Acknowledgements

The authors thank Dr. Swenson-Fields from Kansas University Medical Center, Dr. Seth Alper from Harvard University, and Dr. Purvi Mehrotra from Indiana University School of Medicine for helpful discussions.

Funding

Brazilian agencies CNPq, CAPES, and FAPERGS provided partial support for this project. RMCA acknowledges the kind hospitality of the Biocomplexity Institute, Indiana University, Bloomington. RLB acknowledges support from a Merit Review, BX001736, NIH NIDDK grant R01 DK079312, and a Dr. Ralph and Marian Falk Medical Research Trust Award. An Indiana University Collaborative Research Grant supported the initial collaboration between the RLB and JAG groups. We acknowledge additional generous support from Amgen and Indiana University. RLB thanks the Bloch family for continued support. JAG acknowledges support from NIH NIGMS/NIEHS/NIBIB grants R01 GM11243, R01 GM076692, R01 GM077138, and a Dr. Ralph and Marian Falk Medical Research Trust Award. AWN acknowledges support from NIH NIDDK grant R01 DK050141 and NIH NCI grant P30 CA118100. HHW acknowledges support from NIH NIDDK grant K01 DK097206 and Paul Teschan Research Fund project #3RX05.

Authors' contributions

RMCA performed all calculations for GSEA and transcriptogram analyses and all statistical analyses. RMCA, SGC, JAG, and RLB participated in the design and coordination of the study and writing of the manuscript. BSH, HHW, AWN, and RLB developed the cell lines. WX assisted in the development and maintenance of the cell lines and isolated all RNA samples for these studies. BR, MB, and MD performed the microarray experiments and performed Volcano plots analyses. HHW participated in the initial analyses of the microarray data and made critical suggestions concerning the direction of further analyses. BSH, AWN, and HHW provided critical input for interpretation of the transcriptogram analysis results. RLB oversaw the project. WGR analyzed Agilent human gene array data. SR and PCH analyzed the genetic changes in the HmPKD1 loci in the human cystic epithelial cell lines. All authors read and approved the final manuscript.

Competing interests

The authors declare that they have no competing interests.

Consent for publication

Not applicable.

Author details
[1]Biocomplexity Institute and Department of Physics, Indiana University, Bloomington, IN 47405, USA. [2]Instituto de Física and Instituto Nacional de Ciência e Tecnologia, Universidade Federal do Rio Grande do Sul, 91501-970 Porto Alegre, RS, Brazil. [3]Biocomplexity Institute and Department of Intelligent Systems Engineering, Indiana University, Bloomington, IN 47405, USA. [4]AMGEN Inc., One Amgen Center Drive, Thousand Oaks, CA 91320-1799, USA. [5]Division of Nephrology, Mayo Clinic, 200 First Street SW, Rochester, MN 55905, USA. [6]Department of Medical and Molecular Genetics, Indiana University School of Medicine, Indianapolis, IN 46202, USA. [7]Division of Nephrology, Department of Medicine, Richard Roudebush VAMC and Indiana University School of Medicine, Indianapolis, IN 46202, USA. [8]Department of Pathology MSC08-4640 and Cancer Research and Treatment Center, University of New Mexico Health Sciences Center, Albuquerque, NM 87131, USA. [9]Division of Nephrology, Department of Medicine, University of New Mexico Health Sciences Center, Albuquerque, NM 87131, USA.

References

1. Torres VE, Harris PC, Pirson Y. Autosomal dominant polycystic kidney disease. Lancet. 2007;369(9569):1287–301.
2. Santoro D, Pellicanò V, Visconti L, Trifirò G, Buemi M, Cernaro V. An overview of experimental and early investigational therapies for the treatment of polycystic kidney disease. Expert Opin Investig Drugs. 2015;24(9):1199–218.
3. Qian F, Germino FJ, Cai Y, Zhang X, Somlo S, Germino GG. PKD1 interacts with PKD2 through a probable coiled-coil domain. Nat Genetics. 1997;16(2):179–83.
4. Yoder BK, Hou X, Guay-Woodford LM. The polycystic kidney disease proteins, polycystin-1, polycystin-2, polaris, and cystin, are co-localized in renal cilia.[see comment]. J Am Soc Nephrol. 2002;13(10):2508–16.
5. Gainullin VG, Hopp K, Ward CJ, Hommerding CJ, Harris PC. Polycystin-1 maturation requires polycystin-2 in a dose-dependent manner. J Clin Invest. 2015;125(2):607–20.
6. Praetorius HA, Spring KR. A physiological view of the primary cilium. Annu Rev Physiol. 2005;67:515–29.
7. Hildebrandt F, Benzing T, Katsanis N. Ciliopathies. N Engl J Med. 2011; 364(16):1533–43.
8. Gallagher AR, Hidaka S, Gretz N, Witzgall R. Molecular basis of autosomal-dominant polycystic kidney disease. Cell Mol Life Sci. 2002;59(4):682–93.
9. Walz G, Budde K, Mannaa M, Nürnberger J, Wanner C, Sommerer C, et al. Everolimus in patients with autosomal dominant polycystic kidney disease. N Engl J Med. 2010;363(9):830–40.
10. He Q, Lin C, Ji S, Chen J. Efficacy and safety of mTOR inhibitor therapy in patients with early-stage autosomal dominant polycystic kidney disease: a meta-analysis of randomized controlled trials. Am J Med Sci. 2012;344(6):491–7.
11. Torres VE, Chapman AB, Devuyst O, Gansevoort RT, Grantham JJ, Higashihara E, et al. Tolvaptan in patients with autosomal dominant polycystic kidney disease. N Engl J Med. 2012;367(25):2407–18.
12. Gattone VH, Maser RL, Branden MG, Tiam C, Resenberg J. Collecting duct gene expression and effect of an AVP-V2 receptor antagonist on the progression of PKD in pcy mice. J Am Soc Nephrol. 1998;9:18A.
13. Wang X, Gattone 2nd V, Harris PC, Torres VE. Effectiveness of vasopressin V2 receptor antagonists OPC-31260 and OPC-41061 on polycystic kidney disease development in the PCK rat.[see comment]. J Am Soc Nephrol. 2005;16(4):846–51.
14. Torres VE, Higashihara E, Devuyst O, Chapman AB, Gansevoort RT, Grantham JJ, et al. Effect of tolvaptan in autosomal dominant polycystic kidney disease by CKD stage: results from the TEMPO 3:4 trial. Clin J Am Soc Nephrol. 2016;11(5):803–11.
15. Harris PC, Bae KT, Rossetti S, Torres VE, Grantham JJ, Chapman AB, et al. Cyst number but not the rate of cystic growth is associated with the mutated gene in autosomal dominant polycystic kidney disease. J Am Soc Nephrol. 2006;17(11):3013–9.
16. Waldherr R, Zerres K, Gall A, Enders H. Polycystic kidney disease in the fetus. Lancet. 1989;2(8657):274–5.
17. Song X, Di Giovanni V, He N, Wang K, Ingram A, Rosenblum ND, et al. Systems biology of autosomal dominant polycystic kidney disease (ADPKD): computational identification of gene expression pathways and integrated regulatory networks. Hum Mol Genet. 2009;18(13):2328–43.
18. Surendran K, Selassie M, Liapis H, Krigman H, Kopan R. Reduced Notch signaling leads to renal cysts and papillary microadenomas. J Am Soc Nephrol. 2010;21(5):819–32.
19. Romaker D, Puetz M, Teschner S, Donauer J, Geyer M, Gerke P, et al. Increased expression of secreted frizzled-related protein 4 in polycystic kidneys. J Am Soc Nephrol. 2009;20(1):48–56.
20. Liu M, Shi S, Senthilnathan S, Yu J, Wu E, Bergmann C, et al. Genetic variation of DKK3 may modify renal disease severity in ADPKD. J Am Soc Nephrol. 2010;21(9):1510–20.
21. Hayward P, Kalmar T, Arias AM. Wnt/Notch signalling and information processing during development. Development. 2008;135(3):411–24.
22. da Silva SR, Perrone GC, Dinis JM, de Almeida RM. Reproducibility enhancement and differential expression of non predefined functional gene sets in human genome. BMC Genomics. 2014;15:1181.
23. Rybarczyk-Filho JL, Castro MA, Dalmolin RJ, Moreira JC, Brunnet LG, de Almeida RM. Towards a genome-wide transcriptogram: the Saccharomyces cerevisiae case. Nucleic Acids Res. 2011;39(8):3005–16.
24. de Almeida RMC. The Transcriptogramer: a software for genome wide expression analysis. http://lief.if.ufrgs.br/pub/biosoftwares/transcriptogramer [Available from: lief.if.ufrgs.br/pub/biosoftwares/transcriptogramer. Accessed 14 Nov 2016.
25. Herbert BS, Grimes BR, Xu WM, Werner M, Ward C, Rossetti S, et al. A telomerase immortalized human proximal tubule cell line with a truncation mutation (Q4004X) in polycystin-1. PLoS One. 2013;8(1):e55191.
26. Subramanian A, Tamayo P, Mootha VK, Mukherjee S, Ebert BL, Gillette MA, et al. Gene set enrichment analysis: a knowledge-based approach for interpreting genome-wide expression profiles. Proc Natl Acad Sci U S A. 2005;102(43):15545–50.
27. da Silva SRM, Perrone GC, Dinis JM, de Almeida RMC. Transcriptograms: signal to noise enhancement in transcriptome analysis. BMC Genomics. 2014;15:1181–99.
28. Nauli SM, Alenghat FJ, Luo Y, Williams E, Vassilev P, Li X, et al. Polycystins 1 and 2 mediate mechanosensation in the primary cilium of kidney cells. [comment]. Nat Genetics. 2003;33(2):129–37.
29. Xu C, Shmukler BE, Nishimura K, Kaczmarek E, Rossetti S, Harris PC, et al. Attenuated, flow-induced ATP release contributes to absence of flow-sensitive, purinergic Cai2+ signaling in human ADPKD cyst epithelial cells. Am J Physiol Renal Physiol. 2009;296(6):F1464–76.
30. Ong AC, Ward CJ, Butler RJ, Biddolph S, Bowker C, Torra R, et al. Coordinate expression of the autosomal dominant polycystic kidney disease proteins, polycystin-2 and polycystin-1, in normal and cystic tissue. Am J Pathol. 1999;154(6):1721–9.
31. Ong ACM, Wheatley DN. Polycystic kidney disease—the ciliary connection. Lancet. 2003;361(9359):774–6.
32. Irizarry RA, Wang C, Zhou Y, Speed TP. Gene set enrichment analysis made simple. Stat Methods Med Res. 2009;18(6):565–75.
33. Mootha VK, Lindgren CM, Eriksson KF, Subramanian A, Sihag S, Lehar J, et al. PGC-1alpha-responsive genes involved in oxidative phosphorylation are coordinately downregulated in human diabetes. Nat Genet. 2003; 34(3):267–73.
34. Szklarczyk D, Franceschini A, Wyder S, Forslund K, Heller D, Huerta-Cepas J, et al. STRING v10: protein-protein interaction networks, integrated over the tree of life. Nucleic Acids Res. 2015;43(Database issue):D447–52.
35. Jensen LJ, Kuhn M, Stark M, Chaffron S, Creevey C, Muller J, et al. STRING 8—a global view on proteins and their functional interactions in 630 organisms. Nucleic Acids Res. 2009;37(Database issue):D412–6.
36. Huang dW, Sherman BT, Zheng X, Yang J, Imamichi T, Stephens R, et al. Extracting biological meaning from large gene lists with DAVID. Curr Protoc Bioinformatics. 2009;Chapter 13:Unit 13.1.
37. Huang dW, Sherman BT, Lempicki RA. Bioinformatics enrichment tools: paths toward the comprehensive functional analysis of large gene lists. Nucleic Acids Res. 2009;37(1):1–13.
38. Thomson RB, Mentone S, Kim R, Earle K, Delpire E, Somlo S, et al. Histopathological analysis of renal cystic epithelia in the Pkd2WS25/- mouse model of ADPKD. Am J Physiol Renal Physiol. 2003;285(5):F870–80.
39. Carone FA, Nakamura S, Caputo M, Bacallao R, Nelson WJ, Kanwar YS. Cell polarity in human renal cystic disease. Lab Invest. 1994;70(5):648–55.
40. Yamaguchi T, Reif GA, Calvet JP, Wallace DP. Sorafenib inhibits cAMP-dependent ERK activation, cell proliferation, and in vitro cyst growth of human ADPKD cyst epithelial cells. Am J Physiol Renal Physiol. 2010;299(5):F944–51.
41. Belibi FA, Reif G, Wallace DP, Yamaguchi T, Olsen L, Li H, et al. Cyclic AMP promotes growth and secretion in human polycystic kidney epithelial cells. [see comment]. Kidney Int. 2004;66(3):964–73.
42. Chuang PY, Menon MC, He JC. Molecular targets for treatment of kidney fibrosis. J Mol Med (Berl). 2013;91(5):549–59.

43. Fearn A, Sheerin NS. Complement activation in progressive renal disease. World J Nephrol. 2015;4(1):31–40.
44. Yang W, Yoshigoe K, Qin X, Liu JS, Yang JY, Niemierko A, et al. Identification of genes and pathways involved in kidney renal clear cell carcinoma. BMC Bioinformatics. 2014;15 Suppl 17:S2.
45. Seeger-Nukpezah T, Geynisman DM, Nikonova AS, Benzing T, Golemis EA. The hallmarks of cancer: relevance to the pathogenesis of polycystic kidney disease. Nat Rev Nephrol. 2015;11(9):515–34.
46. Hou J, Rajagopal M, Yu AS. Claudins and the kidney. Annu Rev Physiol. 2013;75:479–501.
47. Yu AS, Kanzawa SA, Usorov A, Lantinga-van Leeuwen IS, Peters DJ. Tight junction composition is altered in the epithelium of polycystic kidneys. J Pathol. 2008;216(1):120–8.
48. Kher R, Sha EC, Escobar MR, Andreoli EM, Wang P, Xu WM, et al. Ectopic expression of cadherin 8 is sufficient to cause cyst formation in a novel 3D collagen matrix renal tubule culture. Am J Physiol Cell Physiol. 2011; 301(1):C99–C105.
49. Roitbak T, Ward CJ, Harris PC, Bacallao R, Ness SA, Wandinger-Ness A. A polycystin-1 multiprotein complex is disrupted in polycystic kidney disease cells. Mol Biol Cell. 2004;15(3):1334–46.
50. Martinez-Hernandez A, Amenta PS. The basement membrane in pathology. Lab Invest. 1983;48(6):656–77.
51. Boone M, Deen PM. Physiology and pathophysiology of the vasopressin-regulated renal water reabsorption. Pflugers Arch. 2008;456(6):1005–24.
52. Nakhoul N, Batuman V. Role of proximal tubules in the pathogenesis of kidney disease. Contrib Nephrol. 2011;169:37–50.
53. Turner CM, Arulkumaran N, Singer M, Unwin RJ, Tam FW. Is the inflammasome a potential therapeutic target in renal disease? BMC Nephrol. 2014;15:21.
54. Du P, Fan B, Han H, Zhen J, Shang J, Wang X, et al. NOD2 promotes renal injury by exacerbating inflammation and podocyte insulin resistance in diabetic nephropathy. Kidney Int. 2013;84(2):265–76.
55. Anders HJ, Lech M. NOD-like and Toll-like receptors or inflammasomes contribute to kidney disease in a canonical and a non-canonical manner. Kidney Int. 2013;84(2):225–8.
56. Palmer BF. Regulation of potassium homeostasis. Clin J Am Soc Nephrol. 2015;10(6):1050–60.
57. Albaqumi M, Srivastava S, Li Z, Zhdnova O, Wulff H, Itani O, et al. KCa3.1 potassium channels are critical for cAMP-dependent chloride secretion and cyst growth in autosomal-dominant polycystic kidney disease. Kidney Int. 2008;74(6):740–9.
58. Rowe I, Chiaravalli M, Mannella V, Ulisse V, Quilici G, Pema M, et al. Defective glucose metabolism in polycystic kidney disease identifies a new therapeutic strategy. Nat Med. 2013;19(4):488–93.
59. Menezes LF, Germino GG. Systems biology of polycystic kidney disease: a critical review. Wiley Interdiscip Rev Syst Biol Med. 2015;7(1):39–52.
60. Menezes LF, Zhou F, Patterson AD, Piontek KB, Krausz KW, Gonzalez FJ, et al. Network analysis of a Pkd1-mouse model of autosomal dominant polycystic kidney disease identifies HNF4α as a disease modifier. PLoS Genet. 2012;8(11):e1003053.
61. Chen WC, Tzeng YS, Li H. Gene expression in early and progression phases of autosomal dominant polycystic kidney disease. BMC Res Notes. 2008;1:131.
62. Gresh L, Fischer E, Reimann A, Tanguy M, Garbay S, Shao X, et al. A transcriptional network in polycystic kidney disease. EMBO J. 2004;23(7):1657–68.
63. Xu C, Rossetti S, Jiang L, Harris PC, Brown-Glaberman U, Wandinger-Ness A, et al. Human ADPKD primary cyst epithelial cells with a novel, single codon deletion in the PKD1 gene exhibit defective ciliary polycystin localization and loss of flow-induced Ca2+ signaling. Am J Physiol Renal Physiol. 2007;292(3):F930–45.
64. Germino GG. Autosomal dominant polycystic kidney disease: a two-hit model. Hosp Pract. 1997;32(3):81–2. 5-8, 91-2 passim.
65. Grantham JJ. Polycystic kidney disease (PKD): neoplasia in disguise. Am J Kidney Dis. 1990;15:110–6.
66. Woo DD, Nguyen DK, Khatibi N, Olsen P. Genetic identification of two major modifier loci of polycystic kidney disease progression in pcy mice. J Clin Invest. 1997;100(8):1934–40.
67. Iakoubova OA, Dushkin H, Beier DR. Genetic analysis of a quantitative trait in a mouse model of polycystic kidney disease. Am J Respir Crit Care Med. 1997;156(4 Pt 2):S72–7.
68. Piontek K, Menezes LF, Garcia-Gonzalez MA, Huso DL, Germino GG. A critical developmental switch defines the kinetics of kidney cyst formation after loss of Pkd1. Nat Med. 2007;13(12):1490–5.
69. Verdeguer F, Le Corre S, Fischer E, Callens C, Garbay S, Doyen A, et al. A mitotic transcriptional switch in polycystic kidney disease. Nat Med. 2010;16(1):106–10.
70. Harris PC, Torres VE. Genetic mechanisms and signaling pathways in autosomal dominant polycystic kidney disease. J Clin Invest. 2014;124(6):2315–24.
71. Zhou Y, Wong CO, Cho KJ, van der Hoeven D, Liang H, Thakur DP, et al. Membrane potential modulates plasma membrane phospholipid dynamics and K-Ras signaling. Science. 2015;349(6250):873–6.
72. Zhou Y, Hancock JF. Ras nanoclusters: versatile lipid-based signaling platforms. Biochim Biophys Acta. 2015;1853(4):841–9.
73. Tanner GA, McQuillan PF, Maxwell MR, Keck JK, McAteer JA. An in vitro test of the cell stretch-proliferation hypothesis of renal cyst enlargement. J Am Soc Nephrol. 1995;6(4):1230–41.
74. Gin E, Tanaka EM, Brusch L. A model for cyst lumen expansion and size regulation via fluid secretion. J Theor Biol. 2010;264(3):1077–88.
75. Sachs F. Stretch-activated ion channels: what are they? Physiology (Bethesda). 2010;25(1):50–6.
76. Sharif-Naeini R, Folgering JH, Bichet D, Duprat F, Lauritzen I, Arhatte M, et al. Polycystin-1 and -2 dosage regulates pressure sensing. Cell. 2009;139(3):587–96.
77. Anders HJ, Muruve DA. The inflammasomes in kidney disease. J Am Soc Nephrol. 2011;22(6):1007–18.
78. Anders HJ, Schaefer L. Beyond tissue injury-damage-associated molecular patterns, toll-like receptors, and inflammasomes also drive regeneration and fibrosis. J Am Soc Nephrol. 2014;25(7):1387–400.
79. Chang A, Ko K, Clark MR. The emerging role of the inflammasome in kidney diseases. Curr Opin Nephrol Hypertens. 2014;23(3):204–10.
80. Darisipudi MN, Knauf F. An update on the role of the inflammasomes in the pathogenesis of kidney diseases. Pediatr Nephrol. 2016;31(4):535–44.
81. Gasse P, Riteau N, Charron S, Girre S, Fick L, Pétrilli V, et al. Uric acid is a danger signal activating NALP3 inflammasome in lung injury inflammation and fibrosis. Am J Respir Crit Care Med. 2009;179(10):903–13.
82. Dawson MJ, Trapani JA. HIN-200: a novel family of IFN-inducible nuclear proteins expressed in leukocytes. J Leukoc Biol. 1996;60(3):310–6.
83. Pichlmair A, Schulz O, Tan CP, Näslund TI, Liljeström P, Weber F, et al. RIG-I-mediated antiviral responses to single-stranded RNA bearing 5'-phosphates. Science. 2006;314(5801):997–1001.
84. Yoneyama M, Kikuchi M, Natsukawa T, Shinobu N, Imaizumi T, Miyagishi M, et al. The RNA helicase RIG-I has an essential function in double-stranded RNA-induced innate antiviral responses. Nat Immunol. 2004;5(7):730–7.
85. Correa-Costa M, Braga TT, Semedo P, Hayashida CY, Bechara LR, Elias RM, et al. Pivotal role of Toll-like receptors 2 and 4, its adaptor molecule MyD88, and inflammasome complex in experimental tubule-interstitial nephritis. PLoS One. 2011;6(12):e29004.
86. Stutz A, Golenbock DT, Latz E. Inflammasomes: too big to miss. J Clin Invest. 2009;119(12):3502–11.
87. Rivers-Auty J, Brough D. Potassium efflux fires the canon: potassium efflux as a common trigger for canonical and noncanonical NLRP3 pathways. Eur J Immunol. 2015;45(10):2758–61.
88. Heid ME, Keyel PA, Kamga C, Shiva S, Watkins SC, Salter RD. Mitochondrial reactive oxygen species induces NLRP3-dependent lysosomal damage and inflammasome activation. J Immunol. 2013;191(10):5230–8.
89. Latz E, Xiao TS, Stutz A. Activation and regulation of the inflammasomes. Nat Rev Immunol. 2013;13(6):397–411.
90. Martinon F. Mechanisms of uric acid crystal-mediated autoinflammation. Immunol Rev. 2010;233(1):218–32.
91. Franchi L, Muñoz-Planillo R, Núñez G. Sensing and reacting to microbes through the inflammasomes. Nat Immunol. 2012;13(4):325–32.
92. de Torre-Minguela C, Barberà-Cremades M, Gómez AI, Martín-Sánchez F, Pelegrín P. Macrophage activation and polarization modify P2X7 receptor secretome influencing the inflammatory process. Sci Rep. 2016;6:22586.
93. Chen K, Zhang J, Zhang W, Yang J, Li K, He Y. ATP-P2X4 signaling mediates NLRP3 inflammasome activation: a novel pathway of diabetic nephropathy. Int J Biochem Cell Biol. 2013;45(5):932–43.
94. Stutz A, Horvath GL, Monks BG, Latz E. ASC speck formation as a readout for inflammasome activation. Methods Mol Biol. 2013;1040:91–101.
95. Schroder K, Tschopp J. The inflammasomes. Cell. 2010;140(6):821–32.
96. Tai YH, Flick J, Levine SA, Madara JL, Sharp GW, Donowitz M. Regulation of tight junction resistance in T84 monolayers by elevation in intracellular Ca2+: a protein kinase C effect. J Membr Biol. 1996;149(1):71–9.

97. Cowley Jr BD, Ricardo SD, Nagao S, Diamond JR. Increased renal expression of monocyte chemoattractant protein-1 and osteopontin in ADPKD in rats. Kidney Int. 2001;60(6):2087–96.
98. Yoo JK, Kwon H, Khil LY, Zhang L, Jun HS, Yoon JW. IL-18 induces monocyte chemotactic protein-1 production in macrophages through the phosphatidylinositol 3-kinase/Akt and MEK/ERK1/2 pathways. J Immunol. 2005;175(12):8280–6.
99. Zheng D, Wolfe M, Cowley BD, Wallace DP, Yamaguchi T, Grantham JJ. Urinary excretion of monocyte chemoattractant protein-1 in autosomal dominant polycystic kidney disease. J Am Soc Nephrol. 2003;14(10):2588–95.
100. Parikh CR, Dahl NK, Chapman AB, Bost JE, Edelstein CL, Comer DM, et al. Evaluation of urine biomarkers of kidney injury in polycystic kidney disease. Kidney Int. 2012;81(8):784–90.
101. Carone FA, Kanwar Y. Pathobiology of tubular basement membranes in renal cystic disease. In: Hatano M, editor. Nephrology. New York: Springer Verlag; 1991. p. 876–84.
102. Norman J. Fibrosis and progression of autosomal dominant polycystic kidney disease. Biochimica et Biophysica Acta (BBA) Mol Basis Dis. 2011;1812(10):1327–36.
103. Swenson-Fields KI, Vivian CJ, Salah SM, Peda JD, Davis BM, van Rooijen N, et al. Macrophages promote polycystic kidney disease progression. Kidney Int. 2013;83(5):855–64.
104. Mekahli D, Parys JB, Bultynck G, Missiaen L, De Smedt H. Polycystins and cellular Ca2+ signaling. Cell Mol Life Sci. 2013;70(15):2697–712.
105. Mekahli D, Sammels E, Luyten T, Welkenhuyzen K, van den Heuvel LP, Levtchenko EN, et al. Polycystin-1 and polycystin-2 are both required to amplify inositol-trisphosphate-induced Ca2+ release. Cell Calcium. 2012;51(6):452–8.
106. Wilson PD, Hovater JS, Casey CC, Fortenberry JA, Schwiebert EM. ATP release mechanisms in primary cultures of epithelia derived from the cysts of polycystic kidneys. J Am Soc Nephrol. 1999;10(2):218–29.
107. Gardner KJ, Burnside J, Elzinga L, Locksley R. Cytokines in fluids from polycystic kidneys. Kidney Int. 1991;39(4):718–24.
108. Carone FA, Kanwar Y. Tubular cell and matrix changes in renal cystic disease. Contrib Nephrol. 1993;101:1–6.
109. Jin H, Carone FA, Nakamura S, Liu ZZ, Kanwar YS. Altered synthesis and intracellular transport of proteoglycans by cyst-derived cells from human polycystic kidneys. J Am Soc Nephrol. 1992;2(12):1726–33.
110. Wilson PD, Norman JT, Kuo NT, Burrow CR. Abnormalities in extracellular matrix regulation in autosomal dominant polycystic kidney disease. Contrib Nephrol. 1996;118:126–34.
111. Woo D. Apoptosis and loss of renal tissue in polycystic kidney diseases. NE J Med. 1995;333:18–25.
112. Kanehisa M, Goto S, Sato Y, Kawashima M, Furumichi M, Tanabe M. Data, information, knowledge and principle: back to metabolism in KEGG. Nucleic Acids Res. 2014;42(Database issue):D199–205.
113. Huang DW, Sherman BT, Tan Q, Collins JR, Alvord WG, Roayaei J, et al. The DAVID Gene Functional Classification Tool: a novel biological module-centric algorithm to functionally analyze large gene lists. Genome Biol. 2007;8(9):R183.
114. Huang dW, Sherman BT, Stephens R, Baseler MW, Lane HC, Lempicki RA. DAVID gene ID conversion tool. Bioinformation. 2008;2(10):428–30.

Transcriptome analysis of bronchoalveolar lavage fluid from children with severe *Mycoplasma pneumoniae* pneumonia reveals novel gene expression and immunodeficiency

Kuo Wang[1†], Man Gao[2†], Mingyue Yang[1], Fanzheng Meng[2], Deli Li[2], Ruihua Lu[2], Yan Wang[2], Huadong Zhuang[2], Mengyao Li[3], Genhong Cheng[1,4] and Xiaosong Wang[1*]

Abstract

Background: A growing number of severe *Mycoplasma pneumoniae* pneumonia (MPP) cases have been reported recently. However, the pathogenesis of severe MPP is not clear. In the current study, transcriptome sequencing was used to identify gene expression and alternative splicing profiles to provide insights into the pathogenesis of severe MPP.

Methods: RNAs of bronchoalveolar lavage fluid (BALF) samples from three severe MPP children and three mild MPP children were analyzed respectively by deep sequencing followed by computational annotation and quantification.

Results: The gene expression analysis revealed 14 up-regulated and 34 down-regulated genes in severe MPP children comparing to mild MPP children. The top 10 most up-regulated genes were *IGHV1-69*, *CH17-472G23.1*, *ATP1B2*, *FCER2*, *MUC21*, *IL13*, *FCRLB*, *CLEC5A*, *FAM124A*, and *INHBA*. The top 10 most down-regulated genes were *OSTN-AS1*, *IL22RA2*, *COL3A1*, *C1orf141*, *IGKV2-29*, *RP11-731F5.2*, *IGHV4-4*, *KIRREL*, *DNASE1L3*, and *COL6A2*. Clustering analysis revealed similar expression pattern of *CLEC5A*, *IL13*, *FCER2*, and *FLT1*. Kyoto Encyclopedia of Genes and Genomes (KEGG) pathway enrichment analyses revealed changes related to primary immunodeficiency in severe MPP children comparing to mild MPP children; the pathway involves *CD19*, *TNFRSF13C*, *CD79A*, and *AICDA* genes. Among the differentially expressed genes, significant alternative splicing events were found in *FCER2* and *FCRLA*.

Conclusions: The current study on RNA sequencing provides novel insights into the pathogenesis of severe MPP in terms of gene expression and alternative splicing. The up-regulation of *IL13*, *FCER2*, *FLT1*, and *CLEC5A* and the down-regulation of *CD79A*, *AICDA*, *CD19*, and *TNFRSF13C* may contribute to the pathogenesis of severe MPP. The differential expressions of *FCER2* and *FCRLA* could be due to their alternative splicing.

Keywords: Severe *Mycoplasma pneumoniae* pneumonia, Children, Bronchoalveolar lavage fluid, Transcriptome sequencing, Gene expression profile, Alternative splicing

* Correspondence: xiaosongwang@jlu.edu.cn
†Equal contributors
[1]Institute of Translational Medicine, the First Hospital of Jilin University, Changchun 130061, China
Full list of author information is available at the end of the article

Background

Mycoplasma pneumoniae pneumonia (MPP), as a common community-acquired pneumonia, counts for 20 to 40% of children pneumonia and may reach 50 to 80% during the time of local outbreak [1, 2]. MPP is usually described as mild and self-limited; however, more and more severe or even fatal cases of MPP with severe complications such as pulmonary necrosis and chronic interstitial fibrosis have been reported recently [3–5]. Macrolide-resistant and excessive immunological inflammation are also commonly found in severe MPP [6]. Therefore, it is essential for pediatricians to recognize severe MPP early, treat it promptly, and prevent the progression of the disease effectively. However, the mechanism and etiology of severe MPP are largely unknown.

Based on published hypotheses, severe MPP is considered as a hyper-immune response that originates from repeated or longer lasting childhood MP infections in the lung [7]; further, severe MPP can be an overactive innate immune response such as macrophage activation via heterodimerization of Toll-like receptors two and six of the bronchoepithelial cells to *M. pneumoniae* lipoproteins [8]. With ELISA and real-time quantitative PCR techniques, researchers have found that the cell-mediated immune response plays an important role in the pathogenesis of MPP [9–11] but the role of humoral-mediated immune response in mild and severe MPP is still unclear.

High-throughput RNA sequencing technology, so called next-generation sequencing, revolutionarily enhanced our understanding on the complexity of eukaryotic transcriptome [12, 13]. It has several key advantages including being independent on the predetermined genome sequences, highly accurate in detecting gene expression with very wide dynamic detection ranges with low background. Thus, RNA sequencing is not only useful to precisely determine gene expression profiles but also particularly powerful to detect novel transcription variants via alternative splicing [12].

In the present study, we observed the transcriptome of bronchoalveolar lavage fluid (BALF) from children with mild MPP and severe MPP. The large sum of novel information on the gene expression profiles as well as novel transcripts through alternative splicing would provide not only insights into the pathogenesis of severe MPP but also as basis for the development of biomarkers and therapeutic targets.

Methods

Study subjects

The current study was conducted at the First Hospital of Jilin University (Changchun City, Jilin Province, People's Republic of China). Six newly diagnosed children (three male and three female) with acute stage of MPP admitted to our hospital were recruited [see Additional file 1: Table S1]. All of the children enrolled in this study had no recurrent severe or unusual infections and had no inflammatory disorders or autoimmunity. Therefore, based on the published diagnostic criteria, they had no history of common variable immunodefiency (CVID) [14]. After admission to our hospital, the levels of immunoglobulins in the blood of these children had been examined; the levels of IgG, IgA, and IgM had been found within normal range published for children [see Additional file 2: Figure S1] [15]. Lymphocyte profiles in the peripheral blood of these children had also been examined, the cell numbers and percentage of T cells, B cells, and natural killer cells had been found within normal range [see Additional file 3: Table S2] [15]. Therefore, the enrolled children had been excluded from having CVID, autosomal recessive agammaglobulinemia [15], or high IgM syndrome [16]. All children did not have untreated metabolic/congenital systemic diseases. The diagnosis of pneumonia was based on clinical manifestations (cough, fever, dry or productive sputum, dyspnea, abnormal breath sound, radiological pulmonary abnormalities). The diagnosis of *Mycoplasma pneumoniae* (MP) infection was based on positive results of serologic test (MP-IgM test ≥1:40) and positive results of MP DNA (>500 copy/L) in BALF with real-time quantitative PCR. MP was the only pathogen identified in all the MPP subjects. The mild and severe community-acquired pneumonia was defined based on the criteria described [17, 18]. Mild group was defined as fever <38.5 °C at any age, tachypnea but respiratory rate <70 breaths/min at age <3 years old or <50 breaths/min at age ≥3 years old, normal food-intake, and no dehydration. Severe group was defined as fever ≥38.5 °C at any age, breathless with respiratory rate ≥70 breaths/min at age <3 years old or ≥50 breaths/min at age ≥3 years old (excluding the reasons of fever and cry), cyanosis, marked retractions, anorexia, and dehydration.

The written informed consents were obtained by care givers of all children. The study was approved by the Institutional Medical Ethics Review Board of the First Hospital of Jilin University in compliance with the Declaration of Helsinki.

Bronchoscopy and bronchoalveolar lavage

Following the guidelines described previously [17], flexible fiber optic bronchoscopy with bronchoalveolar lavage (BAL) was performed within 3 days after the admission. Both groups received similar supportive and symptomatic treatment, including sputum aspiration, nebulization, and fluid therapy. Corticosteroid and the other immune regulation agents were not permitted before bronchoscopy. A 2.8-mm pediatric flexible bronchoscope (Olympus BF-XP60, New Hyde Park, NY) or a

4.0-mm flexible bronchoscope (Olympus P-260, New Hyde Park, NY) was used for children depending on their age and body weight. All of the enrolled subjects had indications for bronchoscopy and BAL: radiologically proven large pulmonary lesions (including atelectasis and consolidation of lung fields). Supplemental oxygen was administered during the procedure. Transcutaneous oxygen saturation and pulse rate (Masimo Radical-7 pulse oximetry, Masimo, CA) were continuously monitored during the bronchoscopy.

Intravenous injection of midazolam (0.1–0.15 mg/kg) was used for sedation; aerosolized lidocaine spraying on the throat insertion was performed 5–10 min before bronchoscope for throat local anesthesia; dripping 2% lidocaine through flexible bronchoscopy was used for the topical anesthesia of the upper and lower airways. BAL was performed in an area most prominently affected based on the chest radiology (MPP groups) by gently wedging the tip of the Bronchoscope in a segmental or subsegmental bronchus. 1 ml/kg sterile saline was instilled through the instrumentation channel. The BALF was gently aspirated and collected in a sterile container and immediately centrifuged. The pallet was resuspended in TRIzol (Life Technologies, CA, USA) and stored in −80 °C freezer. The composition of the nucleated cells in the BALF was counted; results were shown in Additional file 4: Table S3.

RNA preparation and sequencing

Total RNA was extracted using TRIzol according to the manufacturer's instructions. RNA degradation and contamination were monitored on 1% agarose gels. RNA purity was checked using the NanoPhotometer spectrophotometer (IMPLEN, CA, USA). RNA concentration was measured using Qubit RNA Assay Kit in Qubit 2.0 Flurometer (Life Technologies, CA, USA). RNA integrity was assessed using the RNA Nano 6000 Assay Kit of the Bioanalyzer 2100 system (Agilent Technologies, CA, USA).

A total amount of 3 μg RNA per sample was used as input material for the RNA sample preparation. Sequencing libraries were generated using NEBNext® Ultra™ RNA Library Prep Kit for Illumina® (NEB, USA) following the manufacturer's recommendations, and index codes were added to attribute sequences to each sample. The clustering of the index-coded samples was performed on a cBot Cluster Generation System using TruSeq PE Cluster Kit v3-cBot-HS (Illumia) according to the manufacturer's instructions. After cluster generation, the library preparations were sequenced on an Illumina Hiseq platform and 125 bp/150 bp paired-end reads were generated.

Sequencing data analysis

Raw data (raw reads) of fastq format were firstly processed through in-house perl scripts, and clean data (clean reads) were obtained. Index of the reference genome was built using Bowtie v2.2.3, and paired-end clean reads were aligned to the reference genome using TopHat v2.0.12. Only uniquely and properly mapped read pairs were used for further analysis. The differentially expressed genes between BALF samples were identified using the DESeq R package (1.18.0) [19]. Differentially expressed genes were defined as those with changes of at least twofold between samples. The resulting p values were adjusted using the Benjamini and Hochberg approach for controlling the false discovery rate (FDR). Genes with an adjusted p value <0.05 found by DESeq were assigned as differentially expressed. Protein functional classification of differentially expressed genes was performed using the PANTHER classification system [20]. KOBAS software was used to test the statistical enrichment of differential expression genes in KEGG pathways. The significance of enriched KEGG pathways were determined by corrected p value <0.05. Cufflinks v2.1.1 Reference Annotation Based Transcript (RABT) assembly method was used to construct and identify both known and novel transcripts from TopHat alignment results. The analysis of alternative splicing events was performed using MATS and IGV software [21]; alternative splicing events were classified to five basic types by software Asprofile v1.0. The differences in alternative splicing of genes were considered significant with a cutoff of 5% FDR.

Results

RNA sequencing results

Total RNA was extracted from six BALF samples of children with severe MPP or mild MPP [see Additional file 1: Table S1]. Then, mRNAs from each sample were sequenced. After the removal of adaptor sequences, ambiguous reads and low-quality reads, about 40–70 million pairs of clean read, were generated for each sample (Table 1). The percentage of reads mapped to the forward chain was equal to that mapped to the reverse chain. When compared with the reference sequence of the Genome Reference Consortium GRCh37/hg19, more than 85% of total read pairs were uniquely mapped on the human genome (Table 1). A correlation matrix shown a high consistency of measurements within each group, $R^2 > 0.8$ [see Additional file 5: Figure S2A]. Principal component analysis (PCA) was carried out to assess the clustering nature of these samples. Samples of each group had been clustered together; data shown good repeatability and correlation [see Additional file 5: Figure S2B].

Identification and classification of differentially expressed genes between severe MPP and mild MPP

Totally, 48 differentially expressed genes were identified between the severe MPP group and mild MPP group

Table 1 Summary of RNA sequencing read mapping result

Sample number	Mild 202	Mild 224	Mild 247	Severe 177	Severe 223	Severe 324
Total reads	55492664	47186542	64792680	68897254	42136856	46318894
Total mapped	48535137 (87.46%)	40517410 (85.87%)	56013052 (86.45%)	60481397 (87.78%)	36565361 (86.78%)	40224088 (86.84%)
Multiple mapped	844736 (1.52%)	614681 (1.30%)	797662 (1.23%)	881129 (1.28%)	543196 (1.29%)	630869 (1.36%)
Uniquely mapped	47690401 (85.94%)	39902729 (84.56%)	55215390 (85.22%)	59600268 (86.51%)	36022165 (85.49%)	39593219 (85.48%)
Reads map to "+"	23844413 (42.97%)	19967766 (42.32%)	27594117 (42.59%)	29790936 (43.24%)	18008541 (42.74%)	19797319 (42.74%)
Reads map to "−"	23845988 (42.97%)	19934963 (42.25%)	27621273 (42.63%)	29809332 (43.27%)	18013624 (42.75%)	19795900 (42.74%)
Non-splice reads	30580304 (55.11%)	22475106 (47.63%)	34530918 (53.29%)	37577003 (54.54%)	20733762 (49.21%)	24205574 (52.26%)
Splice reads	17110097 (30.83%)	17427623 (36.93%)	20684472 (31.92%)	22023265 (31.97%)	15288403 (36.28%)	15387645 (33.22%)

Total reads: The number of sequence after sequencing data filtering
Total mapped: The number of sequence which can map to the genome
Multiple mapped: The number of sequence which have multiple location on the reference sequencing
Uniquely mapped: The number of sequence which have single location on the reference sequencing
Reads map to "+": The statistics of sequence that were mapped on the "+" chain of the genome
Reads map to "−": The statistics of sequence that were mapped on the "−" chain of the genome

(Fig. 1a). The 14 up-regulated genes listed in Table 2 were *IGHV1-69, CH17-472G23.1, ATP1B2, FCER2, MUC21, IL13, FCRLB, CLEC5A, FAM124A, INHBA, FLT1, APOL4*, and two novel transcripts. These 14 up-regulated genes included cytokine (*IL13*), immunoglobin Fc receptors (*FCER2* and *FCRLB*), and inflammatory response regulator (*CLEC5A*). The top 20 most down-regulated genes were *OSTN-AS1, IL22RA2, COL3A1, C1orf141, IGKV2-29, RP11-731F5.2, IGHV4-4, KIRREL, DNASE1L3, COL6A2, COL6A1, FCRL4, HTRA3, TCL1A, RP11-356K23.1, PLD4, DKK3, UBE2QL1, KLRB1*, and *MS4A1* (Table 3).

Protein functional classification of differentially expressed genes between severe MPP and mild MPP was performed. As a result, the 48 differentially expressed genes were divided into 13 different classes of protein (Fig. 1b). The expression levels of genes classified as signaling molecule (*CLEC5A, IL13, INHBA*), transporter (*ATP1B2*), and transfer/carrier protein (*APOL4*) significantly increased in the severe MPP group comparing to the mild MPP group [see Additional file 6: Table S4]. On the other hand, genes in the categories of nucleic acid binding molecule (*AICDA, PAX5, SPIB, TCF7*), genes encodes defense/immunity protein (*IL22RA2, CD79A*), hydrase (*PLA2G2D, HTRA3, AICDA*), receptor (*MS4A1, IL22RA2*), and transcription factor (*PAX5*), were predominantly expressed in the mild MPP group. Among the cell adhesion molecules, *FCER2* and *FCRLB* were up-regulated in the severe MPP group; *FCRLA* and *FCRL4* were up-regulated in the mild MPP group.

The clustering analysis of differentially expressed genes indicated that *FCER2, FLT1, IL13*, and *CLEC5A* were

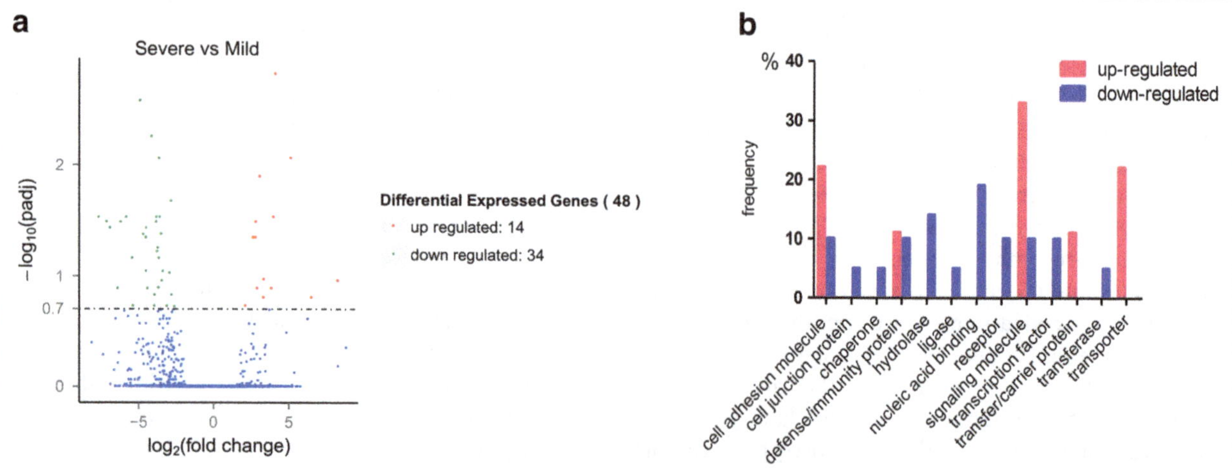

Fig. 1 Differentially expressed genes between the severe MPP group and mild MPP group in BALF. **a** Volcano plot of genes differentially expressed between the severe MPP group and mild MPP group. Each point represents one gene that is detectable in both groups. The *red points* represent significantly up-regulated genes; the *green points* represent significantly down-regulated genes. **b** Protein functional classification of differentially expressed genes has been performed using the PANTHER tool between the severe MPP group and mild MPP group. The protein category is shown on *x*-axis and the gene frequency is shown on *y*-axis

Table 2 Up-regulated genes of the severe MPP group comparing to the mild MPP group

Gene ID	Associated gene name	log_2foldchange	padj	Description
ENSG00000104921	*FCER2*	4.081288	0.001514	Fc fragment of IgE, low affinity II, receptor for (CD23)
ENSG00000129244	*ATP1B2*	5.123508	0.008687	ATPase, Na+/K+ transporting, beta 2 polypeptide
ENSG00000258227	*CLEC5A*	3.046087	0.012798	C-type lectin domain family 5 member A
Novel00326	–	3.957912	0.029750	–
ENSG00000122641	*INHBA*	2.792227	0.032804	Inhibin beta A
ENSG00000102755	*FLT1*	2.773680	0.044977	Fms-related tyrosine kinase 1
Novel00056	–	2.612021	0.044977	–
ENSG00000169194	*IL13*	3.320997	0.107345	Interleukin 13
ENSG00000211973	*IGHV1-69*	8.269132	0.110361	Immunoglobulin heavy variable 1–69
ENSG00000150510	*FAM124A*	2.878502	0.130273	Family with sequence similarity 124 member A
ENSG00000204544	*MUC21*	3.830138	0.130273	Mucin 21, cell surface associated
ENSG00000162746	*FCRLB*	3.307526	0.157765	Fc receptor-like B
ENSG00000274642	*CH17-472G23.1*	6.496741	0.157765	–
ENSG00000100336	*APOL4*	2.103424	0.186854	Apolipoprotein L4

log_2foldchange log_2 (severe MPP/mild MPP), *padj* adjusted *p* value, *Novel* novel gene

up-regulated in the severe MPP group comparing to the mild MPP group (Fig. 2). Similar up-regulation or down-regulation patterns among these genes were identified, which may indicate related local protein functions of these genes under MP infection in children.

Functional annotation of KEGG pathway enrichment analysis revealed changes related to primary immunodeficiency in the BALF of severe MPP children, which was associated with the down-regulation of *CD19, TNFRSF13C, CD79A,* and *AICDA* genes (Table 4). *CD19, TNFRSF13C, CD79A,* and *AICDA* were involved in the B cell differentiation process; down-regulation of these genes may restrain B cell maturation and antibody production (Fig. 3) [22]. Furthermore, *COL6A1, COL6A2, COL5A3, COL3A1,* and *COL1A2* genes were involved in the pathways including protein digestion and absorption, ECM-receptor interaction, P13K-Akt signaling, and focal adhesion; these molecules were found down-regulated in the severe MPP group comparing to the mild MPP group (Table 4). *COL6A1, COL6A2, COL5A3, COL3A1,* and *COL1A2* belong to the collagen super family, which play a role in maintaining the integrity of various tissues including the lung [23]. *FLT1,* which encoded a member of vascular endothelial growth factor receptor (VEGFR) family, was also found significantly increased in the severe MPP group comparing to the mild MPP group in the P13K-Akt signaling and focal adhesion pathways (Tables 2 and 4).

Alternative splicing events between severe MPP and mild MPP

More than 90% of human genes are alternatively spliced through different types of splicing [24]. MATS analysis of the RNA sequencing data significantly revealed 1500 differential alternative splicing events with a cutoff of 5% FDR (Table 5), more than half (50.5%) of them belong to the skipped exon type. Among the differentially expressed genes between the severe MPP group and mild MPP group, *FECR2* and *FCRLA* were identified to have significantly alternative splicing [see Additional file 7: Table S5, Additional file 8: Table S6, Additional file 9: Table S7, Additional file 10: Table S8, and Additional file 11: Table S9].

FCER2 locates on chromosome 19p13.2 (chr 19:7,688,758-7,702,146); its encoding protein is a B cell specific antigen, which is a low-affinity receptor for IgE. This protein plays essential roles in B cell growth, differentiation, and regulation of IgE production. It also exists as a soluble secreted form and acts as a potent mitogenic growth factor. Retained intron (RI) was identified in *FCER2* in some of the samples. RI lies on chr19: 7,698,355-7,698,854; the upstream exon locates on chr19: 7,698,355-7,698,409 and the downstream exon locates on chr19: 7,698,740-7,698,854 [see Additional file 8: Table S6]. Compared to the mild MPP group, the severe MPP group had less RI spliced transcript events of *FCER2,* which could be an explanation for the up-regulation of the *FCER2* in severe MPP children (Fig. 4a).

FCRLA locates on chromosome 1q23.3 (chr 1:161,706,972-161,714,352). This gene encodes a protein similar to Fc receptor of gamma immunoglobulin (IgG), which is selectively expressed in B cells and may be involved in their development. Alternatively, spliced transcript variants of *FCRLA* that encode different protein isoforms have been found in the current study. Two exons of *FCLRA* were involved in mutual exclusive exon (MEX), the first exon starts at 161,710,759 and ends at 161,710,912 and the second exon starts at 161,711,207 and ends at 161,711,474 [see

Table 3 Down-regulated genes of the severe MPP group comparing to the mild MPP group

Gene ID	Associated gene name	log_2foldchange	padj	Description
ENSG00000163687	*DNASE1L3*	−4.90655	0.002613	Deoxyribonuclease I-like 3
ENSG00000166428	*PLD4*	−4.12788	0.005539	Phospholipase D family member 4
ENSG00000269404	*SPIB*	−3.62528	0.008687	Spi-B transcription factor (Spi-1/PU.1 related)
ENSG00000081059	*TCF7*	−2.83313	0.021184	Transcription factor 7 (T cell specific, HMG-box)
ENSG00000156738	*MS4A1*	−3.80125	0.029750	Membrane-spanning 4-domains, subfamily A, member 1
ENSG00000159958	*TNFRSF13C*	−3.59110	0.029750	Tumor necrosis factor receptor superfamily member 13C
ENSG00000233308	*OSTN-AS1*	−7.65241	0.029750	OSTN antisense RNA 1
ENSG00000253364	*RP11-731F5.2*	−5.82530	0.029750	–
ENSG00000111796	*KLRB1*	−3.80851	0.032804	Killer cell lectin-like receptor subfamily B, member 1
ENSG00000164485	*IL22RA2*	−7.13138	0.032804	Interleukin 22 receptor subunit alpha 2
ENSG00000253998	*IGKV2-29*	−6.19209	0.032804	Immunoglobulin kappa variable 2–29 (gene/pseudogene)
ENSG00000168542	*COL3A1*	−6.89272	0.036862	Collagen, type III, alpha 1
ENSG00000170801	*HTRA3*	−4.50354	0.036862	HtrA serine peptidase 3
Novel00339	–	−3.48127	0.041780	–
ENSG00000142173	*COL6A2*	−4.69524	0.042554	Collagen, type VI, alpha 2
ENSG00000100721	*TCL1A*	−4.49274	0.044977	T cell leukemia/lymphoma 1A
ENSG00000142156	*COL6A1*	−4.52065	0.044977	Collagen, type VI, alpha 1
ENSG00000111732	*AICDA*	−3.71025	0.055876	Activation-induced cytidine deaminase
ENSG00000164692	*COL1A2*	−3.75418	0.059895	Collagen, type I, alpha 2
ENSG00000105369	*CD79A*	−3.63713	0.069048	CD79a molecule
ENSG00000276775	*IGHV4-4*	−5.43537	0.069048	Immunoglobulin heavy variable 4-4
ENSG00000080573	*COL5A3*	−3.37399	0.090838	Collagen, type V, alpha 3
ENSG00000163518	*FCRL4*	−4.51056	0.090838	Fc receptor-like 4
ENSG00000196092	*PAX5*	−2.93710	0.093937	Paired box 5
ENSG00000177455	*CD19*	−3.44060	0.110361	CD19 molecule
ENSG00000136573	*BLK*	−3.67317	0.128424	BLK proto-oncogene, Src family tyrosine kinase
ENSG00000203963	*C1orf141*	−6.39692	0.130273	Chromosome 1 open reading frame 141
ENSG00000258752	*RP11-356K23.1*	−4.39265	0.130273	–
ENSG00000167483	*FAM129C*	−2.78386	0.148367	Family with sequence similarity 129 member C
ENSG00000215218	*UBE2QL1*	−3.91473	0.149275	Ubiquitin conjugating enzyme E2Q family-like 1
ENSG00000050165	*DKK3*	−3.95056	0.186854	Dickkopf WNT signaling pathway inhibitor 3
ENSG00000132185	*FCRLA*	−3.11003	0.186854	Fc receptor-like A
ENSG00000183853	*KIRREL*	−5.37583	0.186854	Kin of IRRE like (drosophila)
ENSG00000117215	*PLA2G2D*	−2.60098	0.191201	Phospholipase A2 group IID

log_2foldchange log_2 (severe MPP/mild MPP), *padj* adjusted *p* value, *Novel* novel gene

Additional file 9: Table S7]. The analysis of alternative splicing events indicated that the MEX frequency of the first exon in the severe MPP group was significantly higher than that in the mild MPP group, which may result in the down-regulated expression of *FCRLA* in severe MPP children (Fig. 4b).

Discussion

Recent developments in RNA sequencing technology enabled elaborate analysis of gene expression in numerous human diseases. However, to our best knowledge, no report of RNA-sequencing study on human MPP has been published yet. The current study provides extensive information on gene expression and alternative splicing in the BALF of MPP children through transcriptome analysis, which is crucial for understanding the pathogenesis of severe MPP. The gene expression analysis revealed 14 up-regulated genes and 34 down-regulated genes in severe MPP children comparing to mild MPP children. The top 10 most up-regulated genes are *IGHV1-*

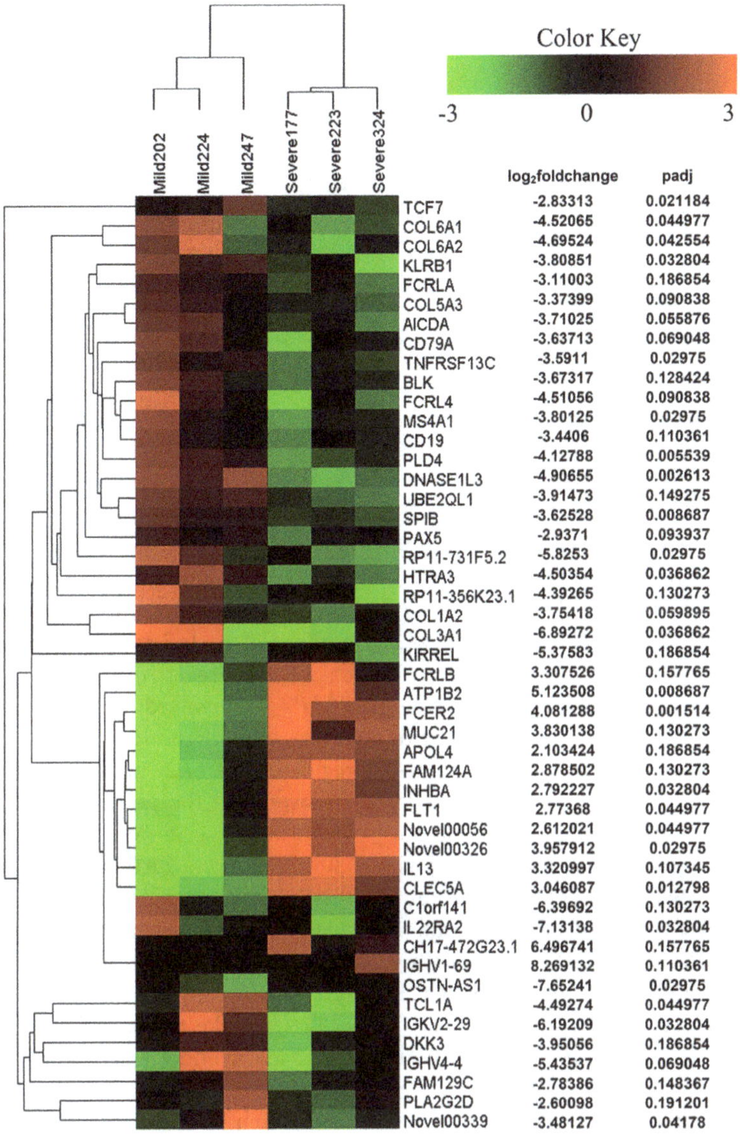

Fig. 2 Cluster of 48 genes showing representative expression patterns between the severe MPP group and mild MPP group. All of the genes that are differentially expressed between the severe MPP group and mild MPP group by $\log_2$ fold change >2 or <−2, adjusted *p* value <0.2, have been selected

Table 4 KEGG pathway enrichment

Term	ID	Adjusted *p* value	Input	KEGG_ID/KO
Protein digestion and absorption	hsa04974	0.000305	*COL6A1*| *COL6A2*| *ATP1B2*| *COL5A3* | *COL3A1*| *COL1A2*	hsa:1291|hsa:1292|hsa:482|hsa:50509 |hsa:1281|hsa:1278|
Primary immunodeficiency	hsa05340	0.001040	*CD19*| *TNFRSF13C*| *CD79A*| *AICDA*	hsa:930|hsa:115650|hsa:973|hsa:57379|
ECM-receptor interaction	hsa04512	0.001350	*COL6A2*| *COL5A3*| *COL6A1* | *COL1A2*| *COL3A1*	hsa:1292|hsa:50509|hsa:1291 |hsa:1278|hsa:1281|
PI3K-Akt signaling pathway	hsa04151	0.003493	*COL6A1*| *TCL1A*| *COL6A2*| *CD19*| *COL5A3* | *COL3A1*| *COL1A2*| *FLT1*	hsa:1291|hsa:8115|hsa:1292|hsa:930 |hsa:50509|hsa:1281|hsa:1278|hsa:2321|
Focal adhesion	hsa04510	0.005512	*COL6A1*| *COL6A2*| *COL5A3*| *COL3A1* | *COL1A2*| *FLT1*	hsa:1291|hsa:1292|hsa:50509|hsa:1281 |hsa:1278|hsa:2321|

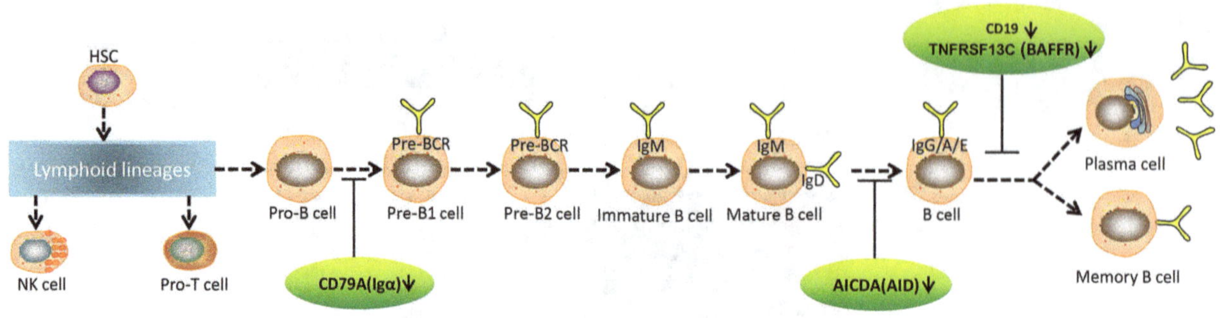

Fig. 3 Model diagram showing primary immunodeficiency. Hematopoietic stem cell (HSC)-derived lymphoid progenitor cells develop into progenitor (pro)-B cells, Pre-B1 cell, Pre-B2 cell, immature B cell, mature B cell, B cell, memory B cell, and plasma cell. The decreased expression of *CD79A* inhibits the differentiation of Pro-B cell into Pre-B1 cell; the decreased expression of *AICDA* inhibits the differentiation of mature B cell into B cell; the decreased expression of *CD19* and *TNFRSF13C* inhibits the differentiation of mature B cell into memory B cell and plasma B cell

69, CH17-472G23.1, ATP1B2, FCER2, MUC21, IL13, FCRLB, CLEC5A, FAM124A, and *INHBA* (Fig. 1a, Table 2). The top 10 most down-regulated genes are *OSTN-AS1, IL22RA2, COL3A1, C1orf141, IGKV2-29, RP11-731F5.2, IGHV4-4, KIRREL, DNASE1L3*, and *COL6A2* (Fig. 1a, Table 3).

Several key genes that are differentially expressed between severe MPP and mild MPP are associated with hyper-immune response and signaling. For example, IL13, a cytokine secreted by T helper type 2 (Th2) cells, can induce many features of allergic lung disease including airway hyper-responsiveness, goblet cell metaplasia, and mucus hyper-secretion, which all contribute to airway obstruction [25, 26]. IL13 is found to cause mucin overproduction through STAT6/EGFR-FOXA2 signaling and mucus plugging formation in MP infection, which results in pulmonary atelectasis or consolidation [27]. These results prove that IL13 play an important role in the airway obstruction of severe MPP. In addition, Wu Q et al. [26] have reported that IL13 can restrain MP clearance by the suppression of Toll-like receptor 2 in mice. Therefore, high levels of IL13 may make severe MPP children lose the ability to eradicate MP from the lung in primary infection, resulting in longer lasting MP infection and a hyper-immune response [7]. Another gene associated with hyper-immune response is *FCER2*. *FCER2* is a B cell specific antigen and a low-affinity receptor for IgE. It has essential roles in B cell growth, differentiation, and the regulation of IgE production. On the basis of study with animal models, *FCER2* has been implicated in IgE-mediated allergic diseases and bronchial hyper-reactivity [28]. It has been proved that *FCER2* is involved in the pharmacogenetic basis for severe exacerbations in children with asthma [29]. Up-regulated *FCER2* in severe MPP children has been discovered in the present study. Similarly, increased IgE levels in the serum of MPP patients have been reported [30]. Therefore, further study will be needed to prove that up-regulated *FCER2* causes the bronchial inflammation and hyper-immune reactivity. Among the up-regulated genes in severe MPP comparing to mild MPP, *FLT1* may also associate with hyper-immune response. *FLT1* (fms-like tyrosine kinase 1) encodes a member of the vascular endothelial growth factor receptor (VEGFR) family. Wu WK et al. demonstrate that Th2-related cytokines, such as IL4 and IL13, could drive the expression of *FLT1* [31]. Moreover, Th2-related cytokines can promote VEGF release in the airway, and VEGF has been proposed to be associated with severe MPP [32, 33]. Therefore, atopic children may be more prone to develop severe pneumonia [34]. We tentatively put forward the hypothesis that *IL13, FCER2*, and *FLT1* may be

Table 5 Summary of the differential alternative splicing event analysis

	Skipped exon	Retained intron	Mutual exclusive exon	Alternative 5′ splicing sites	Alternative 3′ splicing sites
Number of total alternative splicing events (genes)	44856 (11195)	3772 (2353)	6862 (3327)	2793 (2103)	4374 (2874)
Percentage of total alternative splicing event (%)	71.6	6.0	10.9	4.5	7.0
Number of differential alternative splicing events (up-regulation/down-regulation)	758 (398:360)	181 (107:74)	315 (193:122)	101 (74:27)	145 (86:59)
Percentage of total differential alternative splicing event (%)	50.5	12.1	21	6.7	9.7

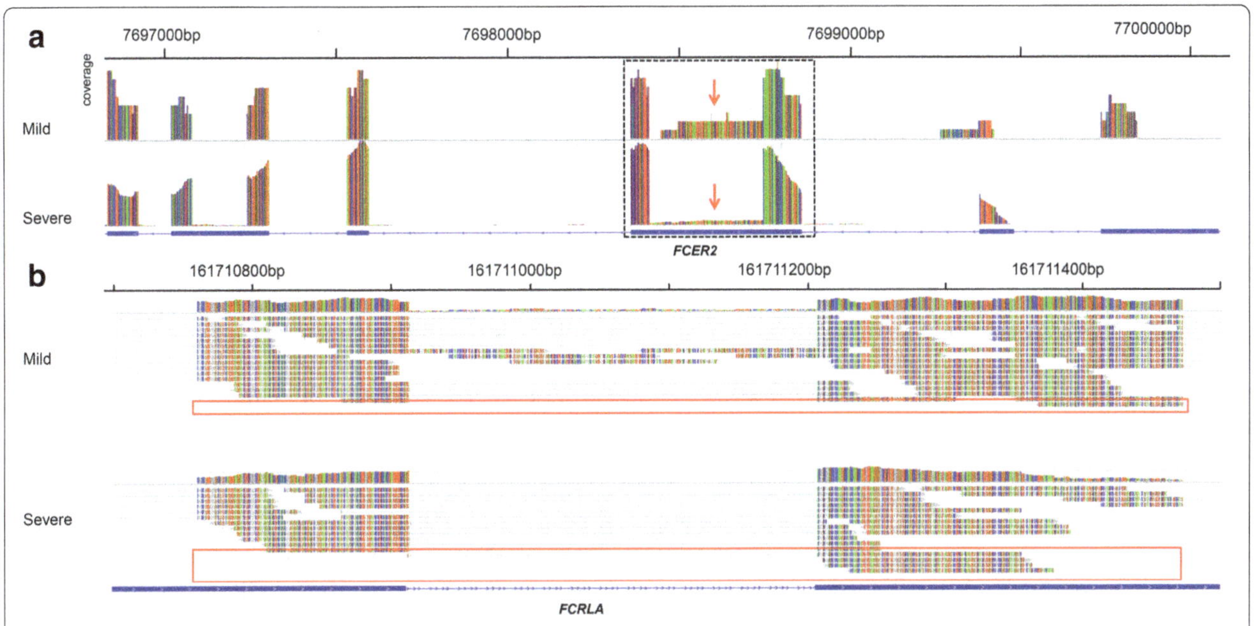

Fig. 4 Differential alternative splicing of *FCER2* and *FCRLA*. **a** Read distribution plot for *FCER2* with differential isoform expression due to retained intron in the mild MPP group is shown. The *black box* and *red arrows* indicated the location of the retained intron. **b** Read distribution plot for *FCRLA* with differential isoform expression due to mutually exclusive exon is shown. The ratio of mutually exclusive exon happened in the severe MPP group is compared with that in the mild MPP group

associated with each other and all of them are involved in the pathogenesis of severe MPP.

Based on our data [see Additional file 4: Table S3] and published results [35], more than half of the nucleated cells in BALF of MPP children without other pathogen infection are macrophages. But it is still unclear how macrophages are involved in the pathogenesis of severe MPP. Clustering analysis of the differentially expressed genes reveals that the expression patterns of *IL13*, *FCER2*, *FLT1*, and *CLEC5A* are similar in the severe MPP group (Fig. 2). One possible mechanism of severe MPP is the overactivation of macrophage in innate immune response [7]. *CLEC5A* (C-type lectin domain family 5, member A) is expressed on alveolar macrophages; it has been demonstrated to mediate macrophage response and play roles in pro-inflammatory cytokine expression and airspace enlargement in a mice model of chronic obstructive pulmonary disease (COPD) [36]. Muro S et al. suggested that MP infection could be an independent risk factor for COPD in the general population [37]. *CLEC5A* encodes a member of the CTL/CTLD (C-type lectin/C-type lectin-like domain) superfamily, which family members play roles in inflammation and immune responses. Teng O et al. have revealed that *CLEC5A*-mediated enhancement of the inflammatory response in myeloid cells contributes to influenza's pathogenicity in vivo [38]. We found significant higher expression levels of *CLEC5A* in the BALF of severe MPP comparing to that of mild MPP. Therefore, our results support the hypothesis that *CLEC5A* is involved in the pathogenesis of severe MPP through the overactivation of macrophage. Protein functional classification of the differentially expressed genes indicates that signaling molecules including *IL13*, *CLEC5A*, and *INHBA* are obviously increased in severe MPP comparing to mild MPP [see Fig. 1b, Additional file 6: Table S4]. *INHBA* (Inhibin beta A) encodes a member of the transforming growth factor superfamily. The encoded preproprotein is proteolytically processed to generate a subunit of the dimeric activin and inhibin protein complexes. Rheumatoid arthritis synovium fluid (RA-SF) promotes *INHBA* production as a pro-inflammatory cytokine from macrophages in vitro [39]. Similarly, *INHBA* is reported to be up-regulated in endometritis by Hoelker M et al. [40]. It is interesting that the current study finds increased levels of *INHBA* in severe MPP. The causal relationship between the up-regulation of *INHBA* and severe MPP requires further investigation.

It is still unclear how B cells are involved in the pathogenesis of severe MPP. In the current study, KEGG pathway enrichment analyses have revealed changes related to primary immunodeficiency in severe MPP patients, which involves *CD79A*, *AICDA*, *CD19*, and *TNFRSF13C* genes (Table 4, Fig. 3) [22]. *CD79A*, *AICDA*, *CD19*, and *TNFRSF13C* are related to the B cell antigen signaling pathway; lower expression of these genes can lead to the deficiency of B cell functions. *CD79A* encodes the Igα protein of the B cell antigen component, which is necessary for expression and function of the B cell antigen receptor. Defected *CD79A* has been discovered in immunodeficiency-related diseases [41]. Similarly, *AICDA* (activation-induced cytidine deaminase) encodes a RNA-editing deaminase, which is expressed in a B cell differentiation stage-specific fashion. *AICDA* is involved in somatic hyper-mutation, gene conversion, and class-switch recombination of immunoglobulin genes [42]. Defects in *AICDA* can cause autosomal recessive hyper-IgM immunodeficiency syndrome type 2 (HIGM2) [43]. *CD19* is a B cell-specific molecule, which serves as a major costimulatory molecule for amplifying B cell receptor (BCR) responses. Morbach H et al. have revealed that *CD19* is required for TLR9-induced B cell activation and CD19/PI3K/AKT/BTK is an essential axis integrating BCRs and TLR9 signaling in human B cells [44]. In addition, biallelic *CD19* gene mutations cause common variable immunodeficiency in human. BCR-induced B cell responses are impaired in most patients with common variable immunodeficiency. *TNFRSF13C* (tumor necrosis factor receptor superfamily member 13C) encodes a receptor for BAFF (B cell activating factor), which enhances B cell survival in vitro and regulates the peripheral B cell population. *TNFRSF13C* is a principal receptor required for BAFF-mediated mature B cell survival and it has been reported to be associated with common variable immunodeficiency [45]. In our study, significantly decreased expression levels of *CD79A*, *AICDA*, *CD19*, and *TNFRSF13C* have been observed in the BALF of the severe MPP group comparing to the mild MPP group. Comparing to the local reduction of *CD79A*, *AICDA*, *CD19*, and *TNFRSF13C* genes found in BALF, these patient's immunoglobulins and lymphocyte profiles in the peripheral blood are normal, which means they do not have any systemic immunodeficiency disease [see Additional file 2: Fig. S1, Additional file 3: Table S2]. We have found these local changes related to primary immunodeficiency in the bronchoalveolar of severe MPP. Local B cell-related immunodeficiency may be involved in the pathogenesis of severe MPP comparing with mild MPP. Figure 3 shows how these molecules are involved in the pathway of B cell differentiation and immunoglobulin gene class switch; down-regulation of these molecules may restrain antibody production and make the MPP children lose the ability to eradicate MP from the lung, which leads to happen of severe MPP [7].

Alternative splicing events of genes are involved in the diversity of proteome as well as genome evolution, control of developmental processes, and physiological regulation of various biological systems [46]. It could be deduced that dysregulation of alternative splicing event is often linked to various human diseases [47]. However, alternative splicing events in the context of MPP have rarely been investigated. The current study discovered significant differential alternative splicing events in *FCER2* and *FCRLA* which could be an explanation for the differential expression of these two genes between severe MPP and mild MPP. The alternative splicing type of *FCER2* is retained intron (RI), which can change the function and expression levels of a gene [48]. Therefore, lower rate of RI in the severe MPP group comparing to the mild MPP group may partly explain the significantly increased expression levels of *FCER2* in the severe MPP group. *FCRLA* is a soluble resident endoplasmic reticulum protein. It is capable of associating with multiple Ig isotypes including IgM, IgG, and IgA, which makes it unique among the large family of Fc receptors. The expression of *FCRLA* is restricted to B lineage and is most abundant in germinal center B lymphocytes [49]. In the present study, the alternative splicing type of *FCRLA* is MEX, which is significantly increased in the severe MPP group comparing to the mild MPP group. According to the literatures [50, 51], alternative splicing may be a causal explanation for the down-regulation of *FCRLA* in the severe MPP group.

Previous studies have found that cell-mediated immune response, specifically Th1-type cytokines such as IL8, IL18, and IFNγ, plays important roles in the mechanism of MPP [9–11, 52]. Most of these studies observed serum levels of Th1 cytokines, but we have chosen BALF to study the local differentially expressed genes. Cytokines may be expressed differently in BALF comparing to that in the peripheral blood; this could partly explain why significant difference of IL8, IL18, and IFNγ was not found in the current study. Additionally, our transcriptome analysis focused on comparing severe MPP with mild MPP in order to study the specific pathogenesis of severe MPP; similar results have been reported by Kang YM et al. group [53]. In their study, higher levels of IFNγ in BALF of MPP patients comparing with that of control children were discovered, but no significant difference of IFNγ was found between the severe MPP group and mild MPP group.

Some limitations of the current study should be discussed. First, this is a small size transcriptome analysis between mild MPP children and severe MPP children; bigger sized analysis would be preferred in future study to support solid conclusions. However, three samples in each group have been chosen carefully to receive next-generation sequencing separately; quality control analysis of the whole process has been greatly satisfied. Correlation matrix shows a high consistency of measurements within each group. Principal component analysis (PCA) shows good repeatability and correlation of these samples. Second, this is a preliminary study on the pathogenesis of severe MPP comparing to mild MPP. Further study will be needed to further prove the hypothesis that gene reduction related to primary immunodeficiency in bronchoalveolar is involved in the pathogenesis of severe MPP. Patient's primary cell culture and in vivo experiments using animal model may help to clarify how these genes and pathways are involved in the pathogenesis of severe MPP in the future.

Conclusions

The current study presented gene expression profiles as well as alternative splicing in BALF samples from MPP patients by next-generation RNA sequencing. This study clearly indicates that the up-regulation of *IL13*, *FCER2*, *FLT1*, and *CLEC5A* and the down-regulation of *CD79A*, *AICDA*, *CD19*, and *TNFRSF13C* may contribute to the pathogenesis of severe MPP or the progression from mild MPP to severe MPP. Furthermore, the differentially expression of *FCER2* and *FCRLA* may be due to the alternative splicing; further studies will be required to confirm this hypothesis.

Additional files

Additional file 1: Table S1. Summary of patients' information.

Additional file 2: Figure S1. The levels of immunoglobulins in the peripheral blood of MPP patients. A. The levels of IgG in each patients. Normal range of 5.09–14.17 g/L is shown as dotted lines. B. The levels of IgA in each patients. Normal range of 0.31–1.92 g/L is shown as dotted lines. C. The levels of IgM in each patient. Normal range of 0.98–2.56 g/L is shown as dotted lines.

Additional file 3: Table S2. Lymphocyte profiles in the peripheral blood of the MPP patients.

Additional file 4: Table S3. Nucleated cell count in the BALF of the MPP patients.

Additional file 5: Figure S2. Evaluation of each sample included in the current study. A. The correlation coefficient heat map. Correlation matrix shows a high consistency of measurements within each group. $R^2 \geq 0.8$ is needed for the up-coming analyzing. B. Principal component analysis (PCA) plot. PCA is conducted to evaluate the clustering nature of the samples. Each point represents one sample. The repeatability of the samples has been shown.

Additional file 6: Table S4. Protein functional classification in differentially expressed genes between severe MPP and mild MPP.

Additional file 7: Table S5. Summary of the differential expressed genes with skipped exon.

Additional file 8: Table S6. Summary of the differential expressed genes with retained intron.

Additional file 9: Table S7. Summary of the differential expressed genes with mutually exclusive exon.

Additional file 10: Table S8. Summary of the differential expressed genes with alternative 5' splice site.

Additional file 11: Table S9. Summary of the differential expressed genes with alternative 3' splice site.

Abbreviations

AICDA: Activation-induced cytidine deaminase; BAFF: B cell activating factor; BAL: Bronchoalveolar lavage; BALF: Bronchoalveolar lavage fluid; BCR: B cell receptor; CAP: Community acquired pneumonia; CLEC5A: C-type lectin domain family 5, member A; COPD: Chronic obstructive pulmonary disease; CTL: C-type lectin; CTLD: C-type lectin-like domain; DNA: Deoxyribonucleic acid; ELISA: Enzyme-linked immunosorbent assay; FDR: False discovery rate; IgA: Immunoglobin A; IgG: Immunoglobin G; IgM: Immunoglobin M; IGV: Integrative Genomics Viewer; Igα: Immunoglobin α; KEGG: Kyoto Encyclopedia of Genes and Genomes; MEX: Mutual exclusive exon; MP: *Mycoplasma pneumoniae*; MPP: *Mycoplasma pneumoniae* pneumonia; PANTHER: Protein analysis through evolutionary relationships; PCR: Polymerase chain reaction; RA-SF: Rheumatoid arthritis synovium fluid; RI: Retained intron; RNA: Ribonucleic acid; Th2: T helper type 2; TNFRSF13C: Tumor necrosis factor receptor superfamily member 13C

Acknowledgements

The authors thank Dr. Aiping Wu from Suzhou Institute of Systems Medicine for the helpful discussions.

Funding

This work was supported by Starting Fund of the First Hospital, Jilin University (2011041).

Authors' contributions

KW collected the samples, performed the experiments, contributed to the interpretation of data, and made the figures and tables. MG determined the clinical status for the participation in the study, contributed to the interpretation of the data, and helped to draft the manuscript with the input from all authors. MY performed the statistical analysis, helped with the experiments, and made the tables. FM participated in the study design and coordination. DL, RL, YW, HZ, and ML provided the samples and collected the clinical information. GC participated in the study design and data analysis. XW designed the study, analyzed the data, finished the manuscript, and approved the final manuscript. All of the authors read and approved the manuscript.

Competing interests

The authors declare that they have no competing interests.

Consent for publication

Not applicable.

Author details

[1]Institute of Translational Medicine, the First Hospital of Jilin University, Changchun 130061, China. [2]Department of Pediatrics, the First Hospital of Jilin University, Changchun 130021, China. [3]Bethune Medical School of Jilin University, Changchun 130021, China. [4]Department of Microbiology, Immunology and Molecular Genetics, University of California Los Angeles, Los Angeles, CA 90095, USA.

References

1. Chaudhry R, Ghosh A, Chandolia A. Pathogenesis of Mycoplasma pneumoniae: an update. Indian J Med Microbiol. 2016;34(1):7–16.
2. Yan C, Sun H, Zhao H. Latest surveillance data on Mycoplasma pneumoniae infections in children, suggesting a new epidemic occurring in Beijing. J Clin Microbiol. 2016;54(5):1400–1.
3. Sawicki GS, Lu FL, Valim C, Cleveland RH, Colin AA. Necrotising pneumonia is an increasingly detected complication of pneumonia in children. Eur Respir J. 2008;31(6):1285–91.

4. Leonardi S, del Giudice MM, Spicuzza L, Saporito M, Nipitella G, La Rosa M. Lung abscess in a child with Mycoplasma pneumoniae infection. Eur J Pediatr. 2010;169(11):1413–5.
5. Hawkins S, Rausch CM, McCanta AC. Constrictive pericarditis secondary to infection with Mycoplasma pneumoniae. Curr Opin Pediatr. 2011;23(1):126–9.
6. Waites KB, Balish MF, Atkinson TP. New insights into the pathogenesis and detection of Mycoplasma pneumoniae infections. Future Microbiol. 2008;3(6):635–48.
7. Izumikawa K. Clinical features of severe or fatal Mycoplasma pneumoniae pneumonia. Front Microbiol. 2016;7:800.
8. Takeuchi O, Kawai T, Muhlradt PF, Morr M, Radolf JD, Zychlinsky A, Takeda K, Akira S. Discrimination of bacterial lipoproteins by Toll-like receptor 6. Int Immunol. 2001;13(7):933–40.
9. Tanaka H, Narita M, Teramoto S, Saikai T, Oashi K, Igarashi T, Abe S. Role of interleukin-18 and T-helper type 1 cytokines in the development of Mycoplasma pneumoniae pneumonia in adults. Chest. 2002;121(5):1493–7.
10. Zhang Y, Zhou Y, Li S, Yang D, Wu X, Chen Z. The clinical characteristics and predictors of refractory Mycoplasma pneumoniae pneumonia in children. PLoS One. 2016;11(5):e0156465.
11. Miyashita N, Kawai Y, Inamura N, Tanaka T, Akaike H, Teranishi H, Wakabayashi T, Nakano T, Ouchi K, Okimoto N. Setting a standard for the initiation of steroid therapy in refractory or severe Mycoplasma pneumoniae pneumonia in adolescents and adults. J Infect Chemother. 2015;21(3):153–60.
12. Wang Z, Gerstein M, Snyder M. RNA-Seq: a revolutionary tool for transcriptomics. Nat Rev Genet. 2009;10(1):57–63.
13. Garber M, Grabherr MG, Guttman M, Trapnell C. Computational methods for transcriptome annotation and quantification using RNA-seq. Nat Methods. 2011;8(6):469–77.
14. Ameratunga R, Woon ST, Gillis D, Koopmans W, Steele R. New diagnostic criteria for common variable immune deficiency (CVID), which may assist with decisions to treat with intravenous or subcutaneous immunoglobulin. Clin Exp Immunol. 2013;174(2):203–11.
15. Jiang YHZ. Zhu Futang's textbook of pediatrics. Beijing: People's Military Medical Publisher; 2003.
16. Qamar N, Fuleihan RL. The hyper IgM syndromes. Clinical reviews in allergy & immunology. 2014;46(2):120–30.
17. Chernick V, Kendig EL. Kendig's disorders of the respiratory tract in children. 7th ed. Philadelphia: Saunders/Elsevier; 2006.
18. Guo L, Liu F, Lu MP, Zheng Q, Chen ZM. Increased T cell activation in BALF from children with Mycoplasma pneumoniae pneumonia. Pediatr Pulmonol. 2015;50(8):814–9.
19. Anders S, Huber W. Differential expression analysis for sequence count data. Genome Biol. 2010;11(10):R106.
20. PANTHER classification system. http://pantherdb.org. Accessed 1 Nov 2016.
21. Shen S, Park JW, Huang J, Dittmar KA, Lu ZX, Zhou Q, Carstens RP, Xing Y. MATS: a Bayesian framework for flexible detection of differential alternative splicing from RNA-Seq data. Nucleic Acids Res. 2012;40(8), e61.
22. KEGG PATHWAY Database. http://www.genome.jp/kegg/pathway.html. Accessed 1 Jan 2017.
23. GeneCards. http://www.genecards.org/. Accessed 11 Nov 2016.
24. Wang ET, Sandberg R, Luo S, Khrebtukova I, Zhang L, Mayr C, Kingsmore SF, Schroth GP, Burge CB. Alternative isoform regulation in human tissue transcriptomes. Nature. 2008;456(7221):470–6.
25. Wills-Karp M, Luyimbazi J, Xu X, Schofield B, Neben TY, Karp CL, Donaldson DD. Interleukin-13: central mediator of allergic asthma. Science. 1998; 282(5397):2258–61.
26. Wu Q, Martin RJ, Lafasto S, Efaw BJ, Rino JG, Harbeck RJ, Chu HW. Toll-like receptor 2 down-regulation in established mouse allergic lungs contributes to decreased mycoplasma clearance. Am J Respir Crit Care Med. 2008; 177(7):720–9.
27. Hao Y, Kuang Z, Jing J, Miao J, Mei LY, Lee RJ, Kim S, Choe S, Krause DC, Lau GW. Mycoplasma pneumoniae modulates STAT3-STAT6/EGFR-FOXA2 signaling to induce overexpression of airway mucins. Infect Immun. 2014; 82(12):5246–55.
28. Sharma V, Michel S, Gaertner V, Franke A, Vogelberg C, von Berg A, Bufe A, Heinzmann A, Laub O, Rietschel E, et al. A role of FCER1A and FCER2 polymorphisms in IgE regulation. Allergy. 2014;69(2):231–6.
29. Tantisira KG, Silverman ES, Mariani TJ, Xu J, Richter BG, Klanderman BJ, Litonjua AA, Lazarus R, Rosenwasser LJ, Fuhlbrigge AL, et al. FCER2: a pharmacogenetic basis for severe exacerbations in children with asthma. J Allergy Clin Immunol. 2007;120(6):1285–91.
30. Ye Q, Xu XJ, Shao WX, Pan YX, Chen XJ. Mycoplasma pneumoniae infection in children is a risk factor for developing allergic diseases. Sci World J. 2014; 2014:986527.
31. Wu WK, Georgiadis A, Copland DA, Liyanage S, Luhmann UF, Robbie SJ, Liu J, Wu J, Bainbridge JW, Bates DO, et al. IL-4 regulates specific Arg-1(+) macrophage sFlt-1-mediated inhibition of angiogenesis. Am J Pathol. 2015; 185(8):2324–35.
32. Choi SH, Park EY, Jung HL, Shim JW, Kim DS, Park MS, Shim JY. Serum vascular endothelial growth factor in pediatric patients with community-acquired pneumonia and pleural effusion. J Korean Med Sci. 2006;21(4):608–13.
33. Shim JY, Park SW, Kim DS, Shim JW, Jung HL, Park MS. The effect of interleukin-4 and amphiregulin on the proliferation of human airway smooth muscle cells and cytokine release. J Korean Med Sci. 2008; 23(5):857–63.
34. Shin JE, Cheon BR, Shim JW, Kim DS, Jung HL, Park MS, Shim JY. Increased risk of refractory Mycoplasma pneumoniae pneumonia in children with atopic sensitization and asthma. Korean J Pediatr. 2014;57(6):271–7.
35. Tang LF, Shi YC, Xu YC, Wang CF, Yu ZS, Chen ZM. The change of asthma-associated immunological parameters in children with Mycoplasma pneumoniae infection. The Journal of asthma : official journal of the Association for the Care of Asthma. 2009;46(3):265–9.
36. Wortham BW, Eppert BL, Flury JL, Garcia SM, Donica WR, Osterburg A, Joyce-Shaikh B, Cua DJ, Borchers MT. Cutting edge: CLEC5A mediates macrophage function and chronic obstructive pulmonary disease pathologies. J Immunol. 2016;196(8):3227–31.
37. Muro S, Tabara Y, Matsumoto H, Setoh K, Kawaguchi T, Takahashi M, Ito I, Ito Y, Murase K, Terao C, et al. Relationship among chlamydia and Mycoplasma pneumoniae seropositivity, IKZF1 genotype and chronic obstructive pulmonary disease in a general Japanese population: the Nagahama study. Medicine (Baltimore). 2016;95(15), e3371.
38. Teng O, Chen ST, Hsu TL, Sia SF, Cole S, Valkenburg SA, Hsu TY, Zheng JT, Tu W, Bruzzone R et al. CLEC5A-mediated enhancement of the inflammatory response in myeloid cells contributes to influenza virus pathogenicity in vivo. J Virol. 2017;91(1):e01813-16.
39. Soler Palacios B, Estrada-Capetillo L, Izquierdo E, Criado G, Nieto C, Municio C, Gonzalez-Alvaro I, Sanchez-Mateos P, Pablos JL, Corbi AL, et al. Macrophages from the synovium of active rheumatoid arthritis exhibit an activin A-dependent pro-inflammatory profile. J Pathol. 2015;235(3):515–26.
40. Salilew-Wondim D, Ibrahim S, Gebremedhn S, Tesfaye D, Heppelmann M, Bollwein H, Pfarrer C, Tholen E, Neuhoff C, Schellander K, et al. Clinical and subclinical endometritis induced alterations in bovine endometrial transcriptome and miRNome profile. BMC Genomics. 2016;17:218.
41. Capello D, Gloghini A, Martini M, Spina M, Tirelli U, Bertoni F, Rinaldi A, Morra E, Rambaldi A, Sinigaglia F, et al. Mutations of CD79A, CD79B and EZH2 genes in immunodeficiency-related non-Hodgkin lymphomas. Br J Haematol. 2011;152(6):777–80.
42. Xu Z, Pone EJ, Al-Qahtani A, Park SR, Zan H, Casali P. Regulation of aicda expression and AID activity: relevance to somatic hypermutation and class switch DNA recombination. Crit Rev Immunol. 2007;27(4):367–97.
43. Trotta L, Hautala T, Hamalainen S, Syrjanen J, Viskari H, Almusa H, Lepisto M, Kaustio M, Porkka K, Palotie A, et al. Enrichment of rare variants in population isolates: single AICDA mutation responsible for hyper-IgM syndrome type 2 in Finland. Eur J Hum Genet. 2016;24(10):1473–8.
44. Morbach H, Schickel JN, Cunningham-Rundles C, Conley ME, Reisli I, Franco JL, Meffre E. CD19 controls Toll-like receptor 9 responses in human B cells. J Allergy Clin Immunol. 2016;137(3):889–98. e886.
45. Boqaert DJ, Dullaers M, Lambrecht BN, Vermaelen KY, De Baere E, Haerynck F. Gene associated with common variable immunodeficiency: one diagnosis to rule them all. J Med Genet. 2016;59:575–90.
46. Gamazon ER, Stranger BE. Genomics of alternative splicing: evolution, development and pathophysiology. Hum Genet. 2014;133(6):679–87.
47. Tazi J, Bakkour N, Stamm S. Alternative splicing and disease. Biochim Biophys Acta. 2009;1792(1):14–26.
48. Li Y, Bor YC, Fitzgerald MP, Lee KS, Rekosh D, Hammarskjold ML. An NXF1 mRNA with a retained intron is expressed in hippocampal and neocortical neurons and is translated into a protein that functions as an Nxf1 cofactor. Mol Biol Cell. 2016;27(24):3903–12.
49. Santiago T, Kulemzin SV, Reshetnikova ES, Chikaev NA, Volkova OY, Mechetina LV, Zhao M, Davis RS, Taranin AV, Najakshin AM, et al. FCRLA is a resident endoplasmic reticulum protein that associates with intracellular Igs, IgM, IgG and IgA. Int Immunol. 2011;23(1):43–53.

50. Kulemzin S, Chikaev N, Volkova O, Reshetnikova E, Taranin A, Najakshin A, Mechetina L. Characterization of human FCRLA isoforms. Immunol Lett. 2013;152(2):153–8.
51. Peng X, Li SS, Gilbert PB, Geraghty DE, Katze MG. FCGR2C polymorphisms associated with HIV-1 vaccine protection are linked to altered gene expression of Fc-gamma receptors in human B cells. PLoS One. 2016;11(3), e0152425.
52. Lee KE, Kim KW, Hong JY, Kim KE, Sohn MH. Modulation of IL-8 boosted by Mycoplasma pneumoniae lysate in human airway epithelial cells. J Clin Immunol. 2013;33(6):1117–25.
53. Kang YM, Ding MJ, Han YL, Wang SF, Ma X, Li H. Th1/Th2 immune response in bronchoalveolar lavage fluid in children with severe Mycoplasma pneumoniae pneumonia. Zhongguo Dang Dai Er Ke Za Zhi. 2011;13(3):188–90.

10

Variant effect prediction tools assessed using independent, functional assay-based datasets: implications for discovery and diagnostics

Khalid Mahmood, Chol-hee Jung, Gayle Philip, Peter Georgeson, Jessica Chung, Bernard J. Pope and Daniel J. Park*

Abstract

Background: Genetic variant effect prediction algorithms are used extensively in clinical genomics and research to determine the likely consequences of amino acid substitutions on protein function. It is vital that we better understand their accuracies and limitations because published performance metrics are confounded by serious problems of circularity and error propagation. Here, we derive three independent, functionally determined human mutation datasets, UniFun, BRCA1-DMS and TP53-TA, and employ them, alongside previously described datasets, to assess the pre-eminent variant effect prediction tools.

Results: Apparent accuracies of variant effect prediction tools were influenced significantly by the benchmarking dataset. Benchmarking with the assay-determined datasets UniFun and BRCA1-DMS yielded areas under the receiver operating characteristic curves in the modest ranges of 0.52 to 0.63 and 0.54 to 0.75, respectively, considerably lower than observed for other, potentially more conflicted datasets.

Conclusions: These results raise concerns about how such algorithms should be employed, particularly in a clinical setting. Contemporary variant effect prediction tools are unlikely to be as accurate at the general prediction of functional impacts on proteins as reported prior. Use of functional assay-based datasets that avoid prior dependencies promises to be valuable for the ongoing development and accurate benchmarking of such tools.

Keywords: Variant effect prediction, Functional datasets, Benchmarking, Mutation assessment, Pathogenicity prediction, Protein function, Functional assays, Genomic screening

Background

Screening the entire protein-coding compartment of the human genome yields thousands of protein amino acid substitutions per individual, the majority of which are present at low frequencies (minor allele frequency (MAF) <0.1%) within the population [1]. Genetic screens typically seek to classify variants and genes of relevance to given phenotypes, including disease states. To this end, it is desirable to know whether a given variant is likely to impact protein function, with the inference being that this might influence phenotypes of interest [2–5]. However, appropriate functional assays exist for only a minority of proteins, and in those cases where functional assays do exist, their associated resource requirements are often prohibitive to routine, large-scale application.

Widely used variant effect prediction methods include SIFT [6, 7], PolyPhen (v2) [8, 9], GERP++ [10, 11], Condel [12], CADD [13], fathmm [14], MutationTaster [15], MutationAssessor [16, 17], GESPA [18] and, more recently, REVEL [19]. These use information, variously, about local sequence phylogenetic conservation, amino acid physicochemical properties, functional domains and structural attributes (Table 1). Ensemble or consensus methods such as fathmm, Condel, CADD and REVEL integrate and weight predictions from collections of tools. Recent approaches to algorithm training have applied machine learning techniques. Training and validation (or 'benchmarking') of these algorithms

* Correspondence: djp@unimelb.edu.au
Melbourne Bioinformatics, The University of Melbourne, Melbourne, Australia

Table 1 Characteristics of the protein variant effect prediction tools assessed in this study. The table indicates their scoring ranges and thresholds, training data, summary information about features and, where applicable, machine learning method

Prediction tool	Score range	Deleterious score cutoff	Training data	Features	Machine learning method
GERP++	−12.0 to 6.17	>0.047	None	Infers conserved or constrained elements from 33 mammalian genomes	–
fitCons	0 to 1	>0.4	None	Functional genomics data mainly sourced from chromatin analysis, e.g. ChIP-seq, and evolutionary conservation data	–
SIFT	1 to 0	<0.05	None	Conservation data (MSA of homologous sequences) and transformed into normalised probability matrix	–
PolyPhen	0 to 1	>0.5	HumVar, HumDiv	Conservation data (MSA of homologous sequences), protein functional domain data and protein structural features	Naïve Bayes classifier
CADD	0 to 35 +	>15	Simulated, Swissvar, HumVar	Integrates several annotations into a single score, e.g. SIFT, GERP++, PolyPhen, CPG distance, GC content	SVM
Condel	0 to 1	>0.5		Builds a unified classification by integration output from a collection of tools, e.g. SIFT, PolyPhen	Weighted average normalised scores
REVEL	0 to 1	>0.5	HGMD, EPS	HGMD and rare EPS variants used for training	Random forest
fathmm	0 to 1	>0.45	HGMD, Swiss-Prot	Combines evolutionary conservation with disease-specific protein weights for intolerance to mutation	Hidden Markov models

has been conducted using datasets that list variants with assigned classifications. Commonly used datasets include HumDiv [20], HumVar [21], Humsavar [22], EPS [23], dbSNP [24] and HGMD [25].

All of the above algorithms have reported potential merit and are widely used in practice. The original publication of REVEL, for example, reported that when this tool was tested against a set of variants from Clinvar, the resulting area under the receiver operating characteristic curve was an impressive 0.96. However, fundamental problems exist with the manner of the training and benchmarking for this and prior tools, centred primarily on the independence and truthfulness of reference sets. Indeed, the authors of REVEL acknowledged that these issues placed potential limitations on their study.

Grimm et al. [20] described the issue of data circularity and its effect on the assessment of prediction algorithms, explaining the importance of the choice and composition of variant datasets used for training and validation. Type 1 circularity results from substantial overlap between training and testing datasets, leading to artificially inflated apparent accuracy in contexts where variants or genes are well represented in training data and to deflated apparent accuracy in settings where they are poorly represented. Type 2 circularity results from all variants in featured genes having been labelled predominantly as either deleterious or benign. Grimm et al. postulated a third type of circularity. In this case, prediction tools contribute to new variant classifications, which, in turn, are used in further benchmarking. Variant classifications within training and benchmarking datasets have been guided substantially by computational predictions, resulting in imperfect 'truth sets'. Disease risk inflation has been observed in the Clinvar and HumVar databases, whereby considerably fewer individuals in the general population are afflicted with given diseases than would be expected based on pathogenicity classifications within these clinical databases [1]. Ideally, mutation effect prediction training data for supervised machine learning methods should have good coverage of the protein landscape and mutation categorisation that is based on strong evidence from protein functional studies [26]. Miosge et al. [27] reported that of all the amino acid-substituting mutations predicted by PolyPhen to be deleterious to the mouse form of the key tumour suppressor, TP53, 42% had no assay-detectable functional consequence. Similarly, 45% of CADD-predicted deleterious mutations conferred no assay-detectable impact on protein function.

In this study, we conduct benchmarking of eight computational variant impact prediction methods. In addition to assessing their performance using commonly used benchmarking variant datasets, we have derived three independent, functional assay-determined datasets that we have called UniFun (UniProt-derived, functionally characterised, based on UniProt mutagenesis data), BRCA1-DMS (based on deep mutational scanning of BRCA1) and TP53-TA (TP53 mutational scanning via transactivation assay). Our findings have important implications with regard to our confidence in variant classifications derived from computational prediction methods and to how we should train and benchmark such methods in the future.

Results

In order to limit problems of circularity and systematic error, we derived three human protein mutation datasets that strive for independence from training data and are characterised by direct functional assays: UniFun, BRCA1-DMS and TP53-TA. UniFun represents 11,519 mutations from UniProt for which categorical assignments of protein functional consequence have been made based on direct assays ('Datasets and methods'). The UniFun variants were sourced from 2209 proteins and exhibit minimal overlap with variants featured in prior disease catalogue datasets (Fig. 1). UniFun is composed of a relatively high percentage of proteins that contribute both deleterious and benign mutations (Additional file 1: Figure S1). BRCA1-DMS (BRCA1 deep mutational scanning) was generated from measured efficiencies of BRCA1 mutants in activities required for efficient homology-directed DNA repair (HDR) and tumour suppression [28]. TP53-TA (TP53 transactivation assay) comprises variants in human TP53 classified by transactivation assay [29] ('Datasets and methods') (Table 2).

Employing the independent, 'functional' datasets UniFun, BRCA1-DMS and TP53-TA alongside four prior datasets, we conducted benchmarking of eight prominent variant effect prediction systems (Fig. 2 and Table 3). For all methods, the choice of benchmarking data influenced measured prediction accuracy markedly. When UniFun was employed across tools, the apparent prediction accuracies were consistently among the lowest two measures when compared to measures derived for all the datasets. BRCA1-DMS also tended to yield relatively low apparent prediction accuracies, although the apparent accuracies for Condel, REVEL and fathmm were somewhat elevated when benchmarked using BRCA1-DMS compared with UniFun (see Fig. 3). Compared with UniFun, the BRCA1-DMS and TP53-TA datasets yielded more variable apparent predictive accuracies, with apparent accuracies tending higher for TP53-TA. The apparent prediction accuracies for UniFun, BRCA1-DMS and TP53-TA were in the ranges 0.52 to 0.63, 0.54 to 0.75 and 0.53 to 0.91, respectively. To highlight the strength of influence that the benchmarking dataset choice can have, the apparent accuracy of REVEL, for example, dropped from AUC = 0.945 to AUC = 0.629 when assessment was conducted using UniFun instead of ClinvarHC. For a majority of tools, there was a general grouping of relatively high measured accuracy for the ClinvarHC, Humsavar and TP53-TA datasets. fathmm exhibited its highest apparent accuracy when benchmarked against Varibench (AUC = 0.936), consistent with the observations of [20], and appeared to perform relatively poorly when benchmarked using any of our functional datasets. Remarkably, when benchmarking was conducted using the most extensive and independent of our functional datasets, UniFun, SIFT achieved the highest measured accuracy score of any method tested, at a level comparable with recent machine learning-based methods.

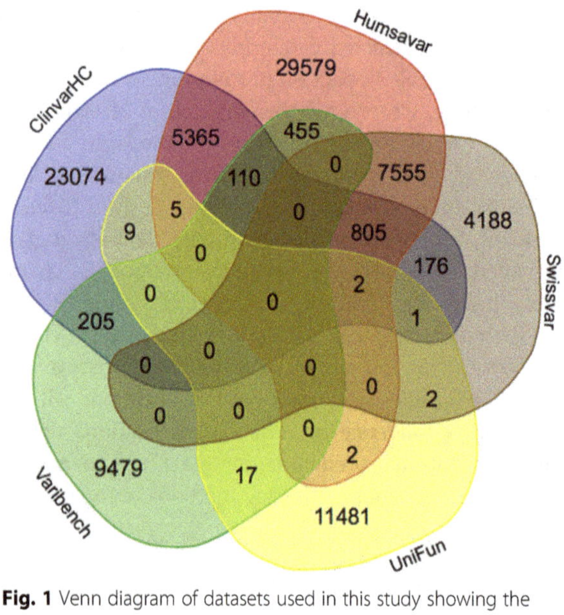

Fig. 1 Venn diagram of datasets used in this study showing the overlaps among the deleterious and benign variants observed in these datasets. Humsavar displays a relatively high degree of overlap with the ClinvarHC and Swissvar datasets. The remaining datasets overlap to relatively small extents

Table 2 Composition of the variant reference datasets used in this study. This table separates mutation catalogues into those derived from clinical databases (disease mutation catalogues) and those derived directly from functional assays (functional mutation catalogues). The table provides summary information for the numbers of proteins and variants of different classifications that have contributed to each dataset. See Additional file 1: Figure S1 and Table S1 for more detailed information

	Total variants	Deleterious	Benign	Total proteins
Disease mutation catalogues				
ClinvarHC	29,752	19,461	10,291	2979
Humsavar	43,878	19,329	24,549	10,231
Swissvar	12,729	4526	8203	5036
Varibench	10,266	4309	5957	4203
Functional mutation catalogues				
TP53-TA	1886	582	1304	1
BRCA1-DMS	1683	408	1275	1
UniFun	11,519	9503	2016	2209

Discussion

We have generated three functional datasets that attempt to better represent the truth with regard to variant classifications, guided by direct in vitro functional assays. They are relatively unrelated to prior variant effect prediction tool training datasets. As such, they promise to be useful for tool benchmarking and training, along with similar, expanded datasets in the future. A potential confounder of our functional datasets (although the same applies to

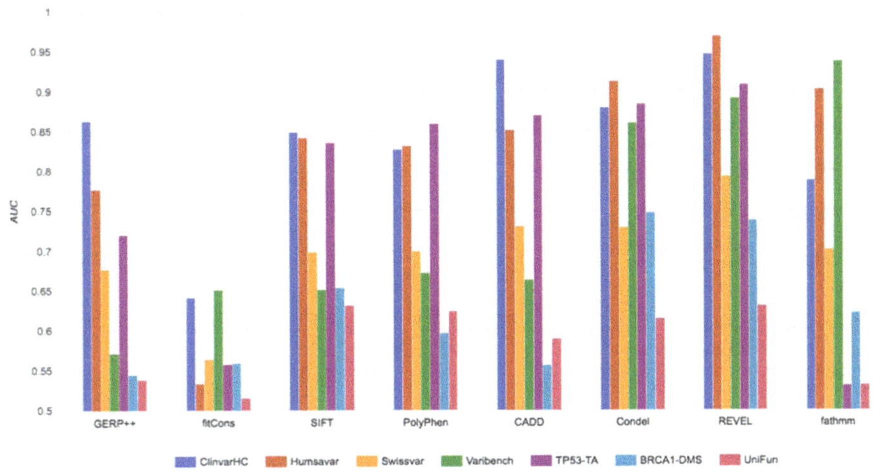

Fig. 2 Histogram depicting apparent accuracies of in silico variant effect predictors based on ROC curve AUCs for the benchmarking datasets used in this study

other datasets) is that we cannot be certain of our variant classifications—despite being guided by dedicated in vitro tests. Although our functional datasets include genetic variants that have not been observed in human populations to date, observations for established pathogenic mutations support their relevance to the disease setting. Starita et al. [28] showed that for ten known disease-causing missense mutations in BRCA1, all were found to be deleterious by functional assay. Since UniFun represents 2209 proteins, it includes a relatively broad sampling of the human protein landscape and should provide a good basis for general variant effect benchmarking, including for proteins that have not been studied in depth previously. The BRCA1-DMS and TP53-TA datasets focus on single proteins. As single-gene datasets, they do not necessarily offer good representation of the broader protein landscape. They are also likely to be confounded by type 1 circularity because BRCA1 and TP53 are relatively highly represented at the protein level, albeit via different collections of variants, in prior training datasets.

Our observations upon benchmarking a range of in silico variant effect prediction tools against different datasets appeared to broadly reflect the properties of the datasets and how the tools had been calibrated. The high variability of observed prediction accuracies (as measured by the AUC) of the various tools depending on the benchmarking dataset casts serious doubts over the interpretation of outputs from and utility of such tools. That the 'conservation-only' tools tended to yield relatively low measured prediction accuracies across datasets is likely due to their comparative naïvety. The low measured prediction accuracies observed when UniFun was used to benchmark machine learning-derived prediction tools are likely to have been influenced by avoidance of circularity problems. This is supported by similar AUC values having been observed by Grimm et al. when they applied their VariBenchSelected and SwissVarSelected

Table 3 Measured accuracies of eight in silico predictors as benchmarked against seven different variant reference datasets. Measured accuracies are calculated as the areas under the respective ROC curves (AUCs) and Matthews correlation coefficients (MCCs). See Additional file 1: Figure S4 for the ROC curve graphs

	ClinvarHC		Humsavar		Swissvar		Varibench		TP53-TA		BRCA1-DMS		UniFun	
	AUC	MCC	AUC	MCC	AUC	MCC	AUC	MCC	AUC	MCC	AUC	MCC	AUC	MCC
GERP++	0.863	0.587	0.777	0.469	0.677	0.286	0.571	0.15	0.719	0.283	0.544	0.069	0.538	0.04
fitCons	0.641	0.3	0.533	0.033	0.564	0.008	0.651	0.024	0.557	0	0.559	0	0.515	0.033
SIFT	0.848	0.489	0.841	0.543	0.698	0.289	0.651	0.228	0.835	0.484	0.653	0.199	0.631	0.184
PolyPhen	0.827	0.447	0.831	0.541	0.699	0.301	0.672	0.256	0.859	0.469	0.596	0.088	0.623	0.168
CADD	0.939	0.731	0.851	0.57	0.73	0.331	0.663	0.25	0.869	0.418	0.556	0.032	0.589	0.119
Condel	0.879	0.51	0.911	0.664	0.728	0.333	0.86	0.57	0.883	0.074	0.747	0.172	0.614	0.098
REVEL	0.945	0.68	0.968	0.83	0.792	0.462	0.89	0.59	0.907	0.465	0.737	0.088	0.63	0.148
fathmm	0.787	0.288	0.902	0.538	0.701	0.253	0.936	0.509	0.53	0	0.621	0	0.531	0.02

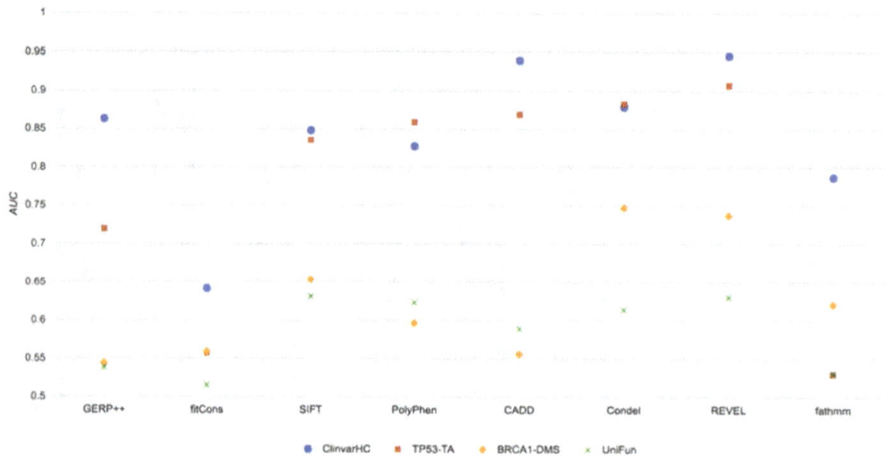

Fig. 3 Apparent prediction accuracies of variant effect prediction tools when assessed using ClinvarHC versus functional mutation derived datasets, reported as AUCs derived from ROC curves

datasets, engineered to avoid circularity, to the benchmarking of a variety of variant effect prediction tools.

The general grouping observed for the ClinvarHC, Humsavar and TP53-TA datasets with respect to apparent accuracies of variant effect prediction tools has likely been influenced by substantial protein representation overlaps between these datasets. Approximately 83% of ClinvarHC proteins overlap with Humsavar variant proteins, and TP53 mutations are represented strongly within each of these (Additional file 1: Table S2 and Figure S3). However, BRCA1 variants are even more strongly represented in ClinvarHC and Humsavar than those of TP53, without BRCA1-DMS displaying similar grouping. It is possible that TP53 behaves as a relatively highly representative protein for these datasets with respect to selected predictive features. We observe that a relatively high proportion of TP53 mutants in ClinvarHC and Humsavar are deleterious (Additional file 1: Figure S3). As inferred by Grimm et al., that fathmm's best apparent performance was observed when benchmarked using Varibench is likely due to type 2 circularity-associated inflation. Varibench contains mutations across 4203 genes, of which only 1.6% have mutations labelled as both benign and deleterious. That SIFT exhibited comparable apparent performance to more recent machine learning-based tools when tested against UniFun may be explained by their training datasets not being conducive to improved general protein effect prediction.

Important to the selection of datasets for training is the issue of whether a prediction tool aims to determine functional consequences generally or only in specific (e.g. particular disease-relevant protein set) contexts. The extent of functional damage conferred by a given variant is an important consideration, which may inform the clinical relevance and preferred classification. Future prediction tools will likely perform best when trained specifically for particular sets of proteins and mutation/variant classes, via multiple partitioned 'sub-tools'. Regardless, in vitro assay-informed datasets similar to UniFun promise to make important contributions by enabling high-confidence protein functional consequence classifications while allowing training and benchmarking independence.

Conclusions

Our findings, consistent with those of Grimm et al. [20], indicate that the accuracies of contemporary variant effect prediction tools are likely to be considerably lower than reported in their original method publications. This has profound implications for how we use such tools in clinical diagnostic and disease-gene discovery programs. Indeed, we should treat the predictions generated by such tools with considerable caution. We offer a new paradigm for benchmarking such tools that avoids many of the prior conflicts with the ideals of machine learning. Use of these, and expansion to similar independent, functionally determined mutation datasets as training and benchmarking datasets, will be extremely valuable to the progression of this field. Investigating the properties of incorrectly classified variants and using the findings to better inform algorithm design should result in improved prediction accuracy in the future.

Datasets and methods

We have employed seven benchmarking datasets (refer to Table 1) to assess the performance of eight amino acid mutation impact prediction methods: GERP++, fitCons, SIFT, PolyPhen, CADD, Condel, REVEL and fathmm. These datasets contain variants classified as *deleterious* (likely significant effect on protein function) or *benign* (unlikely significant effect on protein function). We have used a variety of datasets that can be broadly categorised into two classes: (1) variants sourced from disease variation catalogues and (2) variants sourced from molecular functional analysis experiments. Figure 1 depicts the overlaps between parent datasets used in this study.

Disease variant catalogues

Databases such as the Swiss-Prot/UniProt-based Humsavar and others, including OMIM [30] and HGMD [25], catalogue disease-associated mutations along with relevant evidence, mainly sourced from the literature. Benign mutations are catalogued via a combination of Swiss-Prot classifications and common alleles (MAF > 1%) from population-based variant databases such as dbSNP and 1000 Genomes.

Clinvar is a database to which contributors submit variants and their classifications along with accompanying evidence. Variously, classifications are based on evidence and assertion criteria such as the Emory Genetics Laboratory Classification Definitions and the InSiGHT Variant Interpretation Committee guidelines [31]. For the present study, we have further filtered Clinvar data to include only high-confidence, expert panel-verified variants with clinical significance scores of 2 (CLNSIG = 2), in the case of benign variants, and 5 (CLNSIG = 5), in the case of deleterious mutations. We term this dataset ClinvarHC (Clinvar high confidence). Mutations classified as likely benign, likely deleterious or of uncertain significance were excluded due to insufficient evidence supporting their influence on protein function and disease.

'Functional' mutation catalogues

As indicated previously, the disease mutation catalogues in common use for in silico prediction tool training and benchmarking suffer from circularity through a lack of independence on multiple levels [20]. To address this, we have identified that data relating to biochemical assays of protein function, without significant overlap with disease mutation catalogues, should be highly valuable for variant effect prediction tool assessment (and training). These reflect validated effects on protein function while achieving independence. Since highly curated and accessible databases with these properties are not available, we have engineered three such datasets, based on (1) mining functional mutagenesis data from UniProt, (2) the deep mutational scanning (DMS) protocol applied to *BRCA1* and (3) the assessment of TP53 mutants by transactivation assay.

UniFun dataset

UniFun is derived using protein annotation data from UniProt. In particular, we employed results from human protein mutagenesis experiments in which amino acids had been mutated prior to measuring their effects on protein function. We mined the UniProt data using keywords and the SPARQL querying framework to compose two sets of variants: (1) a 'functional' set containing amino acid mutations that disrupt protein function and (2) a 'non-functional' set of mutations that have no apparent effect on protein function. More details on how we generated this data are presented in Additional file 1: Figure S2.

BRCA1-DMS dataset

This relatively new protocol efficiently analyses the impacts of thousands of missense mutations on a protein's function [32]. Because of the relative recency of this approach, only one publicly available dataset could be sourced [28], derived from measurements of mutated BRCA1 ubiquitin ligase activity and binding to the BARD1 RING domain. Both functions are required for efficient homology-directed DNA repair (HDR) and tumour suppression. The HDR rescue score is used to measure disease risk and is derived from a functional assay to measure the ability of mutant BRCA1 to repair double-stranded DNA breaks. Starita et al. defined an HDR rescue score of 0.53 as the point of inflection between the classifications of deleterious (<0.53) and benign (≥0.53). The authors developed a support vector regression predictor based on both ubiquitin ligase activity and BARD1 RING domain binding to predict the HDR rescue scores for DMS data. In the present study, we employed the conservative approach of categorising variants as 'deleterious' if their associated HDR rescue scores were less than 0.33 (above which, no known pathogenic variant score was recorded) and 'benign' for HDR rescue scores above 0.77 (below which, the scores of no known benign variants were measured).

TP53-TA dataset

We sourced unique TP53 amino acid substitutions that had been deposited in the IARC TP53 database [33] (http://p53.iarc.fr) in accordance with the work of Kato et al. [29]. We defined the TP53-TA dataset to exclude variants exhibiting 'partial' reduction in transactivation and those variants that are present in the Clinvar and Humsavar databases.

Data processing

For consistency, Ensembl Variant Effect Predictor (VEP) [34] was employed to convert all variant datasets into variant call format (VCF), using their HGVS amino acid mutation notations as inputs. The resultant VCF files were then annotated using VEP and SnpEff [35]. Condel and fathmm scores were annotated using the VEP custom annotation tools based on precalculated scores available from FannsDB (http://bg.upf.edu/fannsdb). Similarly, GERP++ and fitCons conservation scores were annotated using custom BED files. CADD scores were annotated using CADD v1.2 (http://cadd.gs.washington.edu/download).

Assessing impact prediction

Prediction performances were evaluated using receiver operating characteristic curves (ROC curves) derived using ratios of true positive rates (TPR or sensitivity) and false positive rates (FPR or 1 – specificity), and the areas under the ROC curves (AUCs) were calculated. AUC values range between 0 and 1, inclusive, where 1 corresponds to a perfect classifier and 0.5 implies a random classification. The Matthews correlation coefficient (MCC) was calculated to measure classifier quality. A score of 1 implies perfect classification and 0 implies random classification.

Additional file

Additional file 1: Figure S1: Proportion of genes represented in both deleterious and benign variant sets for the respective datasets employed in this study. Figure S2: The UniFun variant dataset is derived from UniProt mutagenesis data (http://www.uniprot.org/help/mutagen). Figure S3: Proportion of deleterious variants for TP53, BRCA1 and the per protein mean in ClinvarHC, Humsavar, Swissvar, Varibench and UniFun variant datasets. Figure S4: ROC curves illustrating the measured performance of eight variant effect prediction methods, GERP++, fitCons, SIFT, PolyPhen, CADD, Condel, REVEL and fathmm, evaluated by seven reference variant datasets: (a) ClinvarHC, (b) Humsavar, (c) Swissvar, (d) Varibench, (e) TP53-TA, (f) BRCA1-DMS and (g) UniFun. Table S1: Protein distribution for deleterious and benign variant classifications across datasets. Table S2: Numbers of variants contributed to the ClinvarHC, Humsavar, Swissvar, Varibench and UniFun datasets by BRCA1 and TP53 and the mean per protein for (a) deleterious variants and (b) benign variants.

Abbreviations

AUC: Area under the curve; BED: Browser extensible data; BRCA1-DMS: BRCA1 deep mutational scanning; ClinvarHC: Clinvar high confidence; FPR: False positive rate; HDR: Homology-directed DNA repair; MAF: Minor allele frequency; MCC: Matthews correlation coefficient; OMIM: Online Mendelian Inheritance in Man; ROC: Receiver operating characteristic; SPARQL: SPARQL protocol and RDF query language; TP53-TA: TP53 transactivation assay; TPR: True positive rate; UniFun: UniProt-derived, functionally characterised; VCF: Variant call format

Acknowledgements

This work was supported by Melbourne Bioinformatics through Resource Allocation VR0002.

Funding

The authors are supported by Melbourne Bioinformatics (formerly the Victorian Life Sciences Computation Initiative).

Authors' contributions

KM, DJP and BJP conceived the study and contributed to the study design, analysis and manuscript preparation. C-hJ, GP, PG and JC contributed to the analyses and manuscript preparation. All authors read and approved the final manuscript.

Competing interests

The authors declare that they have no competing interests.

Consent for publication

Not applicable.

References

1. Lek M, Karczewski KJ, Minikel EV, Samocha KE, Banks E, Fennell T, et al. Analysis of protein-coding genetic variation in 60,706 humans. Nature. 2016;536:285–91.
2. Spurdle AB, Healey S, Devereau A, Hogervorst FBL, Monteiro ANA, Nathanson KL, et al. ENIGMA—evidence-based network for the interpretation of germline mutant alleles: an international initiative to evaluate risk and clinical significance associated with sequence variation in BRCA1 and BRCA2 genes. Hum Mutat. 2012;33:2–7.
3. Thompson BA, Spurdle AB, Plazzer J-P, Greenblatt MS, Akagi K, Al-Mulla F, et al. Application of a 5-tiered scheme for standardized classification of 2,360 unique mismatch repair gene variants in the InSiGHT locus-specific database. Nat Genet Nature Research. 2013;46:107–15.
4. Chandler MR, Bilgili EP, Merner ND. A review of whole-exome sequencing efforts toward hereditary breast cancer susceptibility gene discovery. Hum Mutat. 2016;37:835–46.
5. Sullivan PF, Daly MJ, O'Donovan M. Genetic architectures of psychiatric disorders: the emerging picture and its implications. Nat Rev Genet. 2012;13:537–51.
6. Kumar P, Henikoff S, Ng PC. Predicting the effects of coding non-synonymous variants on protein function using the SIFT algorithm. Nat Protoc. 2009;4:1073–81.
7. Ng PC, Henikoff S. Predicting deleterious amino acid substitutions. Genome Res. 2001;11:863–74.
8. Adzhubei IA, Schmidt S, Peshkin L, Ramensky VE, Gerasimova A, Bork P, et al. A method and server for predicting damaging missense mutations. Nat Methods Nature Publishing Group. 2010;7:248–9.
9. Adzhubei I, Jordan DM, Sunyaev SR. Predicting functional effect of human missense mutations using PolyPhen-2. Curr. Protoc. Hum. Genet. 2013;Chapter 7:Unit7.20.
10. Davydov EV, Goode DL, Sirota M, Cooper GM, Sidow A, Batzoglou S. Identifying a high fraction of the human genome to be under selective constraint using GERP++. PLoS Comput Biol. 2010;6, e1001025.
11. Cooper GM, Stone EA, Asimenos G, NISC Comparative Sequencing Program, Green ED, Batzoglou S, et al. Distribution and intensity of constraint in mammalian genomic sequence. Genome Res. 2005;15:901–13.
12. González-Pérez A, López-Bigas N. Improving the assessment of the outcome of nonsynonymous SNVs with a consensus deleteriousness score. Condel Am J Hum Genet. 2011;88:440–9.
13. Kircher M, Witten DM, Jain P, O'Roak BJ, Cooper GM, Shendure J. A general framework for estimating the relative pathogenicity of human genetic variants. Nat Genet. 2014;46:310–5.
14. Shihab HA, Gough J, Cooper DN, Stenson PD, Barker GLA, Edwards KJ, et al. Predicting the functional, molecular, and phenotypic consequences of amino acid substitutions using hidden Markov models. Hum Mutat. 2013; 34:57–65.
15. Schwarz JM, Rödelsperger C, Schuelke M, Seelow D. MutationTaster evaluates disease-causing potential of sequence alterations. Nat Methods Nature Research. 2010;7:575–6.
16. Reva B, Antipin Y, Sander C. Predicting the functional impact of protein mutations: application to cancer genomics. Nucleic Acids Res. 2011;39:e118.
17. Gnad F, Baucom A, Mukhyala K, Manning G, Zhang Z. Assessment of computational methods for predicting the effects of missense mutations in human cancers. BMC Genomics bmcgenomicsbiomedcentralcom. 2013;14 Suppl 3:S7.
18. Khurana JK, Reeder JE, Shrimpton AE, Thakar J. GESPA: classifying nsSNPs to predict disease association. BMC Bioinformatics. 2015;16:228.
19. Ioannidis NM, Rothstein JH, Pejaver V, Middha S, McDonnell SK, Baheti S, et al. REVEL: an ensemble method for predicting the pathogenicity of rare missense variants. Am J Hum Genet. 2016;99:877–85.
20. Grimm DG, Azencott C-A, Aicheler F, Gieraths U, MacArthur DG, Samocha KE, et al. The evaluation of tools used to predict the impact of missense variants is hindered by two types of circularity. Hum Mutat Wiley Online Library. 2015;36:513–23.
21. Capriotti E, Calabrese R, Casadio R. Predicting the insurgence of human genetic diseases associated to single point protein mutations with support vector machines and evolutionary information. Bioinformatics. 2006;22:2729–34.
22. Wu CH, Apweiler R, Bairoch A, Natale DA, Barker WC, Boeckmann B, et al. The Universal Protein Resource (UniProt): an expanding universe of protein information. Nucleic Acids Res. 2006;34:D187–91.

23. Exome Variant Server, NHLBI GO Exome Sequencing Project (ESP) [Internet]. Seattle, WA [cited 2016 Dec 22]. Available from: http://evs.gs.washington.edu/EVS/
24. Sherry ST, Ward M-H, Kholodov M, Baker J, Phan L, Smigielski EM, et al. dbSNP: the NCBI database of genetic variation. Nucleic Acids Res. 2001;29:308–11.
25. Stenson PD, Ball EV, Mort M, Phillips AD, Shiel JA, Thomas NST, et al. Human Gene Mutation Database (HGMD®): 2003 update. Hum Mutat Wiley Subscription Services, Inc, A Wiley Company. 2003;21:577–81.
26. Ionita-Laza I, McCallum K, Xu B, Buxbaum JD. A spectral approach integrating functional genomic annotations for coding and noncoding variants. Nat Genet. 2016;48:214–20.
27. Miosge LA, Field MA, Sontani Y, Cho V, Johnson S, Palkova A, et al. Comparison of predicted and actual consequences of missense mutations. Proc Natl Acad Sci. 2015;112:E5189–98.
28. Starita LM, Young DL, Islam M, Kitzman JO, Gullingsrud J, Hause RJ, et al. Massively parallel functional analysis of BRCA1 RING domain variants. Genetics Genetics Soc America. 2015;200:413–22.
29. Kato S, Han S-Y, Liu W, Otsuka K, Shibata H, Kanamaru R, et al. Understanding the function-structure and function-mutation relationships of p53 tumor suppressor protein by high-resolution missense mutation analysis. Proc Natl Acad Sci U S A. 2003;100:8424–9.
30. Hamosh A, Scott AF, Amberger J, Bocchini C, Valle D, McKusick VA. Online Mendelian Inheritance in Man (OMIM), a knowledgebase of human genes and genetic disorders. Nucleic Acids Res Oxford Univ Press. 2002;30:52–5.
31. Richards S, Aziz N, Bale S, Bick D, Das S, Gastier-Foster J, et al. Standards and guidelines for the interpretation of sequence variants: a joint consensus recommendation of the American College of Medical Genetics and Genomics and the Association for Molecular Pathology. Genet Med. 2015;17:405–24.
32. Fowler DM, Fields S. Deep mutational scanning: a new style of protein science. Nat Methods naturecom. 2014;11:801–7.
33. Bouaoun L, Sonkin D, Ardin M, Hollstein M, Byrnes G, Zavadil J, et al. TP53 variations in human cancers: new lessons from the IARC TP53 database and genomics data. Hum Mutat. 2016;37:865–76.
34. McLaren W, Gil L, Hunt SE, Riat HS, Ritchie GRS, Thormann A, et al. The Ensembl Variant Effect Predictor. Genome Biol. 2016;17:122.
35. Cingolani P, Platts A, Wang LL, Coon M, Nguyen T, Wang L, et al. A program for annotating and predicting the effects of single nucleotide polymorphisms, SnpEff: SNPs in the genome of Drosophila melanogaster strain w1118; iso-2; iso-3. Fly. 2012;6:80–92.

11

Mutational analysis of COL1A1 and COL1A2 genes among Estonian osteogenesis imperfecta patients

Lidiia Zhytnik[1*], Katre Maasalu[1,2], Ene Reimann[3,4], Ele Prans[4], Sulev Kõks[3,4] and Aare Märtson[1,2]

Abstract

Background: Osteogenesis imperfecta (OI) is a rare bone disorder. In 90% of cases, OI is caused by mutations in the *COL1A1/2* genes, which code procollagen α1 and α2 chains. The main aim of the current research was to identify the mutational spectrum of *COL1A1/2* genes in Estonian patients. The small population size of Estonia provides a unique chance to explore the collagen I mutational profile of 100% of OI families in the country.

Methods: We performed mutational analysis of peripheral blood gDNA of 30 unrelated Estonian OI patients using Sanger sequencing of *COL1A1* and *COL1A2* genes, including all intron-exon junctions and 5′UTR and 3′UTR regions, to identify causative OI mutations.

Results: We identified *COL1A1/2* mutations in 86.67% of patients (26/30). 76.92% of discovered mutations were located in the *COL1A1* (n = 20) and 23.08% in the *COL1A2* (n = 6) gene. Half of the *COL1A1/2* mutations appeared to be novel. The percentage of quantitative *COL1A1/2* mutations was 69.23%. Glycine substitution with serine was the most prevalent among missense mutations. All qualitative mutations were situated in the chain domain of pro-α1/2 chains.

Conclusion: Our study shows that among the Estonian OI population, the range of collagen I mutations is quite high, which agrees with other described OI cohorts of Northern Europe. The Estonian OI cohort differs due to the high number of quantitative variants and simple missense variants, which are mostly Gly to Ser substitutions and do not extend the chain domain of *COL1A1/2* products.

Keywords: Osteogenesis Imperfecta, Collagen I, *COL1A1*, *COL1A2*, Sanger sequencing

Background

Despite being a rare genetic bone fragility disorder, osteogenesis imperfecta (OI) is among the most widely occurring of rare congenital skeletal dysplasias [1]. OI prevalence is estimated 1/10,000–20,000 at birth [2, 3]. OI is characterized by low bone mineral density, recurrent fractures, skeletal deformations, and blue eye sclera [2, 4–6]. Other remarkable features of OI include Dentinogenesis Imperfecta, triangular face, hearing loss, joint laxity, short stature, and easy bruising [2, 4–6].

OI has many manifestations and is considered a group of disorders. Phenotypes range from mild osteopenia to severe deformities or even mortality. In 1979, Sillence described four OI types (I–IV) according to phenotype severity [5]. Recent updated classification distinguishes three additional types with specific histologies (V–VII) [4, 7]. Genetic OI classification considers every OI gene as a separate OI type and so far includes OI types I–XVII [4, 8, 9].

The genetics of the disorder reflect the complexity of the OI phenotype range. Up to 21 different genes have been associated with occurrence of OI [10–19]. Previous studies have shown that the primary cause of OI are mutations in the *COL1A1/2* genes, which code procollagen type I α1 and α2 chains, respectively [20]. Despite the approximately 1500 mutations already described in collagen type I genes, investigators continue to report novel mutations [21]. Moreover, there is still some

* Correspondence: Lidiia.Zhytnik@ut.ee
[1]Department of Traumatology and Orthopedics, University of Tartu, Puusepa 8, 51014 Tartu, Estonia
Full list of author information is available at the end of the article

controversy regarding the proportion of collagen mutations reported in different populations, which have ranged from 60 to 95% [9, 10]. In this context, we believe that population-based studies of OI genetics might broaden current knowledge of collagen I mutations and OI.

Due to Estonia's small population (1.3 million) and centered treatment, follow-up, and research of all OI patients at the OI Center of the Traumatology and Orthopedics Clinic, Tartu University (TU) Hospital, it was possible to perform analysis of *COL1A1/2* mutations among the whole Estonian OI population [22]. Herein, we describe for the first time the mutational spectrum of *COL1A1/2* genes among 30 unrelated OI patients, from 30 Estonian OI families, which we estimate to constitute ~ 100% of OI cases in Estonia.

Methods

Subjects

The patients included in the study are treated and followed-up by the OI Center of the Traumatology and Orthopedics Clinic, TU Hospital.

A total of 30 OI patients from 30 unrelated families were included in the study. Data regarding the OI types of the subjects were obtained from the medical records of TU Hospital [23]. All new OI cases across Estonia are registered by and treated at TU Hospital's OI Center. Thus, it can be estimated that as of May 2017, the current patient cohort represented ~ 100% of the Estonian OI population.

No patient came from a consanguineous family. Mutational analysis of the *COL1A1/2* genes was performed on a younger affected member of every OI family included in the study.

In accordance with the Declaration of Helsinki, all patients or their legal representatives signed an informed consent form prior to participation. The study was approved by the University of Tartu's Ethical Review Committee on Human Research (permit no. 221/M-34).

Genealogical description

Genealogical data of OI history in the family, consanguinity, and miscarriages was obtained from each patient or their representative. We constructed pedigree trees per kindred using the "Kinship2" package in R v3.3.2 [24].

Mutational analysis of the *COL1A1/2* genes

Genomic DNA (gDNA) was purified from 3 ml of ethylenediaminetetraacetic acid (EDTA) preserved whole blood samples—stored at −80 °C—using a Gentra Puregene Blood Kit (Quiagen, Germany) following the manufacturer's protocol.

PCR amplification and Sanger sequencing were performed as described previously [25]. Sequence products were analyzed using Applied Biosystems' Sequence Scanner v1.0 and Mutation Surveyor DNA Variant analysis software v5.0.1. (Softgenetics, USA) and aligned to the GenBank human reference genome sequences of *COL1A1* (gDNA NG_007400.1, complementary (cDNA) NM_000088.3), and *COL1A2* (gDNA NG_007405.1, cDNA NM_000089.3). Raw sequencing data are available from the authors upon request. We focused on non-synonymous and splice-site variants absent from the publicly available normal datasets (including dbSNP135 and the 1000 Genomes Project) [26, 27]. We used the PolyPhen-2, SIFT, and MutationTaster software tools to predict the functional effects and pathogenicity of mutations [28–30]. Variants absent from the osteogenesis imperfecta mutation database were considered novel (http://www.le.ac.uk/ge/collagen/) [21, 31].

All statistical analyses were carried out with R v3.3.2. software (R Team, Austria) [32]. To assess the distribution of *COL1A1/2* mutations and compare them to other studied OI populations, percentage differences were used.

Results

Mutational analysis of the *COL1A1/2* genes of Estonian OI patients highlighted OI causative mutations in 26 of 30 patients (86.67%) (Fig. 1a). The number of patients harboring *COL1A1* mutations was 20 (76.92%); *COL1A2* mutations were found in 6 patients (23.08%) (Fig. 1b). A list of the mutations and their characteristics can be found in Table 1.

The number of novel mutations was 13/26 (50%) (Table 1). Half of the *COL1A1* and *COL1A2* mutations appeared to be undescribed in the collagen type I mutation database. Patient EE26 had a heterozygous non-synonymous rs1800215 SNP (p.Ala1075Thr) in the *COL1A1* gene, which was described before as a benign variant (data not shown). [33]

Twenty-five mutations had an autosomal dominant inheritance pattern (Table 1). Of these, eight patients had no previous history of OI in the family. Thus, we assumed that their parents and relatives, who did not have any clinical features of OI, are not carriers of these mutations.

Patient EE07 had a recessive missense mutation. Mutational analysis showed that their parents are not carriers of the mutation, which confirmed the de novo nature of the mutation.

We found 12/26 mutations (46.15%) had altering splice sites, 10 and 2 in the *COL1A1* and *COL1A2* genes, respectively. One of the patients harbored a deletion capturing both coding and intronic sequence, in exon-intron 34 (EE30). Nonsense mutations were present in 6

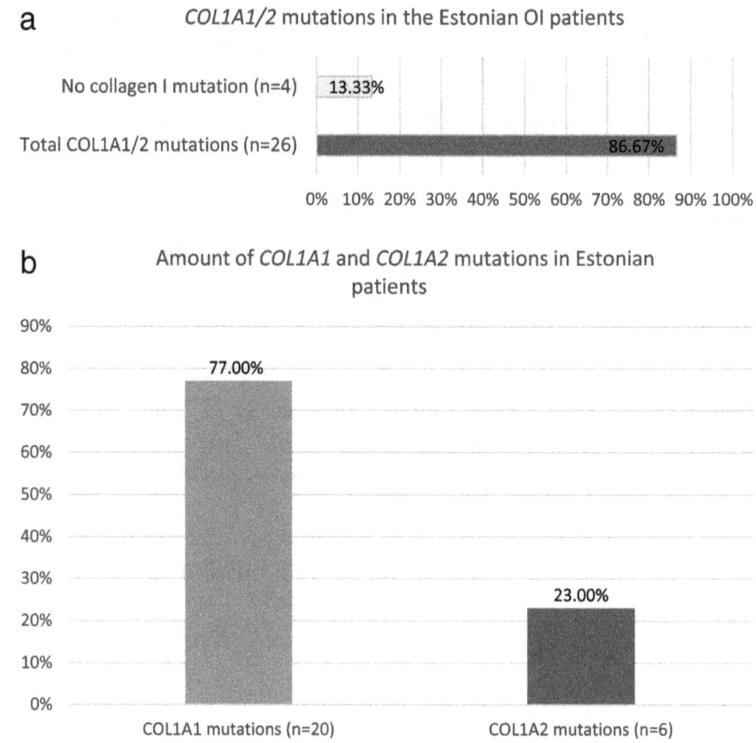

Fig. 1 Diagram of collagen type I mutation distribution Estonian OI patients. **a** Percentage of patients with *COL1A1/2* mutations vs patients negative for collagen I mutations. **b** Percentage of mutations in the *COL1A1* and *COL1A2* genes

patients (23.08%), all in the *COL1A1* gene. Overall, quantitative mutations were present in 18 patients (16 in *COL1A1* and 2 in *COL1A2* genes) (Fig. 2).

Missense mutations, associated with collagen I quality defects, were indicated in eight patients (30.77%), four in *COL1A1* and four in *COL1A2* genes. Of these, seven were Glycine substitutions (four of the *COL1A2* and three of the *COL1A1* missense mutations). In four cases, Glycine was substituted with Serine, two in the *COL1A1* and *COL1A2* genes, respectively (Fig. 2).

A c.3262G>T (*COL1A1*) mutation was detected in two patients (EE21 and EE22), who were thought to be unrelated (Table 1). Investigation of the pedigree trees revealed a distant relationship between the families four generations back, of which the patients were not aware. Two identical splice site mutations at c.1821 + 1G>A (*COL1A1*) in intron 26 were identified in patients EE02 (type III OI) and EE05 (type I OI) (Table 1). This mutation arose independently in the patients and caused phenotypes of different severity.

Discussion

Collagen I mutations were found in 26/30 (87%) studied OI patients. Previous findings have suggested collagen mutations ranging from 60 to 90% among different OI populations and study cohorts [25]. In a Finnish OI study, 90.7% of patients harbored collagen I mutations [34], which is higher than we found among Estonian OI patients. In Pollitt et al.'s study, collagen I mutations were revealed in 75% of OI patients [35], which is slightly lower than our Estonian cohort. Our data is in good agreement with research on the genetic epidemiology of the Swedish OI population, of which 87% had collagen I mutations [36]. The results of our study are also in concordance with Bardai et al.'s recent study of a large number (598) of OI individuals, where collagen type I mutations were found in 86% of OI patients of all types and different ethnic groups [19].

In some population studies, the amount of collagen I mutations were also lower. For example, in 51.4% of Taiwanese patients (N = 72), 52.2% of Korean patients (N = 67), and 59.4% of Vietnamese OI patients (N = 91) [25, 37, 38]. Due to the difficulties in arranging large cross-population studies of a rare disorder in populous countries, results can often be fragmented, which complicates population-wide estimates [39, 40]. However, questions about the lower collagen type I mutational pattern of OI patients from Asian populations remain.

The proportions of *COL1A1* and *COL1A2* in Estonian, Finnish, and Swedish OI populations were surprisingly similar, 77 and 23%, 78 and 22%, and 79 and 21%, respectively [34, 36]. Similar values were reported by Pollitt et al., where 77% of mutations occurred in the *COL1A1* and 23% in the *COL1A2* gene (N = 83) [35]. In

Table 1 Mutational spectrum of the *COL1A1* and the *COL1A2* genes among Estonian OI patients

No	Patient ID	Gene	Mutation	Exon	Mutation type	Protein alteration	Sillence OI type
1	EE01#	COL1A2	c.1630G>GT*	Exon 28	Missense	p.Gly544Cys	III
2	EE02	COL1A1	c.1821 + 1G>GA	Intron 26	Splice site	–	III
3	EE03	COL1A1	c.1897G>GT*	Exon 26	Nonsense	p.Glu633*	IV
4	EE04	COL1A1	c.750 + 2T>TA*	Intron 10	Splice site	–	IV
5	EE05	COL1A1	c.1821 + 1G>GA	Intron 26	Splice site	–	I
6	EE07#	COL1A1	c.2317G>T*	Exon 33_34	Missense	p.Gly773Cys	II
7	EE08	COL1A1	c.3217G>GA*	Exon 45	Missense	p.Gly1073Ser	III
8	EE09	COL1A1	c.1155 + 2T>TG*	Intron 17	Splice site	–	I
9	EE10	COL1A1	c.1128_hetdelT	Exon 17	Frameshift	p.Gly377Alafs*164	I
10	EE11#	COL1A1	c.3235G>GA	Exon 45	Missense	p.Gly1079Ser	I
11	EE13	COL1A1	c.2089C>CT	Exon 31	Nonsense	p.Arg697*	IV
12	EE14#	COL1A1	c.904-9G>GA	Intron 13	Splice site	–	I
13	EE15	COL1A2	c.1009G>GA	Exon 19	Missense	p.Gly337Ser	III
14	EE16#	COL1A2	c.2324G>GA	Exon 38	Missense	p.Gly775Glu	III
15	EE17#	COL1A1	c.3045 + 1G>GA	Intron 42	Splice site	–	IV
16	EE18	COL1A1	c.505G>GA*	Exon 6	Missense	p.Glu169Lys	I
17	EE19	COL1A1	c.299-1G>GC*	Intron 3	Splice site	–	IV
18	EE20	COL1A2	c.937-3C>CT	Intron 18	Splice site	–	I
19	EE21	COL1A1	c.3262G>GT*	Exon 46	Nonsense	p.Gly1088*	IV
20	EE22	COL1A1	c.3262G>GT*	Exon 46	Nonsense	p.Gly1088*	I
21	EE24	COL1A1	c.1767 + 5G>GA*	Intron 25	Splice site	–	IV
22	EE25	COL1A1	c.1354-2A>AG	Intron 20	Splice site	–	I
23	EE27#	COL1A1	c.3208-1G>GA*	Intron 44	Splice site	–	I
24	EE29#	COL1A2	c.865G>AG	Exon 17	Missense	p.Gly289Ser	III
25	EE30	COL1A2	c.2026-1_2031het dup*	Intron-Exon 34	Splice site, frameshift	–	III/IV
26	EE31#	COL1A1	c.1081C>CT	Exon 17	Nonsense	p.Arg361*	I

Patients with de novo mutations and without OI history in the family are marked with an octothorp (#). Novel mutations unreported in the collagen type I variant database (http://www.le.ac.uk/ge/collagen/) are marked with an asterisk (*). In cases of heterozygous mutation, both the wild type and the mutated allele are indicated after an arrow (>)

Bardai et al.'s 2016 study, 69% were *COL1A1* and 31% *COL1A2* mutations, which is similar to the beforementioned results [19].

The Estonian cohort also has a high proportion of quantitative mutations compared to qualitative collagen mutations, 69 and 31%, respectively. In the Finnish OI cohort, 67% of mutations were quantitative and 33% qualitative [34]. In the work of Pollitt et al., 35% of mutations were qualitative and 65% quantitative [35]. In the Swedish population, the proportions were almost equal (53 and 47%) [36]. Interestingly, we found only two quantitative mutations in the *COL1A2* gene, which matches previous reports about comparatively lower numbers of quantitative mutations of this gene [34–36]. Due to the higher number of mutations leading to haploinsufficiency in the *COL1A1* gene compared to the *COL1A2* gene, patients harboring mutations in the *COL1A1* gene had milder phenotypes (I, IV) compared to patients with *COL1A2* mutations (type III, except EE20 who had a splice site mutation and OI type I).

Glycine substitutions composed the vast majority of missense mutations (7 of 8 cases), with serine being the most substituted amino acid (4 of 7 cases), which supports previous findings. Curiously, all missense mutations were situated in triple helical chain domains (aa residues 162–1218 $\alpha1$; aa residues 80–1102 $\alpha2$) of *COL1A1/2* gene products. Only one mutation (patient EE07 with OI type II) altered the "lethal cluster" proposed by Marini et al. [41].

Half of the mutations (50%) we found appeared to be novel. Despite the numerous works on collagen I mutations and a growing list of identified mutations, the number of revealed novel variants was high, which underlines the individual nature of OI mutations [19, 35, 36]. Half of the glycine substitutions (4 of 7) were even absent from the collagen I mutational database.

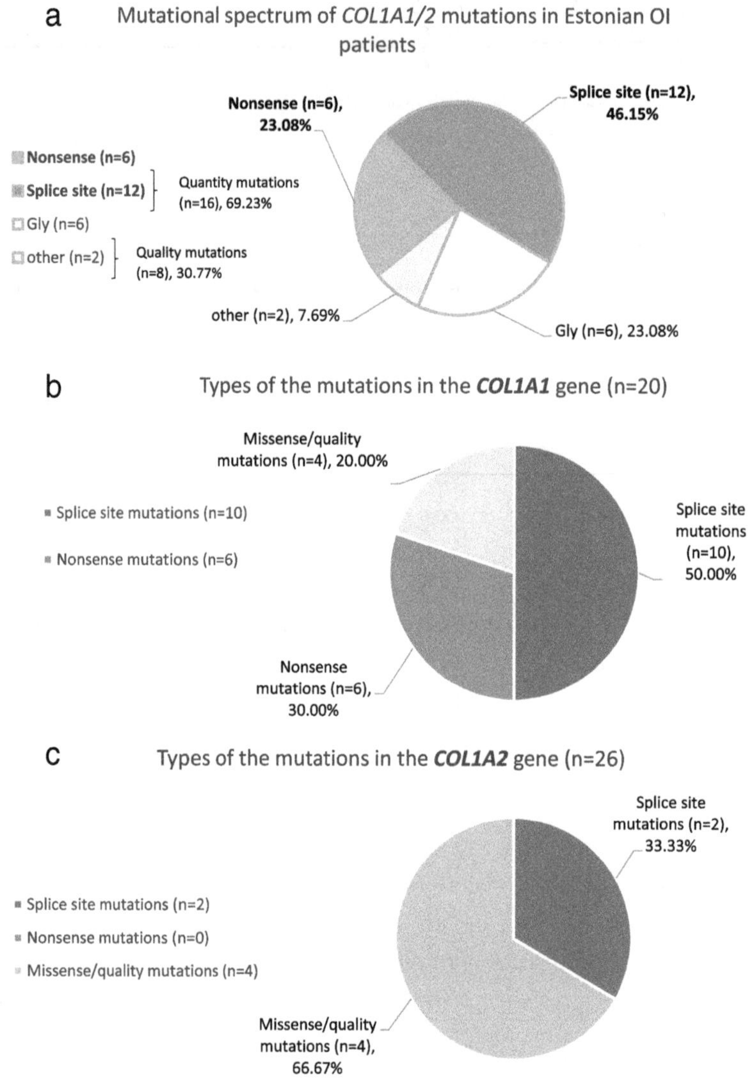

Fig. 2 a Mutational spectrum of *COL1A1/2* mutations in Estonian OI patients. Distribution of the *COL1A1* (**b**) and *COL1A2* (**c**) mutations according to mutation type

Despite sharing of the same mutation, patients may develop different phenotypes, as in the case of patients EE02 and EE05, who had type III and I OI, respectively. Genotype-phenotype correlations remain an unresolved issue in our understanding of OI. Cases of inter- and intra-familial OI diversity are not rare. Not only genetics, but additional factors, such as epigenetics and environment might contribute to the development of specific OI phenotypes. This leads to many questions and the need to further investigate potential OI factors.

Sanger sequencing is a powerful and accurate method of mutational analysis and allows the identification of frameshift, and missense and nonsense mutations in the coding regions of genes. Moreover, due to the special design of the primers distant from intron-exon junction regions, we could asses splice site mutations of the *COL1A1/2* genes, which are the cause of quantitative collagen defects. However, the current study had some limitations. We could not identify whole gene or exon deletions and duplications, which could have slightly reduced the number of discovered *COL1A1/2* mutations. In addition, due to the small population size of Estonia, our cohort was limited. We cannot exclude the possibility that the small sample size might be the cause of differences compared to the results of other studies.

Conclusion

This paper has described the mutational spectrum of *COL1A1/2* genes among 30 Estonian OI patients, which were estimated to represent ~ 100% of OI families in Estonia at the time. We identified collagen I mutations in 87% of Estonian OI families. The number of quantitative mutations (69%) was high compared to other European OI cohorts. All missense mutations of our Estonian patients altered the triple helical chain domain of α1 and α2 procollagen chains. One mutation was situated in the lethal cluster. A normal distribution of novel collagen mutations (50%) among the *COL1A1* (77%) and *COL1A2* (23%) genes, and mostly glycine substitutions were observed, compared to other OI cohorts of Northern Europe. Four patients that showed no collagen type I mutations will be further studied using whole exome sequencing analysis to identify disease causing variants.

Abbreviations

3'UTR: Three prime untranslated region; 5'UTR: Five prime untranslated region; cDNA: Complementary DNA; EDTA: Ethylenediaminetetraacetic acid; gDNA: Genomic DNA; OI: Osteogenesis Imperfecta; TU: University of Tartu

Acknowledgements

We would like to thank the following people and organizations for their help and support with data collection: workers of the Department of Traumatology and Orthopedics and Department of Pathophysiology, University of Tartu, and Ardo Birk and Madis Karu for the development of the online OI database of the Clinic of Traumatology and Orthopedics, TU Hospital.

Funding

This study was supported by the Estonian Science Agency project IUT20-46 (TARBS14046I), the European Regional Development Fund and the Archimedes Foundation to the Centre of Excellence on Translational Medicine, the University of Tartu's Development Fund, University of Tartu's Baseline Funding, and the HypOrth Project funded by the European Union's 7th Framework Programme grant agreement no. 602398.

Authors' contributions

LZ conceived the study, carried out the genetic studies, performed the data analysis, participated in the design of the study, and drafted the manuscript. EP, SK, and ER carried out the genetic studies, performed the data analysis, and helped to draft the manuscript. KM participated in the design of the study, interacted with the patients, coordinated the blood sample collection, and helped to draft the manuscript and perform analysis. SK and AM participated in the designing of the study, coordinated the data interpretation and statistical analysis, and helped to draft the manuscript. All authors read and approved the final manuscript.

Consent for publication

Not applicable.

Competing interests

The authors declare that they have no competing interests.

Author details

[1]Department of Traumatology and Orthopedics, University of Tartu, Puusepa 8, 51014 Tartu, Estonia. [2]Clinic of Traumatology and Orthopedics, Tartu University Hospital, Puusepa 8, 51014 Tartu, Estonia. [3]Centre of Translational Medicine, University of Tartu, Ravila 14a, 50411 Tartu, Estonia. [4]Department of Pathophysiology, University of Tartu, Ravila 19, 50411 Tartu, Estonia.

References

1. Martin E, Shapiro JR. Osteogenesis imperfecta: epidemiology and pathophysiology. Curr Osteoporos Rep. 2009;5(3):91–7. doi:10.1007/s11914-007-0023-z.
2. Byers PH, Steiner RD. Osteogenesis imperfecta. Annu Rev Med. 1992;43:269–82. doi:10.1146/annurev.me.43.020192.001413.
3. Martin E, Shapiro JR. Osteogenesis imperfecta: epidemiology and pathophysiology. Curr Osteoporos Rep. 2007;5(3):91–7. http://www.ncbi.nlm.nih.gov/pubmed/17925189. Accessed 5 Apr 2017
4. Van Dijk FS, Sillence DO. Osteogenesis imperfecta: clinical diagnosis, nomenclature and severity assessment. Am J Med Genet A. 2014;164A(6): 1470–81. doi:10.1002/ajmg.a.36545.
5. Sillence DO, Senn A, Danks DM. Genetic heterogeneity in osteogenesis imperfecta. J Med Genet. 1979;16(2):101–16. http://www.pubmedcentral.nih.gov/articlerender.fcgi?artid=1012733&tool=pmcentrez&rendertype=abstract. Accessed 18 Sept 2014
6. Ben Amor M, Rauch F, Monti E, Antoniazzi F. Osteogenesis imperfecta. Pediatr Endocrinol Rev. 2013;10(Suppl 2):397-405. http://www.ncbi.nlm.nih.gov/pubmed/23858623. Accessed 11 Dec 2014.
7. Fratzl-Zelman N, Misof BM, Roschger P, Klaushofer K. Classification of osteogenesis imperfecta. Wien Med Wochenschr. 2015;165(13-14):264–70. doi:10.1007/s10354-015-0368-3.
8. Home - OMIM - NCBI. http://www.ncbi.nlm.nih.gov/omim. Accessed 18 Feb 2015.
9. Shapiro JR. Clinical and genetic classification of osteogenesis imperfecta and epidemiology. In: Osteogenesis Imperfecta. Elsevier; 2014:15-22. doi:10.1016/B978-0-12-397165-4.00002-2.
10. Cho T-J, Lee K-E, Lee S-K, et al. A single recurrent mutation in the 5'-UTR of IFITM5 causes osteogenesis imperfecta type V. Am J Hum Genet. 2012;91(2): 343–8. doi:10.1016/j.ajhg.2012.06.005.
11. Semler O, Garbes L, Keupp K, et al. A mutation in the 5'-UTR of IFITM5 creates an in-frame start codon and causes autosomal-dominant osteogenesis imperfecta type V with hyperplastic callus. Am J Hum Genet. 2012;91(2):349–57. doi:10.1016/j.ajhg.2012.06.011.
12. Amor IM, Ben F, Rauch K, Gruenwald M, Weis DR, Eyre P. Roughley FH, Glorieux and RM. Severe osteogenesis imperfecta caused by a small in-frame deletion in CRTAP. Am J Med Genet A. 2011;42(11):157–62. doi:10.1002/ajmg.a.34269. Severe.
13. van Dijk FS, Zillikens MC, Micha D, et al. PLS3 mutations in X-linked osteoporosis with fractures. N Engl J Med. 2013;369(16):1529–36. doi:10.1056/NEJMoa1308223.
14. Becker J, Semler O, Gilissen C, et al. Exome sequencing identifies truncating mutations in human SERPINF1 in autosomal-recessive osteogenesis imperfecta. Am J Hum Genet. 2011;88(3):362–71. doi:10.1016/j.ajhg.2011.01.015.
15. Christiansen HE, Schwarze U, Pyott SM, et al. Homozygosity for a missense mutation in SERPINH1, which encodes the collagen chaperone protein HSP47, results in severe recessive osteogenesis imperfecta. Am J Hum Genet. 2010;86(3):389–98. doi:10.1016/j.ajhg.2010.01.034.
16. Willaert a, Malfait F, Symoens S, et al. Recessive osteogenesis imperfecta caused by LEPRE1 mutations: clinical documentation and identification of the splice form responsible for prolyl 3-hydroxylation. J Med Genet. 2009;46: 233–41. doi:10.1136/jmg.2008.062729
17. Marini JC, Reich A, Smith SM. Osteogenesis imperfecta due to mutations in non-collagenous genes: lessons in the biology of bone formation. Curr Opin Pediatr. 2014;26(4):500–7. doi:10.1097/MOP.0000000000000117.
18. Alanay Y, Avaygan H, Camacho N, et al. Mutations in the gene encoding the RER protein FKBP65 cause autosomal-recessive osteogenesis imperfecta. Am J Hum Genet. 2010;86(4):551–9. doi:10.1016/j.ajhg.2010.02.022.
19. Bardai G, Moffatt P, Glorieux FH, Rauch F. DNA sequence analysis in 598 individuals with a clinical diagnosis of osteogenesis imperfecta: diagnostic yield and mutation spectrum. Osteoporos Int. 2016;27(12):3607–13. doi:10.1007/s00198-016-3709-1.

20. van Dijk FS, Cobben JM, Kariminejad A, et al. Osteogenesis imperfecta: a review with clinical examples. Mol Syndromol. 2011;2(1):1–20. doi: 000332228.
21. Dalgleish R. The human collagen mutation database 1998. Nucleic Acids Res. 1998;26(1):253–5. http://www.ncbi.nlm.nih.gov/pubmed/9399846. Accessed 5 Apr 2017
22. Statistics Estonia. The population of Estonia increased last year—statistics Estonia. http://www.stat.ee/news-release-2017-008. Accessed 5 Apr 2017.
23. Maasalu K, Haviko T, Märtson A. Treatment of children with osteogenesis imperfecta in Estonia. Acta Paediatr. 2007;92(4):452–5. doi:10.1111/j.1651-2227.2003.tb00577.x.
24. Sinnwell JP, Therneau TM, Schaid DJ. The kinship2 R package for pedigree data. Hum Hered. 2014;78(2):91–3. doi:10.1159/000363105.
25. Ho Duy B, Zhytnik L, Maasalu K, et al. Mutation analysis of the COL1A1 and COL1A2 genes in Vietnamese patients with osteogenesis imperfecta. Hum Genomics. 2016;10(1):27. doi:10.1186/s40246-016-0083-1.
26. Home - SNP - NCBI. https://www.ncbi.nlm.nih.gov/snp. Accessed 11 Apr 2017.
27. Genomes | A deep catalog of human genetic variation. http://www.internationalgenome.org/. Accessed 11 Apr 2017.
28. Kumar P, Henikoff S, Ng PC. Predicting the effects of coding non-synonymous variants on protein function using the SIFT algorithm. Nat Protoc. 2009;4(7):1073–81. doi:10.1038/nprot.2009.86.
29. Adzhubei IA, Schmidt S, Peshkin L, et al. A method and server for predicting damaging missense mutations. Nat Methods. 2010;7(4):248–9. doi:10.1038/nmeth0410-248.
30. Schwarz JM, Rödelsperger C, Schuelke M, Seelow D. MutationTaster evaluates disease-causing potential of sequence alterations. Nat Methods. 2010;7(8):575–6. doi:10.1038/nmeth0810-575.
31. Dalgleish R. The human type I collagen mutation database. Nucleic Acids Res. 1997;25(1):181–7. http://www.ncbi.nlm.nih.gov/pubmed/9016532. Accessed 5 Apr 2017
32. Chen R, Mias GI, Li-Pook-Than J, et al. Personal omics profiling reveals dynamic molecular and medical phenotypes. Cell. 2012;148(6):1293–307. doi:10.1016/j.cell.2012.02.009.
33. Bodian DL, Chan T-F, Poon A, et al. Mutation and polymorphism spectrum in osteogenesis imperfecta type II: implications for genotype-phenotype relationships. Hum Mol Genet. 2009;18(3):463–71. doi:10.1093/hmg/ddn374.
34. Hartikka H, Kuurila K, Körkkö J, et al. Lack of correlation between the type of *COL1A1* or *COL1A2* mutation and hearing loss in osteogenesis imperfecta patients. Hum Mutat. 2004;24(2):147–54. doi:10.1002/humu.20071.
35. Pollitt R, McMahon R, Nunn J, et al. Mutation analysis of COL1A1 and COL1A2 in patients diagnosed with osteogenesis imperfecta type I–IV. Hum Mutat. 2006;27(7):716. doi:10.1002/humu.9430.
36. Lindahl K, Åström E, Rubin C-J, et al. Genetic epidemiology, prevalence, and genotype–phenotype correlations in the Swedish population with osteogenesis imperfecta. Eur J Hum Genet. 2015;23(8):1042–50. doi:10.1038/ejhg.2015.81.
37. Lin H-Y, Chuang C-K, Su Y-N, et al. Genotype and phenotype analysis of Taiwanese patients with osteogenesis imperfecta. Orphanet J Rare Dis. 2015;10:152. doi:10.1186/s13023-015-0370-2.
38. Lee K-S, Song H-R, Cho T-J, et al. Mutational spectrum of type I collagen genes in Korean patients with osteogenesis imperfecta. Hum Mutat. 2006;27(December 2005):599. doi:10.1002/humu.9423
39. Yang Z, Ke ZF, Zeng C, Wang Z, Shi HJ, Wang LT. Mutation characteristics in type I collagen genes in Chinese patients with osteogenesis imperfecta. Genet Mol Res. 2011;10(1):177–85. doi:10.4238/vol10-1gmr984.
40. Zhang Z-L, Zhang H, Ke Y, et al. The identification of novel mutations in COL1A1, COL1A2, and LEPRE1 genes in Chinese patients with osteogenesis imperfecta. J Bone Miner Metab. 2012;30(1):69–77. doi:10.1007/s00774-011-0284-6.
41. Marini JC, Forlino A, Cabral WA, et al. Consortium for osteogenesis imperfecta mutations in the helical domain of type I collagen: regions rich in lethal mutations align with collagen binding sites for integrins and proteoglycans. Hum Mutat. 2007;28(3):209–21. doi:10.1002/humu.20429.

12

Whole transcriptome analysis of human erythropoietic cells during ontogenesis suggests a role of VEGFA gene as modulator of fetal hemoglobin and pharmacogenomic biomarker of treatment response to hydroxyurea in β-type hemoglobinopathy patients

Vasiliki Chondrou[1], Petros Kolovos[2], Argyro Sgourou[3], Alexandra Kourakli[4], Alexia Pavlidaki[1,8], Vlasia Kastrinou[1], Anne John[5], Argiris Symeonidis[4], Bassam R. Ali[5,6], Adamantia Papachatzopoulou[7], Theodora Katsila[1] and George P. Patrinos[1,5,6*]

Abstract

Background: Human erythropoiesis is characterized by distinct gene expression profiles at various developmental stages. Previous studies suggest that fetal-to-adult hemoglobin switch is regulated by a complex mechanism, in which many key players still remain unknown. Here, we report our findings from whole transcriptome analysis of erythroid cells, isolated from erythroid tissues at various developmental stages in an effort to identify distinct molecular signatures of each erythroid tissue.

Results: From our in-depth data analysis, pathway analysis, and text mining, we opted to focus on the *VEGFA* gene, given its gene expression characteristics. Selected *VEGFA* genomic variants, identified through linkage disequilibrium analysis, were explored further for their association with elevated fetal hemoglobin levels in β-type hemoglobinopathy patients. Our downstream analysis of non-transfusion-dependent β-thalassemia patients, β-thalassemia major patients, compound heterozygous sickle cell disease/β-thalassemia patients receiving hydroxyurea as fetal hemoglobin augmentation treatment, and non-thalassemic individuals indicated that *VEGFA* genomic variants were associated with disease severity in β-thalassemia patients and hydroxyurea treatment efficacy in SCD/β-thalassemia compound heterozygous patients.

Conclusions: Our findings suggest that *VEGFA* may act as a modifier gene of human globin gene expression and, at the same time, serve as a genomic biomarker in β-type hemoglobinopathy disease severity and hydroxyurea treatment efficacy.

Keywords: *VEGFA*, Beta-thalassemia, Transcriptomics, Ontogenesis, Sickle cell disease, Erythroid cell differentiation, Pharmacogenomics, Biomarkers

* Correspondence: gpatrinos@upatras.gr
[1]Department of Pharmacy, School of Health Sciences, University of Patras, University Campus, Rion, GR-265 04 Patras, Greece
[5]Department of Pathology, College of Medicine & Health Sciences, United Arab Emirates University, Al-Ain, United Arab Emirates
Full list of author information is available at the end of the article

Introduction

Hemoglobin is the key tetramer oxygen transport protein of red blood cells, composed of two pairs of identical globin chains (namely, the α-like and β-like chains). Different types of hemoglobin molecules are produced during embryonic, fetal, and adult erythropoiesis at different hematopoietic sites (yolk sac, fetal liver, and bone marrow, respectively) [34]. The differentiation of erythroid progenitors into mature erythrocytes as well as human globin expression needs to be strictly regulated aiming to maintain sufficient oxygen levels in all tissues [11, 20]. There are two developmental switches that occur upon the switch from primitive to definitive hematopoiesis and during the perinatal period. In the latter case, human fetal globin genes (*HBG1* and *HBG2*) that are expressed at high levels during the fetal stage are gradually downregulated, whereas human adult (*HBB* and *HBD*) globin genes are reciprocally upregulated. As a result, fetal hemoglobin (HbF) is expressed at high levels during fetal development and gradually declines to reach less than 2–3% of total hemoglobin levels shortly after birth.

Hemoglobinopathies are the most common single gene disorders and at the same time, one of the most devastating health problems worldwide, as their clinical phenotypes vary from mostly asymptomatic to severe anemia. Hemoglobinopathies are caused by quantitative (α- or β-thalassemia) or qualitative (hemoglobin variants and sickle cell disease, SCD) defects in hemoglobin production [5, 12]. Today, the most common therapeutic interventions for β-type hemoglobinopathies include regular blood transfusions, bone marrow transplantation, and transient pharmacological reactivation of HbF to compensate for the absent or deficient expression of adult hemoglobin. Hydroxyurea or hydroxycarbamide (HU) is the only FDA-approved drug for the treatment of SCD and β-thalassemia patients that transiently increases/reactivates HbF production and hence, ameliorates disease severity. However, HU is less effective in β-thalassemia than in SCD patients, while there is extreme inter-individual variability among β-type hemoglobinopathy patients in response to HU treatment [3, 23].

HbF production as well as the developmental switch from fetal to adult hemoglobin are regulated by various transcription factors and have been the focus of intensive investigations, since our understanding of the molecular mechanisms involved in fetal-to-adult globin gene switching would provide useful insights for β-type hemoglobinopathy therapeutics [19]. It has been proposed that there is a complex interplay between cis-acting elements within the human β-globin gene cluster and transcription factors, such as *MYB*, *BCL11A*, *KLF1* [39, 41], and others, that affect the rate of β-like globin gene transcription. Also, previous studies suggest that genomic loci residing outside the human β-globin gene cluster act as modifier genes to HbF production and are associated with elevated HbF levels and, as such, variable disease severity in β-type hemoglobinopathy patients and HU treatment response rate in SCD/β-thalassemia compound heterozygous patients [18, 25].

We have previously shown that genomic variants in the *MAP3K5*, *KLF10*, *SIN3A*, *NOS1*, *ARG1*, and *ARG2* genes are associated with elevated HbF levels and, hence, milder disease severity in β-type hemoglobinopathy patients and HU treatment response rate in SCD/β-thalassemia compound heterozygous patients [4, 7, 17, 40]. Herein, we adopted a whole transcriptome analysis of erythroid cells derived from human hematopoietic tissues of various developmental stages to identify candidate genes that are differentially expressed at various developmental stages. Following our data analysis coupled to pathway and linkage disequilibrium analyses, we show that selected *VEGFA* genomic variants are associated with β-thalassemia disease severity and HU treatment efficacy in SCD/β-thalassemia compound heterozygous patients, suggesting that *VEGFA* may be considered as a modifier gene for HbF production.

Material and methods

Subjects

For the purpose of microarray-based whole transcriptome analysis, we isolated and cultured erythroid progenitor cells from human fetal liver (n = 4), umbilical cord blood (n = 5), and adult peripheral blood (n = 4) samples, all from unrelated individuals of Caucasian origin. Human umbilical cord blood and fetal liver samples were collected and processed as described previously [24, 43, 44].

For tagSNP genotyping, we exploited a separate set of individuals, namely β-thalassemia major patients, non-transfusion-dependent thalassemia (NTDT) patients, SCD/β-thalassemia compound heterozygous patients, and ethnically matched healthy (non-thalassemic) individuals. β-thalassemia major patients differ from their NTDT counterparts in terms of their clinical phenotype and disease severity. In particular, β-thalassemia major patients require lifelong regular transfusions to survive and avoid disease complications, while NTDT patients present mild anemia (hemoglobin levels ranging from 7.7 to 11.2 g/dl) and need less frequent or no blood transfusions. The clinical phenotype of the NTDT patients included in this study cannot be attributed to α-globin gene variants (α-thalassemia) or hereditary persistence of fetal hemoglobin (HPFH syndrome). SCD/β-thalassemia compound heterozygous patients were systematically administered HU and characterized as "HU-responders" (plateau HbF levels above 20%) or "HU non-responders" (plateau HbF levels below 20%), based on their HbF expression levels following drug administration. All molecular, hematological, and clinical data of patient cohorts have been described in our previously published work [7, 15, 17, 32, 33, 40]. All tagSNP genotyping samples are of Hellenic origin, collected at the Patras University Hospital (Patras, Greece), AHEPA University Hospital (Thessaloniki, Greece), and Ippokrateio General Hospital of Thessaloniki (Thessaloniki, Greece).

Whole transcriptome analysis

Microarray-based whole transcriptome analysis was performed as described previously [4]. In brief, erythroid progenitor cells from fetal liver, umbilical cord blood, and adult peripheral blood samples were isolated and cultured ex vivo. Total RNA was extracted, labeled, and hybridized to the Affymetrix Human Genome Array v2.0 according to manufacturer's instructions (Affymetrix Inc., Santa Carla, CA, USA). Differential expression specifics were set by AltAnalyse. Probe sets were characterized and selected as significant, when their p value was < 0.05. Cluster 3.0 was used for data clustering of the short-listed probe sets [9] and JavaTree View Version 1.1.6r2 for data visualization [35]. A fold-change > 2 (FC > 2) is indicative of gene upregulation, whereas a fold-change < 2 (FC <2) corresponds to gene downregulation.

TagSNP selection and linkage disequilibrium analysis

TagSNP selection across the *VEGFA* gene was carried out by the tagSNP picker program via the International HapMap Project (HapMap data release 27, phase II + III, February 2009, on NCBI36 assembly) and the LD TAG SNP Selection (tagSNP) (National Institute of Environmental Health Sciences) web-based tool. A tagged pairwise method was used with an R-square cutoff value of 0.8 and minor allele frequency (MAF) cutoff value of 0.2 [42, 45]. Pairwise linkage disequilibrium (LD) calculations were based on phase genotyped data (SNAP v2.2) [22], utilizing the HapMap Phase II+III (release 28) [2] and the 1000 Genomes Project (http://www.1000genomes.org) dataset for Caucasians (CEU). Findings were visualized on HaploView 4.2 and by using the LDmatrix module on LDlink web tool [26].

Genotype analysis

Genomic DNA was extracted from whole blood leukocytes collected from healthy individuals and patients using the QIAamp Blood Kit (Qiagen GmbH, Hilden, Germany). Polymerase chain reaction (PCR) was carried out according to the KAPA2G Fast Hot Start protocol (KAPA Biosystems, MA, USA). A detailed description per tagSNP amplification conditions is available upon request. PCR products were purified with NucleoSpin Gel and PCR clean-up kit (Macherey-Nagel, GmbH, Düren, Germany) and subjected to direct DNA sequence analysis on an ABI Prim 3130xl DNA Analyser (Applied Biosystems) using the Big Dye® Terminator v3.1 Cycle Sequencing Kit (Applied Biosystems, CA, USA), according to the manufacturer's instructions.

In silico analyses

Pathway analysis was performed with STRING software v9.1 (http://string-db.org). An emphasis was given to text mining and predicted interactions, both direct (physical) and indirect (functional). Venn diagrams were drawn with VENNY v2.1 (http://bioinfogp.cnb.csic.es/tools/venny/index.html). Gene ontology (GO) term analysis was performed with PANTHER classification system. Molecular function and biological process subcategories were subsequently identified [27]. For our downstream analysis, and to further investigate the role of the *VEGFA* tagSNPs in HU-mediated HbF production, we explored their effect on splicing motifs (including the "accept" and "donor" splice sites), the branch point and auxiliary sequences that enhance (exonic splicing enhancers, ESE) or repress (exonic splicing silencers, ESS) splicing. For this, in silico prediction took place, using Human Splicing Finder (http://www.umd.be/HSF3). This is a system that has quickly become an international reference, as it combines 12 algorithms [10].

Statistical analysis

Hardy-Weinberg equilibrium was explored by Pearson's goodness-of-fit chi-square (degree of freedom = 1), log-likelihood ratio chi-square (degree of freedom = 1), and exact test. De Finetti diagrams were also constructed [37]. Genotype and allele frequencies were evaluated using Fisher's exact test. A two-tailed p value of < 0.05 was considered statistically significant. The R project for statistical computing (R i386 3.2.1) was used.

Results

Transcription profiling of human hematopoietic tissues during ontogenesis

Whole transcriptome analysis was performed to explore the transcription profiles of human hematopoietic tissues at different stages of ontogenesis. A unique molecular signature was obtained, consisting of genes that were differentially expressed among tissues that express (fetal liver, umbilical cord blood) HbF, do not express HbF, or marginally express (adult peripheral blood) HbF. Our comparative analysis includes three different datasets: (i) adult peripheral blood (low HbF) versus umbilical cord blood (high HbF), (ii) adult peripheral blood (low HbF) versus fetal liver (high HbF), and (iii) adult peripheral blood (low HbF) versus umbilical cord blood and fetal liver (high HbF).

When the first comparison was considered, a total of 165 probe sets representing 133 unique genes were differentially expressed (Additional file 1: Figure S1), while the second comparison revealed 1239 probe sets corresponding to 898 unique genes being differentially expressed (Additional file 1: Figure S2). When comparing all tissues (fetal liver and umbilical cord blood) that express high HbF levels versus peripheral blood that does not produce HbF, our analysis revealed 348 probe sets, corresponding to 264 unique genes that were differentially expressed among those tissues (Fig. 1). Data analysis revealed a candidate gene signature of erythropoiesis during human ontogenesis. Next, we focused on the comparison of the gene signature profile of those hematopoietic tissues, being most ontogenically distant, and thus, adult peripheral blood was compared to fetal liver (dataset ii) and/or adult peripheral blood was compared to umbilical cord blood and fetal liver (dataset iii). As indicated in Fig. 2 and Additional file 1: Tables S1 and S2, 103 genes were upregulated and 50 genes were downregulated, when datasets (ii) and (iii) were considered. Data were filtered on the basis of current publicly available literature and experimental evidence regarding gene-to-phenotype associations with β-hemoglobinopathies. We have subsequently performed GO term analysis. Pathway analysis and text mining were carried out for the genes included in the most dominant classifications of the GO term analysis. *VEGFA* was most prevalent in "Binding" (GO: 0005488), "Cellular process" (GO: 0009987), "Developmental process" (GO: 0002376) and "Response to stimulus" (GO: 0050896).

VEGFA was found to be upregulated (FC > 2) in adult peripheral blood (low HbF levels), when compared to umbilical cord blood and fetal liver (high HbF levels). *VEGFA* upregulation was even more profound, when adult peripheral blood was solely compared to fetal liver.

TagSNPs across the *VEGFA* gene are associated with high HbF levels

Three tagSNPs (rs3024997, rs2146323, and rs10434) across the *VEGFA* gene were selected with MAF > 0.2% (CEU population) and explored further for their association with disease severity, attributed to high HbF levels. rs3024997 (G>A) and rs2146323 (C>A) are localized within intron 2, while rs10434 (A>G) within the 3′-untranslated region (3′-UTR) of the *VEGFA* gene. Genotyping data of β-type hemoglobinopathy patients and healthy (non-thalassemic) individuals of Hellenic origin are summarized in Table 1 and Additional file 1: Tables S3 and S4. A strong association for rs3024997 (G > A) with disease severity became evident, when NTDT patients (mild disease phenotype) and β-thalassemia major patients (severe disease phenotype) were compared (p = 0.003), and the same was true when NTDT patients versus non-thalassemic individuals (p = 0.005) were considered. Since

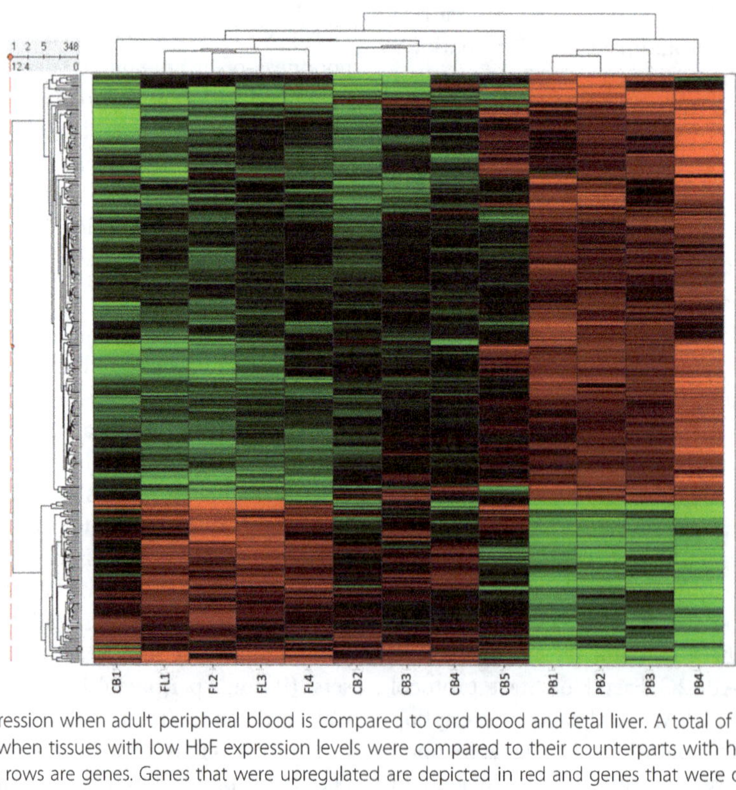

Fig. 1 Differential gene expression when adult peripheral blood is compared to cord blood and fetal liver. A total of 264 genes were up- (FC > 2) or downregulated (FC < 2), when tissues with low HbF expression levels were compared to their counterparts with high HbF expression levels. Columns represent samples; rows are genes. Genes that were upregulated are depicted in red and genes that were downregulated are depicted in green

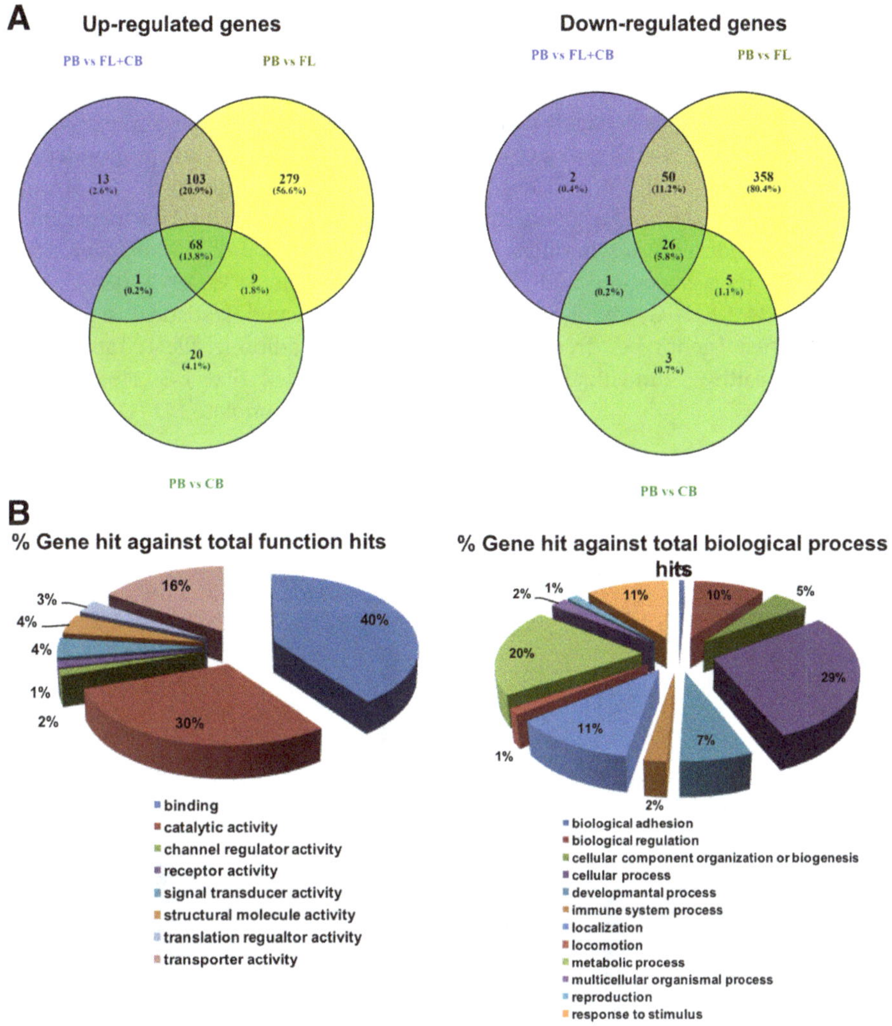

Fig. 2 Common and unique up- and downregulated genes during ontogenesis. **a** The number in each circle represents the number of differentially expressed genes among the groups in question. Common and unique genes are shown. **b** PANTHER analysis outcomes (GO; molecular function and biological process)

Table 1 Summary of our genotype analysis of β-type hemoglobinopathy patients of Hellenic origin and healthy (non-thalassemic) individuals

Study population	Genotype frequency (%)								
	rs3024997 (G>A)			rs2146323 (C>A)			rs10434 (A>G)		
	G/G	A/A	G/A	C/C	A/A	C/A	A/A	G/G	A/G
Healthy individuals	34	21	45	60	9	31	18	31	51
β-thalassemia major patients	26	16	58	51	3	46	21	33	46
NTDT patients	47	6	47	33	11	56	21	29	50
HU responders	26	16	58	43	10	48	26	26	48
HU non-responders	35	12	53	63	17	20	25	29	46

The number of individuals per group (n) is indicated in parentheses per tagSNP: rs3024997 healthy individuals (n = 112), NTDT patients (n = 17), β-thalassemia major patients (n = 112), HU responders (n = 19), HU non-responders (n = 26); rs2146323 healthy individuals (n = 115), NTDT patients (n = 18), β-thalassemia major patients (n = 114), HU responders (n = 21), HU non-responders (n = 30); rs10434 healthy individuals (n = 72), NTDT patients (n = 14), β-thalassemia major patients (n = 105), HU responders (n = 19), HU non-responders (n = 28)

HU hydroxyurea, *NTDT* non-transfusion-dependent thalassemia the homozygous genotype for the rare allele (A) is less frequently found in NTDT patients, the presence of the A allele could be correlated with low HbF levels (Fig. 3a). rs2146323 (C > A) correlates well with disease severity and HbF levels, when (i) NTDT patients versus β-thalassemia major patients (p = 0.009), (ii) NTDT patients versus non-thalassemic individuals (p = 0.0005), and (iii) β-thalassemia major patients (p = 0.03) versus non-thalassemic individuals were considered. Our findings for the rare allele (A) suggest its association with high HbF levels (Fig. 3b). rs10434 (A > G) did not reach statistical significance, when genotype frequencies among patients and healthy individuals were compared.

TagSNPs across the *VEGFA* gene are associated with HU treatment efficacy in SCD/beta-thalassemia compound heterozygous patients

To explore if the selected tagSNPs across the *VEGFA* gene could serve as pharmacogenomic biomarkers, HU-responder and non-responder SCD/β-thalassemia patients were genotyped. A strong association for rs2146323 (C>A) with HU treatment efficacy (elevation of HbF levels) became evident (p = 0.0002), while neither of the rs3024997 (G>A) and rs10434 (A>G) tagSNPs reached statistical significance. As shown in Fig. 4 and Additional file 1: Table S4, pairwise LD calculations revealed that rs3024997 (G>A) and rs2146323 (C>A) are in complete LD (D′ = 1; $R^2 < 1$).

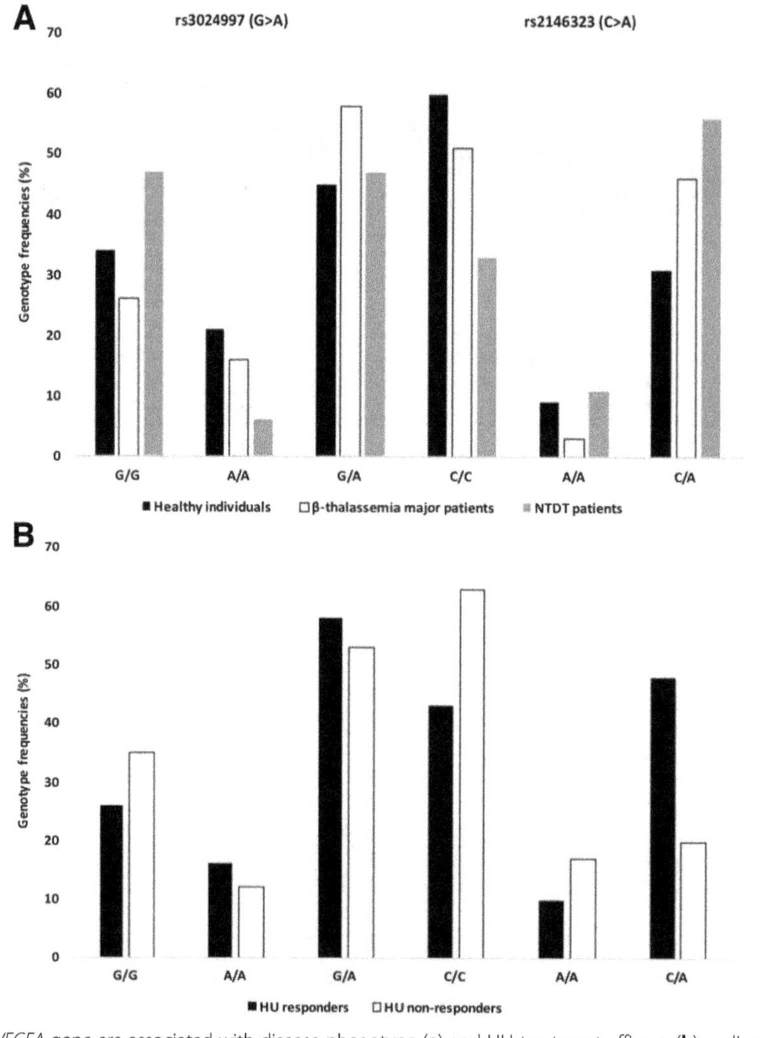

Fig. 3 TagSNPs across the *VEGFA* gene are associated with disease phenotype (**a**) and HU treatment efficacy (**b**). **a** disease phenotype, rs3024997 (G>A; healthy individuals vs. NTDT patients p = 0.005; β-thalassemia major patients vs. NTDT patients p = 0.003) and rs2146323 (C>A; healthy individuals vs. β-thalassemia major patients p = 0.03; healthy individuals vs. NTDT patients p = 0.0005; β-thalassemia major patients vs. NTDT patients p = 0.009). **b** HU treatment efficacy, rs2146323 (C>A; HU responders vs. HU non-responders p = 0.0002). HU: hydroxyurea

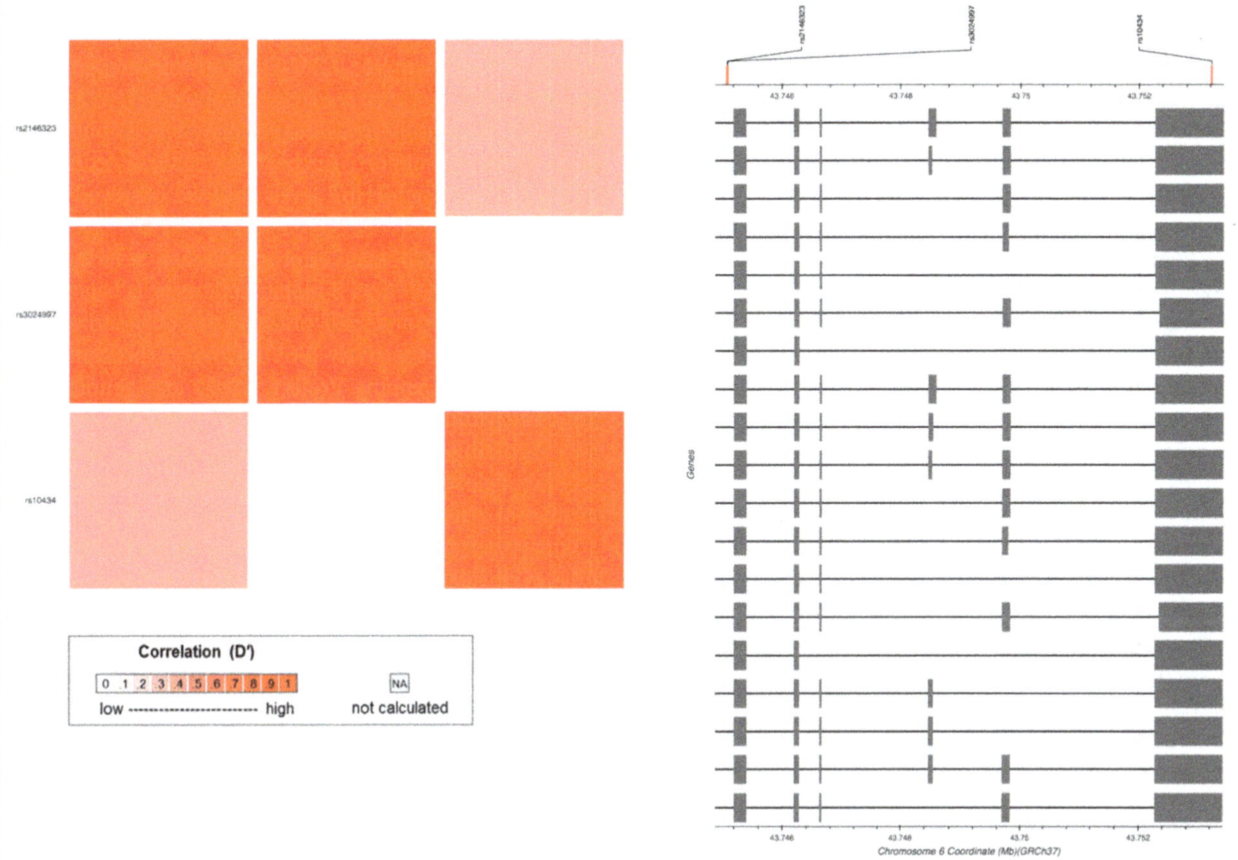

Fig. 4 Pairwise linkage disequilibrium (LD) calculations for the tagSNPs of interest across the *VEGFA* gene (CEU). LD is measured as D′ and R^2 (see also Additional file 1: Table S2)

In silico analyses

According to the Human Splicing Finder prediction algorithm, rs3024997 (G>A) was found to occur in a deep intronic position, resulting on the activation of an intronic cryptic acceptor site and thus, potential alteration of splicing. Yet, the RESCUE ESE, EIEs, PESE Octamers, ESE Finder-SRp40, and ESR Sequences prediction algorithms suggest the creation of an exonic splicing enhancer, probably, with no impact on splicing (Fig. 5). rs2146323 (C>A) causes no significant splicing motif alteration, suggesting that the other co-inherited variants are possibly the key in its association with high HbF levels.

Discussion

In humans, erythropoiesis as well as globin gene expression occurs at different sites during the various developmental

Predicted signal	Prediction algorithm	cDNA Position	Interpretation
New Acceptor Site	1 - HSF Matrices	cttgcctgattcagaagctccaaagagt (390 395 400 405 410 415)	Activation of an intronic cryptic acceptor site. Potential alteration of splicing.
New ESE Site	1 - RESCUE ESE Hexamers 2 - EIEs from Zhang et al. 3 - PESE Octamers from Zhang & Chasin 4 - ESE-Finder - SRp40 5 - ESR Sequences from Goren et al.	cctgattcggaagctccaaa (395 400 405 410)	Creation of an intronic ESE site. Probably no impact on splicing.

Fig. 5 In silico analysis of the role of rs3024997 on splicing. For rs3024997 (G > A), the Human Splicing Finder prediction algorithm supports the activation of an intronic cryptic acceptor site and thus, potential alteration of splicing. Yet, the RESCUE ESE, EIEs, PESE Octamers, ESE Finder-SRp40, and ESR Sequences prediction algorithms suggest the creation of an exonic splicing enhancer, probably, with no impact on splicing. The graphic representation of the region confirms individual outcomes per algorithm considered, each one corresponding at a different color and length. For more information on the data, please visit http://www.umd.be/HSF3/technicaltips.html

stages in a time-specific manner (tissue- and development-specific expression). Hemoglobin switch consists of two separate events; the first event occurs early in endometrial life (embryonic to fetal hemoglobin switch), whereas the second one begins a few weeks before birth and ends ~ 6 months after delivery (fetal-to-adult hemoglobin switch). The understanding of the molecular mechanisms that govern hemoglobin switch holds a great promise for curing β-type hemoglobinopathies [34].

We have previously demonstrated that several genes, residing outside the human β-globin gene cluster, can be held responsible as genes modifying HbF levels in β-type hemoglobinopathy patients, reflecting on the disease severity and HU treatment response [4, 7, 18, 40]. Herein, we adopted a whole transcriptome analysis on tissues that express high and low HbF levels in an effort to identify a unique molecular signature corresponding to high HbF levels.

Following whole transcriptome and pathway analysis, coupled to text mining, we focused on the *VEGFA* gene since it shows a consistent gene expression pattern in most comparisons. We employed linkage disequilibrium analysis to select *VEGFA* genomic variants to further explore their association with elevated HbF levels in β-type hemoglobinopathy patients. In humans, *VEGFA* (belongs to the family of vascular endothelial growth factors, VEGFs) is localized on chromosome 6p21.1 (14 kb), consisting of 8 exons and 7 introns [21]. Studies in knockout mice indicate the role of *VEGFA* in the development of the vascular and hematopoietic tissues. Casella et al. [6] found that *VEGFA* production is crucial for the survival and differentiation of adult hematopoietic stem cells (HSCs), while *VEGFA* has been also shown to participate in hematopoiesis by an internal autocrine loop mechanism and be associated with adult *HBB* gene expression [13, 14]. Nakayama et al. [31] have shown that *VEGFA* synergizes with BMP-4 on the development of hematopoietic cells [31]. The same authors reported that murine embryonic stem cells were white, when grown only in the presence of BMP-4, becoming red, after the addition of *VEGFA* (and stem cell factor (SCF)). A few years later, Adelman et al. [1] showed that the BMP/BMPR/Smad pathway induces the expression of KLF1 and GATA-1 transcription factors during the differentiation of embryonic bodies in mice, yet β-globin expression is only detected, when SCF and *VEGFA* were present [1].

Consistent with this work, our previous findings indicate that at the late stages of human ontogenesis, where HbF levels are low, *VEGFA* mRNA levels are high. In particular, *VEGFA* is upregulated in cultured erythroid progenitor cells derived from adult peripheral blood (low HbF expression levels), when compared to progenitors derived from fetal liver or umbilical cord blood and fetal liver. Furthermore, *VEGFA* is downregulated in erythroblasts, when compared to early (BFU-Es) or late (CFU-Es) erythroid progenitors in hematopoietic tissues expressing high levels of HbF (umbilical cord blood and fetal liver, Kolovos P, unpublished). Such findings support further the inverse correlation between *VEGFA* and HbF levels that we observed during ontogenesis.

High HbF levels may improve disease severity in β-thalassemia and SCD, as β-globin deficiency is balanced by γ-globin synthesis and HbF prevents the polymerization of hemoglobin S, respectively [36]. Following the completion of the Human Genome Project, family and genome-wide association studies reported several SNPs that are associated with high HbF levels or a high proportion of F cells in β-type hemoglobinopathy patients, revealing a relatively large number of genetic modifiers of HbF expression [18, 19].

Today, although several compounds that transiently induce HbF levels (5-azacitidine, dexitabine) have been studied, HU is the only FDA-approved sickle cell disease and β-thalassemia treatment. HU is a cytotoxic antineoplastic agent that was initially administered to patients with myelodysplastic diseases and immune deficiencies as it is an inhibitor of ribonucleotide reductase, an enzyme necessary for DNA synthesis and repair. The drug mechanism towards the induction of HbF is not fully known. In β-thalassemia patients, HU administration leads to a 2- to a ~ 9-fold increase in γ-globin mRNA levels [30]. Inter-individual variability remains an issue and several studies concur that genomic variants residing in genes not only within, but also outside the human β-globin gene cluster, correlate with disease severity and HU treatment efficacy [18, 25].

Interestingly, our whole transcriptome analysis revealed that among those genes with a similar, to *VEGFA*, expression profile, there are genes previously described to be correlated with differentially produced HbF levels and with response to HU treatment in β-type hemoglobinopathy patients [7, 16, 25].

Following our whole transcriptome analysis, we focused on *VEGFA* gene variants and genotyped non--transfusion-dependent β-thalassemia patients, β-thalassemia major patients, and healthy (non-thalassemic) individuals as well as a cohort of compound heterozygous SCD/β-thalassemia patients receiving HU as HbF augmenting therapy. rs3024997 (G>A) was found to be strongly associated with low HbF levels and the severe phenotype of β-thalassemia major. A strong association was also observed between rs2146323 (C>A) and high HbF levels in NTDT patients and hence, a milder clinical phenotype of the disease. rs2146323 (C>A) may also serve as a pharmacogenomic biomarker for HU treatment efficacy. rs10434 (A>G) did not reach statistical significance. Small sample size remains a major limitation in all studies focusing on HU treatment individualization, including ours, especially for NTDT patients, due to the scarcity of such patients. Herein, Fisher's exact test was chosen as the most appropriate test to guarantee type I error control, taking into account small sample sizes (Fisher's exact test is considered more accurate than the chi-square test or G-test of independence in such cases). Yet, the lack of association for rs10434 due to small sample sizes cannot be excluded. *VEFGA* genomic variants have also been found in asymptomatic individuals with high HbF levels (unpublished), suggesting a possible role of *VEGFA* in increasing HbF levels.

According to the outcome of our in silico analyses, rs3024997 (G>A) was found to occur in a deep intronic position, resulting on the activation of an intronic cryptic acceptor site and thus, potential alteration of splicing. Yet, the RESCUE ESE, EIEs, PESE Octamers, ESE Finder-SRp40, and ESR Sequences prediction algorithms suggested the creation of an exonic splicing enhancer, which has probably no impact on splicing. rs2146323 (C>A) causes no significant splicing motif alteration, suggesting that the other co-inherited variants are possibly the key in its association with high HbF levels. No doubt, coupled to the bioinformatics predictions described, functional analysis needs to be performed, such as functional minigene analysis and exon-tiling microarrays to confirm the role of these variants as predicted in silico [8, 28, 29, 38].

Our study has a number of limitations. First of all, we have not managed to isolate fetal tissues from enough number of individuals to replicate our findings and this is subject to future work that is currently ongoing. Secondly, the sample size of the subsequent follow-up study was equally small, due to the lack of sufficient number of well-characterized β-thalassemia/SCD as well as NTDT patients, which are scarce and truly unique to find. Our results are, nevertheless, indicative for future replication work to validate the suggested role of *VEGFA* as possible modifier of HbF levels in adult life.

Conclusion and future perspectives

Human hemoglobin switching still remains a great challenge, when β-type hemoglobinopathy management is considered. In a similar context, HbF production has attracted great interest over the last 50 years towards the amelioration of disease symptoms of β-type hemoglobinopathy patients. Taking into account that HU treatment efficacy exhibits great inter-individual variability, identification, and subsequently validation and clinical implementation of pharmacogenomic biomarkers hold promise for optimum patient stratification and disease management. Herein, our transcriptomics approach provided insights into the differential expression profiles of different erythroid tissues during human ontogenesis and suggested that *VEGFA* genomic variants serve both as genomic biomarkers for β-thalassemia disease severity and pharmacogenomic biomarkers for HU treatment efficacy in β-type hemoglobinopathy patients. In other words, a dual role is implied for *VEGFA* in erythropoiesis and HbF induction, which needs to be further investigated, if the molecular mechanism that delineate human hemoglobin switching is to be better defined and genome-based stratification of β-type hemoglobinopathy patients for HU treatment is to become reality. Notably, not all genomic loci that have been reported to increase HbF levels could be considered as pharmacogenomic biomarkers of HU treatment efficacy, as the clinical features in question, albeit related, are likely controlled by different molecular mechanisms. These findings, in conjunction to previous work conducted by our group and others, hold promise for the identification of pharmacogenomic biomarker for HbF-augmenting therapy, requiring carefully designed prospective clinical studies conducted by large multicenter consortia that include experienced clinicians and researchers from major clinical and academic centers.

Additional file

Additional file 1: Table S1. Upregulated genes when (i) peripheral blood is compared to umbilical cord blood and fetal liver (PB vs CB+FL) and (ii) peripheral blood is compared to fetal liver (PB vs FL). **Table S2.** Downregulated genes when (i) peripheral blood is compared to umbilical cord blood and fetal liver (PB vs CB+FL) and (ii) peripheral blood is compared to fetal liver (PB vs FL). **Table S3.** Statistical and Hardy-Weinberg analyses on the genotyping data of β-type hemoglobinopathy patients of Hellenic origin and healthy (non-thalassemic) individuals. **Table S4.** Pairwise linkage disequilibrium (LD) calculations for the tagSNPs of interest across the *VEGFA* gene (CEU). **Figure S1.** Differential gene expression when adult peripheral blood is compared to cord blood. A total of 135 genes were over- (FC > 2) or downregulated (FC < 2). Columns represent samples; rows are genes. Red, genes that were upregulated; green, genes that were downregulated. **Figure S2.** Differential gene expression when adult peripheral blood is compared to fetal liver. A total of 962 genes were over- (FC > 2) or downregulated (FC < 2). Columns represent samples; rows are genes. Red, genes that were upregulated; green, genes that were downregulated.

Abbreviations

CEU: Caucasian; HbF: Fetal hemoglobin; HPFH: Hereditary persistence of fetal hemoglobin; HU: Hydroxyurea; NTDT: Non-transfusion-dependent thalassemia; SCD: Sickle cell disease

Acknowledgements

The authors are grateful to Dr. Stamatia Theodoridou (Ippokrateio General Hospital Thessaloniki, Thessaloniki, Greece) and Dr. Panagiota Chalkia (AHEPA University Hospital, Thessaloniki, Greece) for their valuable assistance with sample collection.

Funding

This work was partly funded by research grants from the Cypriot Research Promotion Foundation (HU_PHARMGK; RFP_046) and the European Commission (RD-Connect; FP7-305444; U-PGx; H2020-668353) to GPP. BRA is funded by the United Arab Emirates University Center-based grants through Zayed Center for Health Sciences.

Authors' contributions

GPP conceived the study. VC, TK, and GPP designed the study. AK and AS provided the samples. VC, PK, AS, VK, AP, and AJ performed the experiments. VC, PK, and TK analyzed the data. BRA and GPP provided funding for this work. VC, PK, BRA, TK, and GPP wrote the manuscript. All authors read and approved the manuscript.

Consent for publication

Not applicable.

Competing interests

The authors declare that they have no competing interests.

Author details

[1]Department of Pharmacy, School of Health Sciences, University of Patras, University Campus, Rion, GR-265 04 Patras, Greece. [2]Biotech Research and Innovation Centre (BRIC), University of Copenhagen, Copenhagen, Denmark. [3]Hellenic Open University, Patras, Greece. [4]Hematology Division, Department of Internal Medicine, Faculty of Medicine, University of Patras, Patras, Greece. [5]Department of Pathology, College of Medicine & Health Sciences, United Arab Emirates University, Al-Ain, United Arab Emirates. [6]Zayed Bin Sultan Center for Health Sciences, United Arab Emirates University, Al-Ain, United Arab Emirates. [7]Laboratory of General Biology, Faculty of Medicine, University of Patras, Patras, Greece. [8]Present address: Institut de Génétique et de Biologie Moléculaire et Cellulaire IGBMC/CNRS/INSERM/UDS, 67404 ILLKIRCH, BP 10142 CU de Strasbourg, France.

References

1. Adelman CA, Chattopadhyay S, Bieker JJ. The BMP/BMPR/Smad pathway directs expression of the erythroid-specific EKLF and GATA1 transcription factors during embryoid body differentiation in serum-free media. Development. 2002;129:539–49.
2. Barrett JC, Fry B, Maller J, Daly MJ. Haploview: analysis and visualization of LD and haplotype maps. Bioinformatics. 2004;21:263–5.
3. Bordbar MR, Silavizadeh S, Haghpanah S, Kamfiroozi R, Bardestani M, Karimi M. Hydroxyurea treatment in transfusion-dependent β-thalassemia patients. Iran Red Crescent Med J. 2014;16:e18028.
4. Borg J, Phylactides M, Bartsakoulia M, Tafrali C, Lederer C, Felice AE, Papachatzopoulou A, Kourakli A, Stavrou EF, Christou S. KLF10 gene expression is associated with high fetal hemoglobin levels and with response to hydroxyurea treatment in β-hemoglobinopathy patients. Pharmacogenomics. 2012;13:1487–500.
5. Cao A, Galanello R. Beta-thalassemia. Genet Med. 2010;12:61–76.
6. Casella I, Feccia T, Chelucci C, Samoggia P, Castelli G, Guerriero R, Parolini I, Petrucci E, Pelosi E, Morsilli O. Autocrine-paracrine VEGF loops potentiate the maturation of megakaryocytic precursors through Flt1 receptor. Blood. 2003;101:1316–23.
7. Chalikiopoulou C, Tavianatou A-G, Sgourou A, Kourakli A, Kelepouri D, Chrysanthakopoulou M, Kanelaki V-K, Mourdoukoutas E, Siamoglou S, John A. Genomic variants in the ASS1 gene, involved in the nitric oxide biosynthesis and signaling pathway, predict hydroxyurea treatment efficacy in compound sickle cell disease/β-thalassemia patients. Pharmacogenomics. 2016;17:393–403.
8. Cooper DN. Functional intronic polymorphisms: buried treasure awaiting discovery within our genes. Human Genom. 2010;4:284.
9. de Hoon MJ, Imoto S, Nolan J, Miyano S. Open source clustering software. Bioinformatics. 2004;20:1453–4.
10. Desmet F-O, Hamroun D, Lalande M, Collod-Béroud G, Claustres M, Béroud C. Human Splicing Finder: an online bioinformatics tool to predict splicing signals. Nucleic Acids Res. 2009;37:e67.
11. Dzierzak E, Philipsen S. Erythropoiesis: development and differentiation. Cold Spring Harbor Perspect Med. 2013;3:a011601.
12. Galanello R, Origa R. Beta-thalassemia. Orphanet J Rare Dis. 2010;5:11.
13. Gerber H-P, Ferrara N. The role of VEGF in normal and neoplastic hematopoiesis. J Mol Med. 2003;81:20–31.
14. Gerber H-P, Malik AK, Solar GP, Sherman D. VEGF regulates haematopoietic stem cell survival by an internal autocrine loop mechanism. Nature. 2002;417:954.
15. Giannopoulou E, Bartsakoulia M, Tafrali C, Kourakli A, Poulas K, Stavrou EF, Papachatzopoulou A, Georgitsi M, Patrinos GP. A single nucleotide polymorphism in the HBBP1 gene in the human β-globin locus is associated with a mild β-thalassemia disease phenotype. Hemoglobin. 2012;36:433–45.
16. Giardine B, Borg J, Higgs DR, Peterson KR, Philipsen S, Maglott D, Singleton BK, Anstee DJ, Basak AN, Clark B. Systematic documentation and analysis of human genetic variation in hemoglobinopathies using the microattribution approach. Nat Genet. 2011;43:295–301.
17. Gravia A, Chondrou V, Kolliopoulou A, Kourakli A, John A, Symeonidis A, Ali BR, Sgourou A, Papachatzopoulou A, Katsila T. Correlation of SIN3A genomic variants with β-hemoglobinopathies disease severity and hydroxyurea treatment efficacy. Pharmacogenomics. 2016;17:1785–93.
18. Gravia A, Chondrou V, Sgourou A, Papantoni I, Borg J, Katsila T, Papachatzopoulou A, Patrinos GP. Individualizing fetal hemoglobin augmenting therapy for β-type hemoglobinopathies patients. Pharmacogenomics. 2014;15:1355–64.
19. Hagh MF, Fard AD, Saki N, Shahjahani M, Kaviani S. Molecular mechanisms of hemoglobin F induction. Int J Hematol-Oncol Stem Cell Res. 2011;5:5–9.
20. Hattangadi SM, Wong P, Zhang L, Flygare J, Lodish HF. From stem cell to red cell: regulation of erythropoiesis at multiple levels by multiple proteins, RNAs, and chromatin modifications. Blood. 2011;118:6258–68.
21. Holmes DI, Zachary I. The vascular endothelial growth factor (VEGF) family: angiogenic factors in health and disease. Genome Biol. 2005;6:209.
22. Johnson, AD, Handsaker, RE, Pulit, SL, Nizzari, MM, O'donnell, CJ and De Bakker, PI. (2008). SNAP: a web-based tool for identification and annotation of proxy SNPs using HapMap. Bioinformatics 24, 2938-2939.
23. Koren A, Levin C, Dgany O, Kransnov T, Elhasid R, Zalman L, Palmor H, Tamary H. Response to hydroxyurea therapy in β-thalassemia. Am J Hematol. 2008;83:366–70.
24. Leberbauer C, Boulmé F, Unfried G, Huber J, Beug H, Müllner EW. Different steroids co-regulate long-term expansion versus terminal differentiation in primary human erythroid progenitors. Blood. 2005;105:85–94.
25. Ma Q, Wyszynski D, Farrell J, Kutlar A, Farrer L, Baldwin C, Steinberg M. Fetal hemoglobin in sickle cell anemia: genetic determinants of response to hydroxyurea. Pharmacogenom J. 2007;7:386.
26. Machiela MJ, Chanock SJ. LDlink: a web-based application for exploring population-specific haplotype structure and linking correlated alleles of possible functional variants. Bioinformatics. 2015;31:3555–7.
27. Mi H, Muruganujan A, Casagrande JT, Thomas PD. Large-scale gene function analysis with the PANTHER classification system. Nat Protocols. 2013;8:1551–66.
28. Millar DS, Horan M, Chuzhanova NA, Cooper DN. Characterisation of a functional intronic polymorphism in the human growth hormone (GHI) gene. Human Genom. 2010;4:289.
29. Moyer RA, Wang D, Papp AC, Smith RM, Duque L, Mash DC, Sadee W. Intronic polymorphisms affecting alternative splicing of human dopamine D2 receptor are associated with cocaine abuse. Neuropsychopharmacology. 2011;36:753–62.
30. Musallam KM, Taher AT, Cappellini MD, Sankaran VG. Clinical experience with fetal hemoglobin induction therapy in patients with β-thalassemia. Blood. 2013;121:2199–212.
31. Nakayama N, Lee J, Chiu L. Vascular endothelial growth factor synergistically enhances bone morphogenetic protein-4-dependent lymphohematopoietic cell generation from embryonic stem cells in vitro. Blood. 2000;95:2275–83.
32. Papachatzopoulou A, Kaimakis P, Pourfarzad F, Menounos PG, Evangelakou P, Kollia P, Grosveld FG, Patrinos GP. Increased γ-globin gene expression in β-thalassemia intermedia patients correlates with a mutation in 3′ HS1. Am J Hematol. 2007;82:1005–9.
33. Papachatzopoulou A, Kourakli A, Makropoulou P, Kakagianne T, Sgourou A, Papadakis M, Athanassiadou A. Genotypic heterogeneity and correlation to intergenic haplotype within high HbF β-thalassemia intermedia. Eur J Haematol. 2006;76:322–30.
34. Patrinos GP, Antonarakis SE. Human hemoglobin. In: Vogel and Motulsky's human genetics. Vergal Berlin Heidelberg: Springer; 2010. p. 365–401.
35. Saldanha AJ. Java Treeview—extensible visualization of microarray data. Bioinformatics. 2004;20:3246–8.

36. Sankaran VG. Targeted therapeutic strategies for fetal hemoglobin induction. ASH Educ Program Book. 2011;2011:459–65.
37. Sasieni PD. From genotypes to genes: doubling the sample size. Biometrics. 1997:1253–61.
38. Seo S, Takayama K, Uno K, Ohi K, Hashimoto R, Nishizawa D, Ikeda K, Ozaki N, Nabeshima T, Miyamoto Y. Functional analysis of deep intronic SNP rs13438494 in intron 24 of PCLO gene. PLoS One. 2013;8:e76960.
39. Suzuki M, Yamamoto M, Engel JD. Fetal globin gene repressors as drug targets for molecular therapies to treat the β-globinopathies. Mol Cell Biol. 2014;34:3560–9.
40. Tafrali C, Paizi A, Borg J, Radmilovic M, Bartsakoulia M, Giannopoulou E, Giannakopoulou O, Stojiljkovic-Petrovic M, Zukic B, Poulas K. Genomic variation in the MAP3K5 gene is associated with β-thalassemia disease severity and hydroxyurea treatment efficacy. Pharmacogenomics. 2013;14:469–83.
41. Tallack MR, Perkins AC. Three fingers on the switch: Krüppel-like factor 1 regulation of γ-globin to β-globin gene switching. Curr Opin Hematol. 2013;20:193–200.
42. Thorisson GA, Smith AV, Krishnan L, Stein LD. The international HapMap project web site. Genome Res. 2005;15:1592–3.
43. Van Handel, B, Prashad, SL, Hassanzadeh-Kiabi, N, Huang, A, Magnusson, M, Atanassova, B, Chen, A, Hamalainen, EI and Mikkola, HK. (2010). The first trimester human placenta is a site for terminal maturation of primitive erythroid cells. Blood 116, 3321-3330.
44. Xu, J, Shao, Z, Glass, K, Bauer, DE, Pinello, L, Van Handel, B, Hou, S, Stamatoyannopoulos, JA, Mikkola, HK and Yuan, G-C. (2012). Combinatorial assembly of developmental stage-specific enhancers controls gene expression programs during human erythropoiesis. Dev Cell 23, 796-811.
45. Xu Z, Taylor JA. SNPinfo: integrating GWAS and candidate gene information into functional SNP selection for genetic association studies. Nucleic Acids Res. 2009;37:W600–5.

13

Meeting report of the 2017 KidGen Renal Genetics Symposium

Kushani Jayasinghe[1,2*†], Cathy Quinlan[2,3,4†], Zornitza Stark[2,3,5], Chirag Patel[2,6], Matthew G. Sampson[7], Moin Saleem[8], Andrew J. Mallett[2,9,10] and on behalf of the KidGen Collaborative

Abstract

The 2017 KidGen Renal Genetics Symposium was held at the Royal Children's Hospital and Murdoch Children's Research Institute, Melbourne, from 6 to 8 December 2017. This meeting addressed clinical, diagnostic, and research aspects of inherited kidney disease. More than 100 clinicians, researchers, and patient representatives attended the conference. The overall goal was to improve the understanding and direction of genomics in renal medicine in Australia and discuss barriers to the use of genomic testing within this area. It also aimed to strengthen collaborations between local, state, and global research and diagnostic and clinical groups.

Keywords: Inherited kidney disease, Nephrogenetics, Renal genetics

Introduction and background to the meeting

There has been a rapid change and progress in the field of inherited kidney disease and nephrogenetics in recent years, and this has across clinical, diagnostic, and research domains. Within an Australian and Australasian perspective, there have been not only challenges but also opportunities related to this translational process. The obstacles of geography and distance are countered by nationally and regionally coordinated genomic efforts such as Australian Genomics, Melbourne Genomics, and the Queensland Genomic Health Alliance. The annual KidGen Renal Genetics Symposium provides an opportunity to bring together a diversity of clinicians, researchers, and patient representatives from around Australia, Australasia, and the global community. This enables a unique opportunity to better understand the renal genetics implementation landscape while updating on the latest progress within a strong nexus of collaboration focused on this particular emerging subspecialty field.

The renal genetics multidisciplinary workshop

This interactive half-day clinical workshop, convened by Dr. Chirag Patel from Genetic Health Queensland, was designed primarily for nephrologists, geneticists, and genetic counselors new to the clinical practice of renal genetics. Thirty participants attended the workshop, with small groups of six including a facilitator. Participants in each group comprised of a mixture of professionals, which included adult and pediatric nephrologists, genetic counselors, and clinical geneticists, reflecting the typical composition of a multidisciplinary clinic or meeting. Case-based scenarios were discussed including pertinent issues in each case, differential diagnosis, information required, counseling and ethical issues, and genetic testing indications and results. All participants also took part in a survey to evaluate their initial understanding of genomics and confidence in renal genetics cases, and these survey findings will be analyzed as part of an implementation science analysis of renal genetics in Australia.

Providing a map of services available to date

Dr. Andrew Mallett, the National Director of the KidGen Collaborative and the Australian Genomics Health Alliance (AGHA) Renal Genetics Flagship, presented on the renal genetics services and research opportunities in Australia. The KidGen Collaborative continues to grow and evolve. In the last year, services have commenced in South Australia and Western Australia (Fig 1). Multidisciplinary renal genetics clinics will soon be underway in Darwin and Tasmania, with the aim to provide access to 90% of the Australian population over the next 12 months. Dr. Mallett

* Correspondence: kushani.jayasinghe@gmail.com
†Equal contributors
[1]Department of Nephrology, Monash Medical Centre, Melbourne, Australia
[2]KidGen Renal Genetics Flagship, Australian Genomic Health Alliance, Melbourne, Australia
Full list of author information is available at the end of the article

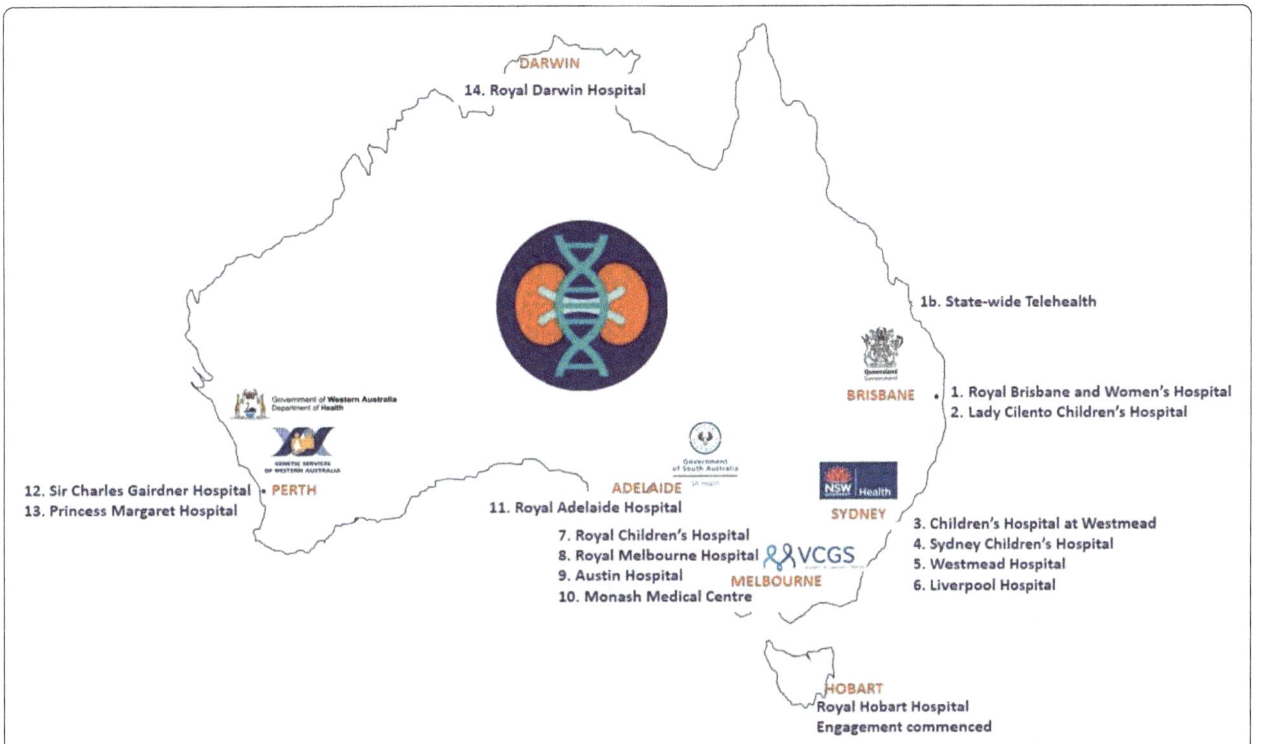

Fig. 1 Location of KidGen-affiliated Renal Genetics Clinics as of 7 December 2017

also described the challenges of recruiting to the Australian Genomics renal flagship. Potential participant recruitment rates have not been as high as projected, and research looking into reasons for this is being conducted via an implementation science project. Another exciting new venture is the Australian Genomics "wHole genome Investigation to iDentify unDEtected Nephropathies (HIDDEN) Flagship" which has recently secured funding to identify undetected genetic nephropathies using whole genome sequencing. Currently, 5% of patients with end-stage kidney disease (ESKD) have an unknown cause of their renal failure. With the cost of genome sequencing decreasing, there is an opportunity to remediate this. The immediate aim is to evaluate 200 participants with unexplained ESKD over the next 24 months. He also highlighted that significant prospective studies evaluating the cost-effectiveness of genomic testing are occurring in Australian cohorts, which will be crucial in securing sustainable funding for genomic testing in routine healthcare.

Rare inherited kidney disease registries

This session focused on the opportunities and challenges of developing rare disease registries. Professor Moin Saleem, Head of Bristol Renal, a world renowned glomerular disease research group, presented on the United Kingdom (UK) approach to rare inherited kidney disease. Rare inherited kidney disease refers to diseases that have a prevalence of 1 in 2000 [1]. Up to 10% of the population will have a rare disease, and 80% of rare diseases will have a genetic basis. The UK renal community has developed perhaps the world leading system for ongoing collation of cohorts of patients with renal rare disease, called renal RaDaR (www.rarerenal.org). This is a web-based and nationally inclusive program, which allows information to build in a bottom-up fashion, driven by interested and enthusiastic stakeholders, professionals, and patients. This registry was developed utilizing the information technology (IT) infrastructure of the UK renal registry. The original target of the registry was to recruit 500 patients, whereas currently, there are over 15,000 patients comprising 25 patient groups and 85 renal units.

Professor Saleem described the importance of understanding rare disease using modern biological advances. In order to stratify and treat patients appropriately, we must move from descriptive classifications to molecular levels of understanding. To do this, it is crucial to recruit as many patients as possible in order to facilitate studies with sufficient analytical power. The RaDaR registry has also provided the opportunity to create rare disease groups and facilitated the development of evidence-based care pathways and further empower patients. There are tremendous opportunities that arise from such registries, and other countries can benefit from the lessons learned from the UK renal registry.

Genomic profiling and molecular insights in nephrotic syndrome

Keynote speakers presented on the benefits of deep clinical and genomic profiling in nephrotic syndrome. Professor Saleem discussed the importance of discovering robust biological biomarkers that identify patients with circulating factor disease. For example, there is strong evidence for a role of a circulating factor in the pathogenesis of idiopathic nephrotic syndrome (iNS) [2, 3]. Previous work has suggested a role for protease-activated receptor (PAR-1) [4]. His group used a model whereby a transgenic mouse was developed that expressed a podocyte-specific constitutively active form of PAR-1 in order to replicate overexposure to a circulating protease. The developmental PAR-1 active mice were born normal and died consistently between the ages of 39 and 45 days. Proteinuria developed from 14 days and markedly increased over time. Electron microscopy (EM) analysis showed a significantly thickened glomerular basement membrane (GBM) and foot process effacement. This demonstrated a clear role for the PAR-1 receptor in proteinuria and strengthened the hypothesis that circulating factor(s) may act via this receptor. Additionally, this is a novel model for circulating factor nephrotic syndrome (NS) to test therapies in vivo. Professor Saleem presented this work at the recent American Society of Nephrology Kidney Week in November 2017.

Dr. Matthew Sampson, a pediatric nephrologist and researcher at the University of Michigan, spoke on the use of population genetics to interrogate monogenic nephrotic syndrome diagnosis. His laboratory combines innovative genomic technologies, statistical genetics, computational genetics, and bioinformatics to elucidate the role of genomic variation in renal disease. Genomic discovery in nephrotic syndrome has allowed insight into biology of disease, clinical correlates such as prognosis and treatments, and prevalence estimates of disease.

Monogenic nephrotic syndrome is a serious form of NS, and these patients often have a continued decline in kidney function that is resistant to immunosuppressive therapy. [5–9]. There are over 60 causative genetic mutations of steroid resistant nephrotic syndrome (SRNS) [10]. Numerous publications have reported robust genotype-phenotype correlations in monogenic NS and their substantial prevalence. Previously, diagnostic genetic screening involved sequencing one or two genes most likely to harbor causal variants in patients with a high pretest probability of having a genetic form of nephrotic syndrome. Once found, other evidence was collected to support causality. Nowadays, genomic technologies are rapidly evolving, enabling sequencing to become much more readily available. Hence, there is a widespread enthusiasm from all stakeholders to expand sequencing efforts in affected patients to make a diagnosis of "monogenic NS." However, there is a need to assess the generalizability of prevalence estimates and clinical correlates previously reported from selected cohorts now that more patients and more genes can be studied. One aspect of this is the recognition from large-scale sequencing projects in reference populations that the prevalence of putatively fully penetrant mutations in the general population can be orders of magnitude higher than the reported disease prevalence.

The NEPTUNE study [11] is a North American cohort of NS patients that provided a laboratory to gain insights on the challenges of making a monogenic diagnosis in previously understudied populations. Patients with NS were enrolled at the time of the first biopsy and independent of age, ancestry, and response to immunosuppression. They were then followed longitudinally. In a paper by Sampson et al. [12], 312 patients underwent targeted sequencing of 21 genes implicated in SRNS. These were compared to the 1000 Genomes Project (1000G) reference population. A typical pathogenicity filter identified causal variants for NS in 4.2% of patients and 5.8% of subjects from the 1000G. The group then devised a more stringent pathogenicity filtering strategy, implicating monogenic NS in 2.9% of NEPTUNE patients and reducing background prevalence of causal variants to 1.5% in the 1000G. Interestingly, patients with putative monogenic NS in NEPTUNE achieved complete remission of proteinuria at similar rates to those without a monogenic diagnosis.

The 1.5% background prevalence suggests that some variants, even if found in patients, might be either incorrectly implicated as pathogenic. In addition, there may be a greater degree of incomplete penetrance of these variants than previously appreciated. Therefore, in an unselected cohort, it may be accurate to consider a monogenic diagnosis from a probabilistic and not a deterministic perspective.

Functional genomics

Professor Melissa Little, the theme Director of Cell Biology at Murdoch Children's Research Institute (MCRI) in Melbourne and program leader of Stem Cells Australia, discussed the clinical and research applications for induced pluripotent stem cells and their application in kidney disease. Advances in next-generation sequencing have improved diagnosis rates for families with inherited kidney disease; however, a causative gene is identified in only 40% of cases [13]. While novel potential causative gene associations are being identified, these still require functional validation. The use of induced pluripotent stem cells (iPSC) is one approach that has the potential to determine the functional significance of previously un-described gene variants. Professor Little and her team developed a protocol for the successful differentiation of human pluripotent stem cells to a kidney organoid [14, 15]. This results in the formation of a complex organoid containing all cellular components anticipated for a first trimester human kidney. Professor Little also presented data illustrating how we can replicate the disease phenotype of an inherited kidney disease. By modeling heritable kidney disease and screening of toxicity and efficacy, we are now able to move towards applying stem cells to cellular therapy. Renal replacement therapy through iPSC-derived cells is still some time away, mainly due to barriers of scale and vascular supply.

Challenges in genomic medicine

This session focused on current challenges in implementing genomic medicine into clinical practice as well as the innovative opportunities and solutions achieved to date. Elly Lynch, a clinical project manager at Melbourne Genomics Health Alliance (MGHA), highlighted the potential health implications from incidental or secondary results that arise from genomic sequencing. This refers to variants found incidentally through genomic sequencing that are not related to the aim of the test but may still have potential health implications and clinical significance [16].

In 2013, the American College of Medical Genetics and Genomics (ACMG) published a policy statement that emphasized the importance of reporting of incidental results [17]. In 2014, the ACMG revised these recommendations to include options for individuals to opt out of being informed of incidental findings. The ACMG Board of Directors created the ACMG Secondary Findings Maintenance Working Group (SFWG) in 2014 to define and implement a process for updating a minimum list of secondary findings that would be updated and refined regularly. The 2016 update statement concluded that "Informed consent is necessary, and reporting of secondary findings should be optional" [18]. However, surprisingly, the research into this area has reflected that often, patients want to be informed of secondary findings, even when limited treatment options are available [19].

Professor Kathryn North, co-chair of the Global Alliance for Genomics and Health (GA4GH) and lead of the Australian Genomics Health Alliance, highlighted the challenges of the implementation of genetic services in Australia. She provided insight into the complex and fragmented structure of the Australian healthcare system. Federal funding for genetic services is currently limited to about 30 tests and genomic testing being supported by clinical services at a state level. This highlighted the importance of linking and collaborating state-based expertise and investment with the formation of national flagships in order to facilitate research, map disparity, and inequity and allow coordinated collaboration between states.

She also highlighted the importance of global collaboration. In October 2017, Australian Genomics was nominated a Driver Project of the GA4GH, an international, nonprofit alliance of over 470 organizations across over 45 countries. Australian Genomics will serve alongside Genomics England and the *All of Us* research program to enable GA4GH to deliver its new 5-year strategic plan to enable the responsible sharing of clinical-grade genomic data by 2022.

The benefits of rapid genomic testing in acute pediatrics

A/Prof Zornitza Stark, clinical geneticist at the Victorian Clinical Genetics Service (VCGS) and clinical research fellow with Australian Genomics, demonstrated the significant clinical and cost benefits from rapid whole exome sequencing (rWES) in a prospective cohort of 40 acutely unwell pediatric patients recruited through the Melbourne Genomics Health Alliance in 2016–2017. In the course of the project, the overall time-to-result decreased tenfold from 109 to 9 days (median 16 days). This required whole-of-system change, with over 20 changes implemented to clinical and laboratory processes to accelerate result delivery. Of the 40 patients who underwent rWES, 52% received a genetic diagnosis, and 57% of those diagnosed had a change in management as a result, including the provision of life-saving treatment, avoidance of invasive biopsies, and redirection towards palliative care. Rapid exome sequencing was also very cost-effective, with cost savings from improved management conservatively estimated to be around AU$550,000 (Stark Z, Lunke S et al: Meeting the challenges of implementing rapid genomic testing in acute pediatric care, submitted).

Genomics in specific ethnic groups

This session focused on genetic variation in patients with chronic kidney disease within Indigenous populations, as well as the lessons learned and challenges of research in various ethnic groups. Matthew Sampson presented on the racial disparity of ESKD in the American population. African-Americans make up only 13% of the US population yet make up 32% of all Americans with ESKD [20]. African-Americans who carry two variant alleles within apolipoprotein L1 (*APOL1*) are classified as having a high-risk (HR) genotype [21]. People with HR genotype have an increased risk of focal segmental glomerulosclerosis and chronic kidney disease compared with those with a low-risk (LR) genotype. Children from two cohorts with HR genotype were characterized (Chronic Kidney Disease in Children (CKiD) and NEPTUNE), which found that children with a HR genotype had a more aggressive form of glomerular disease [22].

William Wong, a pediatric nephrologist at Starship Children's Hospital, Auckland, discussed the congenital nephrotic syndrome in Maori children. Maori children tend to have a milder course compared to infants with Caucasian background. *Nephrin* mutation analysis in 19 surviving CNS patients revealed a variety of different mutations in *NPS1*, with Caucasian infants demonstrating completely different mutations to Maori infants [23].

Madhivanan Sundaram, a nephrologist at Royal Darwin hospital, presented on the practical challenges in the diagnosis and management of inherited kidney disorders in remote Indigenous patients. Due to language barriers, cultural barriers, and scarcity of resources in remote communities, there are many challenges nephrologists face in this population group. Some of these include difficulties in pedigree analysis, obtaining informed consent, and reluctance to participate in research. Some solutions to overcoming these obstacles include involving genetic counselors from indigenous groups, increased use of interpreters, and close links with local community groups and clinics.

Panel discussion: "You can't always get what you want – whole genome sequencing, whole exome sequencing and renal gene panels"

Panelists:

A/Prof Julie McGaughran: Director of Genetic Health Queensland, Royal Brisbane and Women's Hospital, Brisbane

Dr. Cas Simons: Adjunct Senior Fellow, Institute for Molecular Bioscience, University of Queensland, Brisbane

Dr. Amali Mallawaarachchi: Adult Nephrologist and Clinical Genetics Fellow, Liverpool Hospital, Sydney

A/Prof Bruce Bennetts: Associate Professor and Head of Department of Genetic Medicine, Children's Hospital at Westmead, Sydney

Dr. Sebastian Luke: Head of the Translational Genomics Unit, Victorian Clinical Genetics Services and Murdoch Children's Research Institute, Melbourne

A/Prof Zornitza Stark: Clinical Geneticist, Victorian Clinical Genetics Services and Australian Genomics Health Alliance, Melbourne

The panel discussion allowed a passionate group of physicians, geneticists, scientists, and counselors the opportunity to ask thought-provoking questions and participate in open-minded discussions on the major topics surrounding genomics in renal medicine. Urgent unmet needs and challenges in the future were addressed. Issues raised included the "best test" in the eyes of laboratory and research scientists versus clinical geneticists and renal physicians and the balance between cost of sequencing and selecting the optimal test for the patient. Overall, the consensus among panel members was that the current cost of whole genome sequencing is prohibitive to its clinical use and hence does not justify the cost of doing this over whole exome sequencing or targeted panel. Furthermore, we do not know enough about the whole genome yet to be able to fully interpret the sequencing results. It is still unclear who should be the gatekeepers to genetic testing in the future. Should any doctor be able to order genetic tests? Who is responsible for counseling patients? Currently, this differs from state to state, but in general, patients seen in renal genetics clinics are discussed at multidisciplinary meetings to ensure appropriate test ordering. The general consensus was that genetic testing should primarily be ordered if it would change patient management.

Conclusions and outcomes

The KidGen Renal Genetics Symposium is currently one of the few dedicated renal genetics meetings to be held internationally on an annual basis. In 2017, the 5th annual meeting brought together scientific researchers, clinical researchers, adult and pediatric nephrologists, patient representatives, clinical geneticists, and genetic counselors. This model exemplifies how research collaboration should be facilitated, as it brings together the key members and stakeholders that can advance the field of renal genomics. This is of utmost importance to benefit patients and families with inherited kidney disease. The symposium provided not only the increased awareness of the challenges of genomics we face now and into the future but also the promise of insights and advances that are continuously being gained.

Abbreviations

1000G: 1000 Genomes Project; ACMG: American College of Medical Genetics and Genomics; AGHA: Australian Genomics Health Alliance; ESKD: End-stage kidney disease; EM: Electron microscopy; GA4GH: Global Alliance for Genomics and Health; GBM: Glomerular basement membrane; HIDDEN: wHole genome Investigation to iDentify unDEtected Nephropathies; HR: High risk; iPSC: Induced pluripotent stem cells; IT: Information technology; iNS: Idiopathic nephrotic syndrome; LR: Low risk; MCRI: Murdoch Children's Research Institute; MGHA: Melbourne Genomics Health Alliance; NS: Nephrotic syndrome; rWES: Rapid whole exome sequencing; SFWG: Secondary Findings Working Group; SRNS: Steroid resistant nephrotic syndrome; UK: United Kingdom; VCGS : Victorian Clinical Genetics Service

Acknowledgements

The authors and the KidGen Collaborative wish to acknowledge the attendees of the Symposium, Louise Wardrop as the Program Manager of KidGen, and the support given by the Australian Genomics Health Alliance and Melbourne Genomics Health Alliance.

Funding

This symposium was supported in part by untethered educational sponsorship from AGHA, Genome.One, Sanofi-Genzyme, Shire, and Reata Pharmaceuticals. Decisions regarding speakers, topics, and agenda were made by the conference organizers independent of sponsors and sponsorship.

Authors' contributions

All authors were involved in writing and contributing to the manuscript. All authors read and approved the final manuscript.

Consent for publication

Not applicable

Competing interests

The authors declare that they have no competing interests.

Author details

[1]Department of Nephrology, Monash Medical Centre, Melbourne, Australia. [2]KidGen Renal Genetics Flagship, Australian Genomic Health Alliance, Melbourne, Australia. [3]Murdoch Children's Research Institute, Melbourne, Australia. [4]Department of Paediatric Nephrology, Royal Children's Hospital, Melbourne, Australia. [5]Department of Pediatrics, University of Melbourne, Melbourne, Australia. [6]Genetic Health Queensland, Royal Brisbane and Women's Hospital, Brisbane, Australia. [7]Department Of Pediatrics-Nephrology, University of Michigan School of Medicine, Ann Arbor, USA. [8]Bristol Renal, Bristol Medical School, University of Bristol, Bristol, UK. [9]Faculty of Medicine, The University of Queensland, Brisbane, Australia. [10]Kidney Health Service and Conjoint Renal Research Laboratory, Royal Brisbane and Women's Hospital, Butterfield Street, Herston, Brisbane, Queensland 4029, Australia.

References

1. Schieppati A, Henter JI, Daina E, Aperia A. Why rare diseases are an important medical and social issue. Lancet. 2008;371:2039–41.
2. Maas RJ, Deegens JK, Wetzels JF. Serum suPAR in patients with FSGS: trash or treasure? Pediatr Nephrol. 2013;28:1041–8.
3. Savin VJ, Sharma R, Sharma M, et al. Circulating factor associated with increased glomerular permeability to albumin in recurrent focal segmental glomerulosclerosis. N Engl J Med. 1996;334:878–83.
4. Harris JJ, McCarthy HJ, Ni L, Wherlock M, et al. Active proteases in nephrotic plasma lead to a podocin-dependent phosphorylation of VASP in podocytes via protease activated receptor-1. J Pathol. 2013;229:660–71. https://doi.org/10.1002/path.4149.
5. Takasato M, Er PX, Chiu HS, Maier B, Baillie GJ, et al. Kidney organoids from human iPS cells contain multiple lineages and model human nephrogenesis. Nature. 2015;526:564–8.
6. HJ MC, Bierzynska A, Wherlock M, Ognjanovic M, et al. The UK SRNS study group: simultaneous sequencing of 24 genes associated with steroid-resistant nephrotic syndrome. Clin J Am Soc Nephrol. 2013;8:637–48.
7. Lipska BS, Iatropoulos P, Maranta R, et al. PodoNet consortium. Genetic screening in adolescents with steroid-resistant nephrotic syndrome. Kidney Int. 2013;84:206–13.
8. Giglio S, Provenzano A, Mazzinghi B, Becherucci F, et al. Heterogeneous genetic alterations in sporadic nephrotic syndrome associate with resistance to immunosuppression. J Am Soc Nephrol. 2015;26:230-6.
9. Bullich G, Trujillano D, Santín S, Ossowski S, et al. Targeted next-generation sequencing in steroid-resistant nephrotic syndrome: mutations in multiple glomerular genes may influence disease severity. Eur J Hum Genet. 2015;23: 1192–9.
10. Warejko JK, Tan W, Daga A. Whole exome sequencing of patients with steroid-resistant nephrotic syndrome. Clin J Am Soc Nephrol. 2017; https://doi.org/10.2215/CJN.04120417.
11. Gadegbeku CA, Gipson DS, Holzman LB, et al. Design of the Nephrotic Syndrome Study Network (NEPTUNE) to evaluate primary glomerular nephropathy by a multidisciplinary approach. Kidney Int. 2013;83:749–56.
12. Sampson MG, Gillies CE, Robertson CC, Crawford B, et al. Using population genetics to interrogate the monogenic nephrotic syndrome diagnosis in a case cohort. J Am Soc Nephrol. 2016;27:1970–83.
13. Mallet AJ, HJ MC, Ho G, Holman K, et al. Massively parallel sequencing and targeted exomes in familial kidney disease can diagnose underlying genetic disorders. Kidney Int. 2017;92:1493–506.
14. Takasato M, Er PX, Chiu HS, Little MH. Generation of kidney organoids from human pluripotent stem cells. Nat Protoc. 2016;11:1681–92.
15. Sadowski CE, Lovric S, Ashraf S, et al. A single-gene cause in 29.5% of cases of steroid-resistant nephrotic syndrome. J Am Soc Nephrol. 2015;26:1279–89.
16. Tan N, Amendola LM, O'Daniel JM, Burt A, et al. Is "incidental finding" the best term?: a study of patients' preferences. Genet Med. 2017;19:176–81.
17. Green RC, WW BJSG, Kalia SS, et al. ACMG recommendations for reporting of incidental findings in clinical exome and genome sequencing. Genet Med. 2013;15:565–74.
18. Kalia S, Adelman K, Bale SJ, Chung WK, et al. Recommendations for reporting of secondary findings in clinical exome and genome sequencing, 2016 update (ACMG SF v2.0): a policy statement of the American College of Medical Genetics and Genomics. Genet Med. 2017;19:249–55.
19. Stavropoulos DJ, Merico D, Jobling R, Bowdin S, et al. Whole-genome sequencing expands diagnostic utility and improves clinical management in pediatric medicine. Genomic Medicine. 2016; https://doi.org/10.1038/npjgenmed.2015.12.
20. United States Renal Data System 2006 Annual Data Report. Bethesda, MD. National Institutes of Health, National Institute of Diabetes and Digestive and Kidney Diseases. 2006. https://www.usrds.org/2007/pdf/00_intro_07.pdf. Accessed 2 Jan 2018.
21. Genovese G, Friedman DJ, Ross MD, Lecordier L, et al. Association of trypanolytic ApoL1 variants with kidney disease in African Americans. Science. 2010;329:841–5.
22. Ng DK, Robertson CC, Woroniecki RP, Limou S, Gillies CE, et al. APOL1-associated glomerular disease among African-American children: a collaboration of the Chronic Kidney Disease in Children (CKiD) and Nephrotic Syndrome Study Network (NEPTUNE) cohorts. Nephrol Dial Transplant. 2017;32:983–90. https://doi.org/10.1093/ndt/gfw061.
23. Wong W, Morris MC, Kara T. Congenital nephrotic syndrome with prolonged renal survival without renal replacement therapy. Pediatr Nephrol. 2013;28:2313–21.

14

Correlation of gene expression and associated mutation profiles of APOBEC3A, APOBEC3B, REV1, UNG, and FHIT with chemosensitivity of cancer cell lines to drug treatment

Suleyman Vural, Richard Simon and Julia Krushkal*

Abstract

Background: The *APOBEC* gene family of cytidine deaminases plays important roles in DNA repair and mRNA editing. In many cancers, APOBEC3B increases the mutation load, generating clusters of closely spaced, single-strand-specific DNA substitutions with a characteristic hypermutation signature. Some studies also suggested a possible involvement of APOBEC3A, REV1, UNG, and FHIT in molecular processes affecting APOBEC mutagenesis. It is important to understand how mutagenic processes linked to the activity of these genes may affect sensitivity of cancer cells to treatment.

Results: We used information from the Cancer Cell Line Encyclopedia and the Genomics of Drug Sensitivity in Cancer resources to examine associations of the prevalence of APOBEC-like motifs and mutational loads with expression of *APOBEC3A*, *APOBEC3B*, *REV1*, *UNG*, and *FHIT* and with cell line chemosensitivity to 255 antitumor drugs. Among the five genes, *APOBEC3B* expression levels were bimodally distributed, whereas expression of *APOBEC3A*, *REV1*, *UNG*, and *FHIT* was unimodally distributed. The majority of the cell lines had low levels of *APOBEC3A* expression. The strongest correlations of gene expression levels with mutational loads or with measures of prevalence of APOBEC-like motif counts and kataegis clusters were observed for *REV1*, *UNG*, and *APOBEC3A*. Sensitivity or resistance of cell lines to JQ1, palbociclib, bicalutamide, 17-AAG, TAE684, MEK inhibitors refametinib, PD-0325901, and trametinib and a number of other agents was correlated with candidate gene expression levels or with abundance of APOBEC-like motif clusters in specific cancers or across cancer types.

Conclusions: We observed correlations of expression levels of the five candidate genes in cell line models with sensitivity to cancer drug treatment. We also noted suggestive correlations between measures of abundance of APOBEC-like sequence motifs with drug sensitivity in small samples of cell lines from individual cancer categories, which require further validation in larger datasets. Molecular mechanisms underlying the links between the activities of the products of each of the five genes, the resulting mutagenic processes, and sensitivity to each category of antitumor agents require further investigation.

Keywords: APOBEC mutagenesis, Cell line, Chemosensitivity, Gene expression

* Correspondence: julia.krushkal@nih.gov
Computational and Systems Biology Branch, Biometric Research Program, Division of Cancer Treatment and Diagnosis, National Cancer Institute, 9609 Medical Center Dr, Rockville, MD 20850, USA

Background

APOBEC3A and APOBEC3B (apolipoprotein B mRNA-editing enzymes 3A and 3B, catalytic polypeptide-like) are cytosine deaminases from the AID/APOBEC family, members of which play important roles in host immunity against pathogens [1, 2]. The activity of multiple members of the AID/APOBEC family including APOBEC3A but not APOBEC3B has also been linked to epigenetic processes involving DNA demethylation via deamination of 5-hydroxymethyl-cytozine (5-hmC) to 5-hydroxymethyl-uracil (5-hmU) [1, 3, 4]. APOBEC3B is an endogenous mutagen which generates DNA substitutions, most frequently C to T, via a process that involves cytosine to uracil deamination of single-stranded DNA, most commonly in the 5′-TCW-3′ (where W is either A or T) sequence context [2]. In multiple human cancer categories, increased *APOBEC3B* gene expression has been associated with genome-wide hypermutation and with kataegis, a mutagenic process that generates clusters of closely spaced, single-strand-specific DNA substitutions, which are predominantly C to T [5, 6]. Clusters of APOBEC3B mutations are often localized at breakpoints of chromosomal rearrangements [2]. Increased *APOBEC3B* gene expression, germline polymorphisms in the *APOBEC3* genome region, and higher degree of abundance of APOBEC3B mutational signatures have been associated with increased cancer risk and patient survival [5, 7].

APOBEC3B mutagenesis has a characteristic pattern of mutational specificity. It is most commonly represented by the 5′-T(C>T)W-3′ sequence motif [8], where ">" indicates the C to T substitution, and W is an [A or T]. This hypermutation pattern and high mRNA expression levels of *APOBEC3B* have been found in several cancer types [9, 10]. Additional mutation patterns have also been reported for APOBEC3B, although some of these patterns may also be attributed to other APOBEC family members [6, 7, 10, 11]. According to various reports, in addition to the C>T transitions, these patterns may include possible C>G and, in some specific cancer types such as ovarian carcinomas, C>A transversions, as well as a possible 5′-TC(A or G)-3′ sequence context, so that possible mutational motifs could be represented as 5′-T(C>K)W-3′, 5′-T(C>D)R-3′, or 5′-T(C>D)D-3′, where K is [G or T], W is [A or T], R is [A or G], and D is [A or G or T] according to the IUB-IUPAC ambiguity codes [6–8, 11–13]. Below, we present these sequence motifs in the 5′ to 3′ direction as T(C>K)W, T(C>D)R, and T(C>D)D.

While APOBEC3B plays a prominent role in cancer mutagenesis, several other AID/APOBEC family members also have mutagenic roles and affect DNA integrity [9, 14]. Most of them have separate distinct specificities for genome sequence context [2, 8–10, 15, 16]. However, a possible overlap between the activities of APOBEC3B and APOBEC3A has not been fully resolved. The *APOBEC3A* gene is located in proximity to *APOBEC3B* in the *APOBEC* genomic cluster in the chromosomal region 22q13.1 [7]. An *APOBEC3A-APOBEC3B* fusion transcript may be produced due to a germline deletion polymorphism, which results in the complete loss of the coding part of the *APOBEC3B* gene and abolishes *APOBEC3B* gene expression; this deletion polymorphism produces a fusion product of the *APOBEC3A* gene with the 3′-UTR of *APOBEC3B* gene, and it has been associated with an increased risk of several types of cancer [7, 17]. The evidence for a mutagenic role of APOBEC3A so far has been less conclusive than that of APOBEC3B [12, 18]. However, a number of studies suggested that APOBEC3A also acts as an endogenous mutagen that can produce genomic damage, with a mutation signature that may be distinguishable to some extent from that of APOBEC3B [7, 13, 19–25]. In addition to mutagenesis linked to DNA deamination of single-stranded DNA, both APOBEC3B and APOBEC3A can bind RNA, and APOBEC3A has been reported to be involved in both C to U and G to A RNA editing [16, 26].

Based on the strong evidence for APOBEC-associated mutagenesis in a variety of cancer types, it is important to learn whether such mutagenic processes may affect cancer response to therapy, in order to exploit potential pathways involved in sensitivity and to avoid potential mechanisms of resistance. To date, the effect of APOBEC3B-like mutagenic processes on therapeutic response has not been fully understood, with several reports of divergent directions of association. Some studies suggested a potential role of APOBEC mutagenesis in tumor resistance to therapy, with a possible resistance mechanism explained by increased tumor heterogeneity when APOBEC3B activity is elevated [18]. Clinical studies and an analysis of murine xenograft models found an association of increased *APOBEC3B* mRNA expression levels with tamoxifen resistance in estrogen receptor-positive (ER^+) breast cancer [18]. In an analysis of 30 human cell lines, expression levels of the *APOBEC3B* gene were associated with resistance to vinblastine, topotecan, paclitaxel, mitoxantrone, mitomycin C, etoposide, and doxorubicin [27]. In contrast, a study of bladder cancer patients from the Cancer Genome Atlas (TCGA) demonstrated improved survival of those patients who had elevated numbers of APOBEC signature mutations [7]. Experimental in vitro overexpression of *APOBEC3B* in the 293-A3B and 293-GFP cell lines with inactivated p53 resulted in an increase in APOBEC mutagenesis and kataegic events, which were accompanied by cell hypersensitivity to small-molecule DNA damage response inhibitors including ATR (VX-970 and AZD673), CHEK1 (SAR020106), CHEK2 (CCT241553), PARP (olaparib and BMN-673), and WEE1 (AZD1775) inhibitors, as well as by sensitivity to combinations of cisplatin/ATR inhibitor, ATR/PARP inhibitor, and PARP/WEE1 inhibitor [28]. Increased *APOBEC3B* expression in breast cell lines was also correlated with sensitivity to the CHEK1 inhibitor CCT244747 [29]. In contrast, *APOBEC3B* or *APOBEC3A* expression levels were not significantly correlated with sensitivity to any drugs in breast cancer cell lines from the Genomics of Drug Sensitivity in Cancer (GDSC, or GDS1000) dataset [30]; however, they were associated with sensitivity to 38 and 16 agents, respectively, in a joint analysis of all cancer types [31].

At the molecular level, APOBEC3B hypermutation activity has been reported to have a synergistic effect with the absence of the uracil-specific uracil DNA glycosylase (UNG) and to involve molecular steps that require the activity of the translesion synthesis DNA polymerase REV1 [8, 20, 22, 24]. APOBEC mutagenesis may also be increased in case of reduced expression or the loss of protein activity of the tumor suppressor fragile histidine triad protein (FHIT), and higher levels of APOBEC mutagenesis were observed in TCGA lung adenocarcinoma tumors that had both increased *APOBEC3B* expression and the loss of FHIT protein expression [7, 9, 32].

Whereas many studies have focused on the molecular roles of APOBEC3B, and to some extent APOBEC3A, possible cumulative effects of action of APOBEC3A, APOBEC3B, UNG, REV1, and FHIT on generation of APOBEC3B-like mutation motifs and on drug sensitivity in cancer have not been clearly elucidated. To address this question, we investigated the presence of APOBEC3B-like mutational patterns and mRNA expression of the *APOBEC3A*, *APOBEC3B*, *UNG*, *REV1*, and *FHIT* genes in cancer cell lines, in order to identify those cancer cell lines that may have experienced kataegis events. We further examined associations between mutational patterns of APOBEC3 activity, individual cancer types, and chemosensitivity to a variety of antitumor agents. This analysis was carried out using whole-exome sequencing (WES) data, gene expression microarray data, and drug response data for 255 agents from the Cancer Cell Line Encyclopedia (CCLE) [33, 34] and the GDSC resource [30, 35, 36].

Methods

Analysis of whole-exome sequencing data

We downloaded unprocessed WES BAM files, which were available for 325 CCLE cell lines (Fig. 1), from the CCLE project at the National Cancer Institute (NCI) Cancer Genomics Hub; these data are available at the NCI Genomic Data Commons (GDC) data portal [37]. All CCLE WES data had been reported to be sequenced at the Broad Institute using the same version of the Agilent Exome Bait kit, and the same sequencing protocols and data processing pipeline were applied to all samples across all cancer categories [37, 38].

Raw BAM files were preprocessed according to the GATK Best Practices pipeline v. 3.5 as of 15 May 2016 [39–41] using default or recommended parameters for each tool and using Hg19 as the reference human genome assembly. Single nucleotide variant discovery using preprocessed BAM files was carried out with VarScan2 using default parameters [42]. Nucleotide substitutions were filtered by their allele frequencies in the 1000 Genomes Project dataset (August 2015 release), eliminating common population variants with variant allele frequency > 1% in the combined 1000 Genomes Project dataset from all populations [43]. To identify the prevalence of mutation counts, we computed the sum of identified single nucleotide variants across all sequenced exome regions in several separate categories of DNA sequence changes including all SNV mutation counts, as well as C>G, C>T, and C>K counts on one or both genome strands.

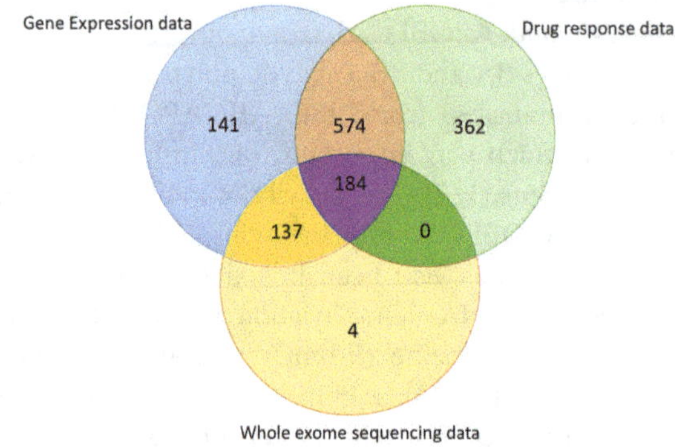

Fig. 1 Venn diagram showing the numbers of CCLE cell lines with available data

We searched the WES nucleotide changes in each cell line for the presence of the three reported APOBEC3B mutation motifs, T(C>K)W, T(C>D)R, or T(C>D)D. This motif representation includes nucleotide IUPAC symbols in three consecutive genome sequence positions, with the two symbols in parenthesis separated by the ">" symbol indicating the direction of nucleotide substitution change. For example, T(C>K)W indicates that the reference genome sequence is 5′-TCA-3′ or 5′-TCT-3′, and an either C>G or C>T substitution was found in the second nucleotide of the triplet. We refer to the three sequence motifs, T(C>K)W, T(C>D)R, and T(C>D)D which were analyzed in this study, as APOBEC-like motifs, in order to distinguish them from the APOBEC mutational signature term, which commonly refers to a matrix of mutational changes that are characteristic of APOBEC activity in the 96-trinucletide format [14, 44]. Both motif and signature formats represent the same patterns of APOBEC mutational activity, and both terms have been used interchangeably in the earlier reports [10].

Because APOBEC activity is characterized by clusters of co-occurring APOBEC motifs with closely spaced mutations on the same genome strands, we further searched each cell line for the presence of kataegis clusters, which were defined using two different but related criteria, either as (a) the same motif occurring on the same genome strand at least five times in a 1000-bp window, to which we refer as 5/1000; or as (b) the same motif occurring on the same genome strand at least six times in a 10,000-bp window, to which we refer as 6/10000. For each cell line, four possible measures of APOBEC-like mutational activity were considered, which defined overall abundance of the APOBEC-like motifs and the abundance and the length of kataegis clusters per WES data of that cell line: (1) the total number of APOBEC-like motifs present in the WES data of each cell line, (2) the number of APOBEC motifs in distinct non-overlapping kataegis regions in WES data of that cell line, (3) the number of distinct non-overlapping kataegis regions in WES data of that cell line, and (4) the total combined length of distinct non-overlapping kataegis regions in WES data of that cell line. We also examined seven overall nucleotide substitution counts for each cell line, including the combined counts of all categories of nucleotide substitutions, and the numbers of C>G, C>T, or C>K substitutions on the reference genome strand and on both genome strands.

Gene expression analysis

Log_2-transformed gene expression levels that were available for 1036 cell lines from the Cancer Cell Line Encyclopedia (Fig. 1) were downloaded from the CCLE web resource of the Broad Institute [34]. These measures had been generated using Affymetrix Human Genome U133 Plus 2.0 microarrays and normalized using the Robust Multi-array Average (RMA) algorithm [33, 45]. We analyzed expression of five genes, *APOBEC3B*, *APOBEC3A*, *REV1*, *UNG*, and *FHIT*, which may be involved in generation of *APOBEC*-like mutation motifs. Gene expression data from multiple microarray probes for each gene were averaged. Microarray-derived gene expression values for each gene analyzed in this study were in strong agreement with RNA-seq gene expression measures which recently became available from the CCLE resource [34], with Spearman correlation coefficient ρ between 0.883 and 0.947 and the correlation p values $\leq 3.33 \times 10^{-144}$ for each of the five genes (data not shown).

To examine possible associations of expression levels of *APOBEC3A* and *APOBEC3B* with the germline *APOBEC3B* gene deletion, we downloaded the copy number status of the *APOBEC3B* gene from the CCLE web resource of the Broad Institute [34]. The copy number data had been generated by the CCLE Consortium using Affymetrix 6.0 SNP arrays, with segmentation of normalized log_2 ratios of the copy number estimates performed using the circular binary segmentation algorithm [34].

Analysis of drug response

The IC50 measures of cell line chemosensitivity, representing the total drug inhibitor concentration that reduced cell activity by 50%, were available for 24 drug agents from the Cancer Cell Line Encyclopedia [33] (Fig. 1). These data were downloaded from the CCLE web resource of the Broad Institute [34]. In addition, chemosensitivity values for 251 drug agents for the same cell lines were available from the Genomics of Drug Sensitivity in Cancer resource [30, 35, 36]. GDSC drug response data, in the ln(IC50) format, were obtained from the supplementary Table 4A of Iorio et al. [30]. All drug sensitivity values derived from the CCLE and GDSC datasets were transformed to the log_{10}(IC50) scale, to which we further refer as log(IC50). Identities of cell lines present in both CCLE and GDSC datasets were verified using information from Cellosaurus [46]. Drug sensitivity measures for 11 agents which were present in both CCLE and GDSC datasets were analyzed separately for the CCLE and GDSC response measures. For those agents that had duplicate measurements within the GDSC dataset [30], we analyzed their drug response by using a combined average of their drug response measurements from separate experiments. The resulting dataset had 275 CCLE and GDSC drug response measures for 255 distinct antitumor agents. The concordance of drug response measures between the CCLE and GDSC datasets has been studied extensively [47, 48] and validated in an independent screening study [49]. While some authors questioned the extent of the agreement between the two sets of measures [48], most studies confirmed that for the majority of the agents, a solid overall agreement was found between the drug response measures, cell line classification as sensitive or resistant, and molecular predictors of drug sensitivity derived from the GDSC and CCLE datasets [47, 49].

Statistical analysis

We examined Spearman rank-order correlation among gene expression values, mutation counts, measures of abundance of motifs and kataegis clusters, and drug sensitivity values (log_{10}(IC50)) in a combined analysis of all cancer types and within individual types of cancer. The p values were adjusted for multiple testing using the Benjamini and Hochberg method of adjustment for false discovery rate, or FDR [50], accounting for 275 drug sensitivity measures, 3 APOBEC-like motifs, 7 different categories of mutation counts, and expression levels of 5 candidate genes. Correlations with FDR adjusted $p < 0.05$ were considered statistically significant. In this report, ρ denotes the Spearman correlation coefficient, p is a p value prior to FDR adjustment, p_{adj} is an FDR-adjusted p value, N_{tests} is the number of correlation tests for which the FDR adjustment of p values was made, and n is the sample size (the number of cell lines used in estimation or the number of pairs included in the correlation analysis). We focused our discussion on statistically significant moderate or strong correlation results with $p_{adj} < 0.05$ and the absolute value of Spearman correlation coefficient $|\rho| > 0.25$.

Analyses of candidate gene expression levels, motif and kataegis cluster abundance, and correlation analyses were performed both in a combined dataset of all cell lines from different cancer types (pan-cancer analysis), and also within 32 individual cancer categories (Table 1). Many cancer categories were based on TCGA definitions. However, some cancer types from the same organ were grouped in broader categories in order to allow for an inclusion of a broader range of the cell lines than those defined by the TCGA enrollment criteria, and additional categories were included with several cancer types not presented in TCGA (e.g., small cell lung cancer and pediatric tumor categories). These categories are described in Table 1 and in the list of abbreviations. Only those cancer types for which at least 5 cell lines had pairs of available matching data (e.g., WES and expression, expression and drug response, or WES and drug response information) were included in the stratified correlation analyses of individual cancer categories. Accordingly, adjustment for false discovery rate in correlation analyses accounted for 23 cancer categories with ≥ 5 cell lines per category for gene expression comparisons, 17 cancer categories with ≥ 5 cell lines that had both expression and WES data, 26 cancer histologies with expression and chemosensitivity data, and 26 cancer types with ≥ 5 cell lines that had both drug sensitivity data and counts of specific APOBEC-like motif counts derived from WES data. All cell lines with available data were included in the pan-cancer correlation analysis combining all cancer categories. To examine the possible effect of the estrogen receptor status on drug sensitivity of breast cancer cell lines, we performed an additional stratified analysis of ER^+ and ER^- breast cancer cell lines, with their estrogen receptor status defined based on available literature reports [51–54].

Bioinformatic and statistical analyses were performed using Python v. 2.7 and R v. 3.4.

Results

Candidate gene expression patterns

Table 1 provides expression levels of each candidate gene in the cell lines from individual cancer types as well as average gene expression levels in the pan-cancer dataset. Examination of gene expression measures in the pan-cancer dataset showed a bimodal distribution of *APOBEC3B* expression (Fig. 2b), whereas *APOBEC3A*, *REV1*, *UNG*, and *FHIT* had unimodal distributions of their expression measures (Fig. 2a, c–e). Analysis of the *APOBEC3B* copy number status showed that low levels of *APOBEC3B* expression were observed both in the samples with the *APOBEC3B* gene loss due to the *APOBEC3B* germline deletion polymorphism and in a number of samples without the loss of the *APOBEC3B* gene (Fig. 2f). The expression of *APOBEC3A* was low in many of the cell lines (mean = 3.89; Table 1; Fig. 2a), in agreement with an earlier study [7].

When compared to the mean *APOBEC3A* and *APOBEC3B* gene expression levels in the pan-cancer dataset (Table 1; mean expression values of 3.89 and 8.43, respectively), cell lines from the following cancer categories had elevated expression values of both *APOBEC3A* and *APOBEC3B*: bladder (mean values of 4.11 and 9.59, respectively), head and neck (HNSC; 4.93 and 9.54), chronic myelogenous leukemia (LCML; 6.20 and 12.56), and multiple myeloma (MM; 4.12 and 9.52). Several other cancer types had increased levels of expression of the *APOBEC3B* gene, but their mean expression levels of *APOBEC3A* were comparable to the mean *APOBEC3A* expression across all cancer types. Among the cancer categories with ≥ 5 cell lines, these included acute myeloid leukemia (LAML; mean *APOBEC3B* expression of 9.44) and melanoma (MEL; 9.81).

Our findings of elevated *APOBEC3B* and *APOBEC3A* expression in cell lines from several cancer types presented in Table 1 were consistent with earlier studies of patient-based samples. Many earlier studies reported elevated expression and activity of *APOBEC3B* and *APOBEC3A* in bladder cancer and of *APOBEC3B* in head and neck cancer patients [5, 6, 9, 55, 56]. APOBEC-derived mutagenesis is considered to be the predominant mutation source in 65% of invasive bladder cancers in the TCGA dataset [57]. Similarly, a genomic signature attributed to APOBEC3 activity was reported in a subset of patients with all melanoma subtypes, although C>T transitions attributed to APOBEC activity could be confounded with UV-induced substitutions in many melanoma cells [12, 57, 58]. Increased expression and activity of both *APOBEC3A* and *APOBEC3B* were also reported in multiple myeloma patients, most commonly in those with the t(14:16) translocation, which was associated with poor survival [56, 59, 60].

Elevated levels of *UNG* expression, but not of other candidate genes, were found in the prostate adenocarcinoma (PRAD; 10.15) and small cell lung cancer (SCLC; 10.10) cell lines (Table 1). Clusters of single-strand mutation patterns suggestive of APOBEC activity were previously reported in prostate cancer [56], and it may be possible that increased *UNG* expression may contribute to mutagenesis in that cancer category. Because abrogated FHIT activity may increase the levels of mutagenesis both as a standalone mechanism and synergistically with APOBEC3B [7, 9, 32], we note that cell lines from several cancer types including head and neck (4.85) and sarcoma (4.87) had a considerably lower mean *FHIT* expression than the pan-cancer average (5.74). Therefore, both high levels of *APOBEC3B* and *APOBEC3A* and low levels of *FHIT* expression may influence APOBEC mutagenesis in the head and neck cancer.

Table 1 Expression of the five candidate genes in cell lines from different cancer types

Cancer type	n	*APOBEC3A*		*APOBEC3B*		*UNG*		*REV1*		*FHIT*	
		Range	Mean ± SD	Range	Mean ± SD	Range	Mean ± SD	Range	Mean ± SD	Range	Mean ± SD
ALL	2	3.40–3.75	3.58 ± 0.25	3.72–9.33	6.53 ± 3.97	10.04–10.56	10.3 ± 0.37	7.52–7.56	7.54 ± 0.03	4.68–7.33	6.01 ± 1.87
BLADDER	27	3.49–6.87	4.11 ± 0.74	3.60–11.51	9.59 ± 1.64	7.86–10.93	9.7 ± 0.81	5.86–8.21	7.01 ± 0.50	4.27–7.10	5.14 ± 0.70
BREAST	59	3.11–6.18	3.88 ± 0.47	3.13–11.28	8.78 ± 2.07	7.00–11.16	9.62 ± 0.82	5.89–8.31	6.98 ± 0.40	4.29–7.26	5.66 ± 0.82
CESC	22	3.14–4.81	3.79 ± 0.33	3.29–10.98	8.87 ± 2.15	8.28–10.39	9.62 ± 0.63	6.45–8.1	7.09 ± 0.45	4.29–7.73	5.87 ± 1.1
CLLE	78	3.29–6.63	3.87 ± 0.46	3.06–11.46	8.01 ± 2.39	7.37–11.50	9.7 ± 0.72	6.53–8.18	7.4 ± 0.36	4.46–10.24	6.59 ± 1.51
COAD/READ	62	3.22–4.54	3.81 ± 0.33	3.02–11.91	8.70 ± 2.30	7.67–10.97	9.75 ± 0.69	6.23–7.76	7.07 ± 0.29	4.30–7.81	6.05 ± 0.89
DA	2	3.36–3.37	3.36 ± 0.01	3.41–3.56	3.49 ± 0.11	9.36–9.95	9.66 ± 0.42	6.97–7.19	7.08 ± 0.16	4.75–4.96	4.85 ± 0.15
EC	26	3.34–5.21	3.90 ± 0.46	3.03–11.81	8.80 ± 2.39	8.51–10.64	9.69 ± 0.55	6.19–7.79	7.06 ± 0.38	4.49–8.34	5.29 ± 0.90
GLIOMA	79	3.27–4.44	3.76 ± 0.25	3.07–11.45	8.42 ± 2.71	7.82–11.09	9.34 ± 0.64	6.32–8.03	7.00 ± 0.34	4.08–7.33	5.13 ± 0.63
HNSC	33	3.34–11.29	4.93 ± 1.86	6.51–11.66	9.54 ± 1.27	7.82–10.35	9.01 ± 0.68	6.25–8.18	7.24 ± 0.45	4.26–6.06	4.85 ± 0.34
LAML	5	3.53–4.74	3.96 ± 0.47	8.14–10.67	9.44 ± 1.06	8.35–10.43	9.67 ± 0.82	7.22–7.69	7.47 ± 0.21	5.80–7.53	6.67 ± 0.80
LCML	1	6.20	6.20	12.56	12.56	9.79	9.79	6.54	6.54	7.69	7.69
LIHC	34	3.34–4.64	3.82 ± 0.3	3.34–12.42	8.39 ± 2.62	7.82–10.72	9.55 ± 0.67	6.07–8.02	6.88 ± 0.39	4.26–7.48	5.33 ± 0.74
MATBCL	60	3.36–5.15	3.84 ± 0.34	3.31–11.76	7.09 ± 2.68	5.81–10.69	9.33 ± 1.1	6.45–8.05	7.27 ± 0.44	4.34–10.67	6.35 ± 1.38
MB	2	3.48–3.83	3.65 ± 0.25	3.48–5.86	4.67 ± 1.68	7.69–9.75	8.72 ± 1.45	6.77–6.94	6.85 ± 0.12	6.00–7.68	6.84 ± 1.19
MEL	59	3.45–4.35	3.87 ± 0.21	3.47–11.81	9.81 ± 1.52	7.32–10.51	9.12 ± 0.62	6.41–7.91	6.91 ± 0.3	4.34–7.67	5.55 ± 0.78
MEN	3	3.65–4.05	3.85 ± 0.20	8.78–9.64	9.08 ± 0.48	8.69–9.72	9.15 ± 0.53	6.47–6.93	6.76 ± 0.25	4.84–5.96	5.25 ± 0.62
MESO	2	3.80–3.95	3.88 ± 0.11	9.92–11.05	10.48 ± 0.79	9.32–9.58	9.45 ± 0.19	6.61–6.8	6.71 ± 0.14	4.18–5.80	4.99 ± 1.15
MGCT	3	3.37–3.62	3.53 ± 0.14	7.19–9.23	8.28 ± 1.03	7.33–8.09	7.77 ± 0.40	6.40–6.73	6.60 ± 0.17	4.73–5.86	5.27 ± 0.57
MM	28	3.46–5.61	4.12 ± 0.48	2.96–12.09	9.52 ± 2.54	7.10–10.85	9.42 ± 0.91	5.83–7.31	6.68 ± 0.36	4.99–8.74	6.96 ± 1.00
NSCLC	186	3.06–7.82	3.79 ± 0.52	3.04–11.92	7.98 ± 2.59	7.85–11.31	9.67 ± 0.64	5.98–8.28	7.08 ± 0.45	4.14–8.11	5.43 ± 0.80
OVARIAN	51	3.31–4.46	3.72 ± 0.24	3.09–10.98	8.06 ± 2.3	7.32–10.71	9.35 ± 0.72	6.29–7.99	7.00 ± 0.32	4.26–8.38	5.79 ± 0.97
PAAD	44	3.28–6.13	3.89 ± 0.50	3.10–11.66	8.95 ± 2.31	7.50–10.95	9.54 ± 0.8	6.48–8.42	7.19 ± 0.36	4.43–7.44	5.34 ± 0.72
PNET	3	3.21–3.59	3.45 ± 0.21	2.94–3.50	3.21 ± 0.28	9.16–10.09	9.54 ± 0.49	6.57–7.58	7.06 ± 0.51	4.43–6.97	5.58 ± 1.29
PRAD	7	3.58–4.07	3.81 ± 0.19	3.33–9.99	8.10 ± 2.18	9.49–11.20	10.15 ± 0.67	6.48–7.65	6.98 ± 0.43	5.04–7.38	5.94 ± 1.01
RCC	36	3.23–4.17	3.70 ± 0.22	3.17–11.25	8.87 ± 1.97	7.70–9.98	9.18 ± 0.51	6.52–7.59	6.96 ± 0.25	4.57–7.05	5.7 ± 0.73
SAR	43	3.38–4.29	3.74 ± 0.23	3.15–11.24	8.37 ± 2.37	7.57–10.73	9.26 ± 0.79	6.48–7.95	7.03 ± 0.39	4.14–6.36	4.87 ± 0.49
SCLC	7	3.01–4.11	3.67 ± 0.39	3.28–11.28	7.38 ± 3.16	9.54–10.60	10.10 ± 0.45	6.88–8.02	7.49 ± 0.41	5.07–6.6	5.71 ± 0.55
STAD	38	3.16–4.58	3.72 ± 0.27	3.21–11.68	7.88 ± 2.68	8.51–10.38	9.53 ± 0.52	5.97–7.75	7.01 ± 0.44	4.35–7.81	5.62 ± 0.9
THCA	13	3.37–4.28	3.66 ± 0.22	3.87–10.97	8.57 ± 2.14	8.07–10.31	9.21 ± 0.62	6.32–7.67	6.94 ± 0.36	4.34–7.63	5.49 ± 0.98
UCEC	6	3.40–4.05	3.66 ± 0.26	3.81–10.99	8.84 ± 2.63	9.36–10.14	9.82 ± 0.32	6.18–7.28	6.78 ± 0.45	4.53–8.11	5.82 ± 1.32
MISC	15	3.36–6.68	4.01 ± 0.80	4.50–11.28	8.83 ± 1.80	7.18–10.42	9.11 ± 1.07	6.47–8.38	7.28 ± 0.53	4.17–6.90	5.26 ± 0.74
Pan-cancer	1036	3.23–8.48	3.89 ± 0.61	3.02–12.42	8.43 ± 2.43	7.00–11.50	9.41 ± 0.78	5.83–8.18	7.05 ± 0.42	4.14–10.67	5.74 ± 1.16

n number of cell lines for each cancer type with available Affymetrix U133 2.0 plus microarray expression data, *SD* standard deviation, *ALL* acute lymphocytic leukemia, *BLADDER* bladder cancer, *BREAST* breast cancer, *CESC* cervical squamous cell carcinoma and endocervical adenocarcinoma, *CLLE* chronic lymphocytic leukemia, *COAD/READ* colon adenocarcinoma and rectum adenocarcinoma, *DA* duodenal adenocarcinoma, *EC* esophageal cancer, *GLIOMA* glioma brain tumors, *HNSC* head and neck squamous cell carcinoma, *LAML* acute myeloid leukemia, *LCML* chronic myelogenous leukemia, *LIHC* liver hepatocellular carcinoma, *MATBCL* mature B cell lymphoma, *MB* medulloblastoma, *MEL* melanoma, *MEN* meningioma, *MESO* mesothelioma, *MGCT* malignant giant cell tumor of bone, *MM* multiple myeloma, *NSCLC* non-small cell lung cancer, *OVARIAN* ovarian cancer, *PAAD* pancreatic adenocarcinoma, *PNET* primitive neuroectodermal tumors, *PRAD* prostate adenocarcinoma, *RCC* renal cell carcinoma, *SAR* sarcoma, *SCLC* small cell lung cancer, *STAD* stomach adenocarcinoma, *THCA* thyroid carcinoma, *UCEC* uterine corpus endometrial carcinoma, *MISC* other miscellaneous categories of cancer including rare cancers or cancers with unspecified information, *Pan-cancer* combined analysis of all cancer categories

Expression levels of *APOBEC3B* showed strong and statistically significant positive correlation with *APOBEC3A* expression in 21 cancer categories (Table 2; ρ between 0.576 and 1.000; $p_{adj} < 0.05$). These categories (NSCLC, LAML, GLIOMA, COAD/READ, MATBCL, STAD, OVARIAN, RCC, MEL, CLLE, SAR, BREAST, BLADDER, LIHC, EC, PAAD, HNSC, CESC, MM, THCA, and UCEC; see legend of Table 1 and the list of abbreviations for their description) included both solid tumors and hematological malignancies. A strong positive and highly significant

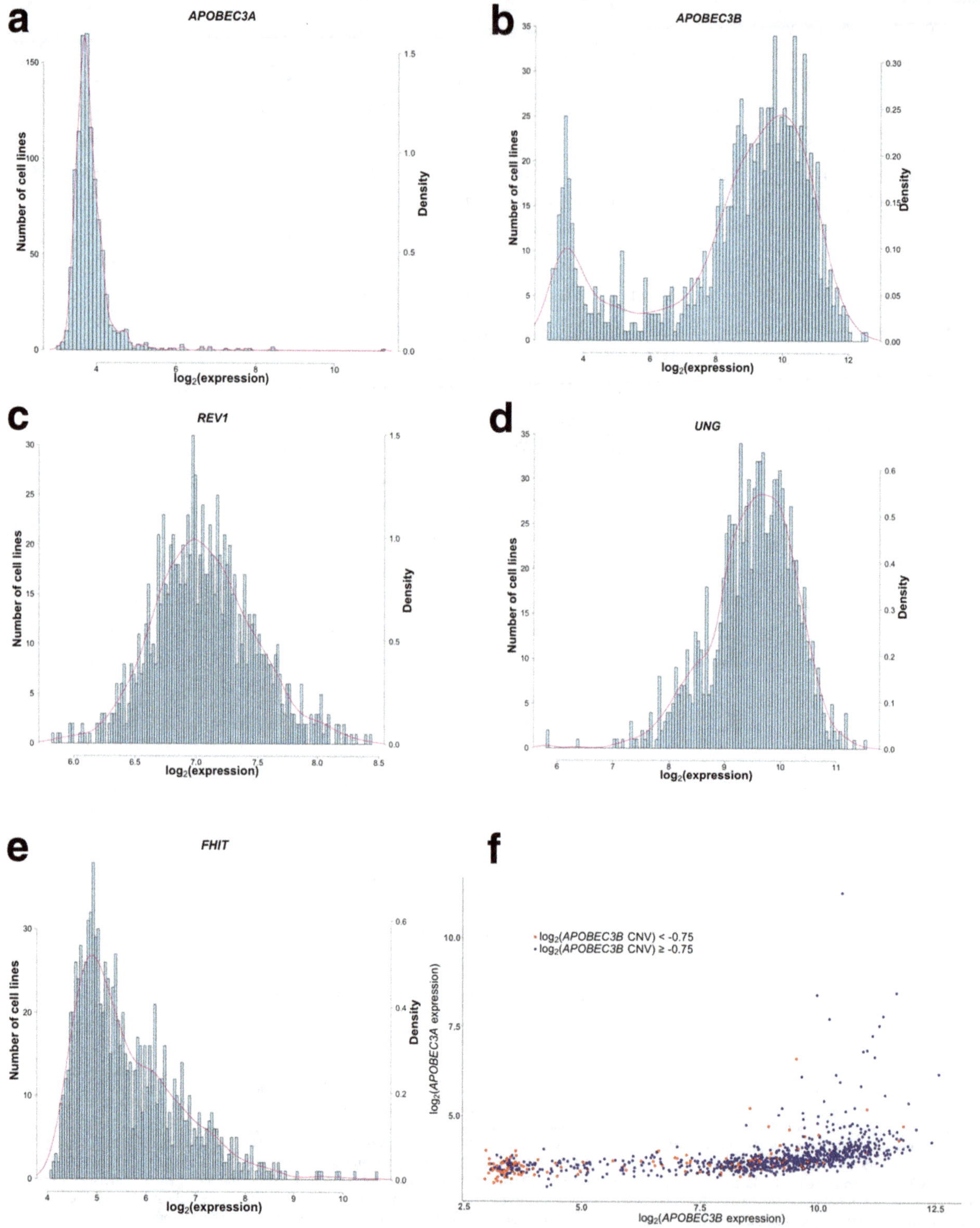

Fig. 2 a–e Histograms and density functions showing the distributions of expression of the five candidate genes in the cell lines. **a** *APOBEC3A*. **b** *APOBEC3B*. **c** *REV1*. **d** *UNG*. **e** *FHIT*. Horizontal scale represents $\log_2$-transformed gene expression values. The left vertical scale represents cell line counts, whereas the right vertical scale represents density values. **f** A scatterplot of *APOBEC3B* vs *APOBEC3A* expression in 1012 cell lines from the CCLE microarray expression dataset which shows the copy number status of the *APOBEC3B* gene according to the CCLE data [33]. Cell lines with $\log_2$(normalized ratio of *APOBEC3B* copy number estimate) ≥ -0.75 are shown in blue, whereas those with $\log_2$(normalized ratio of *APOBEC3B* copy number estimate) < -0.75 are shown in red

Table 2 Significant correlations among candidate gene expression levels

Gene 1	Gene 2	n	ρ	p	p_{adj}	Cancer category
Within individual cancer categories						
APOBEC3B	*APOBEC3A*	186	0.741	1.15×10^{-33}	2.64×10^{-31}	NSCLC
APOBEC3B	*APOBEC3A*	5	1.000	1.40×10^{-24}	1.61×10^{-22}	LAML
APOBEC3B	*APOBEC3A*	62	0.759	8.88×10^{-13}	6.81×10^{-11}	COAD/READ
APOBEC3B	*APOBEC3A*	78	0.690	2.83×10^{-12}	1.44×10^{-10}	CLLE
APOBEC3B	*APOBEC3A*	79	0.686	3.12×10^{-12}	1.44×10^{-10}	GLIOMA
APOBEC3B	*APOBEC3A*	38	0.811	6.60×10^{-10}	2.53×10^{-8}	STAD
APOBEC3B	*APOBEC3A*	51	0.712	4.82×10^{-9}	1.58×10^{-7}	OVARIAN
APOBEC3B	*APOBEC3A*	44	0.746	6.12×10^{-9}	1.76×10^{-7}	PAAD
APOBEC3B	*APOBEC3A*	60	0.651	1.73×10^{-8}	4.43×10^{-7}	MATBCL
APOBEC3B	*APOBEC3A*	59	0.612	2.65×10^{-7}	6.09×10^{-6}	BREAST
APOBEC3B	*APOBEC3A*	26	0.805	7.04×10^{-7}	1.47×10^{-5}	EC
UNG	*REV1*	186	0.344	1.56×10^{-6}	2.98×10^{-5}	NSCLC
APOBEC3B	*APOBEC3A*	59	0.576	1.81×10^{-6}	3.20×10^{-5}	MEL
APOBEC3B	*APOBEC3A*	27	0.773	2.30×10^{-6}	3.78×10^{-5}	BLADDER
APOBEC3B	*APOBEC3A*	43	0.639	3.95×10^{-6}	6.06×10^{-5}	SAR
APOBEC3B	*APOBEC3A*	36	0.637	3.00×10^{-5}	0.0004	RCC
APOBEC3B	*APOBEC3A*	34	0.645	3.83×10^{-5}	0.0005	LIHC
APOBEC3B	*APOBEC3A*	22	0.747	6.48×10^{-5}	0.0008	CESC
APOBEC3B	*APOBEC3A*	33	0.636	6.87×10^{-5}	0.0008	HNSC
APOBEC3B	*FHIT*	79	−0.407	0.0002	0.0022	GLIOMA
APOBEC3B	*APOBEC3A*	28	0.632	0.0003	0.0034	MM
APOBEC3B	*APOBEC3A*	13	0.769	0.0021	0.0221	THCA
APOBEC3B	*UNG*	60	−0.372	0.0034	0.0342	MATBCL
APOBEC3A	*UNG*	78	−0.324	0.0039	0.0369	CLLE
APOBEC3B	*APOBEC3A*	6	0.943	0.0048	0.0442	UCEC
Across all cancer categories						
APOBEC3B	*APOBEC3A*	1036	0.714	1.91×10^{-162}	1.91×10^{-161}	Pan-cancer
UNG	*REV1*	1036	0.189	8.04×10^{-10}	4.02×10^{-9}	Pan-cancer
APOBEC3B	*REV1*	1036	−0.118	0.0001	0.0005	Pan-cancer
APOBEC3B	*FHIT*	1036	−0.088	0.0046	0.0115	Pan-cancer
APOBEC3B	*UNG*	1036	−0.070	0.0251	0.0426	Pan-cancer
APOBEC3A	*UNG*	1036	−0.068	0.0291	0.0426	Pan-cancer
UNG	*FHIT*	1036	0.068	0.0298	0.0426	Pan-cancer

Listed are significant correlations with $p_{adj} < 0.05$. The p values were adjusted for false discovery rate accounting for five genes ($N_{tests} = 10$). Among individual cancer categories, FDR adjustment also accounted for 23 cancer categories with ≥ 5 cell lines with available expression data in both genes ($N_{tests} = 230$). Abbreviations of cancer categories are provided in the legend of Table 1

n sample size for correlation analysis, ρ Spearman correlation coefficient, p p value prior to FDR adjustment, p_{adj} FDR-adjusted p value

correlation between *APOBEC3B* and *APOBEC3A* expression was also observed in the pan-cancer analysis (Table 2; $\rho = 0.714$, $p_{adj} < 0.001$, $n = 1036$, $N_{tests} = 10$). Interestingly, breast cancer cell lines were among the cancer types with positive correlation between *APOBEC3A* and *APOBEC3B* expression (Table 2). Earlier studies found strong evidence for increased *APOBEC3B* activity and mutagenesis in a subset of breast cancers [7, 20, 21, 61] and with APOBEC signature enrichment in the HER2 breast cancer subtype and in triple negative breast cancer (TNBC) [6, 62]; however, a study of breast cancer cell lines found generally low levels of *APOBEC3A* expression [29]. Possible molecular impact of coordinated expression levels of *APOBEC3A* and *APOBEC3B* in the breast cancer cell lines analyzed in our study is of interest and requires further investigation.

Expression of *APOBEC3B* was significantly negatively correlated with *FHIT* expression in glioma cell lines ($\rho = -0.407$, $p_{adj} = 0.0022$, $n = 79$, $N_{tests} = 230$). This negative correlation is notable because low levels of the *FHIT* gene expression or the loss of FHIT function have been reported to have a cooperative effect with APOBEC3B in mutagenesis, even though *APOBEC3B* overexpression and DNA damage induced by the replication stress caused by the loss of FHIT have been proposed to occur independently from each other [7, 9, 32]. Negative correlation between *APOBEC3B* and *FHIT* expression levels could potentially produce hypermutated clusters in those cells where *APOBEC3B* expression were elevated and *FHIT* expression were diminished. However, this did not appear to be the case because in our analysis of glioma cell lines, which included astrocytoma, lower-grade glioma, and glioblastoma multiforme cell lines, mean APOBEC3B and *FHIT* expression levels were comparable to those in the pan-cancer dataset (Table 1). Such expression levels were consistent with earlier studies [12, 63], which had reported low levels of *APOBEC3B* in lower-grade glioma TCGA patient samples and had suggested that mutation processes in glioma tumors could be caused by mechanisms other than APOBEC mutagenesis.

UNG expression was negatively correlated with *APOBEC3B* expression in mature B cell lymphoma cell lines (MATBCL; $\rho = -0.372$, $p_{adj} = 0.034$, $n = 60$, $N_{tests} = 230$) and with *APOBEC3A* expression in chronic lymphocytic leukemia cells (CLLE; $\rho = -0.324$, $p_{adj} = 0.037$, $n = 78$, $N_{tests} = 230$). Expression levels of *UNG* and *REV1* were significantly positively correlated in non-small cell lung cancer cell lines (NSCLC; $\rho = 0.344$, $p_{adj} = 2.98 \times 10^{-5}$, $n = 186$, $N_{tests} = 230$).

APOBEC-like mutation motifs and mutation loads in cancer cell lines

Prevalence of mutation counts and single nucleotide positions in the combined analysis of all cancer categories and within individual cancer types in the 325 cell lines with available WES data is provided in Table 3. Because some individual cancer categories had small sample sizes of the

Table 3 Prevalence of mutation counts in the whole-exome sequencing data

		C>G		C>T		C>K		All SNV counts	
Cancer type	*n*	Range	Mean ± SD	Range	Mean ± SD	Range	Mean ± SD	Range	Mean ± SD
BLADDER	6	5297–7790	6564 ± 968	19,570–28,590	24,077 ± 3408	24,867–36,380	30,640 ± 4373	54,376–78,947	66,878 ± 9294
BREAST	14	6141–8460	6860 ± 566	22,789–33,262	25,705 ± 2548	28,930–41,722	32,564 ± 3102	63,719–89,515	71,153 ± 6292
CESC	15	6309–7994	7095 ± 530	23,581–34,126	28,889 ± 3587	29,890–41,452	35,984 ± 3926	65,633–101,318	79,411 ± 9753
COAD/READ	16	5332–7595	6657 ± 664	20,925–36,866	25,962 ± 3970	26,257–44,461	32,620 ± 4555	59,552–89,617	70,796 ± 8093
EC	3	6703–7357	6954 ± 353	24,685–27,760	25,752 ± 1740	31,486–35,117	32,706 ± 2088	68,907–76,008	71,472 ± 3940
GLIOMA	18	5833–7682	6713 ± 458	21,183–28,151	24,924 ± 1644	27,016–35,833	31,637 ± 2096	60,001–78,102	69,420 ± 4414
HNSC	18	5195–7378	6714 ± 467	20,073–27,050	25,054 ± 1618	25,268–34,428	31,768 ± 2074	55,628–75,813	69,801 ± 4531
CLLE	42	4235–8400	6974 ± 723	17,410–32,021	26,545 ± 2888	21,645–40,010	33,520 ± 3549	47,685–86,517	72,972 ± 7267
LIHC	17	5864–8444	7007 ± 497	22,051–30,565	25,793 ± 1781	27,915–39,009	32,800 ± 2266	61,208–85,224	72,102 ± 4850
MATBCL	29	6350–8912	7209 ± 593	23,674–33,141	27,029 ± 2170	30,125–42,053	34,239 ± 2751	66,014–91,667	74,874 ± 5935
MEL	17	5722–8448	6759 ± 631	22,174–31,819	25,874 ± 2324	27,896–40,267	32,633 ± 2945	60,650–87,815	70,805 ± 6434
MESO	1	6112	6112	21,790	21,790	27,902	27,902	62,016	62,016
MM	17	6187–8662	6840 ± 628	22,773–32,455	25,456 ± 2338	28,960–41,117	32,296 ± 2961	63,335–88,898	70,785 ± 6192
NSCLC	36	5509–8739	6927 ± 768	20,710–32,767	25,641 ± 2666	26,219–41,506	32,567 ± 3424	57,506–90,159	71,563 ± 7520
OVARIAN	15	5951–7461	6682 ± 503	22,453–27,222	25,077 ± 1500	28,433–34,683	31,760 ± 1988	62,699–75,986	69,753 ± 4383
PAAD	16	5011–7432	6640 ± 588	19,327–27,658	24,801 ± 2144	24,338–35,090	31,441 ± 2725	53,010–76,653	68,905 ± 5941
PRAD	4	5699–6889	6423 ± 512	20,538–28,059	25,092 ± 3450	26,237–34,948	31,515 ± 3947	57,717–74,831	68,722 ± 8018
RCC	8	6521–7566	6980 ± 411	24,508–27,801	26,133 ± 1383	31,082–35,264	33,114 ± 1783	68,091–77,777	72,638 ± 4113
SAR	12	6336–7808	6968 ± 423	23,647–29,155	26,129 ± 1610	29,983–36,963	33,098 ± 2027	65,833–81,175	72,342 ± 4357
STAD	16	5861–7530	6807 ± 448	21,971–28,460	25,305 ± 1763	27,832–35,741	32,112 ± 2199	61,311–79,632	70,672 ± 4843
THCA	3	5811–6918	6463 ± 579	22,080–25,849	24,363 ± 2007	27,891–32,767	30,826 ± 2586	61,598–71,836	67,720 ± 5406
UCEC	2	6063–6489	6276 ± 301	24,128–24,223	24,176 ± 67	30,286–30,617	30,452 ± 234	66,406–67,542	66,974 ± 803
Pan-cancer	325	4235–8912	6865 ± 618	17,410–36,866	25,867 ± 2575	21,645–44,461	32,732 ± 3139	47,685–101,318	71,661 ± 6693

Shown are counts of C>T, C>G, and C>K substitutions on both genome strands, and of any types of SNV variants representing nucleotide substitutions
K G or T, *SD* standard deviation, *SNV* single nucleotide variant, *n* number of cell lines

cell lines with WES data, not all mutation counts in cell lines were representative of mutation counts in large patient samples for specific cancer types. For example, mutation counts at single nucleotide positions in the bladder cancer category, which included six cell lines, were lower than the typically high mutation rates that are commonly seen in bladder cancer patients [12, 57, 64]. However, clusters of mutations in genome regions have been reported to provide a more robust representation of mutational processes in tumor genomes that do average mutation rates at single positions [13]. As discussed below, the prevalence of APOBEC-like motifs and kataegis clusters (Fig. 3) in bladder cancer cell lines and in cell lines from several other cancer categories of our dataset was generally consistent with the relative ranking of cancer categories previously described using patient data.

Table 4 shows the abundance of the three APOBEC-like motifs and their predicted kataegis clusters in WES sequence data of CCLE cell lines in the combined analysis of all cancer types. Among the three motifs, the commonly reported APOBEC3B motif with narrow specificity, T(C>K)W [7], resulted in the smallest numbers of predicted motifs (mean ± standard deviation of 603.58 ± 121.17) and kataegis clusters (0.12 ± 0.36 clusters of 5 motifs in 1000-bp windows per cell line), followed by higher numbers of motifs (743.51 ± 317.68) and kataegis clusters (0.56 ± 0.77) for the T(C>D)R motif. The highest numbers of APOBEC-like motifs (1184.94 ± 887.46) and clusters (2 ± 1.2 per cell line) were predicted for the least specific motif, T(C>D)D. That motif included possible nucleotide changes of both motifs T(C>K)W and T(C>D)R. Similar patterns were observed for the combined length of the 5/1000 kataegis clusters, the numbers of motifs in distinct 5/1000 clusters, or when considering 6/10000 kataegis clusters (Table 4).

Similar trends in the abundance of motifs and kataegis-like clusters were also observed among individual cancer categories, as presented in Fig. 3, which shows the

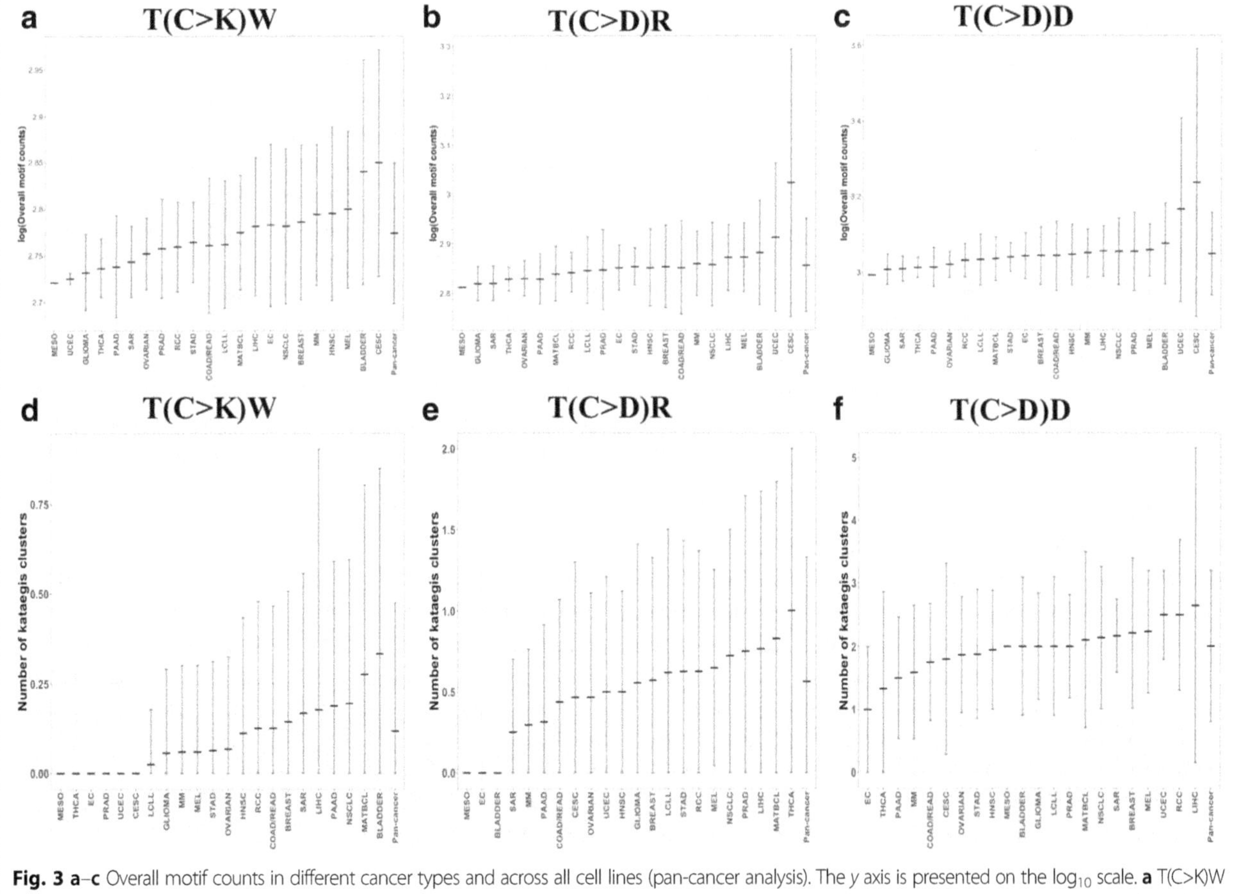

Fig. 3 a–c Overall motif counts in different cancer types and across all cell lines (pan-cancer analysis). The *y* axis is presented on the $\log_{10}$ scale. **a** T(C>K)W motif counts. **b** T(C>D)R motif counts. **c** T(C>D)D motif counts. **d–f** Numbers of distinct, not overlapping 5/1000 kataegis clusters with ≥ 5 motifs on the same genome strand per 1000 bp in different cancer types and in the pan-cancer dataset. **d** T(C>K)W motif counts. **e** T(C>D)R motif counts. **f** T(C>D)D motif counts. Horizontal middle bars show the mean for each cancer category. Vertical bars show mean ± standard deviation. Negative values of (mean – standard deviation) in **d** and **e** were truncated at 0. Cancer categories with no vertical columns had no predicted kataegis clusters (**d–f**) and/or too few cell lines to compute the standard deviation (*n* = 2 for mesothelioma, **a–c**)

Table 4 Prevalence of APOBEC mutation motifs and kataegis clusters in a combined analysis of all cancer categories

Measure	T(C>K)W		T(C>D)R		T(C>D)D	
	Range	Mean ± SD	Range	Mean ± SD	Range	Mean ± SD
Total motif count	381–1369	603.58 ± 121.17	465–4633	743.51 ± 317.68	715–13,461	1184.94 ± 887.46
Predicted non-overlapping kataegis clusters, 5/1000						
Number of motifs in distinct clusters	0–16	0.6 ± 1.87	0–21	2.9 ± 3.99	0–69	10.71 ± 6.8
Number of distinct clusters	0–3	0.12 ± 0.36	0–4	0.56 ± 0.77	0–11	2 ± 1.2
Combined length (bp) of distinct clusters	0–1994	76.95 ± 238.6	0–3148	418.47 ± 615.59	0–7484	1327.31 ± 894.04
Predicted non-overlapping kataegis clusters, 6/10000						
Number of motifs in distinct non-overlapping clusters	0–95	0.87 ± 6.08	0–93	3.93 ± 8.34	0–221	10.26 ± 16.69
Number of distinct non-overlapping clusters	0–10	0.11 ± 0.67	0–8	0.53 ± 0.86	0–18	1.45 ± 1.65
Combined length (bp) of distinct clusters	0–89,163	750.11 ± 5802.03	0–78,974	2997.94 ± 7701	0–147,285	5323.27 ± 12,925.39

Shown are values per cell line, computed using whole-exome sequence data of each cell line

SD standard deviation, *5/1000* a kataegis cluster with ≥ 5 motifs on the same genome strand per 1000 bp, *6/10000* a kataegis cluster with ≥ 6 motifs on the same genome strand per 10,000 bp

distributions of motif counts and numbers of the 5/1000 kataegis clusters among cell lines from different cancer types. For the most specific APOBEC motif, T(C>K)W, the highest mean number of motifs per cell line was observed in cervical squamous cell carcinoma and endocervical adenocarcinoma (CESC; mean = 736 motifs per cell line), followed by bladder cancer (mean = 716 motifs), and melanoma (mean = 642 motifs; Fig. 3a). These categories have been reported to have high levels of APOBEC3 activity [12], although some C>K mutations in melanoma were likely caused by ultraviolet (UV) radiation [10, 14]. The highest mean number of the 5/1000 kataegis clusters with the T(C>K)W motif was observed in bladder cancer (mean = 0.33 clusters per cell line), followed by mature B cell lymphoma (MATBCL; mean = 0.28 clusters), and NSCLC (mean = 0.19 clusters; Fig. 3d). For a less specific motif, T(C>D)R, the three cell line categories with the highest mean numbers of motifs were CESC (mean = 1343 motifs per cell line), uterine corpus endometrial carcinoma (UCEC; mean = 842 motifs), and bladder cancer (mean = 781 motifs; Fig. 3b). While high levels of APOBEC3 activity have been reported in these cancers, additional mechanisms may also be contributing to UCEC mutagenesis [12]; in addition, only two UCEC cell lines had WES data, resulting in a very small sample size. The highest mean number of the 5/1000 kataegis clusters with the T(C>D)R motif was observed for THCA (mean = 1.00 cluster), followed by MATBCL (mean = 0.83 clusters) and the liver hepatocellular carcinoma (LIHC; mean = 0.76; Fig. 3e). The highest counts of the third and the least specific motif, T(C>D)D, were found in CESC (mean = 2744 motifs per cell line), UCEC (mean = 2177 motifs), and bladder cancer cell lines (mean = 1221 motifs; Fig. 3c). These cancer categories been reported to have strong APOBEC3 activity [12]. The highest numbers of 5/1000 kataegis clusters with the T(C>D)D motif were observed in LIHC (mean = 2.65 clusters), renal cell carcinoma (RCC; mean = 2.50 clusters), and UCEC (mean = 2.50 clusters; Fig. 3f). When 6/10000 kataegis clusters (data not shown), the two cancer types with the highest mean numbers of kataegis clusters were LIHC (mean = 0.76 clusters for T(C>K)W, 1.24 clusters for T(C>D)R, and 3.24 clusters for the T(C>D)D motif) and RCC (mean = 0.38, 0. 88, and 2.13 clusters, respectively).

Our findings for bladder cancer, melanoma, non-small cell lung cancer, uterine corpus endometrial carcinoma, and prostate adenocarcinoma were consistent with previous reports which suggested the roles for APOBEC3 mutagenesis in those cancer types [5, 6, 12, 57, 60, 65]. In contrast, APOBEC3B was reported to be less likely to play a role in mutagenesis of renal cell carcinoma cell lines [6, 12, 65], suggesting that high prevalence of mutation clusters in the RCC cell lines observed in our study could be generated by molecular factors other than APOBEC3B. The increased prevalence of mutagenic clusters in mature B cell lymphoma cell lines may be explained by the effects of translesion synthesis DNA polymerase η [13, 66]. It is also possible that some of the mutations in MATBCL could be explained by a partial overlap of the motifs examined in our study with a characteristic signature for another member of the APOBEC family, the activation-induced cytidine deaminase (AID), which has been linked to mutagenesis in MATBCL. However, AID has a distinct preference for the WRCY/RGYW motif, and its mutational signature is distinguishable from that of APOBEC3A/B [9, 10, 16, 67], and therefore, it is less likely that an increased number of APOBEC3-like motifs found in MATBCL could be attributed to AID activity.

The statistically significantly increased *APOBEC3B* gene and protein expression in hepatocellular carcinoma as compared to non-tumor tissues, as well as the high rates of C>D mutation changes in the genomes of hepatocellular carcinoma tumors have been documented previously [68–72], in agreement with an increased prevalence of APOBEC-like motifs in LIHC cell lines in our dataset (Fig. 3). However, the potential role of APOBEC3B in mutagenesis in hepatocellular carcinoma has been controversial, with some studies reporting its tumor-inducing roles and others suggesting that it may play a role in tumor suppression. Mutation signature analysis found the presence of signatures other than those induced by APOBEC3B in patient samples of hepatocellular carcinoma [11]. Other molecular factors such as transcription-coupled repair, inhibition of UNG accompanied by APOBEC3G-induced hypermutation, translesion synthesis by one of the DNA polymerases, or the role of APOBEC1 have been implicated in mutagenesis of hepatocellular carcinomas [10, 17, 69–71, 73, 74], and therefore it may be possible that the increased prevalence of APOBEC-like motif clusters in LIHC cell lines may be caused by factors other than APOBEC3B.

Correlation of gene expression levels with mutation counts and with prevalence of APOBEC-like motifs

Analysis of the pan-cancer dataset showed a very weak correlation ($|r| \leq 0.161$) of expression levels of candidate genes with motif counts, counts of kataegis clusters, and mutation counts in the WES data. None of these correlations were statistically significant ($p_{adj} \geq 0.08$). Among the five candidate genes, the strongest correlations were observed for *APOBEC3A*, *APOBEC3B*, and *REV1*.

Among individual cancer types, we observed a strong (ρ between − 0.738 and − 0.902) and statistically significant ($p_{adj} < 0.05$) negative correlation of the frequencies of C>T, C>G, and C>K substitutions and overall nucleotide substitution counts with *REV1* expression in sarcoma and *UNG* expression in melanoma (Table 5). The third ranking gene for correlations with mutation counts was *APOBEC3A*. Although it did not reach the stringent threshold of FDR adjusted $p < 0.05$, it showed strong positive correlations ($\rho \leq 0.90$, $p_{adj} \geq 0.07$) with several categories of mutation counts in renal cell carcinoma. *APOBEC3B* expression also had the strongest correlation with mutation counts in RCC as opposed to other cancer categories; however, such correlations for *APOBEC3B* were somewhat weaker and less significant ($\rho \leq$ 0.86, $p_{adj} \geq 0.16$) than those for *APOBEC3A* (data not shown). These correlation results suggest a strong contribution of REV1, UNG, and possibly APOBEC3A to overall mutagenesis in sarcoma, melanoma, and renal cell carcinoma, respectively. A large proportion of C>T and C>G substitutions in melanoma cell lines were likely generated via mutagenic processes related to UV radiation exposure [10, 14]. However, the role for APOBEC3 in melanoma mutagenesis has also been established in a subset of melanomas [58], and experimental evidence has suggested an important role of APOBEC3A generating mutations specific to skin lesions [75].

Table 5 Statistically significant correlations of gene expression levels with mutation counts

Gene	Mutation count	n	ρ	p	p_{adj}	Cancer type
REV1	C>K[b]	12	− 0.902	6.00×10^{-5}	0.0114	Sarcoma
REV1	C>K[a]	12	− 0.895	8.37×10^{-5}	0.0114	Sarcoma
REV1	C>T[b]	12	− 0.895	8.37×10^{-5}	0.0114	Sarcoma
REV1	Any	12	− 0.881	0.0002	0.0114	Sarcoma
REV1	C>T[a]	12	− 0.881	0.0002	0.0114	Sarcoma
REV1	C>G[a]	12	− 0.867	0.0003	0.0119	Sarcoma
REV1	C>G[b]	12	− 0.867	0.0003	0.0119	Sarcoma
UNG	C>K[a]	17	− 0.816	6.45×10^{-5}	0.0114	Melanoma
UNG	Any	17	− 0.799	0.0001	0.0114	Melanoma
UNG	C>K[b]	17	− 0.797	0.0001	0.0114	Melanoma
UNG	C>G[a]	17	− 0.787	0.0002	0.0118	Melanoma
UNG	C>T[a]	17	− 0.779	0.0002	0.0119	Melanoma
UNG	C>T[b]	17	− 0.777	0.0002	0.0119	Melanoma
UNG	C>G[b]	17	− 0.738	0.0007	0.0308	Melanoma

Shown are correlations of gene expression levels with overall mutation counts in the WES data with $p_{adj} < 0.05$. These p values were FDR adjusted for multiple comparisons that included 5 candidate genes, 17 cancer categories with ≥ 5 cell lines in each category having both WES and expression data, and 7 categories of mutation counts including C>T, C>G, and C>K on one or both genome strands, as well as overall single nucleotide variant counts (N_{tests} = 595). ">" indicates the direction of substitution change
Any all types of nucleotide substitutions, *K* G or T, *n* sample size for correlation analysis, ρ Spearman correlation coefficient, *p p* value prior to FDR adjustment, p_{adj} FDR-adjusted *p* value
[a]Mutation counts on the reference genome strand only
[b]Mutation counts on both genome strands

Among the correlations of gene expression levels with APOBEC-like motif counts and measures of kataegis, significant or nearly significant correlations were observed for *UNG* expression with kataegis measures (ρ between − 0.81 and − 0.80, $0.039 \leq p_{adj} \leq 0.063$, $n = 17$, $N_{tests} = 475$) of the T(C>D)D motif in melanoma, and for *APOBEC3A* expression with motif counts and kataegis measures in renal cell carcinoma (ρ between 0.93 and 0. 98, $0.008 \leq p_{adj} \leq 0.087$ with $n = 8$ and $N_{tests} = 510$ for the T(C>D)R and T(C>D)D motifs; data not shown).

Correlation of candidate gene expression with chemosensitivity

Table 6 lists the strongest ($|\rho| > 0.25$) statistically significant ($p_{adj} < 0.05$) correlations between candidate gene expression levels and cell line chemosensitivity to drug treatment. Several strong correlations were observed in PAAD, PRAD, CESC, MM, SAR, RCC, NSCLC, MEL, and SCLC cell lines.

In pancreatic adenocarcinoma (PAAD) cell lines, both *APOBEC3A* and *UNG* expression was significantly negatively correlated (Table 6; $\rho \leq -0.819$, $p_{adj} \leq 0.0001$; $n = 28$ for *APOBEC3A* and 5 for *UNG*; $N_{tests} = 26{,}610$) with log(IC50) of the BET inhibitor JQ1 (Fig. 4a). JQ1 has been reported to inhibit

Table 6 Strongest significant correlations between candidate gene expression and drug sensitivity

Cancer category	Gene	Agent	n	ρ	p	p_{adj}	Drug action/alternative name	Reference
PAAD	*APOBEC3A*	JQ1[a]	28	−0.819	9.70×10^{-8}	0.0001	BET inhibitor	[78]
PRAD	*APOBEC3A*	PD-0332991[a]	5	−1.000	1.40×10^{-24}	1.75×10^{-21}	Palbociclib; CDK 4/6 inhibitor	[100]
PRAD	*APOBEC3B*	GDC0941[a]	5	−1.000	1.40×10^{-24}	1.75×10^{-21}	Pictilisib; pan-class I PI3K inhibitor	[101]
PRAD	*APOBEC3B*	KIN001-260[a]	5	−1.000	1.40×10^{-24}	1.75×10^{-21}	IKKb inhibitor	[36]
PRAD	*APOBEC3B*	EHT 1864[a]	5	−1.000	1.40×10^{-24}	1.75×10^{-21}	Rac inhibitor	[102]
PRAD	*APOBEC3B*	Nutlin-3a[a]	5	−1.000	1.40×10^{-24}	1.75×10^{-21}	Inhibitor of MDM2-p53 interaction	[87]
CESC	*APOBEC3B*	ZM-447439[a]	5	−1.000	1.40×10^{-24}	1.75×10^{-21}	Aurora kinase inhibitor	[103]
MM	*APOBEC3B*	QL-VIII-58[a]	5	−1.000	1.40×10^{-24}	1.75×10^{-21}	Inhibitor of mTOR and ATR signaling	[36]
MM	*APOBEC3B*	ZG-10[a]	5	−1.000	1.40×10^{-24}	1.75×10^{-21}	Inhibitor of JNK1 and p38 signaling	[36]
SAR	*APOBEC3B*	TGX221[a]	6	−1.000	$< 4.95 \times 10^{-324}$	$< 4.95 \times 10^{-324}$	PI3Kβ inhibitor	[36]
CESC	*REV1*	MLN4924[a]	5	−1.000	1.40×10^{-24}	1.75×10^{-21}	Pevodenistat; NAE inhibitor	[36]
RCC	*REV1*	XMD8-92[a]	6	−1.000	$< 4.95 \times 10^{-324}$	$< 4.95 \times 10^{-324}$	BMK1/ERK5 inhibitor	[104]
NSCLC	*REV1*	RDEA119[a]	123	0.381	1.35×10^{-5}	0.0153	Refametinib; BAY 86-9766; MEK inhibitor	[83]
NSCLC	*REV1*	PD-0325901[a]	106	0.405	1.64×10^{-5}	0.0179	MEK inhibitor	[81]
NSCLC	*REV1*	AKT inhibitor VIII[a]	121	0.373	2.51×10^{-5}	0.0262	AKT inhibitor	[36]
NSCLC	*REV1*	Embelin[a]	121	0.366	3.61×10^{-5}	0.0349	XIAP inhibitor	[36]
NSCLC	*REV1*	Trametinib[a]	121	0.361	4.71×10^{-5}	0.0436	MEK inhibitor	[84]
NSCLC	*REV1*	AZD6482[a]	130	0.348	4.84×10^{-5}	0.0436	PI3Kβ inhibitor	[36]
NSCLC	*REV1*	PD-0332991[a]	100	0.392	5.41×10^{-5}	0.0471	Palbociclib; CDK 4/6 inhibitor	[100]
PRAD	*REV1*	NSC-207895[a]	5	1.000	1.40×10^{-24}	1.75×10^{-21}	MDMX inhibitor	[105]
PRAD	*REV1*	Piperlongumine[a]	5	1.000	1.40×10^{-24}	1.75×10^{-21}	Piplartine; ROS induction	[36]
PRAD	*UNG*	ZM-447439[a]	5	1.000	1.40×10^{-24}	1.75×10^{-21}	Aurora kinase inhibitor	[103]
PRAD	*UNG*	NU-7441[a]	5	1.000	1.40×10^{-24}	1.75×10^{-21}	DNA-PK inhibitor	[36]
PRAD	*UNG*	CCT007093[a]	5	−1.000	1.40×10^{-24}	1.75×10^{-21}	PPM1D inhibitor	[36]
PRAD	*UNG*	JQ1[a]	5	−1.000	1.40×10^{-24}	1.75×10^{-21}	BET inhibitor	[78]
PRAD	*FHIT*	NVP-BHG712[a]	5	−1.000	1.40×10^{-24}	1.75×10^{-21}	EphB4 inhibitor	[36]
CESC	*FHIT*	MK-2206[a]	5	−1.000	1.40×10^{-24}	1.75×10^{-21}	AKT inhibitor	[36]
MEL	*FHIT*	TAE684[b]	38	0.621	3.24×10^{-5}	0.0325	ALK inhibitor	[36]
SCLC	*FHIT*	ABT-869[a]	6	−1.000	$< 4.95 \times 10^{-324}$	$< 4.95 \times 10^{-324}$	Linifanib; VEGFR/PDGFR family receptor inhibitor	[106]
SCLC	*FHIT*	Mitomycin C[a]	6	−1.000	$< 4.95 \times 10^{-324}$	$< 4.95 \times 10^{-324}$	DNA cross-linking/monoalkylating agent	[36, 107]
Pan-cancer	*APOBEC3B*	17-AAG[a]	536	−0.293	4.25×10^{-12}	5.85×10^{-9}	HSP90 inhibitor	[85]

Shown are statistically significant correlations satisfying $|\rho| > 0.25$, $p_{adj} < 0.05$. The p values were adjusted for false discovery rate accounting for 5 genes and 255 agents with 275 drug sensitivity measures from CCLE or GDSC resources ($N_{tests} = 1375$ for pan-cancer analysis). Among individual cancer categories, FDR adjustment also accounted for 26 cancer categories with ≥ 5 available cell lines in each category with both gene expression and drug sensitivity data for correlation analysis ($N_{tests} = 26{,}110$). Abbreviations of cancer categories are provided in the legend of Table 1

n sample size for correlation analysis, *ρ* Spearman correlation coefficient, *p* *p* value prior to FDR adjustment, p_{adj} FDR-adjusted *p* value, *BET* bromodomain and extraterminal family of proteins, *BRAF* v-raf murine sarcoma viral oncogene homolog B, *CDK* cyclin-dependent kinase, *DNA-PK* DNA-dependent protein kinase, *HDAC* histone deacetylase, *HSP90* molecular chaperone heat shock protein 90, *MEK* mitogen-activated protein kinase kinases, *NAE* NEDD8-activating enzyme E1, *PI3K* phosphatidylinositol-3-kinase, *ROS* reactive oxygen species, *XIAP* X-linked inhibitor of apoptosis

[a]Drug sensitivity data from GDSC [30, 35]

[b]Drug sensitivity data from Cancer Cell Line Encyclopedia (CCLE) [33]

pancreatic cancer cells in vitro and in vivo [76–78]. Correlation of *APOBEC3A* and *UNG* expression with PAAD sensitivity to JQ1 may suggest a possibility that expression of both of these genes may be relevant to the strength of the clinical response to this agent.

Expression of *REV1* in the non-small cell lung cancer cell lines was significantly positively correlated with log(IC50) of MEK (mitogen-activated protein kinase) inhibitors PD-0325901, RDEA119, and trametinib, as well as AKT inhibitor VIII, XIAP inhibitor embelin, PI3Kβ inhibitor AZD6482, and a cyclin-dependent kinase

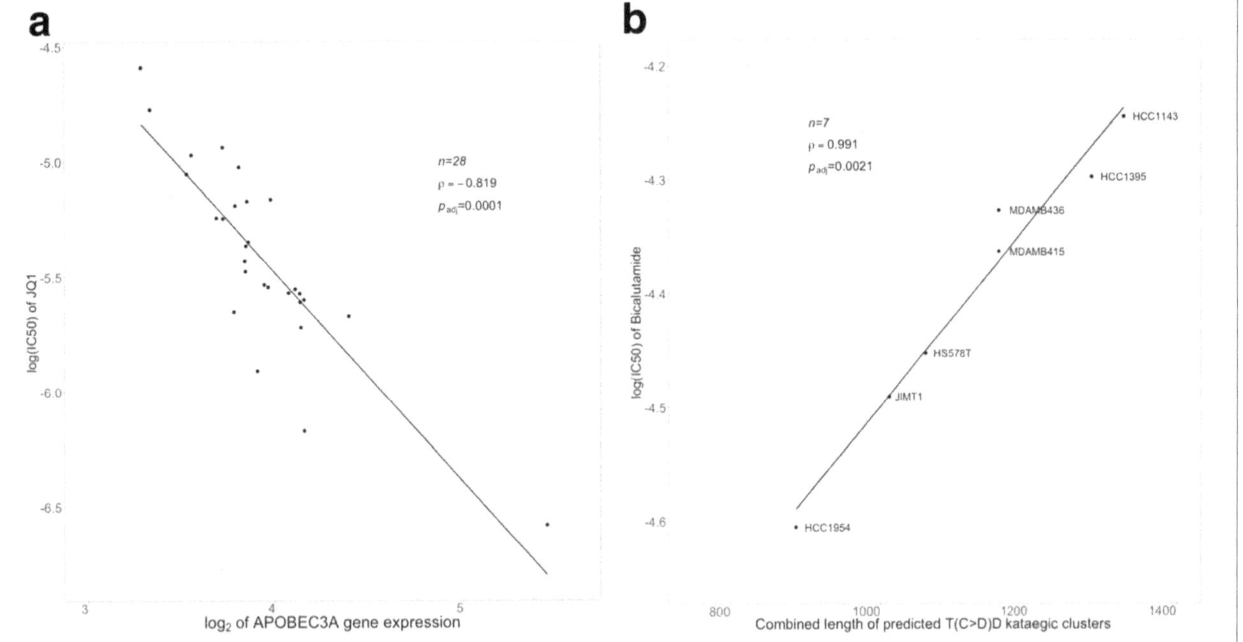

Fig. 4 Scatterplots of drug sensitivity measures from the GDSC dataset in selected cancer types. **a** log(IC50) of JQ1 vs $\log_2$ of the *APOBEC3A* gene expression in pancreatic adenocarcinoma cell lines. **b** log(IC50) of bicalutamide vs the combined length of predicted 5/1000 kataegis clusters with the T(C>D)D motif in breast cancer cell lines. The names of individual breast cancer cell lines are shown. *r* Pearson's correlation coefficient

(CDK) 4/6 inhibitor PD-0332991, or palbociclib (Table 6; $0.348 \le \rho \le 0.405$, $p_{adj} \le 0.0436$, $n \ge 100$, $N_{tests} = 26{,}610$). A number of these agents, e.g., trametinib and its combination with palbociclib, have been used or are under investigation for treatment of NSCLC [79, 80]. PD-0325901 has an in vitro inhibiting effect in NSCLC; however, a phase II clinical trial of that antitumor agent in NSCLC patients did not meet the primary efficacy end point [81, 82]. RDEA119 (refametinib) has antitumor activity in a variety of cancer types including in vitro activity in NCSLC, and it has been under evaluation for its effectiveness in NSCLC [82–84].

In melanoma cell lines, *FHIT* expression was associated with chemoresistance to the ALK inhibitor TAE684 (Table 6; $\rho = 0.621$, $p_{adj} = 0.0326$, $n = 38$, $N_{tests} = 26{,}610$).

Multiple strong significant correlations between expression levels of each of the five candidate genes and sensitivity to multiple agents were found in prostate adenocarcinoma (Table 6); however, the sample size of the PRAD category was small ($n = 5$), and therefore the validity of such correlations may require confirmation in a larger dataset. Similarly, additional correlations found in MM, SAR, CESC, RCC, and SCLC cell lines reported in Table 6 had *n* between 5 and 6 and also require a follow-up confirmation in larger datasets.

In agreement with an earlier report [31], we did not observe an association between *APOBEC3B* expression in breast cancer cell lines and sensitivity to CHK1 inhibitors AZD7762 ($\rho = -0.198$, $p_{adj} = 0.8660$, $n = 33$, $N_{tests} = 26{,}610$) or Calbiochem 681,640 ($\rho = 0.143$, $p_{adj} = 0.933$, $n = 40$, $N_{tests} = 26{,}610$, data not shown), and no other correlations between gene expression and log(IC50) in breast cancer cell lines were statistically significant. Although an association between *APOBEC3B* expression in breast cancer cells and sensitivity to another CHK1 inhibitor, CCT244747, was previously reported [29], that agent was absent from both the CCLE and the GDSC drug sensitivity data sets.

In the pan-cancer analysis, *APOBEC3B* expression was significantly negatively correlated with sensitivity to an HSP90 (molecular chaperone heat shock protein 90) inhibitor 17-AAG (tanespimycin) (Table 6; $\rho = -0.293$, $p_{adj} = 5.85 \times 10^{-9}$, $n = 536$, $N_{tests} = 1375$). Higher levels of *APOBEC3B* expression were associated with higher sensitivity to this agent, which may have a clinical significance. 17-AAG acts in a variety of tumor types [85], and sensitivity to this agent was also correlated with *APOBEC3B* in an earlier analysis of RNA-seq gene expression in the CCLE and GDSC cell lines by Cescon and Haibe-Kains [31].

Some other strong association results did not reach statistical significance, but they had p_{adj} close to 0.05. For example, higher level of expression of *APOBEC3B* in glioma was correlated with increased sensitivity to an HSP90 inhibitor AUY922 ($\rho = -0.556$, $p_{adj} = 0.0701$, $n = 44$, $N_{tests} = 26{,}610$; data not shown). This correlation may have a clinical significance, as this agent has an antitumor effect in glioblastoma [85].

Correlation between the prevalence of kataegis clusters and chemosensitivity

We examined correlations between chemosensitivity to anticancer drugs and the prevalence of predicted kataegis clusters of APOBEC-like motifs which were identified using the 5/1000 criterion. None of the correlations achieved statistical significance in the combined analysis of all cancer cell lines ($p_{adj} > 0.1$ for comparisons). In a stratified analysis among cancer types, a number of statistically significant strong correlations ($0.991 \leq |\rho| \leq 1.0$, $p_{adj} \leq 0.0021$) were observed in BREAST, COAD/READ, GLIOMA, OVARIAN, and PAAD cell lines (Table 7). However, the number of cell lines in each cancer category with significant correlations was small ($n = 5–7$), and therefore, these correlations need future confirmation in larger collections of cell lines of their respective cancer categories. Among notable correlations, the combined length of clusters with the T(C>D)D motif had a strong correlation ($5 \leq n \leq 7$, $N_{tests} = 1834$) with chemoresistance to bicalutamide, a nonsteroidal antiandrogen drug, in the pancreatic adenocarcinoma and breast cancer cell lines (Table 7; Fig. 4b). As discussed above, we did not observe a statistically significant correlation between expression of any candidate gene and the prevalence of T(C>D)D or any other motif in breast cancer cell lines. Sequence variation of breast cancer genomes is shaped by a diversity of mutational processes [86], and further investigation is needed to establish whether the T(C>D) D motif in the breast cancer cell lines is predominantly generated by APOBEC3B and APOBEC3A and/or requires an additional role or REV1, UNG, and FHIT, or whether it involves other molecular mechanisms. Bicalutamide is effective in androgen receptor (AR)-positive breast tumors [87, 88]. Previous studies demonstrated the effectiveness of this agent in triple negative breast tumors [89]. To our knowledge, no relationship between the abundance of APOBEC-like signatures and sensitivity to this agent has been reported, although HER2-enriched cell lines have been reported to have high levels of APOBEC mutagenesis and to be among the breast cancer categories that are likely to be sensitive to bicalutamide [6, 62, 89]. Consistent with an earlier report that suggested the higher prevalence of APOBEC signature in TNBC cells [62], we found that the two TNBC lines with available WES data and bicalutamide sensitivity measures, HCC1395 and MDA-MB-436, had large values of the combined length of the kataegis clusters with the T(C>D)D motif (Fig. 4b). However, both of these cell lines had relatively low sensitivity to bicalutamide in the GDSC dataset (Fig. 4b). We did not find any obvious association between molecular subtypes of the available breast cancer cell lines in our dataset, including their HER2 status [51–53], that could explain the inverse relationship between the length of the T(C>D)D motif clusters and bicalutamide sensitivity presented in Fig. 4b. It is possible that AR-positive status which is associated with bicalutamide sensitivity could affect the expression of genes involved in T(C>D)D motif signature generation; however, the exact molecular mechanisms underlying this relationship remain unclear.

Multiple other strong correlations were observed in different cancer categories. For example, in pancreatic adenocarcinoma cell lines, log(IC50) values of tipifarnib, a farnesyl transferase inhibitor of the Ras pathway [90], the AKT kinase inhibitor VIII, and the IGF1R/insulin receptor inhibitor GSK-1904529A [36] were associated ($|\rho| = 1$, $p_{adj} \leq 5.15 \times 10^{-22}$, $n = 5$, $N_{tests} = 1834$) with the overall counts of the motif T(C>K)W which is commonly attributed to *APOBEC3B* activity. Similarly, log(IC50) of the hedgehog signaling pathway inhibitor vismodegib [91] and of the PPARγ/PPARδ inhibitor FH535 [36] were associated with the overall counts of the T(C>D)R motif. The overall counts of the T(C>D)D motif were associated with log(IC50) of the PKCB inhibitor LY317615 [36], whereas the length of its predicted kataegis regions was associated with log(IC50) of the Aurora kinase A/B inhibitor Genentech Cpd10, a DNA-damaging agent gemcitabine, and, as discussed above, with a nonsteroidal antiandrogen agent bicalutamide (Table 7). While the correlation of these motif counts and kataegis measures with drug sensitivity in PAAD is notable, none of the five candidate genes had significantly associated expression with sensitivity to these agents in PAAD cell lines, although, as discussed above, in the NSCLC cell lines, log(IC50) of AKT inhibitor VIII was correlated with *REV1* expression (Table 6; $\rho = 0.373$, $p_{adj} = 2.51 \times 10^{-5}$, $n = 121$, $N_{tests} = 26{,}610$). Further validation of observations presented in Table 7 is needed in larger datasets of specific cancer types.

Discussion

We observed a bimodal distribution of *APOBEC3B* expression and unimodal distributions of *APOBEC3A*, *REV1*, *UNG*, and *FHIT* in the pan-cancer dataset (Figs. 2a–e). The bimodal distribution of *APOBEC3B* is likely due to several reasons which include previously reported differences in expression levels of this gene among specific cancer types and individual cell lines within specific cancer categories, along with the germline deletion polymorphism that results in the loss the *APOBEC3B* gene in a subset of the samples [7, 11, 17, 43, 58, 92]. The bimodal distribution of *APOBEC3B* expression is of interest since some studies previously suggested the utility of the genes with bimodally distributed expression patterns as diagnostic and prognostic biomarkers within specific cancer types [93, 94].

Table 7 Significant correlations between the measures of prevalence of APOBEC-like motifs or kataegis clusters and drug sensitivity

Motif	Measure	Agent	n	ρ	p	p_{adj}	Cancer type
T(C>K)W	Total number of motifs	WZ3105	5	1.000	1.40×10^{-24}	5.15×10^{-22}	OVARIAN
T(C>K)W	Total number of motifs	XMD15-27	5	−1.000	1.40×10^{-24}	5.15×10^{-22}	OVARIAN
T(C>K)W	Total number of motifs	Tipifarnib	5	1.000	1.40×10^{-24}	5.15×10^{-22}	PAAD
T(C>K)W	Total number of motifs	AKT inhibitor VIII	5	−1.000	1.40×10^{-24}	5.15×10^{-22}	PAAD
T(C>K)W	Total number of motifs	GSK-1904529A	5	1.000	1.40×10^{-24}	5.15×10^{-22}	PAAD
T(C>D)R	Total number of motifs	rTRAIL	6	−1.000	$< 4.95 \times 10^{-324}$	$< 4.95 \times 10^{-324}$	OVARIAN
T(C>D)R	Total number of motifs	WZ3105	5	1.000	1.40×10^{-24}	3.22×10^{-22}	OVARIAN
T(C>D)R	Total number of motifs	XMD15-27	5	−1.000	1.40×10^{-24}	3.22×10^{-22}	OVARIAN
T(C>D)R	Total number of motifs	KIN001-266	5	−1.000	1.40×10^{-24}	3.22×10^{-22}	COAD/READ
T(C>D)R	Total number of motifs	BMS-536924	5	−1.000	1.40×10^{-24}	3.22×10^{-22}	GLIOMA
T(C>D)R	Total number of motifs	HG-5-113-01	5	1.000	1.40×10^{-24}	3.22×10^{-22}	BREAST
T(C>D)R	Total number of motifs	Vismodegib	5	−1.000	1.40×10^{-24}	3.22×10^{-22}	PAAD
T(C>D)R	Total number of motifs	FH535	5	−1.000	1.40×10^{-24}	3.22×10^{-22}	PAAD
T(C>D)D	Total number of motifs	rTRAIL	6	−1.000	$< 4.95 \times 10^{-324}$	$< 4.95 \times 10^{-324}$	OVARIAN
T(C>D)D	Total number of motifs	WZ3105	5	1.000	1.40×10^{-24}	3.22×10^{-22}	OVARIAN
T(C>D)D	Total number of motifs	XMD15-27	5	−1.000	1.40×10^{-24}	3.22×10^{-22}	OVARIAN
T(C>D)D	Total number of motifs	NVP-BEZ235	5	−1.000	1.40×10^{-24}	3.22×10^{-22}	COAD/READ
T(C>D)D	Total number of motifs	T0901317	5	−1.000	1.40×10^{-24}	3.22×10^{-22}	COAD/READ
T(C>D)D	Total number of motifs	RDEA119	5	−1.000	1.40×10^{-24}	3.22×10^{-22}	COAD/READ
T(C>D)D	Total number of motifs	HG-5-113-01	5	1.000	1.40×10^{-24}	3.22×10^{-22}	BREAST
T(C>D)D	Total number of motifs	LY317615	5	1.000	1.40×10^{-24}	3.22×10^{-22}	PAAD
T(C>D)D	Length of kataegis regions	PF-4708671	6	1.000	$< 4.95 \times 10^{-324}$	$< 4.95 \times 10^{-324}$	BREAST
T(C>D)D	Length of kataegis regions	EX-527	5	−1.000	1.40×10^{-24}	2.15×10^{-22}	COAD/READ
T(C>D)D	Length of kataegis regions	KIN001-236	5	−1.000	1.40×10^{-24}	2.15×10^{-22}	COAD/READ
T(C>D)D	Length of kataegis regions	CAL-101	5	−1.000	1.40×10^{-24}	2.15×10^{-22}	COAD/READ
T(C>D)D	Length of kataegis regions	Y-39983	5	−1.000	1.40×10^{-24}	2.15×10^{-22}	COAD/READ
T(C>D)D	Length of kataegis regions	KIN001-270	5	−1.000	1.40×10^{-24}	2.15×10^{-22}	COAD/READ
T(C>D)D	Length of kataegis regions	Ruxolitinib	5	−1.000	1.40×10^{-24}	2.15×10^{-22}	COAD/READ
T(C>D)D	Length of kataegis regions	XMD14-99	5	−1.000	1.40×10^{-24}	2.15×10^{-22}	COAD/READ
T(C>D)D	Length of kataegis regions	QL-VIII-58	5	1.000	1.40×10^{-24}	2.15×10^{-22}	BREAST
T(C>D)D	Length of kataegis regions	Genentech Cpd 10	5	1.000	1.40×10^{-24}	2.15×10^{-22}	PAAD
T(C>D)D	Length of kataegis regions	Gemcitabine	5	1.000	1.40×10^{-24}	2.15×10^{-22}	PAAD
T(C>D)D	Length of kataegis regions	Bicalutamide	5	1.000	1.40×10^{-24}	2.15×10^{-22}	PAAD
T(C>D)D	Length of kataegis regions	Bicalutamide	7	0.991	1.46×10^{-5}	0.0021	BREAST

Shown are statistically significant correlations satisfying $p_{adj} < 0.05$. The p values were adjusted for false discovery rate accounting for 4 measures of abundance of each motif category, 255 agents with 275 drug sensitivity measures, and 26 cancer categories with ≥ 5 available cell lines (N_{tests} between 1358 and 1874). Drug sensitivity data for all significant correlations listed in the table were obtained from GDSC [30, 35]. Abbreviations of cancer categories are provided in the legend to Table 1

n sample size for correlation analysis, ρ Spearman correlation coefficient, p p value prior to FDR adjustment, p_{adj} FDR-adjusted p value

We observed low expression levels of *APOBEC3B* in a subset of cell lines and of *APOBEC3A* in many cell lines (Fig. 2; Table 1). Low pre-treatment levels of *APOBEC3A* have been reported previously, and expression of both *APOBEC3B* and *APOBEC3A* has been reported to increase in response to cancer cell treatment with DNA-damaging agents or as part of cellular interferon-induced transcriptional response to viral infections [7]. Low expression levels of *APOBEC3A* in nearly all cancer categories and of *APOBEC3B* in specific cancer categories may provide high levels of noise in correlation analyses [95], and therefore, association results for these genes should be interpreted with caution.

As shown in Fig. 2f, a strong correlation between *APOBEC3A* and *APOBEC3B* expression levels (Table 2) appeared to be independent from the *APOBEC3B* deletion polymorphism which removes the coding area of the *APOBEC3B* gene and creates a fusion transcript of *APOBEC3A* with the 3′-UTR of the *APOBEC3* gene, although earlier reports suggest that this transcript increases *APOBEC3A* levels due to the increase in stability of the fusion transcript [7, 17, 26]. According to Fig. 2f, the correlation between the *APOBEC3A* and *APOBEC3B* gene expression levels also appears to be independent of the copy number status of the *APOBEC3B* gene. One possible explanation could be a transcriptional co-regulation of these two genes, which are located in proximity of one another in the chromosomal region 22q13.1 [7].

Mutagenesis in cancer cells generated due to the activity of APOBEC family members, and in particular of APOBEC3B, has been a subject of many recent studies. While the contributing role of REV1, UNG, and FHIT activity to mutagenic processes has been well established [8, 9, 14, 20, 24, 66], their contribution to the generation of signatures attributed to APOBEC3B and other APOBEC family members and their possible effects on sensitivity to drug treatment have not been examined in depth. Our analysis of cancer cell lines showed that expression levels of *REV1* and *UNG* were significantly correlated with mutagenesis in sarcoma and melanoma cell lines, respectively (Table 5), and that expression of all the five genes examined in our study was significantly correlated with chemosensitivity to various antitumor agents (Table 6).

We focused our analyses on two members of the AID/APOBEC family, APOBEC3A and APOBEC3B, and on three additional genes which are involved in molecular pathways associated in their mutagenesis. Several other APOBEC family members have been implicated in mutagenic processes, with some of them, e.g., AID, APOBEC3F, and APOBEC3G, showing sequence specificities that are distinct from APOBEC3A and APOBEC3B [9, 10, 16, 96]. However, the full extent of overlap among sequence specificities of different APOBEC family members remains an active research area. While we found an increased number of APOBEC-like motifs in mature B cell lymphoma, we did not include the *AID* gene expression in our analysis because both the mutational sequence specificity of AID and the biological context in which AID mutations occur are different from those of APOBEC3B and APOBEC3A [1, 9, 10, 16]. AID is an important deaminating factor in antigen-dependent antibody diversification process of immunoglobulin (Ig) genes through somatic hypermutation and class-switch recombination, and it has also been suggested to be involved in epigenetic processes of demethylation by deaminating cytosine, 5-methylcytosine (5-mC), or 5-hmC [1, 9, 10, 16, 67]. While translocations involving the Ig genes in B cell lymphomas and off-target hypermutational activity of AID in other genome regions have been found in several other cancer types (e.g., gastric, liver, breast, ovarian, lung, and T cell lymphomas), AID-specific mutational patterns are clearly distinguishable from the APOBEC3B/A signature patterns [9, 10]. AID deaminates cytosines within the characteristic WRC motif, or more broadly the WRCY/RGYW motif, with several other AID motif variants having been reported [1, 9, 10, 16]. The AID-specific motif is different from the three motifs reported for APOBEC3B and APOBEC3A that were analyzed in our study, and AID signature patterns can be distinguished computationally from those of APOBEC3A and APOBEC3B [10, 11]. For that reason, we excluded *AID* gene expression from our analysis.

Cancer cell lines provide a convenient model for a combined analysis of molecular information and drug response to a wide range of antitumor agents which cannot be achieved in a clinical setting. However, additional factors may affect clinical outcomes in vivo, including, for example, the strength of the immune response and interaction of the tumor with surrounding tissues. Expression levels of *APOBEC3A*, *APOBEC3B*, *APOBEC3D*, *APOBEC3G*, and *APOBEC3H* in tumor specimens from cancer patients were associated with varying clinical responses to chemotherapy and with overall patient survival, and possible suggested mechanisms of such associations, which may also involve other *APOBEC* genes, include immune targeting of increased mutation diversity due to higher levels of APOBEC mutagenesis, associated inflammation, PD-L1 expression on tumor-infiltrating mononuclear cells, and the degree of T lymphocyte infiltration [7, 92, 97–99].

Because our study analyzed cell line data, it could examine only cell line response to chemotherapy and did not account for in vivo effects that may also influence therapy response. Several correlations of *APOBEC3B* and *APOBEC3A* expression and of motifs attributed to APOBEC3 activity observed in our study were consistent with drug sensitivity associations with *APOBEC3A* and *APOBEC3B* activity identified in cell line models by a previous study [31]. Our analysis of breast cancer cell lines, however, was not able to replicate the previously reported correlation of *APOBEC3B* expression level in vivo with resistance to tamoxifen in a clinical setting or in murine xenograft models in ER^+ breast cancer [18] due to the lack of statistical significance. We observed ρ between -0.118 and -0.049, $p_{adj} > 0.94$ ($n = 43$, $N_{tests} = 26{,}110$) for correlations of both *APOBEC3B* and *APOBEC3A* expression levels with log(IC50) of tamoxifen in breast cancer cell lines. Stratified analysis of ER^- and ER^+ breast cell lines with available information about their estrogen receptor status showed the absence of association in the ER^- cell lines with log(IC50) of tamoxifen ($-0.083 \leq \rho \leq -0.026$, unadjusted

$p > 0.67$, $n = 28$). In the ER$^+$ cell lines, we observed an association with sensitivity to tamoxifen for both genes (ρ = 0.– 0.362 for *APOBEC3A* and – 0.418 for *APOBEC3B*, n = 13) which was consistent with that of Law et al. [18]; however, the results for both genes in our study were statistically non-significant ($p = 0.157$ for *APOBEC3A* and 0.224 for *APOBEC3B*), possibly due to a small number of ER$^+$ breast cell lines in the dataset. Additionally, the study of Law et al. [18], which reported association of the *APOBEC3B* expression with tamoxifen resistance, included primary breast tumors from hormone therapy-naïve patients, whereas some of the cell lines in our analysis were likely obtained from patients with prior treatment. In our study, none of the correlations of chemosensitivity to tamoxifen with expression of either of the five candidate genes in any cancer category or in the pan-cancer analysis achieved statistical significance. Therefore, while our use of cell line resources was able to draw from a wealth of molecular information and the data on sensitivity to multiple tumor agents, in using the cell line-based approach, we also encountered several limitations including restricted clinical information, much smaller sample sizes than those available for patient-based clinical studies, and the absence of normal tissues from the same patients that could allow for more accurate inference of mutation calls and for tissue-specific normalization of gene expression levels.

Despite these limitations, we observed a number of correlations, e.g., those between *APOBEC3A* and *APOBEC3B* expression levels, that have also been reported in patient tumor samples [7]. In addition, our results presented in Table 6 show that expression of all five candidate genes was correlated with sensitivity to chemotherapy and that log(IC50) of a number of antitumor agents was significantly correlated not only with expression levels of *APOBEC3B*, but also with those of *APOBEC3A*, *REV1 UNG*, and *FHIT*. Three of these genes, *REV1*, *UNG*, and *APOBEC3A*, were also associated with overall mutation activity and/or with prevalence of APOBEC-like motifs and kataegis clusters in specific cancer types. Because APOBEC3A is also involved in RNA editing [26], association of its expression with drug sensitivity might potentially involve the RNA editing mechanism instead of or in addition to DNA mutagenesis; however, both of these mechanisms would require additional experimental validation. Additionally, as APOBEC3A has also been linked to epigenetic processes of DNA demethylation [1, 3, 4], its involvement in epigenetic mechanisms of sensitivity or resistance to cancer treatment cannot be ruled out, even though the associations reported in Tables 6 and 7 involve non-epigenetic agents.

Recent studies suggest that clustered mutations, including those attributed to APOBEC activity, more accurately represent mutagenic processes in tumors than do overall mutation rates [13]. We observed significant correlations of the prevalence of all the three APOBEC-like motifs with chemosensitivity to multiple agents in small groups of cell lines from specific cancer types (Table 7). When using measures of kataegis clusters, we observed correlations of the combined length of kataegis clusters of the least specific T(C>D)D motif with sensitivity to various agents in breast, pancreatic adenocarcinoma, and colon adenocarcinoma and rectum adenocarcinoma cancer cell lines. However, because expression of none of the five candidate genes was significantly associated with the abundance of the T(C>D)D motif or with the clusters containing this motif, further studies are needed to better understand the mutational pathways generating the T(C>D)D motif and to examine whether additional members of the APOBEC family or translesion DNA polymerases may contribute to its occurrence. Molecular mechanisms underlying correlations of cell line response to treatment with specific agents with motif abundance or with expression of *APOBEC3A*, *APOBEC3B*, *REV1*, *UNG*, and *FHIT* also require further investigation. Nevertheless, specific correlations observed in our studies suggest that both expression levels of candidate genes and the prevalence of APOBEC-like motifs and their clusters could potentially be examined for their roles as biomarkers of drug sensitivity to several agents. Association of activity of these genes with drug response could be examined further when significantly associated agents are evaluated in experimental in vitro studies and in a clinical setting.

Conclusions

Our analysis of cancer cell line data identified associations of drug sensitivity with expression levels of *APOBEC3A*, *APOBEC3B*, *REV1*, and *UNG* genes and with abundance of sequence motifs and kataegis clusters attributed to APOBEC activity. The analysis of exome sequence data suggested that expression of *REV1* and *UNG* and to a lesser extent of *APOBEC3A* was correlated with mutation patterns attributed to APOBEC activity, suggesting that APOBEC-like mutagenic patterns may result from the complex interplay among multiple molecular factors. Future studies may examine the biological mechanisms that could explain how each of the five genes associated with APOBEC-like mutagenic processes may contribute to sensitivity or resistance of tumor cells to cancer drug treatment.

Abbreviations

5-hmC: 5-Hydroxymethyl-cytozine; 5-hmU: 5-Hydroxymethyl-uracil; 5-mC: 5-Methylcytosine; ALL: Acute lymphocytic leukemia; APOBEC: Apolipoprotein B mRNA-editing enzyme, catalytic polypeptide-like; BET: Bromodomain and extraterminal family of proteins; BLADDER: Bladder cancer (including the TCGA category of bladder urothelial carcinoma and other types of bladder cancer); BRAF: V-raf murine sarcoma viral oncogene homolog B; BREAST: Breast cancer (including the TCGA category of breast invasive carcinoma and other types of breast carcinomas); CCLE: Cancer Cell Line Encyclopedia; CDK: Cyclin-dependent kinase; CESC: Cervical squamous cell carcinoma and endocervical adenocarcinoma; CLLE: Chronic lymphocytic leukemia; COAD/READ: Colon adenocarcinoma and rectum adenocarcinoma; DA: Duodenal adenocarcinoma; DNA-PK: DNA-dependent protein kinase;

EC: Esophageal cancer (including esophageal carcinoma and Barrett adenocarcinoma); ER$^-$: Estrogen receptor-negative; ER$^+$: Estrogen receptor-positive; FDR: False discovery rate; FHIT: Fragile histidine triad protein; GDSC: Genomics of Drug Sensitivity in Cancer; GLIOMA: Glioma brain tumors (including astrocytoma, lower-grade glioma, and glioblastoma multiforme); HDAC: Histone deacetylase; HNSC: Head and neck squamous cell carcinoma; HSP90: Molecular chaperone heat shock protein 90; Ig: Immunoglobulin; IGF1R: Insulin-like growth factor 1 receptor; IR: Insulin receptor; LAML: Acute myeloid leukemia; LCML: Chronic myelogenous leukemia; LIHC: Liver hepatocellular carcinoma; MATBCL: Mature B cell lymphoma (including lymphoid neoplasm diffuse large B cell lymphoma, Burkitt lymphoma, and other categories); MB: Medulloblastoma; MEK: Mitogen-activated protein kinase kinase; MEL: Melanoma; MEN: Meningioma; MESO: Mesothelioma; MGCT: Malignant giant cell tumor of bone; MISC: Miscellaneous categories of cancer including rare cancers or cancers with unspecified information; MM: Multiple myeloma; NAE: NEDD8-activating enzyme E1; NCI: National Cancer Institute; NSCLC: Non-small cell lung cancer (including also lung adenocarcinoma and lung squamous cell carcinoma); OVARIAN: Ovarian cancer (including the TCGA category of ovarian serous cyctadenocarcinoma and other categories); PAAD: Pancreatic adenocarcinoma; Pan-cancer: Combined analysis of all cancer categories; PI3K: Phosphatidylinositol-3-kinase; PKCB: Protein kinase C β type; PNET: Primitive neuroectodermal tumors (including neuroblastoma and other categories); PPAR: Peroxisome proliferator-activated receptor; PRAD: Prostate adenocarcinoma; RCC: Renal cell carcinoma (including kidney clear cell carcinoma, kidney papillary carcinoma, and other categories); ROS: Reactive oxygen species; SAR: Sarcoma; SCLC: Small cell lung cancer; SD: Standard deviation; STAD: Stomach adenocarcinoma; TCGA: The Cancer Genome Atlas; THCA: Thyroid carcinoma; TNCB: Triple negative breast cancer; UCEC: Uterine corpus endometrial carcinoma; UNG: Uracil-specific uracil DNA glycosylase; WES: Whole-exome sequencing; XIAP: X-linked inhibitor of apoptosis

Acknowledgements

We are grateful to the editor, Dr. Vasilis Vasiliou, and two anonymous reviewers for their helpful suggestions which improved the manuscript. We also thank Drs. Johanna Shih, Anne Monks, Hossein Hamed, Lisa McShane, and Yingdong Zhao for the helpful discussions and suggestions.

Funding

Not applicable.

Authors' contributions

JK and SV conceived the study and drafted the manuscript. SV carried out the computational analyses including the prediction of locations of APOBEC-like motifs and correlations among expression of candidate genes, APOBEC motifs prevalence, and cell line drug sensitivity. RS oversaw the statistical design and analysis of the data. JK provided biological interpretation of the study design and results and oversaw bioinformatic aspects of data analysis. All authors edited the manuscript and read and approved the final manuscript.

Consent for publication

Not applicable.

Competing interests

The authors declare that they have no competing interests.

References

1. Franchini DM, Petersen-Mahrt SK. AID and APOBEC deaminases: balancing DNA damage in epigenetics and immunity. Epigenomics. 2014;6(4):427–43.
2. Kuong KJ, Loeb LA. APOBEC3B mutagenesis in cancer. Nat Genet. 2013; 45(9):964–5.
3. Lauschke VM, Barragan I, Ingelman-Sundberg M. Pharmacoepigenetics and toxicoepigenetics: novel mechanistic insights and therapeutic opportunities. Annu Rev Pharmacol Toxicol. 2018;58:161–85.
4. Guo JU, Su Y, Zhong C, Ming GL, Song H. Hydroxylation of 5-methylcytosine by TET1 promotes active DNA demethylation in the adult brain. Cell. 2011;145(3):423–34.
5. Zou J, Wang C, Ma X, Wang E, Peng G. APOBEC3B, a molecular driver of mutagenesis in human cancers. Cell Biosci. 2017;7:29.
6. Roberts SA, Lawrence MS, Klimczak LJ, Grimm SA, Fargo D, Stojanov P, Kiezun A, Kryukov GV, Carter SL, Saksena G, et al. An APOBEC cytidine deaminase mutagenesis pattern is widespread in human cancers. Nat Genet. 2013;45(9):970–6.
7. Middlebrooks CD, Banday AR, Matsuda K, Udquim KI, Onabajo OO, Paquin A, Figueroa JD, Zhu B, Koutros S, Kubo M, et al. Association of germline variants in the APOBEC3 region with cancer risk and enrichment with APOBEC-signature mutations in tumors. Nat Genet. 2016;48(11):1330–8.
8. Harris RS. Molecular mechanism and clinical impact of APOBEC3B-catalyzed mutagenesis in breast cancer. Breast Cancer Res. 2015;17:8.
9. Rebhandl S, Huemer M, Greil R, Geisberger R. AID/APOBEC deaminases and cancer. Oncoscience. 2015;2(4):320–33.
10. Roberts SA, Gordenin DA. Hypermutation in human cancer genomes: footprints and mechanisms. Nat Rev Cancer. 2014;14(12):786–800.
11. Alexandrov LB, Nik-Zainal S, Wedge DC, Aparicio SA, Behjati S, Biankin AV, Bignell GR, Bolli N, Borg A, Borresen-Dale AL, et al. Signatures of mutational processes in human cancer. Nature. 2013;500(7463):415–21.
12. Burns MB, Temiz NA, Harris RS. Evidence for APOBEC3B mutagenesis in multiple human cancers. Nat Genet. 2013;45(9):977–83.
13. Supek F, Lehner B. Clustered mutation signatures reveal that error-prone DNA repair targets mutations to active genes. Cell. 2017;170(3):534–47. e23
14. Helleday T, Eshtad S, Nik-Zainal S. Mechanisms underlying mutational signatures in human cancers. Nat Rev Genet. 2014;15(9):585–98.
15. Fruman DA, O'Brien S. Cancer: a targeted treatment with off-target risks. Nature. 2017;542(7642):424–5.
16. Siriwardena SU, Chen K, Bhagwat AS. Functions and malfunctions of mammalian DNA-cytosine deaminases: the known knowns and the known unknowns. Chem Rev. 2016;116(20):12688–710.
17. Zhang T, Cai J, Chang J, Yu D, Wu C, Yan T, Zhai K, Bi X, Zhao H, Xu J, et al. Evidence of associations of APOBEC3B gene deletion with susceptibility to persistent HBV infection and hepatocellular carcinoma. Hum Mol Genet. 2013;22(6):1262–9.
18. Law EK, Sieuwerts AM, LaPara K, Leonard B, Starrett GJ, Molan AM, Temiz NA, Vogel RI, Meijer-van Gelder ME, Sweep FC, et al. The DNA cytosine deaminase APOBEC3B promotes tamoxifen resistance in ER-positive breast cancer. Sci Adv. 2016;2(10):e1601737.
19. Chan K, Roberts SA, Klimczak LJ, Sterling JF, Saini N, Malc EP, Kim J, Kwiatkowski DJ, Fargo DC, Mieczkowski PA, et al. An APOBEC3A hypermutation signature is distinguishable from the signature of background mutagenesis by APOBEC3B in human cancers. Nat Genet. 2015;47(9):1067–72.
20. Taylor BJ, Nik-Zainal S, Wu YL, Stebbings LA, Raine K, Campbell PJ, Rada C, Stratton MR, Neuberger MS. DNA deaminases induce break-associated mutation showers with implication of APOBEC3B and 3A in breast cancer kataegis. elife. 2013;2:e00534.
21. Burns MB, Lackey L, Carpenter MA, Rathore A, Land AM, Leonard B, Refsland EW, Kotandeniya D, Tretyakova N, Nikas JB, et al. APOBEC3B is an enzymatic source of mutation in breast cancer. Nature. 2013;494(7437):366–70.
22. Nik-Zainal S, Alexandrov LB, Wedge DC, Van Loo P, Greenman CD, Raine K, Jones D, Hinton J, Marshall J, Stebbings LA, et al. Mutational processes molding the genomes of 21 breast cancers. Cell. 2012;149(5):979–93.
23. Landry S, Narvaiza I, Linfesty DC, Weitzman MD. APOBEC3A can activate the DNA damage response and cause cell-cycle arrest. EMBO Rep. 2011;12(5):444–50.
24. Suspene R, Aynaud MM, Guetard D, Henry M, Eckhoff G, Marchio A, Pineau P, Dejean A, Vartanian JP, Wain-Hobson S. Somatic hypermutation of human mitochondrial and nuclear DNA by APOBEC3 cytidine deaminases, a pathway for DNA catabolism. Proc Natl Acad Sci U S A. 2011;108(12):4858–63.
25. Bohn MF, Shandilya SMD, Silvas TV, Nalivaika EA, Kouno T, Kelch BA, Ryder SP, Kurt-Yilmaz N, Somasundaran M, Schiffer CA. The ssDNA Mutator APOBEC3A is regulated by cooperative dimerization. Structure. 2015;23(5):903–11.

26. Salter JD, Bennett RP, Smith HC. The APOBEC protein family: united by structure, divergent in function. Trends Biochem Sci. 2016;41(7):578–94.
27. Gyorffy B, Surowiak P, Kiesslich O, Denkert C, Schafer R, Dietel M, Lage H. Gene expression profiling of 30 cancer cell lines predicts resistance towards 11 anticancer drugs at clinically achieved concentrations. Int J Cancer. 2006; 118(7):1699–712.
28. Nikkila J, Kumar R, Campbell J, Brandsma I, Pemberton HN, Wallberg F, Nagy K, Scheer I, Vertessy BG, Serebrenik AA, et al. Elevated APOBEC3B expression drives a kataegic-like mutation signature and replication stress-related therapeutic vulnerabilities in p53-defective cells. Br J Cancer. 2017;117(1): 113-23.
29. Kanu N, Cerone MA, Goh G, Zalmas LP, Bartkova J, Dietzen M, McGranahan N, Rogers R, Law EK, Gromova I, et al. DNA replication stress mediates APOBEC3 family mutagenesis in breast cancer. Genome Biol. 2016;17(1):185.
30. Iorio F, Knijnenburg TA, Vis DJ, Bignell GR, Menden MP, Schubert M, Aben N, Goncalves E, Barthorpe S, Lightfoot H, et al. A landscape of pharmacogenomic interactions in cancer. Cell. 2016;166(3):740–54.
31. Cescon DW, Haibe-Kains B. DNA replication stress: a source of APOBEC3B expression in breast cancer. Genome Biol. 2016;17(1):202.
32. Waters CE, Saldivar JC, Amin ZA, Schrock MS, Huebner K. FHIT loss-induced DNA damage creates optimal APOBEC substrates: insights into APOBEC-mediated mutagenesis. Oncotarget. 2015;6(5):3409–19.
33. Barretina J, Caponigro G, Stransky N, Venkatesan K, Margolin AA, Kim S, Wilson CJ, Lehar J, Kryukov GV, Sonkin D, et al. The Cancer Cell Line Encyclopedia enables predictive modelling of anticancer drug sensitivity. Nature. 2012;483(7391):603–7.
34. CCLE Cancer Cell Line Encyclopedia. http://www.broadinstitute.org/ccle. Accessed 22 Sept 2016.
35. Garnett MJ, Edelman EJ, Heidorn SJ, Greenman CD, Dastur A, Lau KW, Greninger P, Thompson IR, Luo X, Soares J, et al. Systematic identification of genomic markers of drug sensitivity in cancer cells. Nature. 2012;483(7391):570–5.
36. Genomics of Drug Sensitivity in Cancer. http://www.cancerrxgene.org/. Accessed 22 Sept 2016.
37. National Cancer Institute GDC Legacy Archive. https://portal.gdc.cancer.gov/legacy-archive. Accessed 10 Mar 2018.
38. Chang LC, Vural S, Sonkin D. Detection of homozygous deletions in tumor-suppressor genes ranging from dozen to hundreds nucleotides in cancer models. Hum Mutat. 2017;38(11):1449–53.
39. DePristo MA, Banks E, Poplin R, Garimella KV, Maguire JR, Hartl C, Philippakis AA, del Angel G, Rivas MA, Hanna M, et al. A framework for variation discovery and genotyping using next-generation DNA sequencing data. Nat Genet. 2011;43(5):491–8.
40. McKenna A, Hanna M, Banks E, Sivachenko A, Cibulskis K, Kernytsky A, Garimella K, Altshuler D, Gabriel S, Daly M, et al. The Genome Analysis Toolkit: a MapReduce framework for analyzing next-generation DNA sequencing data. Genome Res. 2010;20(9):1297–303.
41. Van der Auwera GA, Carneiro MO, Hartl C, Poplin R, Del Angel G, Levy-Moonshine A, Jordan T, Shakir K, Roazen D, Thibault J, et al. From FastQ data to high confidence variant calls: the genome analysis toolkit best practices pipeline. Curr Protoc Bioinformatics. 2013;11(1110):11.10.1–11.10.33.
42. Koboldt DC, Zhang Q, Larson DE, Shen D, McLellan MD, Lin L, Miller CA, Mardis ER, Ding L, Wilson RK. VarScan 2: somatic mutation and copy number alteration discovery in cancer by exome sequencing. Genome Res. 2012;22(3):568–76.
43. Auton A, Brooks LD, Durbin RM, Garrison EP, Kang HM, Korbel JO, Marchini JL, McCarthy S, McVean GA, Abecasis GR. A global reference for human genetic variation. Nature. 2015;526(7571):68–74.
44. Alexandrov LB, Nik-Zainal S, Wedge DC, Campbell PJ, Stratton MR. Deciphering signatures of mutational processes operative in human cancer. Cell Rep. 2013;3(1):246–59.
45. Irizarry RA, Hobbs B, Collin F, Beazer-Barclay YD, Antonellis KJ, Scherf U, Speed TP. Exploration, normalization, and summaries of high density oligonucleotide array probe level data. Biostatistics. 2003;4(2):249–64.
46. The Cellosaurus: a cell line knowledge resource. http://web.expasy.org/cellosaurus/. Accessed 25 Apr 2017.
47. Cancer Cell Line Encyclopedia C, Genomics of Drug Sensitivity in Cancer C: Pharmacogenomic agreement between two cancer cell line data sets. Nature 2015;528(7580):84–87.
48. Safikhani Z, Smirnov P, Freeman M, El-Hachem N, She A, Rene Q, Goldenberg A, Birkbak NJ, Hatzis C, Shi L, et al. Revisiting inconsistency in large pharmacogenomic studies. F1000Res. 2016;5:2333.
49. Haverty PM, Lin E, Tan J, Yu Y, Lam B, Lianoglou S, Neve RM, Martin S, Settleman J, Yauch RL, et al. Reproducible pharmacogenomic profiling of cancer cell line panels. Nature. 2016;533(7603):333–7.
50. Benjamini Y, Hochberg Y. Controlling the false discovery rate: a practical and powerful approach to multiple testing. J R Statist Soc. 1995;B57:289–300.
51. Lehmann BD, Bauer JA, Chen X, Sanders ME, Chakravarthy AB, Shyr Y, Pietenpol JA. Identification of human triple-negative breast cancer subtypes and preclinical models for selection of targeted therapies. J Clin Invest. 2011;121(7):2750–67.
52. Conley SJ, Bosco EE, Tice DA, Hollingsworth RE, Herbst R, Xiao Z. HER2 drives Mucin-like 1 to control proliferation in breast cancer cells. Oncogene. 2016;35(32):4225–34.
53. Neve RM, Chin K, Fridlyand J, Yeh J, Baehner FL, Fevr T, Clark L, Bayani N, Coppe JP, Tong F, et al. A collection of breast cancer cell lines for the study of functionally distinct cancer subtypes. Cancer Cell. 2006;10(6):515–27.
54. Kao J, Salari K, Bocanegra M, Choi YL, Girard L, Gandhi J, Kwei KA, Hernandez-Boussard T, Wang P, Gazdar AF, et al. Molecular profiling of breast cancer cell lines defines relevant tumor models and provides a resource for cancer gene discovery. PLoS One. 2009;4(7):e6146.
55. Hayes DN, Van Waes C, Seiwert TY. Genetic landscape of human papillomavirus-associated head and neck cancer and comparison to tobacco-related tumors. J Clin Oncol. 2015;33(29):3227–34.
56. Roberts SA, Sterling J, Thompson C, Harris S, Mav D, Shah R, Klimczak LJ, Kryukov GV, Malc E, Mieczkowski PA, et al. Clustered mutations in yeast and in human cancers can arise from damaged long single-strand DNA regions. Mol Cell. 2012;46(4):424–35.
57. Kim J, Akbani R, Creighton CJ, Lerner SP, Weinstein JN, Getz G, Kwiatkowski DJ. Invasive bladder cancer: genomic insights and therapeutic promise. Clin Cancer Res. 2015;21(20):4514–24.
58. Hayward NK, Wilmott JS, Waddell N, Johansson PA, Field MA, Nones K, Patch AM, Kakavand H, Alexandrov LB, Burke H, et al. Whole-genome landscapes of major melanoma subtypes. Nature. 2017;545(7653):175–80.
59. Manier S, Salem KZ, Park J, Landau DA, Getz G, Ghobrial IM. Genomic complexity of multiple myeloma and its clinical implications. Nat Rev Clin Oncol. 2017;14(2):100–13.
60. Walker BA, Wardell CP, Murison A, Boyle EM, Begum DB, Dahir NM, Proszek PZ, Melchor L, Pawlyn C, Kaiser MF, et al. APOBEC family mutational signatures are associated with poor prognosis translocations in multiple myeloma. Nat Commun. 2015;6:6997.
61. Nik-Zainal S, Davies H, Staaf J, Ramakrishna M, Glodzik D, Zou X, Martincorena I, Alexandrov LB, Martin S, Wedge DC, et al. Landscape of somatic mutations in 560 breast cancer whole-genome sequences. Nature. 2016;534(7605):47–54.
62. Jiang T, Shi W, Wali VB, Pongor LS, Li C, Lau R, Gyorffy B, Lifton RP, Symmans WF, Pusztai L, et al. Predictors of chemosensitivity in triple negative breast cancer: an integrated genomic analysis. PLoS Med. 2016; 13(12):e1002193.
63. Swanton C, McGranahan N, Starrett GJ, Harris RS. APOBEC enzymes: mutagenic fuel for cancer evolution and heterogeneity. Cancer Discov. 2015;5(7):704–12.
64. Weinstein JN, Akbani R, Broom BM, Wang W, Verhaak RGW, McConkey D, Lerner S, Morgan M, Creighton CJ, Smith C, et al. Comprehensive molecular characterization of urothelial bladder carcinoma. Nature. 2014;507(7492):315–22.
65. Lawrence MS, Stojanov P, Polak P, Kryukov GV, Cibulskis K, Sivachenko A, Carter SL, Stewart C, Mermel CH, Roberts SA, et al. Mutational heterogeneity in cancer and the search for new cancer-associated genes. Nature. 2013; 499(7457):214–8.
66. Sale JE. Translesion DNA synthesis and mutagenesis in eukaryotes. Cold Spring Harb Perspect Biol. 2013;5(3):a012708.
67. Dominguez PM, Shaknovich R. Epigenetic function of activation-induced cytidine deaminase and its link to lymphomagenesis. Front Immunol. 2014;5:642.
68. Gao Q, Wang ZC, Duan M, Lin YH, Zhou XY, Worthley DL, Wang XY, Niu G, Xia Y, Deng M, et al. Cell culture system for analysis of genetic heterogeneity within hepatocellular carcinomas and response to pharmacologic agents. Gastroenterology. 2017;152(1):232–42. e4
69. Wu PF, Chen YS, Kuo TY, Lin HH, Liu CW, Chang LC. APOBEC3B: a potential factor suppressing growth of human hepatocellular carcinoma cells. Anticancer Res. 2015;35(3):1521–7.
70. Totoki Y, Tatsuno K, Yamamoto S, Arai Y, Hosoda F, Ishikawa S, Tsutsumi S, Sonoda K, Totsuka H, Shirakihara T, et al. High-resolution characterization of a hepatocellular carcinoma genome. Nat Genet. 2011;43(5):464–9.

71. Kitamura K, Wang Z, Chowdhury S, Simadu M, Koura M, Muramatsu M. Uracil DNA glycosylase counteracts APOBEC3G-induced hypermutation of hepatitis B viral genomes: excision repair of covalently closed circular DNA. PLoS Pathog. 2013;9(5):e1003361.
72. Luo X, Huang Y, Chen Y, Tu Z, Hu J, Tavis JE, Huang A, Hu Y. Association of hepatitis B virus covalently closed circular DNA and human APOBEC3B in hepatitis B virus-related hepatocellular carcinoma. PLoS One. 2016;11(6): e0157708.
73. Fujimoto A, Totoki Y, Abe T, Boroevich KA, Hosoda F, Nguyen HH, Aoki M, Hosono N, Kubo M, Miya F, et al. Whole-genome sequencing of liver cancers identifies etiological influences on mutation patterns and recurrent mutations in chromatin regulators. Nat Genet. 2012;44(7):760–4.
74. Totoki Y, Tatsuno K, Covington KR, Ueda H, Creighton CJ, Kato M, Tsuji S, Donehower LA, Slagle BL, Nakamura H, et al. Trans-ancestry mutational landscape of hepatocellular carcinoma genomes. Nat Genet. 2014;46(12): 1267–73.
75. Pham P, Landolph A, Mendez C, Li N, Goodman MF. A biochemical analysis linking APOBEC3A to disparate HIV-1 restriction and skin cancer. J Biol Chem. 2013;288(41):29294–304.
76. Garcia PL, Miller AL, Kreitzburg KM, Council LN, Gamblin TL, Christein JD, Heslin MJ, Arnoletti JP, Richardson JH, Chen D, et al. The BET bromodomain inhibitor JQ1 suppresses growth of pancreatic ductal adenocarcinoma in patient-derived xenograft models. Oncogene. 2016;35(7):833–45.
77. Mazur PK, Herner A, Mello SS, Wirth M, Hausmann S, Sanchez-Rivera FJ, Lofgren SM, Kuschma T, Hahn SA, Vangala D, et al. Combined inhibition of BET family proteins and histone deacetylases as a potential epigenetics-based therapy for pancreatic ductal adenocarcinoma. Nat Med. 2015;21(10): 1163–71.
78. Leal AS, Williams CR, Royce DB, Pioli PA, Sporn MB, Liby KT. Bromodomain inhibitors, JQ1 and I-BET 762, as potential therapies for pancreatic cancer. Cancer Lett. 2017;394:76–87.
79. Tao Z, Le Blanc JM, Wang C, Zhan T, Zhuang H, Wang P, Yuan Z, Lu B. Coadministration of trametinib and palbociclib radiosensitizes KRAS-mutant non-small cell lung cancers in vitro and in vivo. Clin Cancer Res. 2016;22(1):122–33.
80. Zhao Y, Adjei AA. The clinical development of MEK inhibitors. Nat Rev Clin Oncol. 2014;11(7):385–400.
81. Ishida N, Fukazawa T, Maeda Y, Yamatsuji T, Kato K, Matsumoto K, Shimo T, Takigawa N, Whitsett JA, Naomoto Y. A novel PI3K inhibitor iMDK suppresses non-small cell lung Cancer cooperatively with A MEK inhibitor. Exp Cell Res. 2015;335(2):197–206.
82. Zhou X, Yang XY, Popescu NC. Preclinical evaluation of combined antineoplastic effect of DLC1 tumor suppressor protein and suberoylanilide hydroxamic acid on prostate cancer cells. Biochem Biophys Res Commun. 2012;420(2):325–30.
83. Adjei AA. Other signal transduction agents. In: Pass HI, Carbone DP, Johnson DH, MD JDM, Scagliotti GV, III ATT, editors. Principles and practice of lung cancer: the official reference text of the International Association for the Study of Lung Cancer (IASLC). 4th ed. Philadelphia, PA: Wolters Kluwer Health/Lippincott Williams & Wilkins; 2010. p. 739–52.
84. Akinleye A, Furqan M, Mukhi N, Ravella P, Liu D. MEK and the inhibitors: from bench to bedside. J Hematol Oncol. 2013;6:27.
85. Gaspar N, Sharp SY, Eccles SA, Gowan S, Popov S, Jones C, Pearson A, Vassal G, Workman P. Mechanistic evaluation of the novel HSP90 inhibitor NVP-AUY922 in adult and pediatric glioblastoma. Mol Cancer Ther. 2010;9(5):1219–33.
86. Morganella S, Alexandrov LB, Glodzik D, Zou X, Davies H, Staaf J, Sieuwerts AM, Brinkman AB, Martin S, Ramakrishna M, et al. The topography of mutational processes in breast cancer genomes. Nat Commun. 2016;7:11383.
87. Yang P, Chen W, Li X, Eilers G, He Q, Liu L, Wu Y, Wu Y, Yu W, Fletcher JA, et al. Downregulation of cyclin D1 sensitizes cancer cells to MDM2 antagonist Nutlin-3. Oncotarget. 2016;7(22):32652–63.
88. Arce-Salinas C, Riesco-Martinez MC, Hanna W, Bedard P, Warner E. Complete response of metastatic androgen receptor-positive breast cancer to bicalutamide: case report and review of the literature. J Clin Oncol. 2016; 34(4):e21–4.
89. Prat A, Pineda E, Adamo B, Galvan P, Fernandez A, Gaba L, Diez M, Viladot M, Arance A, Munoz M. Clinical implications of the intrinsic molecular subtypes of breast cancer. Breast. 2015;24(Suppl 2):S26–35.
90. Asati V, Mahapatra DK, Bharti SK. K-Ras and its inhibitors towards personalized cancer treatment: pharmacological and structural perspectives. Eur J Med Chem. 2017;125:299–314.
91. Sandhiya S, Melvin G, Kumar SS, Dkhar SA. The dawn of hedgehog inhibitors: Vismodegib. J Pharmacol Pharmacother. 2013;4(1):4–7.
92. Cescon DW, Haibe-Kains B, Mak TW. APOBEC3B expression in breast cancer reflects cellular proliferation, while a deletion polymorphism is associated with immune activation. Proc Natl Acad Sci U S A. 2015;112(9):2841–6.
93. Kernagis DN, Hall AH, Datto MB. Genes with bimodal expression are robust diagnostic targets that define distinct subtypes of epithelial ovarian cancer with different overall survival. J Mol Diagn. 2012;14(3):214–22.
94. Hellwig B, Hengstler JG, Schmidt M, Gehrmann MC, Schormann W, Rahnenfuhrer J. Comparison of scores for bimodality of gene expression distributions and genome-wide evaluation of the prognostic relevance of high-scoring genes. BMC Bioinformatics. 2010;11:276.
95. McClintick JN, Edenberg HJ. Effects of filtering by Present call on analysis of microarray experiments. BMC Bioinformatics. 2006;7:49.
96. Ebrahimi D, Alinejad-Rokny H, Davenport MP. Insights into the motif preference of APOBEC3 enzymes. PLoS One. 2014;9(1):e87679.
97. Mullane SA, Werner L, Rosenberg J, Signoretti S, Callea M, Choueiri TK, Freeman GJ, Bellmunt J. Correlation of Apobec Mrna expression with overall survival and pd-l1 expression in urothelial carcinoma. Sci Rep. 2016;6:27702.
98. Leonard B, Starrett GJ, Maurer MJ, Oberg AL, Van Bockstal M, Van Dorpe J, De Wever O, Helleman J, Sieuwerts AM, Berns EM, et al. APOBEC3G expression correlates with T-cell infiltration and improved clinical outcomes in high-grade serous ovarian carcinoma. Clin Cancer Res. 2016;22(18):4746–55.
99. Lan H, Jin K, Gan M, Wen S, Bi T, Zhou S, Zhu N, Teng L, Yu W. APOBEC3G expression is correlated with poor prognosis in colon carcinoma patients with hepatic metastasis. Int J Clin Exp Med. 2014;7(3):665–72.
100. Finn RS, Dering J, Conklin D, Kalous O, Cohen DJ, Desai AJ, Ginther C, Atefi M, Chen I, Fowst C, et al. PD 0332991, a selective cyclin D kinase 4/6 inhibitor, preferentially inhibits proliferation of luminal estrogen receptor-positive human breast cancer cell lines in vitro. Breast Cancer Res. 2009; 11(5):R77.
101. Sarker D, Ang JE, Baird R, Kristeleit R, Shah K, Moreno V, Clarke PA, Raynaud FI, Levy G, Ware JA, et al. First-in-human phase I study of pictilisib (GDC-0941), a potent pan-class I phosphatidylinositol-3-kinase (PI3K) inhibitor, in patients with advanced solid tumors. Clin Cancer Res. 2015;21(1):77–86.
102. Shutes A, Onesto C, Picard V, Leblond B, Schweighoffer F, Der CJ. Specificity and mechanism of action of EHT 1864, a novel small molecule inhibitor of Rac family small GTPases. J Biol Chem. 2007;282(49):35666–78.
103. Umene K, Banno K, Kisu I, Yanokura M, Nogami Y, Tsuji K, Masuda K, Ueki A, Kobayashi Y, Yamagami W, et al. Aurora kinase inhibitors: potential molecular-targeted drugs for gynecologic malignant tumors. Biomed Rep. 2013;1(3):335–40.
104. Yang Q, Deng X, Lu B, Cameron M, Fearns C, Patricelli MP, Yates JR 3rd, Gray NS, Lee JD. Pharmacological inhibition of BMK1 suppresses tumor growth through promyelocytic leukemia protein. Cancer Cell. 2010;18(3):258–67.
105. Wang H, Ma X, Ren S, Buolamwini JK, Yan C. A small-molecule inhibitor of MDMX activates p53 and induces apoptosis. Mol Cancer Ther. 2011;10(1):69–79.
106. Albert DH, Tapang P, Magoc TJ, Pease LJ, Reuter DR, Wei RQ, Li J, Guo J, Bousquet PF, Ghoreishi-Haack NS, et al. Preclinical activity of ABT-869, a multitargeted receptor tyrosine kinase inhibitor. Mol Cancer Ther. 2006;5(4): 995–1006.
107. Li VS, Tang MS, Kohn H. The effect of C(5) cytosine methylation at CpG sequences on mitomycin-DNA bonding profiles. Bioorg Med Chem. 2001; 9(4):863–73.

15

Integrating rare genetic variants into pharmacogenetic drug response predictions

Magnus Ingelman-Sundberg, Souren Mkrtchian, Yitian Zhou and Volker M. Lauschke*

Abstract

Background: Variability in genes implicated in drug pharmacokinetics or drug response can modulate treatment efficacy or predispose to adverse drug reactions. Besides common genetic polymorphisms, recent sequencing projects revealed a plethora of rare genetic variants in genes encoding proteins involved in drug metabolism, transport, and response.

Results: To understand the global importance of rare pharmacogenetic gene variants, we mapped the variability in 208 pharmacogenes by analyzing exome sequencing data from 60,706 unrelated individuals and estimated the importance of rare and common genetic variants using a computational prediction framework optimized for pharmacogenetic assessments. Our analyses reveal that rare pharmacogenetic variants were strongly enriched in mutations predicted to cause functional alterations. For more than half of the pharmacogenes, rare variants account for the entire genetic variability. Each individual harbored on average a total of 40.6 putatively functional variants, rare variants accounting for 10.8% of these. Overall, the contribution of rare variants was found to be highly gene- and drug-specific. Using warfarin, simvastatin, voriconazole, olanzapine, and irinotecan as examples, we conclude that rare genetic variants likely account for a substantial part of the unexplained inter-individual differences in drug metabolism phenotypes.

Conclusions: Combined, our data reveal high gene and drug specificity in the contributions of rare variants. We provide a proof-of-concept on how this information can be utilized to pinpoint genes for which sequencing-based genotyping can add important information to predict drug response, which provides useful information for the design of clinical trials in drug development and the personalization of pharmacological treatment.

Keywords: Pharmacogenetics, Personalized medicine, ADME genes, Genetic variability, Drug response

Background

The response of patients to medical treatment is influenced by a variety of physiological, pathological, environmental, and genetic factors [1]. These inter-individual differences can lower treatment efficacy or manifest in adverse drug reactions (ADRs), which are estimated to cause around 6.5% of all hospital admissions [2]. Overall, the genetic makeup of a patient accounts for 20–30% of the inter-individual variability in drug response [3], but for certain clinically important drugs, such as metoprolol and torsemide, twin studies suggested genetic contributions to the variability in their pharmacokinetics of up to 90% [4].

Genetic variability in phase I and phase II enzymes, transporters, cytochrome reductases, and nuclear receptors, hereafter jointly termed pharmacogenes, can modulate drug absorption, distribution, metabolism, and excretion (ADME), thereby shaping human drug response and the risk of ADRs. Prominent examples include associations of common *TPMT* variants with hematological toxicity of 6-mercaptopurines, ultrarapid metabolism of CYP2D6 with codeine toxicity, and effects of specific *CYP2C19* polymorphisms on the response to clopidogrel or proton pump inhibitors [5]. Yet, a substantial fraction of the heritable variability in drug response cannot be explained by these common variants, suggesting that other genetic factors are

* Correspondence: volker.lauschke@ki.se
Department of Physiology and Pharmacology, Section of Pharmacogenetics, Karolinska Institutet, SE-171 77 Stockholm, Sweden

important contributors. In recent years, increasing capacities and decreasing costs of next-generation sequencing (NGS) platforms have facilitated large-scale studies of genetic variation and NGS assays are becoming increasingly implemented in clinical diagnostics [6]. Importantly, NGS-based analyses revealed that over 90% of the overall genetic variability in pharmacogenes is allotted to rare genetic variants, but the impact of rare genetic variability on drug pharmacokinetics has not been systematically evaluated (Additional file 1: Table S1) [7–10].

We therefore analyzed the distribution of rare and common gene variants in the 208 clinically most relevant pharmacogenes of 60,706 unrelated individuals and leveraged these genetic variability profiles to predict the relevance of rare SNVs for the pharmacokinetics or ADR risks for several clinically important drugs of diverse therapeutic areas. Based on these analyses, we conclude that the contribution of rare genetic variants is gene- and drug-specific and can account for a substantial part of the unexplained genetic inter-individual variability in drug response. Furthermore, we highlight genes for which comprehensive NGS-based genotyping instead of candidate SNP interrogations can reveal important additional information to personalize pharmacological treatment strategies. The presented data incentivizes the consideration of rare pharmacogenetic variants for the guidance of personalized drug therapy and holds important implications for the design of clinical trials.

Methods

Data sources

Human sequencing data from 60,706 unrelated individuals was obtained from the Exome Aggregation Consortium (ExAC) database [11], a platform that provides summary frequency information of exonic genetic variants from 17 large-scale sequencing projects. Notably, consistency of the individual data sets is assured by reprocessing of all raw data through the same bioinformatic pipelines. We complemented the obtained variants with six non-exonic variants from the 1000 Genomes Project [12] that define *CYP1A2*1C* (rs2069514), *CYP1A2*1F* (rs762551), *CYP2C19*17* (rs12248560), *CYP3A4*22* (rs35599367), *CYP3A5*3* (rs776746), and *UGT1A1*28* (rs8175347). Variants with less than 10,000 called high-quality alleles were not considered. Novel variants were defined relative to dbSNP release 135.

Definitions

Loss-of-function (LoF) intolerance scores were provided by Lek et al. based on the expectation-maximization algorithm [11]. In brief, low scores (< 0.1) indicate that the number of protein-truncating variants is similar to what is expected by chance, whereas high scores (> 0.9) indicate much fewer of such variants are observed than would be expected, suggesting haploinsufficiency. Aggregated functional variant frequency is defined as the sum of MAFs of all variants predicted to be deleterious. Variants with MAF ≤ 0.01 were considered as rare, and variants with MAF > 0.01 were considered as common.

Variant analyses and computational functionality predictions

Computational algorithms mostly use evolutionary conservation as a metric to predict whether a given variant likely has functional effects. Importantly, we previously evaluated 18 current functionality prediction methods and found that their predictive performance was low for poorly conserved genes, such as cytochrome P450s [13].

Here, we therefore used a functionality prediction method that we previously developed [13]. In brief, using high-quality experimental data for 123 pharmacogenetic alleles, Zhou et al. tailored the parameterization of 18 different algorithms specifically for ADME genes and integrated the results of multiple prediction methods into an ADME-optimized prediction framework [13]. Finally, the model's performance was validated in an independent validation cohort of additional 121 experimentally characterized variants. Overall, the model achieved 92% sensitivity and 95% specificity for loss-of-function and functionally neutral variants, respectively, thereby substantially outperforming previous computational tools on pharmacogenomics data sets.

Results

Analysis of the genetic landscape in 208 human pharmacogenes

We analyzed the genetic variability in 208 genes with importance for drug ADME using exome sequencing data from 60,706 unrelated individuals. In total, we identified 69,923 variants distributed across transporter genes (33,792 variants in 73 genes), genes encoding phase 1 (21,161 variants in 71 genes) and phase 2 enzymes (10,411 variants in 46 genes), nuclear receptors (2338 variants in 9 genes), and other pharmacogenes with miscellaneous functions (2221 variants in 6 genes; Fig. 1a). Notably, 57,773 (83%) of these 69,923 variants we identified were novel as compared to dbSNP release 135 (Fig. 1b).

Evolutionary constraints in transporters as well as in phase 1 and phase 2 drug-metabolizing genes were low as judged by the large numbers of loss-of-function variants identified in these genes (LoF intolerance score $= 0.08 \pm 0.02$ SEM; see the "Methods" section for details). In contrast, nuclear receptors and other selected genes with importance for drug response were highly LoF-intolerant (LoF intolerance score $= 0.53 \pm 0.11$ SEM), comparable to values observed across haploinsufficient genes (LoF intolerance score > 0.5; Fig. 1c) [11]. Importantly, the vast majority of variants were rare (98.5%; MAF < 1%) or very rare (96.2%; MAF < 0.1%) and

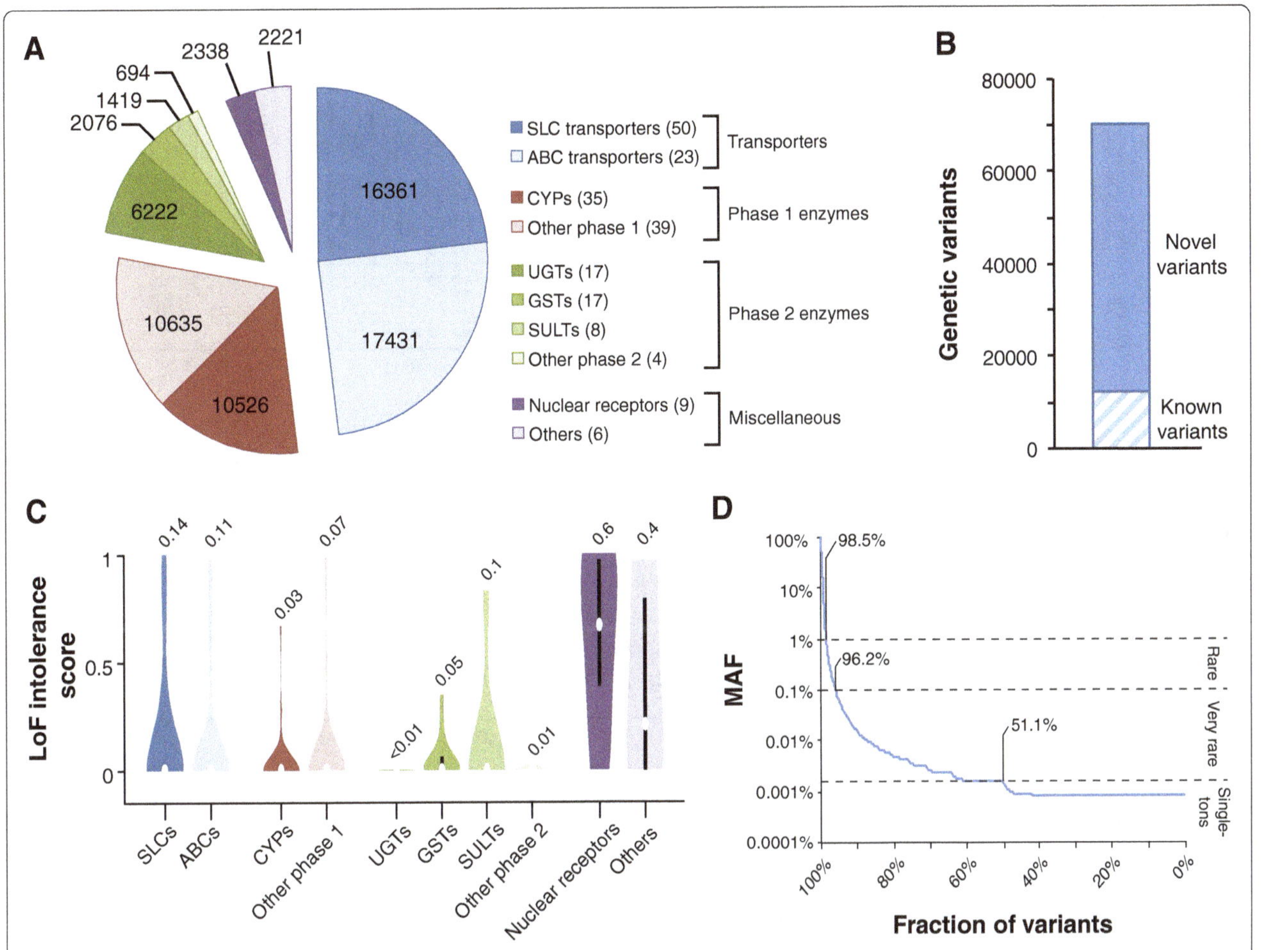

Fig. 1 The landscape of pharmacogenomic variability. **a** Pie chart showing the distribution of the identified 69,923 variants across transporters (blue), phase 1 (red) and phase 2 (green) enzymes, and other pharmacogenes (purple). **b** 57,723 (83%) of the identified 69,923 pharmacogenetic variants were novel as compared to dbSNP release 135. **c** Violin plots showing the evolutionary constraint on loss-of-function (LoF) alleles. High scores indicate significantly less LoF variants than expected by chance. Details regarding the statistical framework are given in Lek et al. [11]. Violin plots were generated using BoxPlotR [50]. **d** Of the identified variants, 98.5 and 96.2% were rare (MAF < 1%) or very rare (MAF < 0.1%), respectively, and 51.1% of all variants were only found in a single individual

more than half (51.1%) of all variants were only detected in a single individual, highlighting the genetic diversity in human pharmacogenes (Fig. 1d).

Rare variants contribute substantially to functional variability

To evaluate the functional importance of rare pharmacogenetic variants, we computed functionality assessments of each SNV using a computational assessment model specifically optimized for the assessment of pharmacogenes (see the "Methods" section for details). We then aggregated frequencies of frameshift, splice, start-lost, stop-gain, and putatively deleterious missense variants and found that the pattern and distribution of genetic variability differed substantially across the 208 pharmacogenes analyzed. Genetic variability with functional impact was governed by few high-frequency variants for some genes, including *ABCB5*, *SLC22A10*, *CYP1A2*, *CYP2C8*, or *GSTT2* (Fig. 2a). In contrast, the functionality of the majority of pharmacogenes, including *ABCB1*, *SLC10A1*, and *CYP3A7*, is dominated by rare genetic variants. The frequency of genetic variants predicted to affect the functionality of the gene product differed more than 1000-fold between genes. The most highly variable genes were *SLC22A10* (aggregated functional variant frequency 1.08), *ABCB5* (0.91), and *FMO2* (0.86), whereas the lowest numbers of functional variants were observed for *GSTT1* (0.0006), *RXRA* (0.0007), *PPARD* (0.0011), and *CYP17A1* (0.0014; Fig. 2a).

Notably, rare pharmacogenetic variants were strongly enriched in mutations predicted to cause functional alterations (Fig. 2b), consistent with previous reports [12, 14, 15]. In the 208 pharmacogenes combined, each individual harbored on average a total of 40.6 putatively functional variants (Fig. 2c). Rare variants accounted for 4.4 (10.8%) of these functional variants, of which 1.8, 1.7,

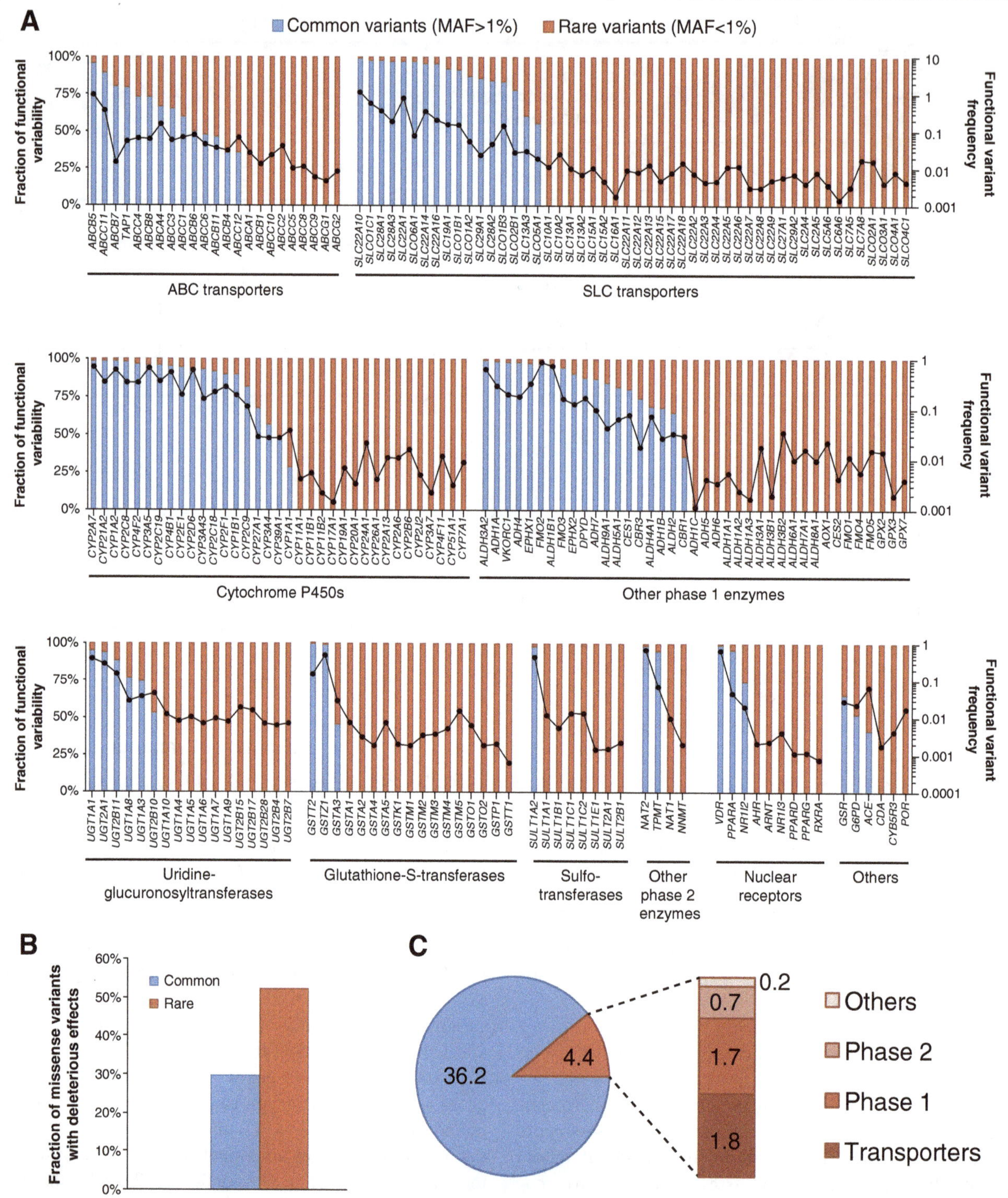

Fig. 2 Rare genetic variants contribute substantially to pharmacogenomic variability. **a** The frequency of putatively functional variants is plotted in log scale and indicated as dots connected by the black line for each of the 208 pharmacogenes analyzed (right *y*-axis). The fraction of this functional variability that is allotted to common (blue) or rare (red) variants is indicated on the left *y*-axis. Importantly, overall genetic variability as well as the fraction of functional variation that is allotted to rare variants differs considerably between genes. **b** Rare genetic polymorphisms in pharmacogenes are enriched in variants predicted to cause functional alterations. **c** Across the 208 ADME genes analyzed, each individual was found to harbor on average 4.4 rare functional variants (frameshift, splice, start-lost, stop-gain, and putatively functional missense variants). Of these, 1.8, 1.7, 0.7, and 0.2 are allotted to transporters, phase 1 and phase 2 enzymes, and other pharmacogenes, respectively

0.7, and 0.2 were allotted to transporters, phase 1, phase 2, and other pharmacogenes, respectively (Fig. 2c).

Prediction of the importance of rare genetic variants for drug response

Given the significant contribution of rare genetic variants to the functional variability in pharmacogenes, we considered it of importance to include rare variants into predictions of drug response. Using the genetic information as template, we analyzed the contribution of rare genetic variants for drug pharmacokinetics and/or drug response, focusing on five drugs with well-characterized pharmacology and substantial unexplained inter-individual variability. Specifically, we evaluated the relevance of rare SNVs for the anticoagulant warfarin, the HMG-CoA reductase inhibitor simvastatin, the antifungal voriconazole, the antipsychotic olanzapine, and the antineoplastic agent irinotecan (Additional file 2: Table S2). We first estimated the relative importance of different genetic factors for drug metabolism phenotypes of the specific drugs based on extensive literature analysis. Subsequently in a second step, we integrated these evaluations with our genetic variability data to derive assessments of the impact of rare genetic variants on the pharmacokinetics of or response to the given drug.

Warfarin response

Warfarin is a racemic mixture of the R- and S-stereoisomers of which the S-form is at least five times more potent. Warfarin response is influenced by common genetic polymorphisms in *CYP2C9*, *CYP4F2*, and *VKORC1*, which jointly explain up to 45% of warfarin dose requirements [16]. Yet also other genes, such as *CYP3A4*, *CYP1A2*, *EPHX1*, and *ABCB1*, have been implicated in warfarin pharmacokinetics [17–19]. However, despite this extensive knowledge of warfarin transport and metabolism, around 40% of the variability in warfarin dose requirements remains unexplained by common genetic variants and other patient-specific factors [20].

Our analyses predict that rare genetic variants contribute only minorly to the metabolism of the pharmacologically less potent R-enantiomer of warfarin (Fig. 3a–c). Similarly, their contribution to warfarin pharmacodynamics by alterations in CYP4F2 (3.6%) and VKORC1 (2%) function is expected to be relatively low. Importantly however, rare SNVs have a major impact on hepatic S-warfarin metabolism. Overall, 2.1% of *CYP2C9* alleles are predicted to harbor rare variants with deleterious effects, accounting for 18.4% of the genetically encoded functional differences in CYP2C9 activity (Fig. 3b). Moreover, our analyses predict rare variants with functional consequences in 1.3% of *ABCB1* alleles, encoding the P-gp/MDR1 transporter that is implicated in warfarin clearance, whereas no common deleterious variants were identified (Fig. 3b). However, given the controversy regarding the functional impacts of common *ABCB1* variants, such as rs1045642 and rs2032582, future research is necessary to delineate associations between *ABCB1* genotypes and factors related to P-gp/MDR1 activity [21]. Combined, our analyses pinpoint *CYP2C9* and *ABCB1* as loci for which comprehensive NGS profiling can likely reveal substantial additional information regarding the unexplained variability in warfarin dose requirements.

Simvastatin myopathy

ADRs related to high-dose simvastatin therapy are strongly linked to the common (12.9% MAF) genetic variant rs4149056 in *SLCO1B1* (encoding the transporter OATP1B1) with an odds ratio of 4.5 per copy of the risk allele [22]. Toxicity is caused by an impaired hepatic uptake of the drug that results in elevated plasma concentrations of simvastatin acid, which have been shown to cause myotoxicity in vitro [23] (Fig. 3d). In our analyses, we correctly predicted the functional impact of rs4149056 and did not find additional common variants with reduced functionality. However, we identified rare deleterious variants with an aggregated frequency of 1.2%, which are estimated to jointly explain 8.7% of the genetic basis of *SLCO1B1* variability (Fig. 3e). Similarly, rare variants are expected to contribute substantially to the metabolism and transport of simvastatin with an aggregated rare functional variant frequency of 1.3, 1.1, and 0.8% for *ABCB1*, *CYP3A4*, and *ABCG2*, respectively (Fig. 3f).

Voriconazole efficacy and ADRs

Voriconazole is a triazole antifungal agent exhibiting large inter-individual variability in serum concentrations that is a common reason for therapeutic failure or the manifestation of ADRs. Voriconazole is extensively metabolized by various CYPs (CYP2C19, CYP2C9, and CYP3A4) and FMOs (FMO1, FMO3, and FMO5) accounting for 75 and 25% of its hepatic metabolism, respectively (Fig. 4a) [24, 25]. Genetic polymorphisms in *CYP2C19* have been reproducibly linked to differences in voriconazole serum levels and jointly explain around 50% of the inter-individual variability in voriconazole metabolism ([26] and references therein). In addition to *CYP2C19* alleles, clinical pharmacogenetic studies also implicated reduced functionality variants of *CYP2C9* (*CYP2C9*2*) and *CYP3A4* (rs4646437) in differences in voriconazole pharmacokinetics [27, 28]. For *CYP2C19*, our analyses identified rare deleterious variants with an aggregated frequency of 1.6%, whereas the common functional *CYP2C19* alleles *CYP2C19*2* and *CYP2C19*17* showed frequencies of 18.5 and 15.3%, respectively (Fig. 4b). Consequently, rare variants are estimated to account for 4.4% of the overall genetic variability of CYP2C19 function. Furthermore, rare alleles contributed substantially to the variability in other genes implicated in voriconazole efficacy

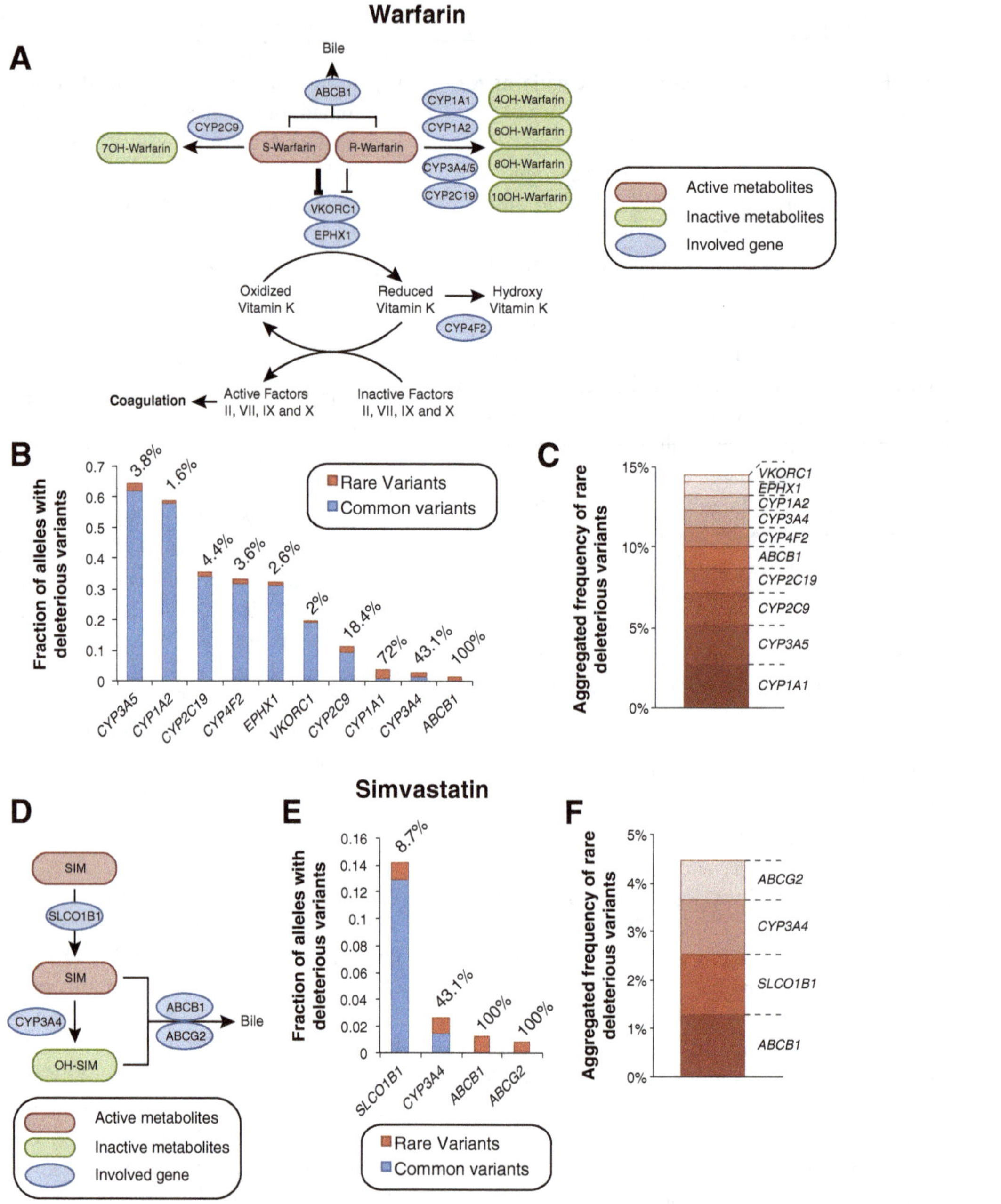

Fig. 3 The relevance of rare genetic variants for warfarin response and simvastatin-related myotoxicity. **a** Scheme depicting the metabolism and therapeutic action of warfarin. The less potent R-enantiomer of warfarin is metabolized by CYP1A1, CYP1A2, CYP3A, and CYP2C19, whereas the more potent S-enantiomer is inactivated by CYP2C9. Warfarin inhibits the VKOR complex, which reduces vitamin K, an essential factor for the formation of functional coagulation factors. See www.pharmgkb.org/pathway/PA145011113 and www.pharmgkb.org/pathway/PA145011114 for further information. **b** Overview of the aggregated frequencies of common (MAF ≥ 1%, blue) and rare deleterious genetic variants (MAF < 1%, red) in genes involved in warfarin pharmacokinetics or pharmacodynamics. Values next to the columns indicate the relative contribution of rare genetic variants. **c** Stacked column plot showing the aggregated frequency of deleterious rare variants of potential relevance for warfarin action. **d** Scheme depicting metabolites and genetic factors involved in the hepatic uptake, metabolism, and excretion of simvastatin. See www.pharmgkb.org/pathway/PA145011109 for further information. **e** Overview of the aggregated frequencies of common (MAF ≥ 1%, blue) and rare deleterious genetic variants (MAF < 1%, red) in genes implicated in simvastatin ADME. Values next to the columns indicate the relative contribution of rare genetic variants. **f** Stacked column plot showing the aggregated frequency of deleterious rare variants of potential relevance for simvastatin pharmacokinetics

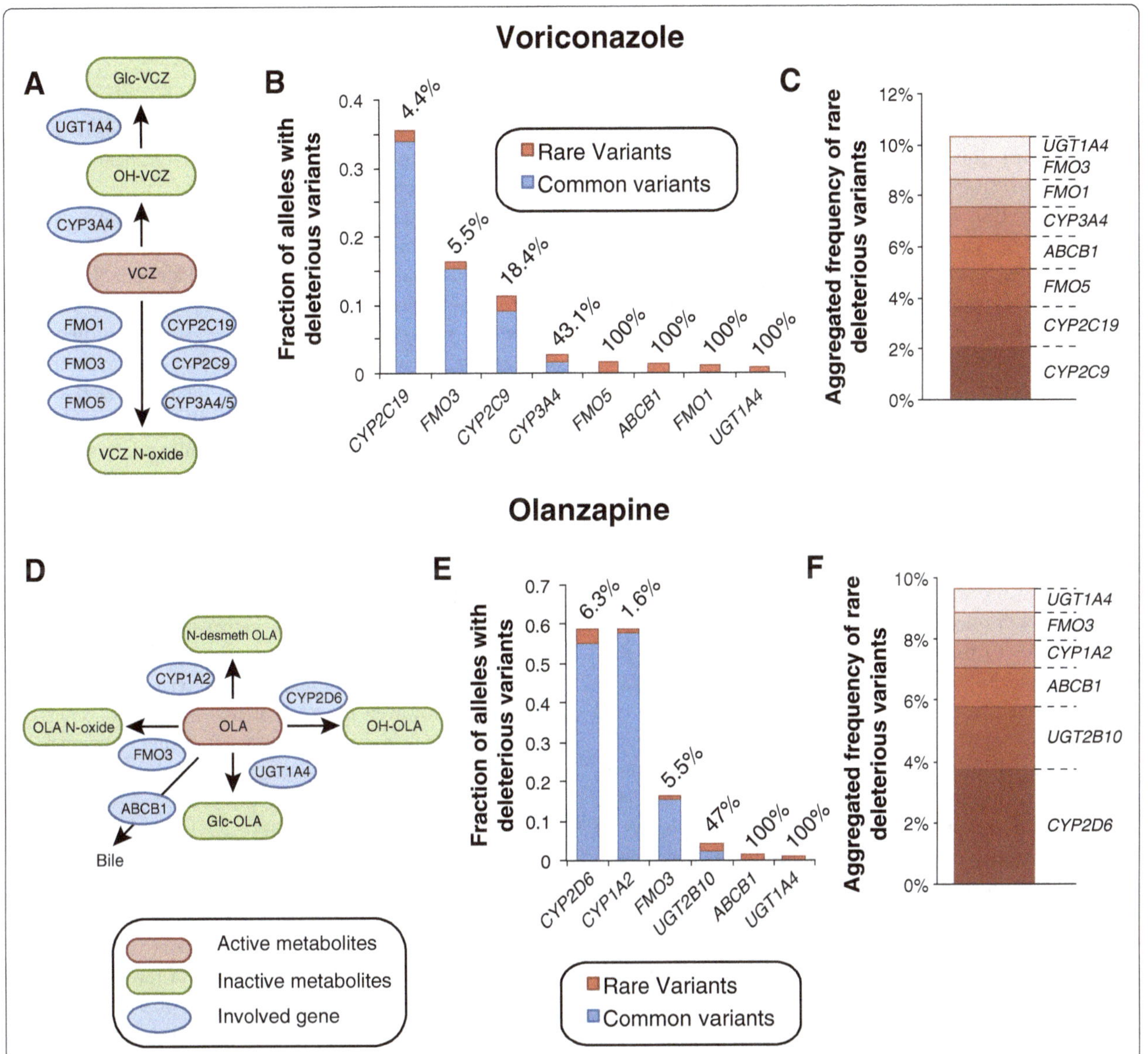

Fig. 4 Evaluation of the role of rare genetic variants for voriconazole and olanzapine pharmacokinetics. **a** Schematic depiction of key events in voriconazole metabolism. See www.pharmgkb.org/pathway/PA166160640 for further information. **b** Overview of the aggregated frequencies of common (MAF ≥ 1%, blue) and rare deleterious genetic variants (MAF < 1%, red) in genes involved in voriconazole metabolism. Values next to the columns indicate the relative contribution of rare genetic variants. **c** Stacked column plot showing the aggregated frequency of deleterious rare variants of potential relevance for voriconazole metabolism. **d** Schematic showing steps involved in the pharmacokinetics of the antipsychotic olanzapine. See www.pharmgkb.org/pathway/PA166165056 for further information. **e** Overview of the aggregated frequencies of common (MAF ≥ 1%, blue) and rare deleterious genetic variants (MAF < 1%, red) in genes implicated in olanzapine clearance. Values next to the columns indicate the relative contribution of rare genetic variants. **f** The aggregated frequency of deleterious rare variants of potential relevance for olanzapine metabolism is shown

and ADRs, including *FMO1* (100% contribution), *FMO5* (100%), *CYP3A4* (43.1%), and *CYP2C9* (18.4%; Fig. 4b, c).

Serum olanzapine levels

The therapeutic benefits for schizophrenic or bipolar patients when treated with the antipsychotic olanzapine are limited by extensive inter-individual variability in olanzapine serum concentrations, which can result in exposure levels outside the therapeutic interval [29]. As olanzapine serum levels are directly linked to the likelihood of therapeutic success [30] and the risk of ADRs [31, 32], an individualization of dosing regimens promises to increase treatment success rates.

While the metabolism of olanzapine is well characterized, the influence of genetic factors is more controversial (Fig. 4d). CYP2D6 and UGT2B10 hydroxylate or glucuronidate olanzapine, respectively, but so far, no study demonstrated clinically relevant effects of haplotypes of these genes on olanzapine exposure. In contrast, multiple clinical association studies found that genetic variants in *CYP1A2*, *FMO3*, and *UGT1A4* could explain up to 50% of differences in olanzapine serum levels, whereas other studies failed to replicate such associations ([33] and references therein). Rare variants substantially contribute to *UGT1A4* and *UGT2B10* variability and are predicted to account for 100 and 47% of the genetically encoded inter-individual variability in the functionality of these genes (Fig. 4e, f). On the contrary, we estimate that rare variants only explain 6.3, 5.5, and 1.6% of the variability in *CYP2D6*, *FMO3*, and *CYP1A2*, respectively.

Irinotecan toxicity

Irinotecan is a topoisomerase inhibitor prodrug that is used in combination therapy for advanced colorectal, lung, and other cancers. Irinotecan has a narrow therapeutic window and, as a consequence, up to 36% of patients suffer from dose-limiting toxicities [34]. Irinotecan is subjected to a complex interplay of competing metabolic activation and inactivation pathways (Fig. 5a). Around 97% of irinotecan is metabolized by CYP3A4 and CYP3A5 to the pharmacologically inactive metabolites APC and NPC, while only 3% become metabolically activated into SN-38 by the carboxylesterases CES1 and CES2. Subsequently, SN-38 is detoxified by glucuronidation mediated by UGT1A1 and, to a lesser extent, UGT1A9. Irinotecan and its metabolites are excreted into the bile and intestine via multiple transporters of the ABC family. Importantly, the β-glucuronidase enzymes of the intestinal microflora can re-activate glucuronidated SN-38 resulting in diarrhea and damage to all segments of the intestine [35].

Genetic variants in *UGT1A1* have been reproducibly linked to neutropenia and diarrhea toxicity in various ethnicities and dosing regimens [36]. Furthermore, multiple polymorphisms in the transporter genes *ABCB1*, *ABCC1*, *ABCC2*, *ABCG2*, and *SLCO1B1* have been implicated in irinotecan clearance and/or risk of toxicity [37–40]. While associations between *CYP3A* genotype and irinotecan pharmacokinetics are controversial, incorporation of CYP3A activity data into dosing calculations have resulted in reduced incidence of severe neutropenia [41].

Interestingly, our computational analyses of population-scale sequencing data indicate that rare genetic variants are important factors for irinotecan activation and transport (Fig. 5b). The aggregated frequency of rare deleterious alleles in *CES1* and *CES2* were 1.5 and 0.4%, respectively, accounting for 19.6 and 100% of the functional genetic variants in these genes. Similarly, for *SLCO1B1* and *ABCC1*, 8.7 and 40.5% of all deleterious variants were assigned to rare variants, while for *ABCB1*, *ABCC2*, and *ABCG2*, no common variants with functional consequences were identified. Notably though, we do not consider here variants with functional impacts that do not result in changes of the gene product, such as the synonymous variants rs1045642 (*ABCB1* I1145I) and rs1128503 (*ABCB1* G412G) or the UTR variant rs717620 in *ABCC2*. In contrast, inter-individual variability in UGT1A1 is primarily due to common polymorphisms, such as *UGT1A1**28*, and only an estimated 4.5% are allotted to rare SNVs.

Combined, our evaluations indicate that rare genetic variants in pharmacogenes have the potential to explain a substantial part of the unexplained genetic variability in drug metabolism phenotypes. Examples were selected for which gene-drug interactions were well studied, and we speculate that the relative importance of rare variants is even higher for less extensively characterized drugs. Furthermore, we give indications about the extent of genetically encoded functional variability that would be missed when only considering common genetic variants, thereby providing guidance for the optimal drug-specific choice of genotyping strategy.

Discussion

From a drug development perspective, an appropriate pharmacokinetic profile is of key importance to achieve the desired spatial and temporal exposure pattern of a given drug of interest. However, genetic variants in ADME genes encoding for transporters, drug-metabolizing enzymes, or nuclear receptors modulate drug pharmacokinetics and thus impact treatment efficacy and the risk of ADRs. Consequently, 190 drugs approved by the US Food and Drug Administration (FDA) and 155 drugs approved by EMA currently contain pharmacogenetic information in their labels, of which many are related to drug pharmacokinetics [42, 43]. Besides well-characterized common polymorphisms, ADME genes harbor a plethora of rare genetic variants that are not interrogated by current pharmacogenomic genotyping panels. By leveraging large-scale whole-exome sequencing data from 60,706 individuals, we present here the first analysis in which we systematically integrated information about rare genetic variability into predictions of pharmacokinetic variability (Additional file 2: Table S2).

Individual in silico functionality prediction algorithms distinguish deleterious from neutral variants with sensitivities and specificities between 60 and 90%. Furthermore, by using computational methods optimized for the evaluation of pharmacogenes with low evolutionary constraints, we were able to show that up to 92% sensitivity and 95% specificity can be achieved for loss-of-function and functionally neutral variants, respectively [13]. Furthermore, rare copy number variations in pharmacogenes, accounting for up to 1% of all loss-of-function alleles, are an additional source of genetic variability with relevance for drug metabolism phenotypes that are commonly not considered by computational functionality prediction algorithms [44].

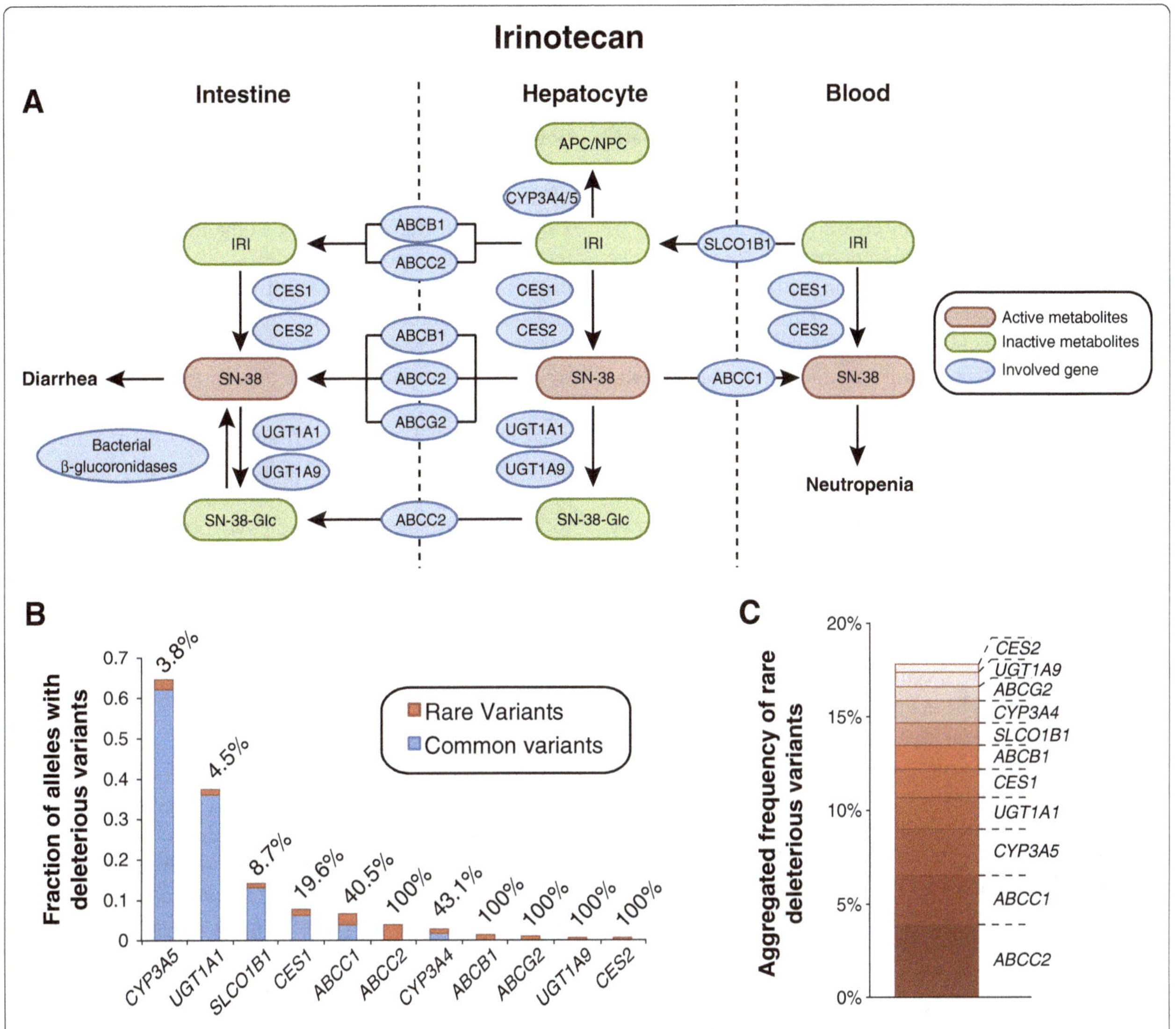

Fig. 5 Analysis of genetic factors contributing to dose-limiting irinotecan toxicity. **a** Scheme showing tissue specific involvement of gene products in the irinotecan pathway. See www.pharmgkb.org/pathway/PA2001 for further information. **b** Overview of the aggregated frequencies of common (MAF ≥ 1%, blue) and rare deleterious genetic variants (MAF < 1%, red) in genes implicated in irinotecan metabolism and transport. Values next to the columns indicate the relative contribution of rare genetic variants. **c** Stacked column plot showing the aggregated frequency of deleterious rare variants involved in irinotecan ADME

Notably, genetic variability in non-coding regions has been demonstrated to have important influence on phenotypic traits [45]. However, while promising progress has been made regarding the prediction of the effects of those variants based on DNA sequence [46], no current prediction framework can reliably predict the functionality of non-coding genetic variation, such as synonymous variants or variants located in UTRs, promoters, or enhancers. With respect to *CYP* alleles, such mutations represent < 1% of all functionally important variant alleles described (https://www.pharmvar.org/genes). We therefore restricted our analyses to the evaluation of LOF variants and variants that directly affect the amino acid sequence of their respective gene products.

Thus, while the predictive power of current functionality prediction methods is still not sufficient to support a recommendation of these tools for genetic counseling of individual patients, our data indicate however that leveraging of NGS technology can yield significant amounts of additional information for pharmacogenomic predictions on a population scale. Accordingly, we advocate for the development of a widened perspective in which conclusions about the functionality of a gene product are not solely based on the interrogation of few common variants. Rather, we recommend that the entire spectrum of genetic variability, including rare or novel variants, should be considered and integrated into gene activity scores. This holistic perspective is especially important as rare polymorphisms are enriched in variants that alter the functionality of the gene product and are the sole genetic factors for variability of more than 50% of the pharmacogenes analyzed (Fig. 2b).

Relating the functional inventory of pharmacogenetic variability to the pharmacology of selected drugs of interest can provide important insights into predicted hotspots of unexplained inter-individual differences in drug metabolism-related phenotypes. In this work, we estimated the relative contribution of rare genetic variants to the variability in pharmacokinetics and/or ADR risk of five clinically important drugs from different therapeutic areas. Rare variants are estimated to contribute significantly to the inter-individual variability of warfarin pharmacokinetics and irinotecan toxicity accounting for 18.4% of deleterious *CYP2C9* alleles and > 40% of the variability in irinotecan transport (Figs. 3a and 5). In contrast, the relative importance of rare variants is expected to be lower for the metabolism of simvastatin, voriconazole, and olanzapine for which rare variants only contribute between 1.6 and 8.7% of the key metabolic and/or transport processes. Thus, we find that the relevance of rare genetic variants is highly drug-specific, depending on the gene products involved. These findings suggest that it is likely that the inter-individual variability in pharmacokinetics and response for certain drugs is to a large extent determined by rare genetic variability, which is important to consider particularly in drug development. Integrating pharmacological information of the drug of interest with information about the distribution of rare variants in pharmacogenes can guide the design of the genotyping strategy most suitable to reveal important additional genetic factors that improve the prediction of drug metabolism phenotypes.

For many drugs, genetic variability cannot be directly translated into effectiveness or ADR susceptibility due to the interdependency of different metabolic pathways. For instance, genetic or pharmacological inhibition of the major pathway of a given drug can result in a shunt to an alternative otherwise negligible metabolic route, as observed for oxycodone [47]. To date, data regarding the effects of such gene-gene or gene-drug interactions is sparse, which complicates predictions of drug effectiveness or safety even when rare genetic variants are incorporated into the analyses. Thus, while the consideration of pharmacogenomic information including rare genetic variants promises to improve ADME predictions, further work particularly in physiologically based pharmacokinetic (PBPK) modeling is necessary to reliably predict treatment outcomes for the individual patient.

Currently, genotyping is largely based on the interrogation of well-characterized, common polymorphisms. This strategy neglects the impacts of rare variants as experimental in vitro or in vivo data that demonstrate their functional impact is not available. Yet, due to rapidly decreasing sequencing times and costs, we suggest that current NGS technology in combination with more advanced computational prediction methods could already today facilitate the refinement of individualized predictions regarding drug efficacy and its propensity to cause ADRs and thereby to contribute to the implementation of pharmacogenetic markers into routine care [48, 49]. Furthermore, the multitude of ongoing sequencing projects on unprecedented scale, such as the 100K Genomes Project run by the British Department of Health and the 1 Million Genomes project as part of the Chinese Precision Medicine Initiative, will soon provide a wealth of information about non-transcribed, regulatory regions and improve linkage information between variants, which will allow to expand the scope of computational analyses from variants to haplotypes. For the field of pharmacogenomics, these developments hold promise to further increase the predictive power of gene-drug response predictions and to allow more accurate estimates of drug response across more narrowly stratified subpopulations.

Conclusions

We present results suggesting that integration of rare pharmacogenomic variability can improve predictions of drug pharmacokinetics compared to the use of candidate variants. This information is important for drug development and clinical care as well as for future preemptive pharmacogenomic advice. Furthermore, these data incentivize the design of prospective trials using NGS-based genotyping for specific medications, such as warfarin and irinotecan, to assess whether clinical outcomes can be improved.

Acknowledgements

The authors would like to thank the Exome Aggregation Consortium and the groups that provided exome variant data for comparison.

Funding

This study was supported by the European Union's Horizon 2020 research and innovation program U-PGx (grant agreement no. 668353), by the Swedish Research Council (grant agreement numbers 2015-02760, 2016-01153, and 2016-01154), and by the Lennart Philipson Foundation.

Authors' contributions

MI-S and VML designed the study. YZ collected the exome sequencing data. VML devised and conducted the data analysis. SM, MI-S, and VML wrote the manuscript. All authors discussed and agreed on the final version of the manuscript.

Competing interests
The authors declare that they have no competing interests.

References

1. Lauschke VM, Ingelman-Sundberg M. The importance of patient-specific factors for hepatic drug response and toxicity. Int J Mol Sci. 2016;17(10): 1714–27. https://doi.org/10.3390/ijms17101714.
2. Pirmohamed M, James S, Meakin S, et al. Adverse drug reactions as cause of admission to hospital: prospective analysis of 18 820 patients. BMJ. 2004; 329(7456):15–9. https://doi.org/10.1136/bmj.329.7456.15.
3. Sim SC, Kacevska M, Ingelman-Sundberg M. Pharmacogenomics of drug-metabolizing enzymes: a recent update on clinical implications and endogenous effects. Pharmacogenomics J. 2012;13(1):1–11. https://doi.org/10.1038/tpj.2012.45.
4. Matthaei J, Brockmöller J, Tzvetkov MV, et al. Heritability of metoprolol and torsemide pharmacokinetics. Clin Pharmacol Ther. 2015;98(6):611–21. https://doi.org/10.1002/cpt.258.
5. Lauschke VM, Milani L, Ingelman-Sundberg M. Pharmacogenomic biomarkers for improved drug therapy-recent progress and future developments. AAPS J. 2017;20(1):4. https://doi.org/10.1208/s12248-017-0161-x.
6. Singh RR, Luthra R, Routbort MJ, et al. Implementation of next generation sequencing in clinical molecular diagnostic laboratories: advantages, challenges and potential. Exp Rev Precision Med Drug Dev. 2016;1(1):109–20. https://doi.org/10.1080/23808993.2015.1120401.
7. Gordon AS, Tabor HK, Johnson AD, et al. Quantifying rare, deleterious variation in 12 human cytochrome P450 drug-metabolism genes in a large-scale exome dataset. Hum Mol Genet. 2014;23(8):1957–63. https://doi.org/10.1093/hmg/ddt588.
8. Fujikura K, Ingelman-Sundberg M, Lauschke VM. Genetic variation in the human cytochrome P450 supergene family. Pharmacogenet Genomics. 2015;25(12):584–94. https://doi.org/10.1097/FPC.0000000000000172.
9. Kozyra M, Ingelman-Sundberg M, Lauschke VM. Rare genetic variants in cellular transporters, metabolic enzymes, and nuclear receptors can be important determinants of interindividual differences in drug response. Genet Med. 2017;19(1):20–9. https://doi.org/10.1038/gim.2016.33.
10. Bush WS, Crosslin DR, Owusu-Obeng A, et al. Genetic variation among 82 pharmacogenes: the PGRNseq data from the eMERGE network. Clin Pharmacol Ther. 2016;100(2):160–9. https://doi.org/10.1002/cpt.350.
11. Lek M, Karczewski KJ, Minikel EV, et al. Analysis of protein-coding genetic variation in 60,706 humans. Nature. 2016;536(7616):285–91. https://doi.org/10.1038/nature19057.
12. Abecasis GR, Chakravarti A, Donnelly P, et al. A global reference for human genetic variation. Nature. 2015;526(7571):68–74. https://doi.org/10.1038/nature15393.
13. Zhou Y, Mkrtchian S, Kumondai M, et al. An optimized prediction framework to assess the functional impact of pharmacogenetic variants. Pharmacogenomics J. (In review)
14. Nelson MR, Wegmann D, Ehm MG, et al. An abundance of rare functional variants in 202 drug target genes sequenced in 14,002 people. Science. 2012;337(6090):100–4. https://doi.org/10.1126/science.1217876.
15. Tennessen JA, Bigham AW, O'Connor TD, et al. Evolution and functional impact of rare coding variation from deep sequencing of human exomes. Science. 2012;337(6090):64–9. https://doi.org/10.1126/science.1219240.
16. Johnson JA, Cavallari LH. Warfarin pharmacogenetics. Trends Cardiovasc Med. 2015;25(1):33–41. https://doi.org/10.1016/j.tcm.2014.09.001.
17. Kaminsky LS, Zhang Z-Y. Human P450 metabolism of warfarin. Pharmacol Ther. 1997;73(1):67–74. https://doi.org/10.1016/s0163-7258(96)00140-4.
18. Wadelius M, Sörlin K, Wallerman O, et al. Warfarin sensitivity related to CYP2C9, CYP3A5, ABCB1 (MDR1) and other factors. Pharmacogenomics J. 2003;4(1):40–8. https://doi.org/10.1038/sj.tpj.6500220.
19. Pautas E, Moreau C, Gouin-Thibault I, et al. Genetic factors (VKORC1, CYP2C9, EPHX1, and CYP4F2) are predictor variables for warfarin response in very elderly, frail inpatients. Clin Pharmacol Ther. 2009;87(1):57–64. https://doi.org/10.1038/clpt.2009.178.
20. The International Warfarin Pharmacogenetics Consortium, Klein TE, Altman RB, et al. Estimation of the warfarin dose with clinical and pharmacogenetic data. N Engl J Med. 2009;360(8):753–64. https://doi.org/10.1056/NEJMoa0809329.
21. Hodges LM, Markova SM, Chinn LW, et al. Very important pharmacogene summary: ABCB1 (MDR1, P-glycoprotein). Pharmacogenet Genomics. 2011; 21(3):152–61. https://doi.org/10.1097/FPC.0b013e3283385a1c.
22. SEARCH Collaborative Group, Link E, Parish S, et al. SLCO1B1 variants and statin-induced myopathy—a genomewide study. N Engl J Med. 2008;359(8): 789–99. https://doi.org/10.1056/NEJMoa0801936.
23. Kobayashi M, Chisaki I, Narumi K, et al. Association between risk of myopathy and cholesterol-lowering effect: a comparison of all statins. Life Sci. 2008;82(17–18):969–75. https://doi.org/10.1016/j.lfs.2008.02.019.
24. Hyland R, Jones BC, Smith DA. Identification of the cytochrome P450 enzymes involved in the N-oxidation of voriconazole. Drug Metab Dispos. 2003;31(5):540–7.
25. Yanni SB, Annaert PP, Augustijns P, et al. Role of flavin-containing monooxygenase in oxidative metabolism of voriconazole by human liver microsomes. Drug Metab Dispos. 2008;36(6):1119–25. https://doi.org/10.1124/dmd.107.019646.
26. Owusu Obeng A, Egelund EF, Alsultan A, et al. CYP2C19 polymorphisms and therapeutic drug monitoring of voriconazole: are we ready for clinical implementation of pharmacogenomics? Pharmacotherapy. 2014;34(7):703–18. https://doi.org/10.1002/phar.1400.
27. Niwa T, Hata T. The effect of genetic polymorphism on the inhibition of azole antifungal agents against CYP2C9-mediated metabolism. J Pharm Sci. 2016;105(3):1345–8. https://doi.org/10.1016/j.xphs.2016.01.007.
28. He HR, Sun JY, Ren XD, et al. Effects of CYP3A4 polymorphisms on the plasma concentration of voriconazole. Eur J Clin Microbiol Infect Dis. 2014; 34(4):811–9. https://doi.org/10.1007/s10096-014-2294-5.
29. Patel MX, Bowskill S, Couchman L, et al. Plasma olanzapine in relation to prescribed dose and other factors. J Clin Psychopharmacol. 2011;31(4):411–7. https://doi.org/10.1097/JCP.0b013e318221b408.
30. Perry PJ, Lund BC, Sanger T, et al. Olanzapine plasma concentrations and clinical response: acute phase results of the North American Olanzapine Trial. J Clin Psychopharmacol. 2001;21(1):14–20.
31. Perry PJ, Argo TR, Carnahan RM, et al. The association of weight gain and olanzapine plasma concentrations. J Clin Psychopharmacol. 2005;25(3):250–4. https://doi.org/10.1097/01.jcp.0000162800.64378.82.
32. Kinon BJ, Volavka J, Stauffer V, et al. Standard and higher dose of olanzapine in patients with schizophrenia or schizoaffective disorder. J Clin Psychopharmacol. 2008;28(4):392–400. https://doi.org/10.1097/JCP.0b013e31817e63a5.
33. Söderberg MM, Dahl M-L. Pharmacogenetics of olanzapine metabolism. Pharmacogenomics. 2013;14(11):1319–36. https://doi.org/10.2217/pgs.13.120.
34. Fuchs CS, Moore MR, Harker G, et al. Phase III comparison of two irinotecan dosing regimens in second-line therapy of metastatic colorectal cancer. J Clin Oncol. 2003;21(5):807–14. https://doi.org/10.1200/JCO.2003.08.058.
35. Brandi G, Dabard J, Raibaud P, et al. Intestinal microflora and digestive toxicity of irinotecan in mice. Clin Cancer Res. 2006;12(4):1299–307. https://doi.org/10.1158/1078-0432.CCR-05-0750.
36. Campbell JM, Stephenson MD, Bateman E, et al. Irinotecan-induced toxicity pharmacogenetics: an umbrella review of systematic reviews and meta-analyses. Pharmacogenomics J. 2017;17(1):21–8. https://doi.org/10.1038/tpj.2016.58.
37. Han J-Y, Lim H-S, Yoo Y-K, et al. Associations of ABCB1, ABCC2, and ABCG2 polymorphisms with irinotecan-pharmacokinetics and clinical outcome in patients with advanced non-small cell lung cancer. Cancer. 2007;110(1):138–47. https://doi.org/10.1002/cncr.22760.
38. Han J-Y, Lim H-S, Park YH, et al. Integrated pharmacogenetic prediction of irinotecan pharmacokinetics and toxicity in patients with advanced non-small cell lung cancer. Lung Cancer. 2009;63(1):115–20. https://doi.org/10.1016/j.lungcan.2007.12.003.
39. Innocenti F, Kroetz DL, Schuetz E, et al. Comprehensive pharmacogenetic analysis of irinotecan neutropenia and pharmacokinetics. J Clin Oncol. 2009; 27(16):2604–14. https://doi.org/10.1200/JCO.2008.20.6300.
40. Li M, Seiser EL, Baldwin RM, et al. ABC transporter polymorphisms are associated with irinotecan pharmacokinetics and neutropenia. Pharmacogenomics J. 2018;18(1):35–42. https://doi.org/10.1038/tpj.2016.75.
41. van der Bol JM, Mathijssen RHJ, Creemers GJM, et al. A CYP3A4 phenotype-based dosing algorithm for individualized treatment of irinotecan. Clin Cancer Res. 2010;16(2):736–42. https://doi.org/10.1158/1078-0432.CCR-09-1526.
42. https://www.fda.gov/Drugs/ScienceResearch/ResearchAreas/Pharmacogenetics/ucm083378.htm. Accessed 20 May 2017.
43. Ehmann F, Caneva L, Prasad K, et al. Pharmacogenomic information in drug labels: European Medicines Agency perspective. Pharmacogenomics J. 2015; 15(3):201–10. https://doi.org/10.1038/tpj.2014.86.
44. Santos M, Niemi M, Hiratsuka M, et al. Novel copy-number variations in pharmacogenes contribute to interindividual differences in drug

pharmacokinetics. Genet Med. 2017; https://doi.org/10.1038/gim.2017.156. [Epub ahead of print]

45. Maurano MT, Humbert R, Rynes E, et al. Systematic localization of common disease-associated variation in regulatory DNA. Science. 2012;337(6099): 1190–5. https://doi.org/10.1126/science.1222794.
46. Lee D, Gorkin DU, Baker M, et al. A method to predict the impact of regulatory variants from DNA sequence. Nat Genet. 2015;47(8):955–61. https://doi.org/10.1038/ng.3331.
47. Samer CF, Daali Y, Wagner M, et al. The effects of CYP2D6 and CYP3A activities on the pharmacokinetics of immediate release oxycodone. Br J Pharmacol. 2010;160(4):907–18. https://doi.org/10.1111/j.1476-5381.2010.00673.x.
48. Lauschke VM, Ingelman-Sundberg M. How to consider rare genetic variants in personalized drug therapy. Clin Pharmacol Ther. 2018;19:20. https://doi.org/10.1002/cpt.976.
49. Lauschke VM, Ingelman-Sundberg M. Precision medicine and rare genetic variants. Trends Pharmacol Sci. 2016;37(2):85–6. https://doi.org/10.1016/j.tips.2015.10.006.
50. Spitzer M, Wildenhain J, Rappsilber J, et al. BoxPlotR: a web tool for generation of box plots. Nat Methods. 2014;11(2):121–2. https://doi.org/10.1038/nmeth.2811.

16

Impact of ZBTB7A hypomethylation and expression patterns on treatment response to hydroxyurea

Vasiliki Chondrou[1†], Eleana F. Stavrou[1†], Georgios Markopoulos[2], Alexandra Kouraklis-Symeonidis[3], Vasilios Fotopoulos[4], Argiris Symeonidis[5], Efthymia Vlachaki[6], Panagiota Chalkia[7], George P. Patrinos[8], Adamantia Papachatzopoulou[9] and Argyro Sgourou[1*]

Abstract

Background: We aimed to clarify the emerging epigenetic landscape in a group of genes classified as "modifier genes" of the β-type globin genes (*HBB* cluster), known to operate *in trans* to accomplish the two natural developmental switches in globin expression, from embryonic to fetal during the first trimester of conception and from fetal to adult around the time of birth. The epigenetic alterations were determined in adult sickle cell anemia (SCA) homozygotes and SCA/β-thalassemia compound heterozygotes of Greek origin, who are under hydroxyurea (HU) treatment. Patients were distinguished in HU responders and HU non-responders (those not benefited from the HU) and both, and in vivo and in vitro approaches were implemented.

Results: We examined the CpG islands' DNA methylation profile of *BCL11A*, *KLF1*, *MYB*, *MAP3K5*, *SIN3A*, *ZBTB7A*, and *GATA2*, along with γ-globin and LRF/*ZBTB7A* expression levels. In vitro treatment of hematopoietic stem cells (HSCs) with HU induced a significant DNA hypomethylation pattern in *ZBTB7A* (p^*, 0.04) and *GATA2* (p^*, 0.03) CpGs exclusively in the HU non-responders. Also, this group of patients exhibited significantly elevated baseline methylation patterns in *ZBTB7A*, before the HU treatment, compared to HU responders (p^*, 0.019) and to control group of healthy individuals (p^*, 0.021) , which resembles a potential epigenetic barrier for the γ-globin expression. γ-Globin expression in vitro matched with detected HbF levels during patients' monitoring tests (in vivo) under HU treatment, implying a good reproducibility of the in vitro HU epigenetic effect. LRF/*ZBTB7A* expression was elevated only in the HU non-responders under the influence of HU.

Conclusions: This is one of the very first pharmacoepigenomic studies indicating that the hypomethylation of *ZBTB7A* during HU treatment enhances the LRF expression, which by its turn suppresses the HbF resumption in the HU non-responders. Its role as an epigenetic regulator of hemoglobin switching is also supported by the wide distribution of *ZBTB7A*-binding sites within the 5′ CpG sequences of all studied human *HBB* cluster "modifier genes." Also, the baseline methylation level of selective CpGs in *ZBTB7A* and *GATA2* could be an indicator of the negative HU response among the β-type hemoglobinopathy patients.

Keywords: SCA homozygotes, SCA/β-thal heterozygotes, Hydroxyurea treatment, HbF induction, *HBB* cluster "modifying genes", Epigenetic regulation

* Correspondence: sgourou@eap.gr
†Vasiliki Chondrou and Eleana F. Stavrou contributed equally to this work.
[1]School of Science and Technology, Biology Laboratory, Hellenic Open University, Patras, Greece
Full list of author information is available at the end of the article

Introduction

Thalassemias and sickle cell anemia (SCA) are still of the most common genetic disorders among human population even after many decades of worldwide prenatal control attempts. Furthermore, the combination of β^s allele, as a consequence of the SCA genotype with β-thalassemic alleles (SCA/β-thal), appears with an evenly severe clinical phenotype. Clinical practice has shown that, despite identical disease-causing mutations, the pathological phenotype of disease varies enormously between individual patients. This is partly related to genetic variants of the genetic loci coding for the hemoglobin subunits alpha and beta (*HBA* and *HBB*) including their remote regulatory regions (LCRs—locus control regions) [1, 2] and the co-interaction with other parameters such as epigenetic regulatory mechanisms [3].

These genetic disorders have an early onset, within a few months after birth, which is accompanied by high financial burdens to healthcare systems due to the expensive therapeutic protocols applied to patients. Apart from the regular blood transfusions and iron-chelating agents, an alternative widely used therapeutic approach is the induction of fetal hemoglobin (HbF) expression that ameliorates their pathological phenotype [4, 5]. Hydroxyurea (HU) or hydroxycarbamide is the major therapeutic agent identified as a potent HbF inducer and has been used for the management of patients with SCA and SCA/β-thal, since its FDA approval in1998 [6, 7]. The main mechanism of HU action is the inhibition of the ribonucleotide reductase (RR), which pauses the DNA synthesis. The in vivo effects of HU in mammalian systems are transient, as a consequence from the rapid absorption, metabolism, and excretion of the drug. Once-daily dosing of HU presumably causes an intermittent cytotoxic effect resulting in stress erythropoiesis and increased HbF levels [8]. Patients administered with HU show elevated HbF levels within the first 3 to 6 months of treatment, with further improvements up to 12 months, where patients reach a plateau with the maximum HbF expression levels and the corresponding maximum mean erythrocyte corpuscular volume (MCV) [9]. However, HbF levels do not present a uniform increase in all patients, whereas long-term use of HU sometimes leads to the loss of its initial beneficial action [10, 11]. The underlying precise molecular mechanism of the HU action and the variance of treatment results remain still elusive, though a concealed epigenetic effect of its action is highly suspected.

Epigenetic modifications, such as DNA methylation and histone methylation/acetylation, constitute an additional layer of gene expression regulation and affect phenotypic heterogeneity of human diseases and drug responses [12, 13]. DNA methylation mainly occurs in the context of CG dinucleotides (CpGs) and has traditionally been associated with gene repression [14].

This study concerns the methylation alterations, induced by HU treatment on known β-type globin genes (*HBB* cluster) "modifier genes":erythroid-specific transcription factors (*KLF1*, *GATA1*, and *GATA2*), regulators of hematopoiesis and erythropoiesis (*MYB*, *SOX6*, *SIN3A*), members of the MAPK signaling pathway (MAP3K5), and HbF repressors (*BCL11A*, *ZBTB7A*) [15–28], in terms of contributing to knowledge on the molecular epigenetic regulation of embryonic HbF ($\alpha_2\gamma_2$) reactivation during the human progenitor cells' exposure to HU. Though *SOX6* and GATA*1* bared no CpG islands within neighboring sequences, indicating that they are alternatively regulated and were excluded from the study, CpG islands' quantitative analysis of hyper- or hypomethylation status within the *HBB* cluster "modifier genes" has been elaborated both in patients comprised within a long-term treatment and newly introduced to HU. The epigenetic landscape of these genes has also been studied during cultivation and erythroid differentiation of human-induced hematopoietic pluripotent stem cells derived from healthy donors' and patients' peripheral blood, cord blood, and bone marrow, under the pressure of HU to simulate in vitro the pharmacological induction of HbF and the corresponding cell molecular responses.

The aim of our study was to depict and highlight changes in the DNA methylation pattern at genomic loci unlinked to the *HBB* cluster on chromosome 11, which may influence the HbF induction in adults, to distinguish the different epigenetic regulatory nuclear mechanisms acting among responders and non-responders to treatment with HU and to contribute to the development of a clinical algorithm for improved prediction of the patients' response to HU treatment.

Material and methods

Bioinformatics analysis and CpG islands' selection

Candidate disease identified "modifier loci," encoding β-type globin gene regulators were: *BCL11A*, *KLF1*, *MYB*, *MAP3K5*, *SOX6*, *SIN3A*, *ZBTB7A*, *GATA1*, and *GATA2* [15–28]. CpG islands of all genes were retrieved by the UCSC genome browser (genome.ucsc.edu) [29]. Selected CpG islands for the study are located at areas flanking genes' promoter or within downstream 5′ UTR regions and gene bodies. Respective data for gene locations and CpG islands analyzed are presented in Table 1. All include sites for CTCF and/or ZBTB7A transcription factors' commitment (Fig. 1). Genes and/or CpG sites that did not preserve these characteristics were excluded from the study.

Transcription factor binding sites for CTCF and ZBTB7A were extracted from ENCODE project Chip-Seq data [30] and visualized in the UCSC genome browser.

Table 1 Chromosomal locations of all CpG islands analyzed

Gene	Location of CpG island	CTCF-binding site	ZBTB7A-binding site
BCL11A	CpG 120	+	-
	Chr2: 60554555-60554409		
	Chr2: 60554304-60554174		
BCL11A	CpG 115	+	+
	Chr 2: 60550535-60550416		
KLF1	CpG 98	+	-
	Chr 19: 12885764-12885569		
	Chr 19: 12885322-12885477		
MYB	CpG 216	-	-
	Chr 6: 135181253-135181153		
	Chr 6: 13518140-135181107		
SIN3A	CpG 401	+	+
	Chr 15: 75454578-75454439		
ZBTB7A	CpG 326	-	+
	Chr 19: 4067422-4067286		
	Chr 19: 4066671-4066789		
GATA2	CpG 515	-	+
	Chr 3: 128488082-128487980		
MAP3K5	CpG 172	+	+
	Chr 6: 136792589-136792545		

Sample collection

Patients were selected based on the existence of homozygosity to HbS (SCA) or compound heterozygosity to SCA and β-thalassemia (SCA/β-thal). All patients were adults, either treated for long-term with HU or for immediate treatment initiation, due to life-threatening disease-related symptoms. For the newly introduced patients to HU therapy, the mean dosage of HU administered was 20 mg/kg and the mean follow-up time was 5–6 months. Upon arrival to the plateau phase, where maximum HbF was produced, patients continued to be monitored annually. HbF levels at baseline and 5–6 months after initiation of HU treatment were estimated in all patients participating in this study with the high-performance liquid chromatography (HPLC) method, HbA_2/HbA_{1c} dual program (VARIANT™ II Beta-Thalassemia, Bio-Rad) (Additional file 1: Figure S1). Patients' hematological data are presented in Additional file 1: Table S1.

Blood samples of SCA, SCA/β-thal, and healthy donors have been included in the study. Experimental procedures have been applied both in vivo and in vitro.

Samples analyzed in vivo were group I—30 peripheral blood samples from SCA and SCA/β-thal patients, sub-categorized to responders and non-responders to HU (Additional file 1: Table S1), and group II—20 peripheral blood samples from healthy donors to act as reference group.

Samples analyzed in vitro were as follows: Group III—burst-forming unit-erythroid (BFU-E) cell populations from hematopoietic progenitor human cells acquired from the peripheral blood of selected SCA/β-thal patients who were undergoing HU therapy for the first time. Total samples cultivated derived from five responders (III R1–R5) and for non-responders (III NR1–NR4). Their characterization as responsive or not to the HU treatment was done later, when they had reached the plateau phase (5–6 months). III NR3 and NR4 were sisters and brothers. Group IV—BFU-E colonies acquired from peripheral blood of the control group (four samples IV CG1–CG4), from the bone marrow (four samples, IV BM1–BM4), and from the umbilical cord blood (four samples, IV UCB1–UCB4), all coming from healthy donors (Table 2).

Responders and non-responders to HU were clinically distinguished in relevance to their hematological parameters before and after administration of HU, their transfusion needs, and the capability to ameliorate anemia symptoms. For the present study, which focused on the epigenetic regulatory differences among the *HBB* cluster "modifier genes" and their influence in HbF induction, the strict clinical evaluation of

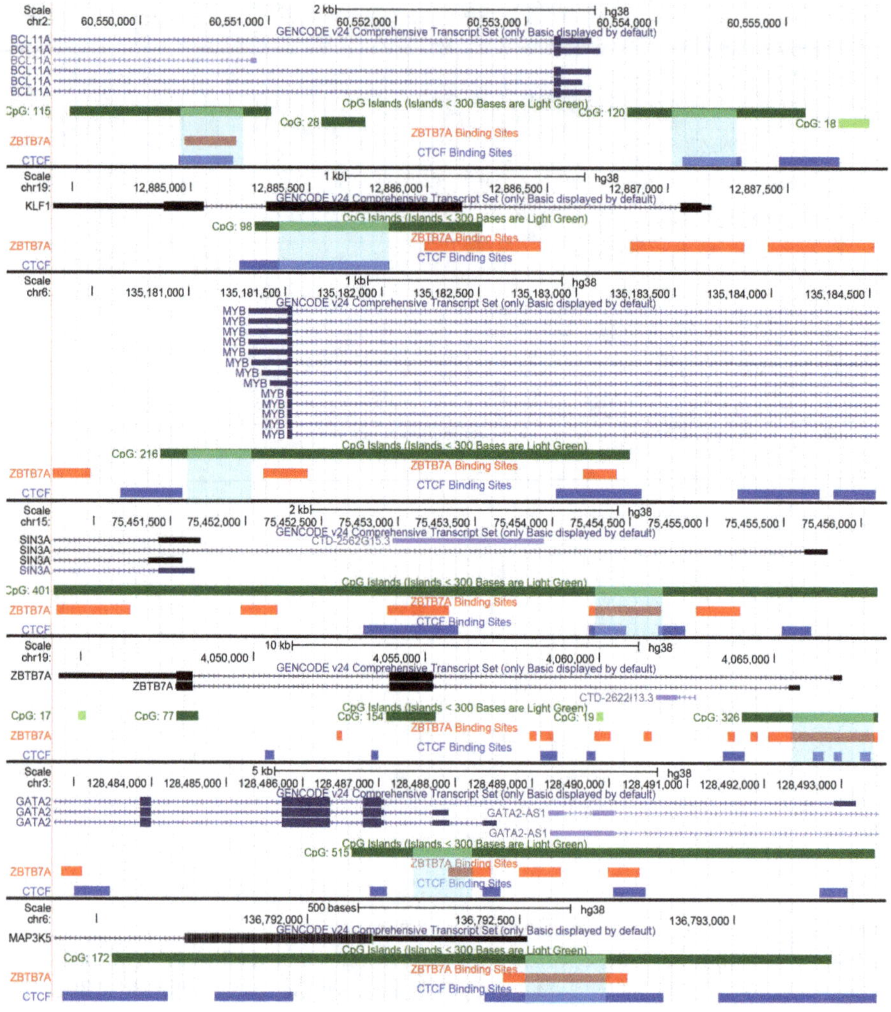

Fig. 1 Epigenetic features of promoter regions of genes analyzed in this study. The promoter regions and sequence features of *BCL11A*, *KLF1*, *MYB*, *SIN3A*, *ZBTB7A*, *GATA2*, and *MAP3K5* respectively are presented in parallel tracks, from top to bottom: scale, chromosomal location, gene transcript from Gencode v.24 (exons are represented as boxes and introns as lines with arrows indicating the 5′ towards the 3′ region), CpG islands (boxes in green color), LRF/*ZBTB7A*-binding sites (boxes in red color), and CTCF-binding sites (boxes in blue color). Chromosomal locations of interest in each promoter region are highlighted with light blue transparent boxes

patients has not been applied. Responders were considered the patients with an overall improved disease course and a ≥ 2.5-fold HbF increase.

Hematopoietic stem cells from categories III and IV have been cultivated simultaneously in the presence and absence of HU (50–100 μM).

Hematopoietic pluripotent stem cell cultures

The hematopoietic pluripotent stem cells derived from human blood samples support an in vitro clonogenic culture system, known as colony-forming unit assay (CFU), simulating the in vivo erythropoiesis in the bone marrow. The cell colonies of the different morphology finally obtained by this type of cultures are the CFU-E (colony-forming unit-erythroid) and the BFU-E (burst-forming unit-erythroid), which are apparent after 14–16 days of continuous culture (Fig. 2).

Peripheral blood (PBMCs) and cord blood mononuclear cells, enriched in $CD34^+$, were isolated with Histopaque-1077 (Sigma-Aldrich) following the vendor's protocol. Single cell common myeloid progenitors (isolated from bone marrow aspirates) were also induced for erythrocyte expansion and differentiation in the same culture conditions. In all cases, 10^5 cells were cultivated in the semi-solid culture media (MethoCultt GF+ H4435, StemCell Technologies), containing the appropriate cytokine cocktail plus erythropoietin.

At day 13, culture medium was supplemented with the pharmacological factor HU (Sigma), freshly prepared, at

Table 2 In vitro samples (III and IV)

Sample ID	In vitro γ-globin (+HU/−HU)	Baseline HbF (−HU)	Plateau HbF (+HU)	In vivo HbF (+HU)/(−HU)
IV CG1	1.75	x	x	x
IV CG2	1.38	x	x	x
IV CG3	1.26	x	x	x
IV CG4	1.69	x	x	x
III NR1	1.35	3.4	4.6	1.35
III NR2	1.54	2.5	2.9	1.16
III NR3	2.12	0.6	1	1.67
III NR4	1.43	2.1	2.9	1.38
III R1	1.09	6.1	22.6	3.7
III R2	3.66	6.7	16.4	2.5
III R3	2.31	10.7	31	2.89
III R4	2.56	9.8	24.5	2.5
III R5	1.87	2.7	15.1	5.6
IV UCB1	2.02	x	x	x
IV UCB2	2.57	x	x	x
IV UCB3	1.96	x	x	x
IV UCB4	2.34	x	x	x
IV BM1	5.58	x	x	x
IV BM2	4.44	x	x	x
IV BM3	3.25	x	x	x
IV BM4	5.02	x	x	x

concentrations between 50 and 100 mM for monitoring the effect of the pharmaceutical agent. In parallel, CFUs were carried under the same conditions apart from the addition of HU. At day 16, when cells reached the BFU-E stage of differentiation, cultures were terminated. Viability of the cells was checked by trypan blue dye exclusion test. Single BFU-E colonies were randomly picked under an inverted microscope (Leica DMI), whereas the rest of the colonies (derived from the same plating) were collectively pooled and used for DNA/RNA extraction. Genetic

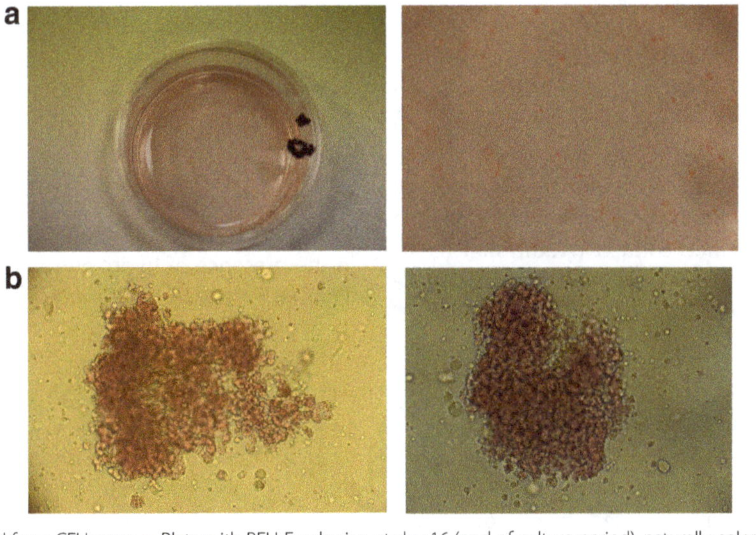

Fig. 2 BFU-E colonies derived from CFU assay. **a** Plate with BFU-E colonies, at day 16 (end of culture period), naturally colored red due to hemoglobin synthesis. **b** Two representative BFU-E colonies, observed under the inverted microscope (× 100)

material from BFU-Es was processed to bisulphite treatment followed by pyrosequencing methylation assays and RNA to qPCR experiments.

Detection of relative gene expression by RNA quantification (qRT-PCR)

In quantitative PCRs, the amount of target cDNA (either γ-globin or LRF/*ZBTB7A*) was compared and normalized to the amount of *GAPDH* reference gene expression. cDNAs were amplified using QuantiFast SYBR Green PCR (Qiagen) and the ECO (Illumina) instrument. The target and internal reference gene were run in separate duplicate or triplicate reactions using primers reported at Table 3. γ-Globin, towards *GAPDH* reaction conditions, were as follows: 10 s at 95 °C, 30 s at 58 °C, 40 cycles (Additional file 1: Figure S1), and LRF/*ZBTB7A* to *GAPDH* were done according to Shen et al. [31] (Fig. 5).

Gene expression in BFU-E colonies was calculated as relative expression of treated compared to untreated with HU colonies, using the formula $2^{(-\Delta Ct)}$ and normalized to the reference *GAPDH* gene.

Methylation analysis

The methylation status of all CpG DNA sequences was determined with the Pyrosequencing CpG assay methodology in duplicate or triplicate analysis indicating a good technical reproducibility and validation of the method. To achieve the complete conversion of the unmethylated cytosines (existing as CpG dinucleotides) to uraciles, bisulphite method (Qiagen) was utilized. Pyrosequencing reactions were performed with the PyroMark Q24 MDx technology (Qiagen). Methylated and unmethylated (bisulphite converted) human DNAs plus unmethylated (physiological) human DNA were used as internal controls in every round of pyrosequencing reactions. Different sequencing primers, specific for the methylation analysis of each DNA CpG sequence, were designed as well as all PCR primers sets with the PyroMark Assay Design Software, version 2.0 (Qiagen) (Table 3). Variation in methylation status of various CpG sites was detected and presented in a sequence context (Additional file 1: Figure S2, S3). Quality controls for the bisulphite conversion efficiency were introduced in every Pyrosequencing run set.

Sodium bisulphite treatment modification for the single-colony CpG assays

Before DNA methylation analysis, normal cytosine residues, existing as CpG dinucleotides, were completely converted to uracil residues while 5-methylocytosine residues remained unchanged through sodium bisulphite conversion reaction. In this study, a modified protocol for bisulphite treatment of single colonies of human erythroid progenitor cells was developed bypassing the DNA extraction step and based on the standard protocol of EpiTect Bisulphite kit (Qiagen, Hilden, Germany) for sodium bisulphite conversion of unmethylated cytosines in DNA from low-concentration solutions. In particular, for the preparation of bisulphite reactions, a single colony of each sample (of maximum 10^6 cells per colony) was stored at − 80 °C for at least 2 h to obtain cell membrane damage. After thawing, 40 μl of DNase-free water was added, mixed by vigorous pipetting, and the protocol for the low concentration solutions of DNA was followed. The eluted (treated) DNA per single colony was stored at − 20 °C until use.

Statistical analysis and correlation of methylation and expression results

Statistical analysis was performed for all data collected regarding percentage of methylation per CpG site and mRNA levels. Results were correlated either to the corresponding gene expression percentages or to the methylation/hypomethylation impact of the CpG islands of all studied genes before and after the HU treatment.

The results of the methylation analysis were presented as mean ratio of the methylation levels at CpG sites within gene loci of interest. Statistical analysis and boxplots were performed using SPSS software version 20. Depending on the normality tests of datasets, independent sample *t* test or Mann-Whitney test was used to compare untreated (−HU) single BFU-E colonies and single BFU-E colonies treated with HU (+HU) between each group. Also, the one-way ANOVA or the Kruskal-Wallis test for not normally distributed data was used for the comparison of methylation status between both untreated single BFU-E colonies and in vivo samples in all subgroups.

In all cases, p values less than 0.05 were considered statistically significant.

Results

Detection and recording of γ-globin expression (in vitro) in the presence of hydroxyurea

Total RNA collected from CFU cultures was subjected to a quantitative PCR (qPCR) assay to detect γ-globin mRNA expression profile. Variation in γ-globin levels were observed in biological replicate experiments with CFU cultures from the same donor, which prompted us to refine the HU concentrations used in culture conditions (50–100 μM). Finally, culture media was supplemented with the maximum cell-tolerated HU dose (100 μM) and subsequently the effects on γ-globin gene expression were normalized, to wit γ-globin level

Table 3 Pyrosequencing and qPCR primer sets

Gene	CpG islands	Sequence	Primers
BCL11A	CpG 120	5′ GTTGTTTTGGAGTGGGAG 3′	Forward
		5′ CAAATTAAAAACTAAACCTCCAAATTAC 3′	Reverse 5′-biotin labeled
		5′ TTTTTTTTTTGAGATTTTTAGGAGT 3′	Forward/Pyrosequencing
		5′ATTACTCCCCAACACCCTCCT 3′	Reverse 5′-biotin labeled
		5′ TTTTATTTTTTTTAGTTAGTTG 3′	Pyrosequencing
	CpG 115	5′ GTTAGTTTGGGAGGGGGTGA 3′	Forward
		5′ AAACCAAATACAAACTTACCATATCC 3′	Reverse 5′-biotin labeled
		5′ GTTATGTGGGTTGAATG 3′	Pyrosequencing
KLF1	CpG 98	5′ GGTTAGGGGTTGGTGGTTGG 3′	Forward
		5′ AACCCCCCCCCCTCACCTATA 3′	Reverse 5′-biotin labeled
		5′ TGGGTTTAGTTTTGGTTTTA 3′	Pyrosequencing
		5′ GAGGATTTAGGTGTGA 3′	Pyrosequencing
MYB	CpG 216	5′ GATAGTGAGTGGGAGTTGGAGGA 3′	Forward
		5′ CCATCAAACAAAAAACTTTAAACACT 3′	Reverse 5′-biotin labeled
		5′ GGAGGAGAGAGAGTAGAATGGGAG 3′	Pyrosequencing
		5′ GGTTTGTTTAGGAAAAGG 3′	Pyrosequencing
SIN3A	CpG 401	5′ AGGGGGTGGTTTGAAAGG 3′	Forward
		5′ ATATCATCCAATCCACATCCAAAA 3′	Reverse 5′-biotin labeled
		5′ GGGAAAAGGAAATGTATTAG 3′	Pyrosequencing
ZBTB7A	CpG 326	5′ GTAGATTTTTTTGTGTTAAGGA 3′	Forward
		5′ AACAAACCCCCAACCTCTAC 3′	Reverse 5′-biotin labeled
		5′ GGGATTTTTATAGTTTTATTTTTAA 3′	Pyrosequencing
		5′ GGGTTTTGGTTGTATTGTATAGTTAT 3′	Forward
		5′ CTCATACACTTAACCCCCAAT 3′	Reverse 5′-biotin labeled
		5′ GAGGGAGAGATTAGGGTA 3′	Pyrosequencing
GATA2	CpG 515	5′ ATTGTTAGGGAGGTTTAGAGTAT 3′	Forward
		5′ ACTCTCAAACCCCAAACTT 3′	Reverse 5′-biotin labeled
		5′ GAGAGAGTAGGGAGGGGGT 3′	Pyrosequencing
MAP3K5	CpG 172	5′ GTGGTGGAGAGGGAGAGAGTTTGTAAG 3′	Forward
		5′ CTAACCAACCACAACTCCAAACTACTCC 3′	Reverse 5′-biotin labeled
		5′ GTTTTTTTTGGTTTTTTTTAGA 3′	Pyrosequencing
		qPCR primer sets	
HBG	–	5′-GAC AAG CTG CAT GTG GAT CCT-3′	Forward
		5′-CCG AAA TGG ATT GCC AAA AC-3′	Reverse
ZBTB7A	–	5′-CAT CTG CGA GAA GGT CAT CC-3′	Forward
		5′-TGT CCT GCC TGG TGA AGC-3′	Reverse
GAPDH	–	5′-CCA TGT TCG TCA TGG GTG TGA-3′	Forward
		5′CAT GGA CTG TGG TCA TGA GT-3′	Reverse

variations between sister CFU cultures from the same donor were of no statistical significance.

BFU-E cell colonies grown at 100 μM HU showed, with no exception, an increase in γ-globin calculated as relative expression. Non-responders (III NR1–4) showed a maximum of 2.1-fold increase while responders (III R1–5) a 3.66-fold, all compared to their related untreated cells (–HU) (Additional file 1: Figure S1). BFU-Es from healthy donors (IV CG1–4, UCB1–4, and BM1–4) showed a 1.3–5.6-fold increase in γ-globin expression.

Correlation of γ-globin induction (in vitro) with HbF levels (in vivo) upon HU treatment

The elevated γ-globin gene expression obtained from the ex vivo culture system (CFU) was compared to the corresponding in vivo HbF levels determined among patients (responders and non-responders) at relevant time points, namely, at baseline, before HU treatment, and at the plateau phase (after 5–6 months of continuous HU treatment). HbF levels were detected during regular preset patients' hematological tests at the Hematology Division of the Patras' University Hospital with the HPLC method. Responders (III R1–5) showed augmented HbF percentage, within a range of 2.5–5.6-fold, while non-responders (III NR1–4) exhibited an increased HbF percentage, always lower than 2.5-fold difference (1.1–1.7) from baseline. Increased γ-globin gene expression (ex vivo) under the presence of HU was well correlated with HbF expression levels in patients at the plateau phase (in vivo) confirming experimental culture conditions and concentrations of HU added (Table 2).

In vivo methylation levels within CpG islands of *HBB* cluster "modifier genes" among non-responders and responders receiving HU treatment and control group

Methylation profiles of the selected CpGs were tested in genomic material derived from peripheral mononuclear blood cells (PBMCs) of non-responders (I NR1–11) and responders (I R1–19) under long and continuous HU therapy, and of the control group (II CG1–20) (Additional file 1: Table S1). CpGs tested were CpG120 and CpG115 of *BCL11A*, CpG98 of *KLF1*, CpG216 of *MYB*, CpG172 of *MAP3K5*, CpG401 of *SIN3A*, CpG326 of *ZBTB7A*, and CpG515 of *GATA2* (Table 1).

DNA from PBMCs showed an extensive heterogeneity of the methylation levels of CpG islands, and non-significant results were recorded apart from the *SIN3A* CpG 401. *SIN3A* CpG 401 was deferentially methylated between non-responders (I NR1–11) and responders (I R1–19) (p^*, 0.024), with the non-responders exhibiting higher methylation rates across the entire CpG DNA sequence (data not shown). Since it is not a tissue-specific factor [32], the statistically significant differentiation of *SIN3A* methylation with a consequent differential expression of its protein product within PBMCs was not an unexpected result.

KLF1 CpG98, *ZBTB7A* CpG326, and *GATA2* CpG515 did not alter significantly their methylation levels compared to all subgroups, before and after HU treatment. *MYB* CpG216, *MAP3K5* CpG172, and *BCL11A* CpG120 had an established intrinsic methylation level of less than 10% among all groups; therefore, we concluded that we could not deliver reliable results of the HU effect on their methylation status.

Differentiation of methylation profiles of *HBB* cluster "modifier genes" caused by HU treatment in single BFU-E colonies derived from non-responders, responders, and control groups

To further explore the potential epigenetic influence of HU and to particularize it on cells of the erythroid lineage, we isolated well-defined single BFU-E colonies (screened under an inverted microscope) [33] and determined hyper-/hypomethylation status of all CpGs in every single colony based on a slightly diverged bisulphite conversion protocol (described in the "Material and methods" section) before and after the HU treatment of the cells. Although an inter-individual character between BFU-E-matured cells within a single colony could not be excluded, uniform distribution of methylation profiles was observed in experimental replicates of individual samples and among two or three (2–3) different BFU-E colonies tested from the same donor.

Regarding the healthy control group, pluripotent hematopoietic stem cells from the peripheral (IV CG1-CG4) and umbilical cord blood (IV UCB1-UCB4) as well as from bone marrow aspirations (IV BM1-BM4) were included, to explore possible fundamental epigenetic similarities with hematopoietic pluripotent stem cells derived from the patient's groups (III NR1-NR4 and III R1-R5). Responders (III R1-R5) and non-responders (III NR1-NR4) were also included in the in vitro assays, but had not entered the HU treatment regimen yet (in vitro samples, Table 2). Assortment of Rs and NRs was done long after the HU treatment initiation, based on their clinical characteristics and HbF induction at plateau phase. Hematopoietic pluripotent stem cells from all different tissues were expanded as described in the "Material and methods" section both without (–HU) and with (+HU) HU addition (100 μM), and at the BFU-E stage, two to three single colonies from every sample were isolated separately and subjected to methylation assay.

The methylation status of all *HBB* cluster "modifier genes" showed mean values below 50–60% along the entire CpG sequences and exhibited hypomethylation in the presence of HU among all different groups of BFU-Es tested, which is consistent with the results from whole genome methylation assays during cell transition from early hematopoietic $CD34^+$ to erythroid lineage committed cells [34].

MYB CpG216, *MAP3K5* CpG172, and *BCL11A* CpG120 had the exact negligible methylation level of less than 10% before (–HU) and after the addition of the drug (+HU), as mentioned in the in vivo methylation reactions; therefore, statistical analysis of these areas was not performed either (Additional file 1: Figure S3).

To the rest of the studied CpGs, the addition of HU (100 μM) caused a general mild decrease in CpG methylation status with minor exceptions. Differential baseline methylation patterns within the CpG islands were obtained, before the HU treatment, between the differently originated descendants (BFUEs: IV CG1–4, III R1–5, III NR1–4, IV UCB1–4, and IV BM1–4). This observation suggests that HU action exhibits epigenetic diversity towards individual primary cell types. Statistically significant differences in the baseline methylation levels were recorded from *ZBTB7A* CpG326 between both BM (p^*, 0.013) and UCB (p^*, 0.016) with CG and between NR with CG (p^*,0.021) and NR with R (p^*, 0.019). Similar results were obtained from *KLF1* CpG98 between BM and UCB (p^*, 0.038) (Fig. 3).

Statistically significant hypomethylation was obtained in the *ZBTB7A* (p^*, 0.047) and *GATA2* (p^*, 0.038) CpG islands only in the NR group of patients after HU treatment (Fig. 4a). BFU-Es derived from the non-responders showed the same trend of a mild hypomethylation profile in *KLF1, SIN3A*, and *BCL11A* CpGs, but of no statistical significance (Fig. 4b) (Additional file 1: Figure S2).

The hypomethylation status of the *ZBTB7A* CpG326 located at the gene's proximal promoter region could lead to a possible elevated expression of LRF (leukemia/lymphoma-related factor) and the protein product of *ZBTB7A* gene and could have emerged the failure of γ-globin induction above the limit of the 2.1-fold (maximum observed γ-globin relative expression), on account of the erythropoietic cells' exposure to the HU agent among non-responders. This observation led us to trace LRF/*ZBTB7A* expression levels among responders and non-responders.

Detection and recording of LRF/*ZBTB7A* mRNA levels

Specific primers to detect the LRF mRNA were designed (Table 3) and subjected to qPCR to quantitate its expression profile before and after the HU addition to cultivated cells. Total RNA for qPCR experiments was extracted from 30 to 50 characterized BFU-E colonies for each sample, to ensure that the LRF/*ZBTB7A* expression levels represent cells of the erythroid lineage and are consistent to similar methylation results obtained from single BFU-E colonies. LRF expression was calculated as previously described ("Materials and methods" section). Relative LRF expression was elevated only in NR group (1.1 to1.4-fold increase) in the presence of HU, which was in consistency with the hypomethylation results obtained in *ZBTB7A* CpG326 among the same group (NRs) (Fig. 5a, b). Similar studies delineate the expression of LRF/*ZBTB7A* at a more mature stage of red cell differentiation, after the proerythroblast stage [35]; hence, its expression at BFU-E colonies is at a minimum detectable level and only upon the simultaneous treatment of cells with the HU.

Discussion

The fine regulation of the *HBB* cluster "modifier genes" caused by their natural epigenetic variations on DNA methylation profile and/or by HU medication widely used to treat β-hemoglobinopathies has been the target of investigation in the present study. CpG islands

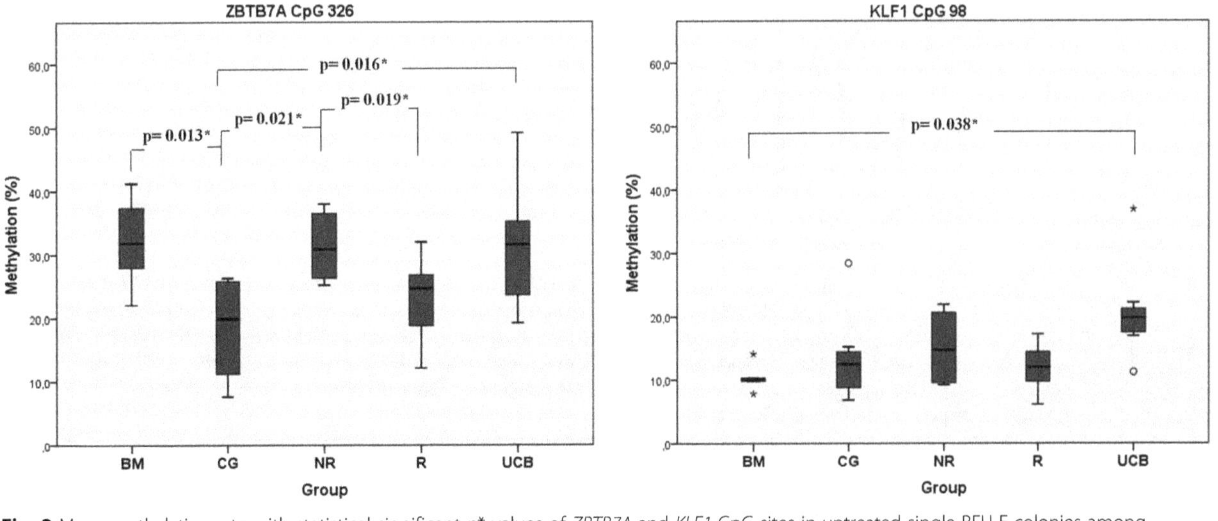

Fig. 3 Mean methylation rate with statistical significant p^* values of *ZBTB7A* and *KLF1* CpG sites in untreated single BFU-E colonies among different groups from Table 2 (in vitro samples). Data derived from single BFU-E colonies before the addition of HU are presented as boxplots. Boxes represent the 25th and the 75th percentiles of total values. They include the maximum and minimum values, the median value of the data set (lines inside the boxes), the most extreme values (*), the outliers (°), and the significant p^* values. BM, CG, NR, R, and UCB indicate bone marrow, control group, HU non-responders, HU responders, and umbilical cord blood respectively

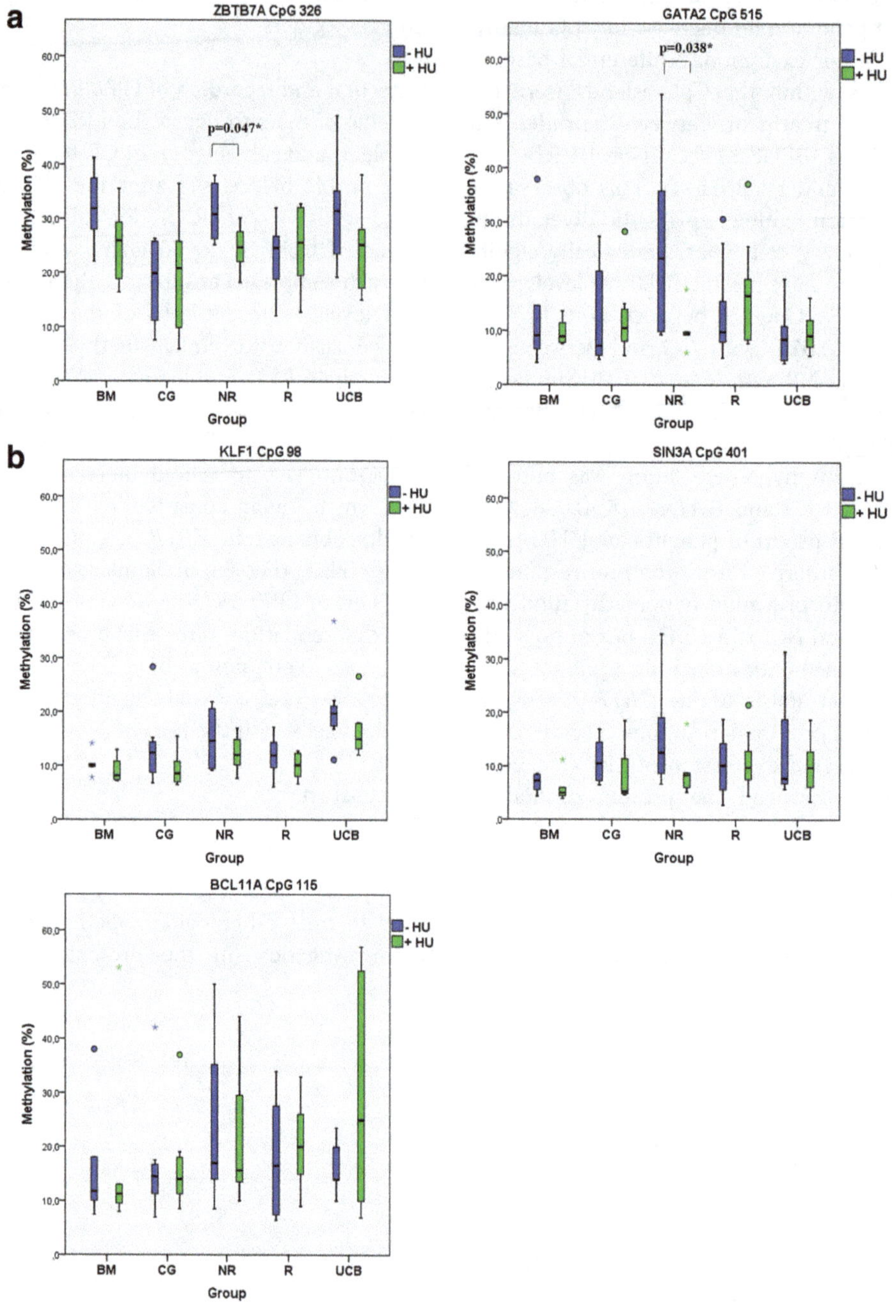

Fig. 4 Mean methylation rate of CpG sites in single BFU-E colonies before and after HU treatment among all in vitro groups of samples (Table 2). **a** *ZBTB7A* CpG 326 and *GATA2* CpG 515 showed a significant hypomethylation profile in non-responders (NRs). **b** *SIN3A* CpG 401, *KLF1* CpG 98, and *BCL11A* CpG 115 showed hypomethylation trend in NRs, though not of statistical significance. Data are presented as boxplots. Boxes represent the 25th and the 75th percentiles of total values. They include the maximum and minimum values, the median value of the data set (lines inside the boxes), the most extreme values (*), the outliers (°), and the significant *p** values recorded. BM, CG, NR, R, and UCB indicate BFU-Es derived from bone marrow, control group, HU non-responders, HU responders, and umbilical cord blood respectively

included in the study were the *BCL11A*, *KLF1*, *MYB*, *MAP3K5*, *SIN3A*, *ZBTB7A*, and *GATA2*, which are known to influence the natural developmental switch in hemoglobin expression, from fetal to adult. Nuclear factors and their genetic variations have long been investigated, but whether and to what extent they cooperate with epigenetic signals in fetal globin repression/induction is not yet fully understood.

The CpG sites selected for the present study bared factors involved in chromatin remodeling, such as the CCCT C-binding factor, known as *CTCF* and the leukemia/lymphoma-related factor (LRF/*ZBTB7A*). *CTCF* is a chromatin

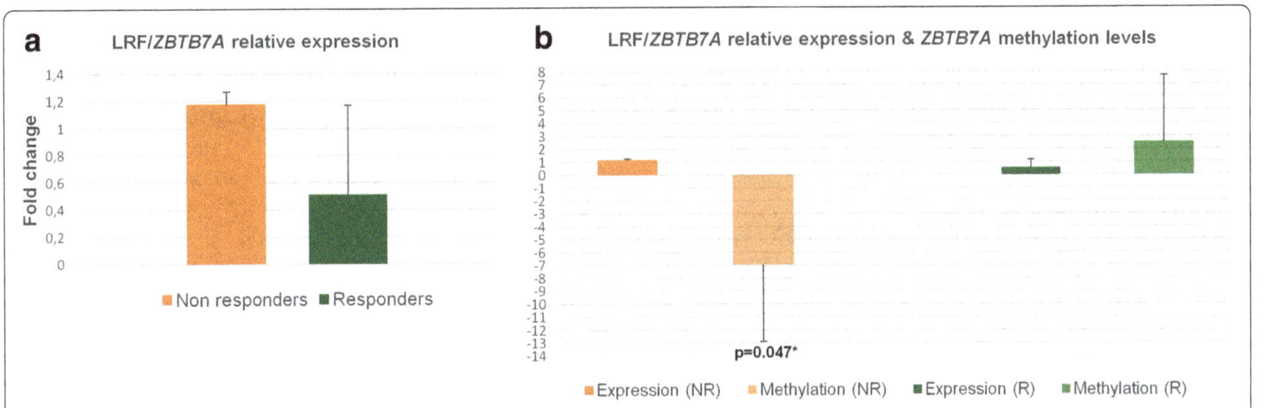

Fig. 5 Relative expression of LRF/*ZBTB7A* and statistical correlations between gene's methylation and expression. **a** Relative expression of LRF/*ZBTB7A* in BFU-E colonies of responders and non-responders (III R1–5, III NR1–4) after HU treatment. **b** Correlation between methylation and gene expression results in responders and non-responders (III R1–5, III NR1–4). Hypomethylation results in *ZBTB7A* CpG 326 were in line with the higher expression of *ZBTB7A* observed in non-responders. Opposite results were detected in the responders' group

structural factor that plays a key role in gene expression through the activation or repression of gene promotes, the insulation of enhancers, and the regulation of distant chromatin interactions [36]. Binding of CTCF on DNA can be altered by DNA methylation. Especially, when CTCF-binding sites contain CpG dinucleotides, binding could be methylation specific, suggesting a role for *CTCF* in epigenetic regulatory mechanisms [37]. Our findings in respect to the methylation repertory of the *HBB* cluster "modifier genes" within the CpG regions encompassing CTCF-binding sites showed that it was normally distributed along the CpG island. These results indicated that the CTCF factor did not preserve any insulating function (at least for the genes studied) that could prevent the hypo- or hyper-methylation spreading across the specific CpG genome sequences, in the presence of HU.

The LRF/*ZBTB7A* is a member of the POK (POZ/BTB and Krüppel) protein family, which binds to CG-rich regions and recruits histone deacetylases to gene promoters leading to a closed chromatin conformation that prevents transcription [38]. The bioinformatics analysis showed that recognition binding sites for *CTCF* and *ZBTB7A* factors were settled at contiguous DNA sequences, while *ZBTB7A*-binding sites were apparent in all CpG areas selected for this study (Fig. 1). LRF/*ZBTB7A* factor has been characterized as an HbF repressor that acts independently from the known fetal globin repressor *BCL11A*, by recruitment of the NuRD complex [39, 40]. Another study has uncovered the combined action of *KLF1* with *ZBTB7A* to depress HbF [41].

Results from the in vitro methylation assays performed in this study clearly showed a hypomethylating trend in non-responders (III NR in Fig. 4) in the presence of HU, which reached a statistical significance for the *ZBTB7A* (–HU/+HU, p^*, 0.047) and the *GATA2* (–HU/+HU, p^*, 0.038) CpGs. Parallel gene expression experiments with RNA isolated from BFU-Es of the same cultures allowed us to directly correlate changes in methylation to gene expression. Hypomethylation of the *ZBTB7A* CpG326 was associated with higher levels of LRF/*ZBTB7A* expression in non-responders (III NR), up to 1.4-fold (Fig. 5). Hypomethylation of *GATA2* CpG515 potentially enhances the GATA2 protein expression too, but levels of GATA2 mRNA were not targeted in this study. The GATA2 high expression was considered assured as premature erythroid cells (and BFU-Es) are known to express higher levels of GATA2, which in later stages of maturation switches to GATA1 [28, 42].

The HU hypomethylation effect was also visible in *KLF1* CpG98, *SIN3A* CpG401, and *BCL11A* CpG115, but not at significant rates, whereas *MYB* CpG216, *MAP3K5* CpG172, and *BCL11A* CpG120 were methylated at nugatory values before and after HU. The detected minor changes in their methylation profiles were likely to be borderline, and thus, statistical analysis of these areas was not performed. Furthermore, the non-responder group of patients (III NR) had an established baseline higher methylation profile in CpG326 of *ZBTB7A*, in the absence of HU, compared to responders (III R) (p^*, 0.019) and healthy donors (IV CG) (p^*, 0.021) (Fig. 3), suggesting an underlying epigenetic mechanism of HU action by the methylation modulation of the *ZBTB7A*, leading to an amplitude modulation of its expression. The LRF encoded by the *ZBTB7A* gene preferentially binds methylated CpGs and acts as a γ-globin repressor [39]. This is in accordance with our results derived from the HU non-responders. Probably, their higher baseline methylation status along the *HBB* "modifier gene loci" favors the LRF binding, leading to a hardly irreversible suppression of the HbF production even under the HU influence.

Additionally, there were statistically significant differences in the CpG326 of *ZBTB7A* among IV CG and IV UCB (p^*, 0.016) and IV CG and IV BM (p^*, 0.013). Evidence from human systems indicates that pluripotent hematopoietic stem cells exhibit an epigenetic memory, related to their donor cell type of origin [43], and our results support these observations.

Results of the present study indicate that HU resets the methylation status and eventually the basal program of expression for several factors and definitely to loci unlinked to the *HBB* cluster. The HU non-responders demonstrated an extra barrier of epigenetic regulation for the γ-globin reactivation. Even though HU provoked a similar terminal hypomethylation status to both the HU non-responders and HU responders, (Fig. 4a), the γ-globin expression was not ultimately prevailed in the HU non-responders. The most likely explanation is that expression of the β- and γ-globin genes is still inherently unstable at the BFU-E stage and that micro-environmental conditions persisting during the erythroid differentiation determine whether β- or γ-globin expression will be favored.

Previous attempts to detect DNA methylation changes in CpG sequences lying at neighboring areas to the γ^G-globin promoter have not achieved any informative insights [44]. Also, the HU epigenetic effect is manifested only in *HBB* modifier factors, derived from cells of the erythroid lineage, which was apparent from our study. A considerable heterogeneity on the epigenetic effect detected at the in vivo samples was attributed to the different origins and the subsistence of mixed cell populations within PBMCs. On the contrary, BFUEs (in vitro samples) consist of a cell population obtained from cell/tissue culture systems, uniformly differentiated towards the erythropoietic lineage, albeit PBMCs isolated from blood samples included a mixture of all mononuclear blood cells, which although they were exposed to the daily dose of HU, they seem not to have responded homogeneously. The methylation profile of all CpG islands gave significant results only when the research focused on well-characterized single erythroid colonies (BFU-Es), with the unique exception of the *SIN3A* CpG 401, which is not an erythroid tissue-specific factor. The SIN3A protein consists of multiple protein interaction domains and contacts a variety of binding partners to perform its biological function, whereas it is considered to co-operate with histone-modifying complexes exhibiting a global transcription regulatory property [32]. Hence, *SIN3A* was differentially methylated (p^*, 0.024) between the in vivo samples (PBMCs) of HU non-responders and HU responders.

The role of *ZBTB7A* as an HbF repressor is fully supported by our data, due to its broad existence as a binding factor to all CpG islands selected and analyzed in this study, its significant hypomethylation, and the elevated levels (although modest) of LRF/*ZBTB7A* expression in non-responders treated with HU (Fig. 5). On the contrary, the baseline hypomethylated ZBTB7A-binding sites in the HU responder group of patients either do not show preference for the LRF binding or LRF is produced at adverse levels unable to force the γ-globin repression.

The present epigenetic analysis of the *HBB* cluster "modifier genes" provides some valuable information related to the heterogeneous response to HU, in an effort to predict patients' response to treatment. We evaluated the HU potential as a hypomethylating agent although HU has not been previously associated with epigenetic responses, other than enhancing the expression of specific miRNAs [45–47]. Several miRNAs have been highlighted as epigenetic regulators of erythroid differentiation that influence HbF production (miR-26b, miR-151-3p, miR210) upon HU treatment. In contrast to fixed genome sequence, epigenetic patterns are plastic; thus, correcting aberrant, disease-causing epigenetic marks holds considerable therapeutic promise.

Conclusions and future perspectives

A drawback to current HU treatment for the SCA and SCA/β-thal patients is its non-specific effects. Our pharmacoepigenomic study reveals the epigenetic pharmacological activity of HU distinguishes the different epigenetic regulatory nuclear mechanisms acting among HU responders and HU non-responders and contributes to the development of a clinical algorithm for improved prediction of the patients' response to HU treatment.

The *ZBTB7A* appears as an emerging epigenetic regulator of the HbF induction bypassing the already known repressors of γ-globin expression. *ZBTB7A* possibly exerts its repressing function to the γ-globin gene through a chromatin remodeling pathway, which is supported by the broad existence of its multiple recognition binding sites close to all *HBB* cluster "modifier loci" tested. The *ZBTB7A*/LRF epigenetically induced binding to preconfigured *HBB* cluster "modifier genes" promoters should also be investigated, to uncover the vital changes to promoter accessibility and subsequent motivations for gene activation or repression.

Moreover, the methodology of the single-colony (BFU-E) DNA methylation analysis, developed by our lab, seems to be mostly appropriate and informative for the specific cell epigenetic responses towards the HbF re-induction pathway during treatment with HU. In addition to our results, it would be very interesting to investigate the epigenetic marks of reprogrammed erythroid progenitors further, under the influence of HU or other HbF inductive agents in immature proerythroblasts and other subpopulations of the hematopoietic cell lineage. Critical questions such as whether CpG islands of different tissues are uniformly targeted by the epigenetic machinery components or some are "safe-guarded" by nuclear factors and remain unaffected need further insight.

Contemporary medication focused on the *HBB* locus-specific modifiers, used in conjunction with epigenetic biomarkers of response, as *ZBTB7A* CpG326 and *GATA2* CpG515, highlighted in this study, will enable truly precision interventions.

Additional file

Additional file 1: Table S1. Hematological data of HU responders (R) and HU non-responders (NR) used as in vivo samples. Figure S1 In vivo HbF levels and γ-globin expression in vitro before and after HU treatment. (a) III NR2 and (b) III NR4 patients (Table 2) at baseline of HbF expression before HU treatment (c) III NR2, (d)III NR4 and (e) III R5 patients at the plateau phase, with maximum detected HbF expression levels. Arrows show the HbF curve. (f) γ-globin gene expression in BFU-E colonies calculated as relative expression of treated compared to untreated with HU colonies, using the formula $2^{(-\Delta Ct)}$ and normalized to the reference *GAPDH* gene. Figure S2 DNA methylation levels estimated by the pyrosequencing CpG assay. Typical pyrograms displaying DNA methylation analyses before and after cells' treatment with HU of: (a) *ZBTB7A* CpG 326, (b) *GATA2* CpG 515, (c) *KLF1* CpG 98, (d) *SIN3A* CpG 401, (e) *BCL11A* CpG 115. Figure S3 DNA methylation levels less than 10% either with or without the addition of HU, estimated using the pyrosequencing CpG assay. Typical pyrograms displaying DNA methylation levels of (a) *BCL11A* CpG 120, and (b) *MYB* CpG 216.

Abbreviations

BFU-E: Burst-forming unit-erythroid; BM: Bone marrow; CFU: Colony-forming unit assay; CFU-E: Colony-forming unit-erythroid; CG: Control group; HbF: Fetal hemoglobin; HU: Hydroxyurea; NR: Non-responders; PBMCs: Peripheral blood mononuclear cells; R: Responders; SCA: Sickle cell anemia; UCB: Umbilical cord blood

Acknowledgements

The authors wish to thank all patients and donors for providing samples for the completion of this research. We would like to thank Vassiliki Pesli, who performed all venipunctures to patients and controls for blood collection, and Constantina Argyropoulou, who performed the HPLC for HbF estimations. We also acknowledge George Georgis from HOU for providing technical assistance with the figures.

Funding

This research was financially supported by PENER_EAP_2016 grant of the Hellenic Open University.

Authors' contributions

VC designed and performed all methylation assays and was responsible for the CFU cultures. EFS designed and performed qPCRs and was also responsible for the CFU cultures. AKS, ArSy, EV, and PC were responsible for monitoring of the patients, collection of their hematological data, and revision of the manuscript. GM did all the bioinformatics analysis. VF performed the statistical analysis. GPP, AP, and ArSg designed the study, elaborated the data, and reviewed the manuscript. ArSg supervised the whole research project and wrote the manuscript. All authors read and approved the final manuscript.

Ethics approval and consent to participate

The whole process of sample collection (peripheral blood and bone marrow aspirations) was carried in accordance to ethical guidelines and under the supervision of the Thalassemia & Hemoglobinopathies Unit, Division of Hematology of the Patras' University Hospital. The study has been approved by the Patras' University Hospital Ethical and Scientific Committee, and a written informed consent to participation from all patients and healthy donors was obtained. Fresh umbilical cord blood samples were collected from the Hellenic Cord Blood Bank (HCBB) of the Biomedical Research Foundation Academy of Athens from healthy donors after their positive response to donate a portion of the sample (2–3 ml) for scientific research purposes.

Consent for publication

Not applicable.

Competing interests

The authors declare that they have no competing interests.

Author details

[1]School of Science and Technology, Biology Laboratory, Hellenic Open University, Patras, Greece. [2]Faculty of Medicine, Biology Laboratory, University of Ioannina, Ioannina, Greece. [3]Thalassemia and Hemoglobinopathies Unit, Hematology Division, Department of Internal Medicine, General University Hospital of Patras, Patras, Greece. [4]School of Science and Technology, Digital Systems and Media Computing Laboratory, Hellenic Open University, Patras, Greece. [5]Medical School, Hematology Division, Department of Internal Medicine, University of Patras, Patras, Greece. [6]Thalassemia Unit, "Hippokrateio" General Hospital of Thessaloniki, Thessaloniki, Greece. [7]Thalassemia and Sickle Cell Unit, AHEPA University General Hospital of Thessaloniki, Thessaloniki, Greece. [8]School of Health Sciences, Department of Pharmacy, Laboratory of Pharmacogenomics and Individualized Therapy, University of Patras, Patras, Greece. [9]Medical Faculty, Laboratory of General Biology, University of Patras, Patras, Greece.

References

1. Taher AVE, Musallam K, Cappellini MD, Viprakasit V. Guidelines for the management of non transfusion dependent thalassaemia (NTDT). Nicosia Cyprus: Thalassaemia International Federation; 2013.
2. Giannopoulou E, Bartsakoulia M, Tafrali C, Kourakli A, Poulas K, Stavrou EF, et al. A single nucleotide polymorphism in the HBBP1 gene in the human beta-globin locus is associated with a mild beta-thalassemia disease phenotype. Hemoglobin. 2012;36(5):433–45. https://doi.org/10.3109/03630269.2012.717515.
3. Lessard S, Beaudoin M, Benkirane K, Lettre G. Comparison of DNA methylation profiles in human fetal and adult red blood cell progenitors. Genome Med. 2015;7(1):1. https://doi.org/10.1186/s13073-014-0122-2.
4. Lavelle DE. The molecular mechanism of fetal hemoglobin reactivation. Semin Hematol. 2004;41(4 Suppl 6):3–10.
5. Gravia A, Chondrou V, Sgourou A, Papantoni I, Borg J, Katsila T, et al. Individualizing fetal hemoglobin augmenting therapy for beta-type hemoglobinopathies patients. Pharmacogenomics. 2014;15(10):1355–64. https://doi.org/10.2217/pgs.14.101.
6. Kolliopoulou A, Stratopoulos A, Siamoglou S, Sgourou A, Ali BR, Papachatzopoulou A, et al. Key pharmacogenomic considerations for sickle cell disease patients. OMICS. 2017;21(6):314–22. https://doi.org/10.1089/omi.2017.0058.
7. Platt OS, Orkin SH, Dover G, Beardsley GP, Miller B, Nathan DG. Hydroxyurea enhances fetal hemoglobin production in sickle cell anemia. J Clin Invest. 1984;74(2):652–6. https://doi.org/10.1172/JCI111464.
8. Mabaera R, West RJ, Conine SJ, Macari ER, Boyd CD, Engman CA, et al. A cell stress signaling model of fetal hemoglobin induction: what doesn't kill red blood cells may make them stronger. Exp Hematol. 2008;36(9):1057–72. https://doi.org/10.1016/j.exphem.2008.06.014.
9. Musallam KM, Taher AT, Cappellini MD, Sankaran VG. Clinical experience with fetal hemoglobin induction therapy in patients with beta-thalassemia.

Blood. 2013;121(12):2199–212; quiz 372. https://doi.org/10.1182/blood-2012-10-408021.

10. Rigano P, Pecoraro A, Calzolari R, Troia A, Acuto S, Renda D, et al. Desensitization to hydroxycarbamide following long-term treatment of thalassaemia intermedia as observed in vivo and in primary erythroid cultures from treated patients. Br J Haematol. 2010;151(5):509–15. https://doi.org/10.1111/j.1365-2141.2010.08397.x.
11. Mancuso A, Maggio A, Renda D, Di Marzo R, Rigano P. Treatment with hydroxycarbamide for intermedia thalassaemia: decrease of efficacy in some patients during long-term follow up. Br J Haematol. 2006;133(1):105–6. https://doi.org/10.1111/j.1365-2141.2006.06002.x.
12. Gluckman PD, Hanson MA, Buklijas T, Low FM, Beedle AS. Epigenetic mechanisms that underpin metabolic and cardiovascular diseases. Nat Rev Endocrinol. 2009;5(7):401–8. https://doi.org/10.1038/nrendo.2009.102.
13. Tang J, Xiong Y, Zhou HH, Chen XP. DNA methylation and personalized medicine. J Clin Pharm Ther. 2014;39(6):621–7. https://doi.org/10.1111/jcpt.12206.
14. Bird A. DNA methylation patterns and epigenetic memory. Genes Dev. 2002;16(1):6–21. https://doi.org/10.1101/gad.947102.
15. Sheehan VA, Luo Z, Flanagan JM, Howard TA, Thompson BW, Wang WC, et al. Genetic modifiers of sickle cell anemia in the BABY HUG cohort: influence on laboratory and clinical phenotypes. Am J Hematol. 2013;88(7):571–6. https://doi.org/10.1002/ajh.23457.
16. Liu P, Keller JR, Ortiz M, Tessarollo L, Rachel RA, Nakamura T, et al. Bcl11a is essential for normal lymphoid development. Nat Immunol. 2003;4(6):525–32. https://doi.org/10.1038/ni925.
17. Tafrali C, Paizi A, Borg J, Radmilovic M, Bartsakoulia M, Giannopoulou E, et al. Genomic variation in the MAP3K5 gene is associated with beta-thalassemia disease severity and hydroxyurea treatment efficacy. Pharmacogenomics. 2013;14(5):469–83. https://doi.org/10.2217/pgs.13.31.
18. Gravia‡ A, Chondrou‡ V, Kolliopoulou A, Kourakli A, John A, Symeonidis A, Ali BR, Sgourou A, Papachatzopoulou A, Katsila T, Patrinos GP. "Correlation of SIN3A genomic variants with β-hemoglobinopathies disease severity and hydroxyurea treatment efficacy". Pharmacogenomics. 2016;17(16). https://doi.org/10.2217/pgs-2016-0076, https://www.ncbi.nlm.nih.gov/pubmed/27767389.
19. Uda M, Galanello R, Sanna S, Lettre G, Sankaran VG, Chen W, et al. Genome-wide association study shows BCL11A associated with persistent fetal hemoglobin and amelioration of the phenotype of beta-thalassemia. Proc Natl Acad Sci U S A. 2008;105(5):1620–5. https://doi.org/10.1073/pnas.0711566105.
20. Zhou D, Liu K, Sun CW, Pawlik KM, Townes TM. KLF1 regulates BCL11A expression and gamma- to beta-globin gene switching. Nat Genet. 2010;42(9):742–4. https://doi.org/10.1038/ng.637.
21. Zhang JS, Moncrieffe MC, Kaczynski J, Ellenrieder V, Prendergast FG, Urrutia R. A conserved alpha-helical motif mediates the interaction of Sp1-like transcriptional repressors with the corepressor mSin3A. Mol Cell Biol. 2001;21(15):5041–9. https://doi.org/10.1128/MCB.21.15.5041-5049.2001.
22. Wahlberg K, Jiang J, Rooks H, Jawaid K, Matsuda F, Yamaguchi M, et al. The HBS1L-MYB intergenic interval associated with elevated HbF levels shows characteristics of a distal regulatory region in erythroid cells. Blood. 2009;114(6):1254–62. https://doi.org/10.1182/blood-2009-03-210146.
23. Kawata H, Yamada K, Shou Z, Mizutani T, Yazawa T, Yoshino M, et al. Zinc-fingers and homeoboxes (ZHX) 2, a novel member of the ZHX family, functions as a transcriptional repressor. Biochem J. 2003;373(Pt 3):747–57. https://doi.org/10.1042/BJ20030171.
24. Sankaran VG, Xu J, Ragoczy T, Ippolito GC, Walkley CR, Maika SD, et al. Developmental and species-divergent globin switching are driven by BCL11A. Nature. 2009;460(7259):1093–7. https://doi.org/10.1038/nature08243.
25. Dumitriu BB, Dy P, Huang P, Quayum Y, Jensen N, Lefebvre J. Sox6 is necessary for efficient erythropoiesis in adult mice under physiological and anemia-induced stress conditions. PLoS One. 2010;5(8):e12088. https://doi.org/10.1371/journal.pone.0012088.
26. Borg J, Papadopoulos P, Georgitsi M, Gutierrez L, Grech G, Fanis P, et al. Haploinsufficiency for the erythroid transcription factor KLF1 causes hereditary persistence of fetal hemoglobin. Nat Genet. 2010;42(9):801–5. https://doi.org/10.1038/ng.630.
27. Borg J, Patrinos GP, Felice AE, Philipsen S. Erythroid phenotypes associated with KLF1 mutations. Haematologica. 2011;96(5):635–8. https://doi.org/10.3324/haematol.2011.043265.
28. Suzuki M, Yamamoto M, Engel JD. Fetal globin gene repressors as drug targets for molecular therapies to treat the beta-globinopathies. Mol Cell Biol. 2014;34(19):3560–9. https://doi.org/10.1128/MCB.00714-14.
29. Kent WJ, Sugnet CW, Furey TS, Roskin KM, Pringle TH, Zahler AM, et al. The human genome browser at UCSC. Genome Res. 2002;12(6):996–1006. https://doi.org/10.1101/gr.229102.
30. Consortium. EP. An integrated encyclopedia of DNA elements in the human genome. Nature. 2012;489(7414):57–74. https://doi.org/10.1038/nature11247.
31. Shen Y, Cao R, Liu W, Zhou Y, Wu Y, Tan J, et al. Negative feedback loop between ZBTB7A and TGF-beta in breast cancer. Oncol Lett. 2017;14(2):1403–10. https://doi.org/10.3892/ol.2017.6291.
32. Chaubal A, Pile LA. Same agent, different messages: insight into transcriptional regulation by SIN3 isoforms. Epigenetics Chromatin. 2018;11(1):17. https://doi.org/10.1186/s13072-018-0188-y.
33. Nissen-Druey CT, A. Meyer-Monard, S. Human hematopoietic colonies in health and disease.; 2005.
34. Yu Y, Mo Y, Ebenezer D, Bhattacharyya S, Liu H, Sundaravel S, et al. High resolution methylome analysis reveals widespread functional hypomethylation during adult human erythropoiesis. J Biol Chem. 2013;288(13):8805–14. https://doi.org/10.1074/jbc.M112.423756.
35. Maeda T. Regulation of hematopoietic development by ZBTB transcription factors. Int J Hematol. 2016;104(3):310–23. https://doi.org/10.1007/s12185-016-2035-x.
36. Kim S, Yu NK, Kaang BK. CTCF as a multifunctional protein in genome regulation and gene expression. Exp Mol Med. 2015;47:e166. https://doi.org/10.1038/emm.2015.33.
37. Filippova GN. Genetics and epigenetics of the multifunctional protein CTCF. Curr Top Dev Biol. 2008;80:337–60. https://doi.org/10.1016/S0070-2153(07)80009-3.
38. Lunardi A, Guarnerio J, Wang G, Maeda T, Pandolfi PP. Role of LRF/Pokemon in lineage fate decisions. Blood. 2013;121(15):2845–53. https://doi.org/10.1182/blood-2012-11-292037.
39. Masuda T, Wang X, Maeda M, Canver MC, Sher F, Funnell AP, et al. Transcription factors LRF and BCL11A independently repress expression of fetal hemoglobin. Science. 2016;351(6270):285–9. https://doi.org/10.1126/science.aad3312.
40. Vinjamur DS, Bauer DE, Orkin SH. Recent progress in understanding and manipulating haemoglobin switching for the haemoglobinopathies. Br J Haematol. 2018;180(5):630–43. https://doi.org/10.1111/bjh.15038.
41. Norton LJ, APW F, Burdach J, Wienert B, Kurita R, Nakamura Y, et al. KLF1 directly activates expression of the novel fetal globin repressor ZBTB7A/LRF in erythroid cells. Blood Adv. 2017;1(11):685–92. https://doi.org/10.1182/bloodadvances.2016002303.
42. Anguita E, Hughes J, Heyworth C, Blobel GA, Wood WG, Higgs DR. Globin gene activation during haemopoiesis is driven by protein complexes nucleated by GATA-1 and GATA-2. EMBO J. 2004;23(14):2841–52. https://doi.org/10.1038/sj.emboj.7600274.
43. Kim K, Zhao R, Doi A, Ng K, Unternaehrer J, Cahan P, et al. Donor cell type can influence the epigenome and differentiation potential of human induced pluripotent stem cells. Nat Biotechnol. 2011;29(12):1117–9. https://doi.org/10.1038/nbt.2052.
44. Walker AL, Steward S, Howard TA, Mortier N, Smeltzer M, Wang YD, et al. Epigenetic and molecular profiles of erythroid cells after hydroxyurea treatment in sickle cell anemia. Blood. 2011;118(20):5664–70. https://doi.org/10.1182/blood-2011-07-368746.
45. Bianchi N, Zuccato C, Lampronti I, Borgatti M, Gambari R. Expression of miR-210 during erythroid differentiation and induction of gamma-globin gene expression. BMB Rep. 2009;42(8):493–9.
46. Svasti S, Masaki S, Penglong T, Abe Y, Winichagoon P, Fucharoen S, et al. Expression of microRNA-451 in normal and thalassemic erythropoiesis. Ann Hematol. 2010;89(10):953–8. https://doi.org/10.1007/s00277-010-0980-7.
47. Lulli V, Romania P, Morsilli O, Cianciulli P, Gabbianelli M, Testa U, et al. MicroRNA-486-3p regulates gamma-globin expression in human erythroid cells by directly modulating BCL11A. PLoS One. 2013;8(4):e60436. https://doi.org/10.1371/journal.pone.0060436.

17

Identification of drug repurposing candidates based on a miRNA-mediated drug and pathway network for cardiac hypertrophy and acute myocardial infarction

Jiantao Sun[1], Jiemei Yang[1], Jing Chi[1], Xue Ding[1] and Nan Lv[2*]

Abstract

Background: Cardiac hypertrophy and acute myocardial infarction (AMI) are two common heart diseases worldwide. However, research is needed into the exact pathogenesis and effective treatment strategies for these diseases. Recently, microRNAs (miRNAs) have been suggested to regulate the pathological pathways of heart disease, indicating a potential role in novel treatments.

Results: In our study, we constructed a miRNA-gene-drug network and analyzed its topological features. We also identified some significantly dysregulated miRNA-gene-drug triplets (MGDTs) in cardiac hypertrophy and AMI using a computational method. Then, we characterized the activity score profile features for MGDTs in cardiac hypertrophy and AMI. The functional analyses suggested that the genes in the network held special functions. We extracted an insulin-like growth factor 1 receptor-related subnetwork in cardiac hypertrophy and a vascular endothelial growth factor A-related subnetwork in AMI. Finally, we considered insulin-like growth factor 1 receptor and vascular endothelial growth factor A as two candidate drug targets by utilizing the cardiac hypertrophy and AMI pathways.

Conclusion: These results provide novel insights into the mechanisms and treatment of cardiac hypertrophy and AMI.

Keywords: Drug repurposing, miRNAs, Pathway, Cardiac hypertrophy, Acute myocardial infarction

Background

Cardiovascular disease, especially coronary heart disease and stroke, remains the leading cause of death and disability-adjusted life years for all regions worldwide [1]. Cardiac hypertrophy and acute myocardial infarction (AMI) are two types of common cardiovascular diseases. Cardiac hypertrophy is the heart's response to a variety of extrinsic and intrinsic stimuli that impose increased biomechanical stress [2]. AMI is a common disease with serious consequences in mortality, morbidity, and cost to society [3]. Over the past several years, numerous studies have enhanced our understanding of the mechanism and treatment of cardiovascular health. However, divergent results have created confusion among patients. Drug treatment options and reduction of side effects remain urgent problems for studies of heart disease.

Recent studies have revealed that microRNAs (miRNAs) play essential roles in cardiovascular diseases, including cardiac hypertrophy and AMI. For example, miR-378 suppresses myocardial fibrosis through a paracrine mechanism at the early stage of cardiac hypertrophy following mechanical stress [4]. miR-133 is downregulated in thyroid hormone-mediated cardiac hypertrophy partially via the type 1 angiotensin II receptor [5]. Wei et al. identified miR-101 as an important regulator of cardiac hypertrophy and suggested its potential application in therapy for cardiac hypertrophy [6]. Additionally, many studies have suggested important roles in AMI. For instance, circulating miR-1 and miR-499 have potential as novel biomarkers for AMI [7, 8]. miR-214 inhibits left ventricular remodeling in AMI by suppressing cellular apoptosis via the

* Correspondence: 13936538221@163.com
[2]Department of Obstetrics, the Second Affiliated Hospital, Harbin Medical University, 246 XueFu Road, Harbin 150086, Heilongjiang, People's Republic of China
Full list of author information is available at the end of the article

phosphatase and tensin homolog [9]. In addition, high-throughput microarray and sequencing experiments have identified numerous novel microRNAs in cardiovascular diseases, such as cardiac hypertrophy and AMI [10, 11]. However, many valuable and significant data available for cardiac hypertrophy and AMI had not been abundantly utilized.

Integration of mRNA and miRNA double expression profiles can provide novel insights into research of the mechanisms underlying cardiac hypertrophy and AMI. For example, Yang et al. combined miRNA and mRNA sequencing to identify the protective transcriptome signature of enhanced PI3K signaling in the context of pathological hypertrophy; the results demonstrated that regulation of TGF/miR-21 contributed to the protection of enhanced PI3K signaling against cardiac hypertrophy [12]. Santana et al. compared mRNA and miRNA expression profiles to identify transcriptional and post-transcriptional changes in AMI [13]. Moreover, a network-based method is an effective approach to globally identify biomarkers of disease. For example, Song et al. constructed and analyzed a cardiac hypertrophy-associated long non-coding RNA-mRNA network based on competitive endogenous RNA and revealed functional lncRNAs involved in cardiac hypertrophy. However, these networks have almost exclusively integrated mRNA, miRNA, or lncRNA expression and have lacked drug information.

Research into and development of novel drugs for cardiac hypertrophy and AMI are time-consuming and labor-intensive processes. Recently, drug repurposing has become an essential part of drug discovery that can uncover novel indications for existing drugs [14]. Donner et al. used deep embeddings of gene expression profiles for drug repurposing [15]. Drug repurposing has been successfully used in Parkinson's disease and cancer [16, 17]. However, few studies have focused on drug repurposing for cardiac hypertrophy and AMI.

In this study, we used heart disease-related genes to construct a miRNA-gene-drug network and analyzed its topological features. We also developed a computational approach to identify candidate risk miRNA-gene-drug triplets (MGDTs) based on mRNA and miRNA expression data. The candidate risk MGDTs hold specific and strong activity score profiles in cardiac hypertrophy and AMI. We also extracted an insulin-like growth factor 1 receptor-related subnetwork in cardiac hypertrophy and a vascular endothelial growth factor A-related subnetwork in AMI. Finally, we utilized pathways to explore the mechanisms underlying cardiac hypertrophy and AMI and to identify candidate drugs for these diseases. These results provide novel insights into the underlying mechanisms and treatment of cardiac hypertrophy and AMI.

Results

Global properties of the MGDT network in heart disease

We used cardiovascular disease-associated genes and experimentally verified interactions to construct a MGDT network (Fig. 1a). The MGDT network consisted of 2709 nodes (329 genes, 452 miRNAs, and 928 drugs) and 4571 edges (Fig. 1b). We found that the whole MGDT network showed a scale-free distribution ($R^2 = 0.917$) that was close to that of the majority of biological networks (Fig. 1c). In addition, this result suggested that this MGDT network was similar to a small-world network [18]. Moreover, we found that the degree increased when the topological coefficient decreased, which indicated that the MGDT network showed a hierarchical modularity phenomenon (Fig. 1d). Other types of regulatory networks, such as the ceRNA network in cancer, showed similar topological characteristics [19, 20]. We found that miRNAs in the MGDT network held a higher degree than genes and drugs. The average degrees of the genes, miRNAs, and drugs were 13.85, 4.32, and 1.36, respectively (Fig. 1e). These results indicated that although the miRNAs did not encode proteins, they exhibited more specific topological properties than the mRNAs in the MGDT network. The highest degree nodes were CA2, DRD2, and ESR1 (Fig. 1f). These high degree nodes all play essential roles in biological processes. The above results indicated that the MGDT network showed special features of a regulatory network and might provide an effective background for drug repurposing for cardiac hypertrophy and AMI.

Some MGDTs are specific for cardiac hypertrophy and AMI

We found 15,696 MGDTs in the whole network. We identified 644 and 1029 significantly dysregulated MGDTs in cardiac hypertrophy and AMI, respectively. Then, we constructed cardiac hypertrophy- and AMI-specific networks (Fig. 2a, b). The cardiac hypertrophy-specific network consisted of 374 nodes, 373 edges, 42 genes, 73 miRNAs, and 259 drugs. The AMI-specific network consisted of 701 nodes, 794 edges, 92 genes, 44 miRNAs, and 566 drugs (Fig. 2c). A total of 4.01% of the MGDTs were significantly dysregulated in cardiac hypertrophy, and 6.56% of the MGDTs were significantly dysregulated in AMI (Fig. 2d). We also discovered 80 common MGDTs between cardiac hypertrophy and AMI (Fig. 2e). In total, we found 564 cardiac hypertrophy-specific MGDTs and 949 AMI-specific MGDTs. Then, we constructed a common MGDT network to explore the mechanisms underlying cardiac hypertrophy and AMI (Fig. 2f). The common MGDT network consisted of 91 nodes and 88 edges.

Activity profiles of MGDTs for cardiac hypertrophy and AMI

To characterize the compactness of MGDTs for cardiac hypertrophy and AMI, we evaluated the score values of all MGDTs. We evaluated four types of scores (the last

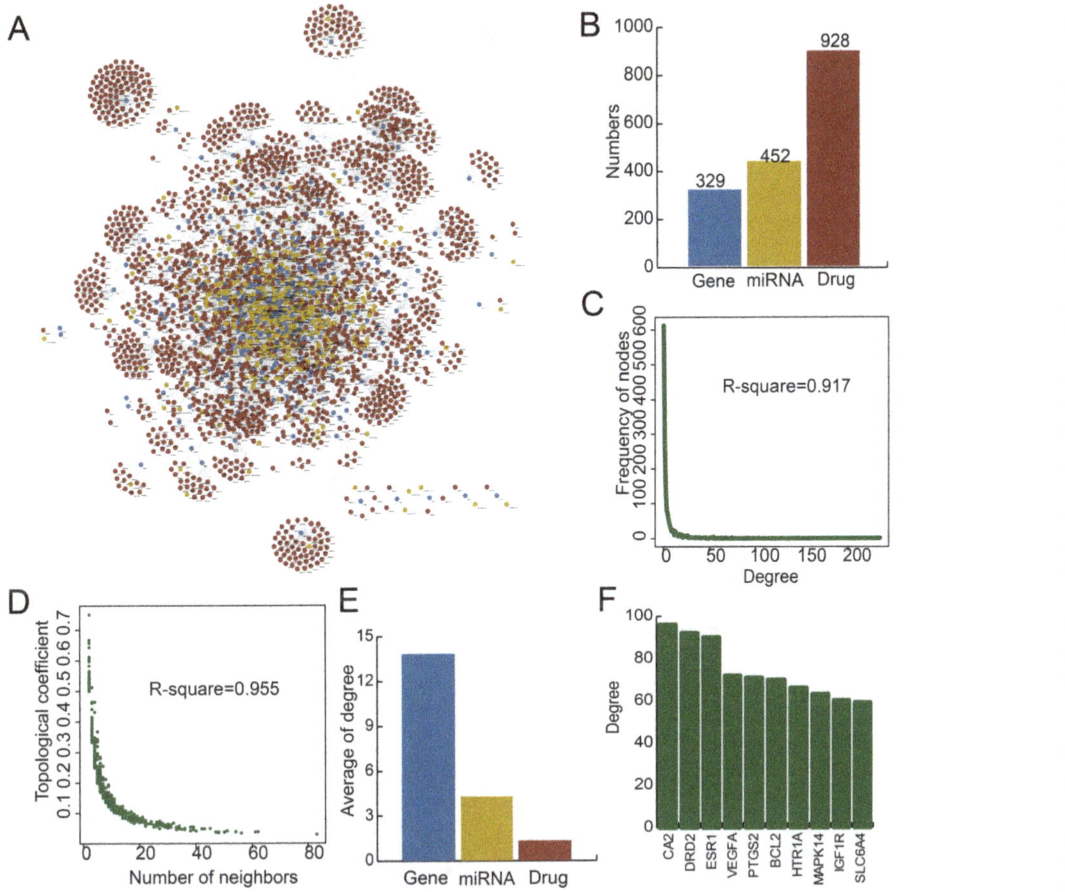

Fig. 1 Construction and global characteristics of the MGDT networks for cardiac hypertrophy and AMI. **a** A global MGDT network for cardiac hypertrophy and AMI. Blue, yellow, and red represent coding genes, miRNAs, and drugs, respectively. **b** A bar plot showing the numbers of coding genes, miRNAs, and drugs. **c** Degree distribution of all nodes in the MGDT network. **d** Topological coefficient of all nodes in the MGDT network. **e** A bar plot showing the average degrees of coding genes, miRNAs, and drugs. **f** The degrees of nodes with the highest degrees in the whole network

score, risk score, score_p, and score_cor) for cardiac hypertrophy and AMI. We found that the density curves for these four types of scores were not all similar (Fig. 3a). For example, most last score values of these dysregulated MGDTs were concentrated between 0.01 and 0.015, and the results indicated that these dysregulated MGDTs all had strong dysregulated features. In addition, we discovered some distinctions for score_p and score_cor between cardiac hypertrophy and AMI (Fig. 3b). Although the MGDTs for cardiac hypertrophy had stronger score_cor values than those of AMI, the MGDTs for cardiac hypertrophy also had weaker score_p values. For cardiac hypertrophy, the highest MGDT score was obtained for miR-449a/MAP2K1/arsenic trioxide. miR-449a and MAP2K1 were both significantly differentially expressed ($P = 0.001$ and 0.039, respectively) (Fig. 3c). For AMI, the highest MGDT score was obtained for miR-140-3p/NRIP1/4-HYDROXY-N'-BENZOHYDRAZIDE. miR-140-3p and NRIP1 were both significantly differentially expressed ($P = 0.09$ and < 0.001, respectively) (Fig. 3d). These results indicated that dysregulated MGDTs in cardiac hypertrophy and AMI all had strong dysregulated levels.

Functional analyses and strong MGDTs in cardiac hypertrophy and AMI

To explore the underlying mechanisms and identify drug repurposing candidates for cardiac hypertrophy and AMI, we performed functional analyses for all genes in the two significant dysregulated networks. We discovered that the genes in the cardiac hypertrophy and AMI networks were all enriched in some basic biological processes (Fig. 4a, b). Specifically, the genes in the cardiac hypertrophy network were enriched in the HIF-1 signaling pathway. P53-induced inhibition of HIF-1 can cause cardiac dysfunction during pressure overload [21]. The genes in the AMI network were enriched in the FOXO signaling pathway. FOXO transcription factors regulate cardiomyocyte proliferation and myocardial growth during development [22]. In addition, the genes in the cardiac hypertrophy and

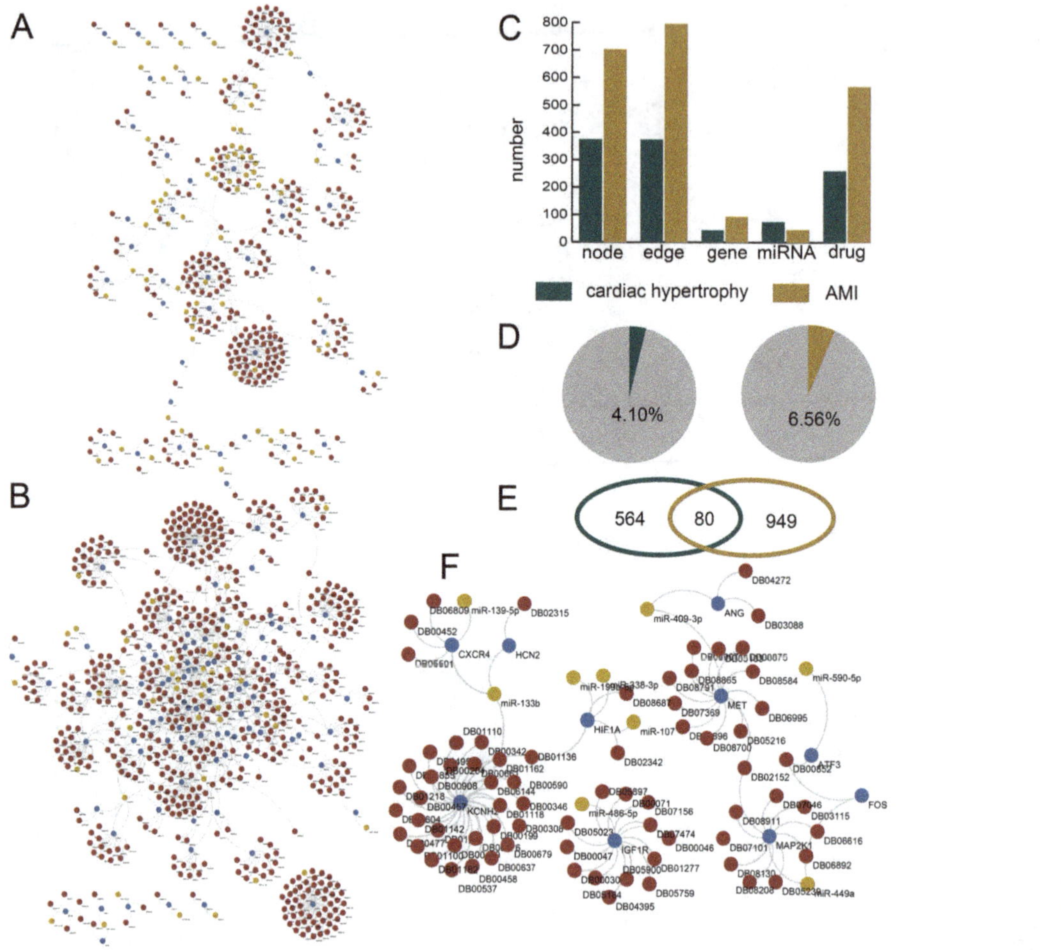

Fig. 2 The significantly dysregulated MGDTs in the cardiac hypertrophy and AMI networks. **a** The significantly dysregulated MGDTs in the cardiac hypertrophy network. **b** The significantly dysregulated MGDTs in the AMI network. **c** The numbers of nodes, edges, genes, miRNAs, and drugs in the cardiac hypertrophy and AMI networks. **d** Pie charts showing the percentages of significantly dysregulated MGDTs out of all MGDTs in the cardiac hypertrophy and AMI networks. **e** Venn diagram showing the common dysregulated MGDTs between the cardiac hypertrophy and AMI networks. **f** The common dysregulated MGDTs in the networks

AMI network were enriched in a pathway named the AGE-RAGE signaling pathway, which is involved in diabetic complications. This pathway is a well-studied cascade in many different disease states, particularly diabetes. We also explored candidate drugs in the two MGDT networks. We extracted two candidate drugs that participated in most dysregulated MGDTs in cardiac hypertrophy and AMI. In cardiac hypertrophy, the drug that participated in most of the dysregulated MGDTs was ATL1101, which is a second-generation antisense drug designed to block the synthesis of the IGF-1 receptor (IGF1R), a protein involved in the regulation of cell overgrowth in psoriasis. (Fig. 4c). IGF1R plays an important role in the growth and continues to anabolic effects in adults; thus, it can induce hypertrophy of skeletal muscle and other target tissues. We also constructed an IGF1R-centered subnetwork (Fig. 4d). The network consisted of one drug, one gene, and 19 miRNAs. We found that the direct target of ATL1101 was the IGF1R gene, which was regulated by some miRNAs. We inferred that ATL1101 influenced cardiac hypertrophy via IGF1R and some essential miRNAs. In AMI, the drug that participated in most of the dysregulated MGDTs was carvedilol, which is a non-selective beta blocker indicated in the treatment of mild to moderate congestive heart failure. Its direct target is VEGFA which is a dimeric glycoprotein that plays a significant role in neurons and is considered the main and dominant inducer of blood vessel growth (Fig. 4e). We also constructed a VEGFA-centered subnetwork (Fig. 4f). The network consisted of one drug, one gene, and 7 miRNAs. Most of the miRNAs in the two subnetworks were differentially expressed. The two heatmaps showed differences between the disease and control samples in the cardiac hypertrophy and AMI networks (Fig. 4g). Some of the other top drugs in the cardiac hypertrophy network were Insulin Human, Insulin Lispro, and Insulin Pork. These top drugs

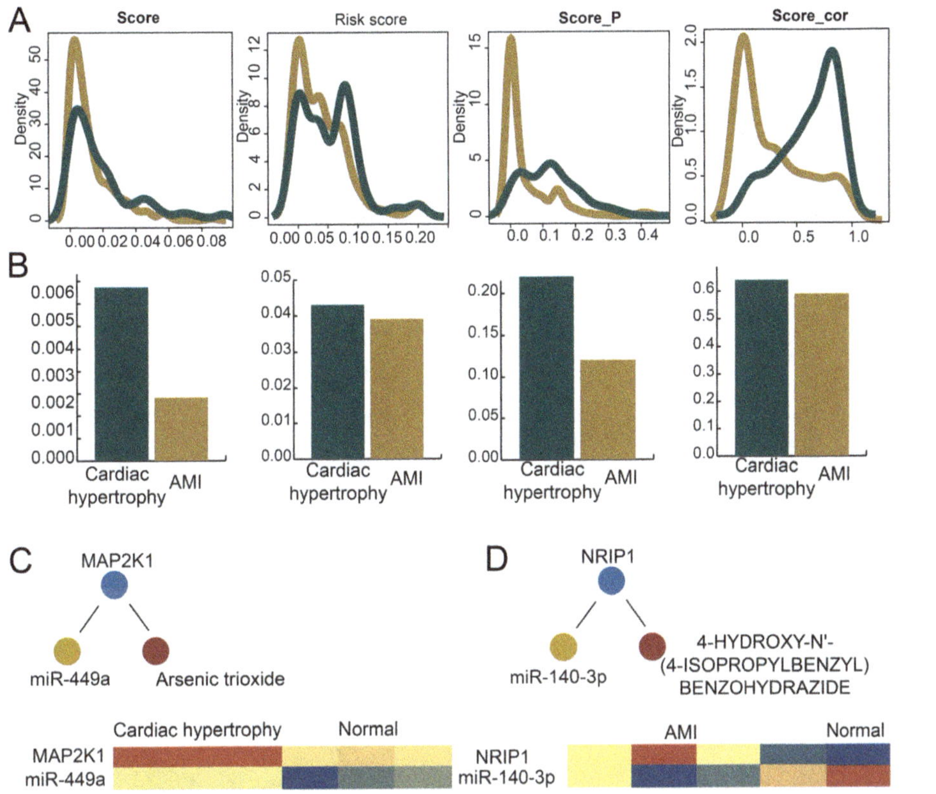

Fig. 3 Construction of an activity score profile for MGDTs in the cardiac hypertrophy and AMI networks. **a** The density distribution curves of the last score, risk score, score_p, and score_cor. **b** Bar plots showing the four types of scores in the cardiac hypertrophy and AMI networks. **c**, **d** The top-ranked MGDTs with the highest scores in the cardiac hypertrophy and AMI networks. The heat map shows miRNA and mRNA expression

were all related with insulin and indicated insulin maybe play an essential role in cardiac hypertrophy. In the AMI network, some of the other top drugs were minocycline, vandetanib, and acetylsalicylic acid.

Identification of novel drug repurposing candidates for cardiac hypertrophy and AMI based on the miRNA-regulated drug pathway

To obtain novel drug repurposing candidates for cardiac hypertrophy and AMI, we identified miRNA-associated pathways based on the miRNA target genes. We used the target genes of each miRNA in the subnetwork to identify miRNA-associated pathways. We discovered different multiple target genes for each miRNA in the two subnetworks. miR-181b-5p had the most target genes for the IGF1R-centered subnetwork for cardiac hypertrophy (Fig. 5a). miR-199a-5p had the most target genes for the VEGFA-centered subnetwork for AMI (Fig. 5b). We also constructed a miRNA-mediated pathway and drug network. In the cardiac hypertrophy network, IGF1R was a target of ATL1101 and 19 other miRNAs (Fig. 5c). We used all target genes of these miRNAs to perform pathway enrichment. We extracted some common enrichment pathways for these miRNAs, including the FOXO and Rap1 signaling pathways. A similar regulatory relationship was also constructed for AMI (Fig. 5d). VEGFA was a target of drug carvedilol and 7 miRNAs. Pathway enrichment was also performed for all of the target genes of these miRNAs. Some common enrichment pathways, such as the mTOR signaling pathway, were extracted. We considered that these two candidate drugs were associated with cardiac hypertrophy and AMI because these common pathways were related to biological processes involved in heart disease. For example, the FOXO signaling pathway was a common enrichment pathway for cardiac hypertrophy in our analyses. We discovered that IGF1R was an upstream gene of the FOXO signaling pathway. FOXO is a key gene in the FOXO signaling pathway, and inactivation of the FOXO protein governs cell growth in the heart and thus contributes to cardiac hypertrophy [23]. Additionally, we found that the insulin signaling pathway was an essential part of the FOXO signaling pathway. Insulin-like growth factor 1 receptor can induce physiological heart growth via the phosphoinositide 3-kinase (p110a) pathway [24]. Insulin-like growth factor 1 receptor in muscle is critical for glucose homeostasis, and signaling from these receptors, particularly the insulin receptor, is required for normal cardiac metabolism and function [25].

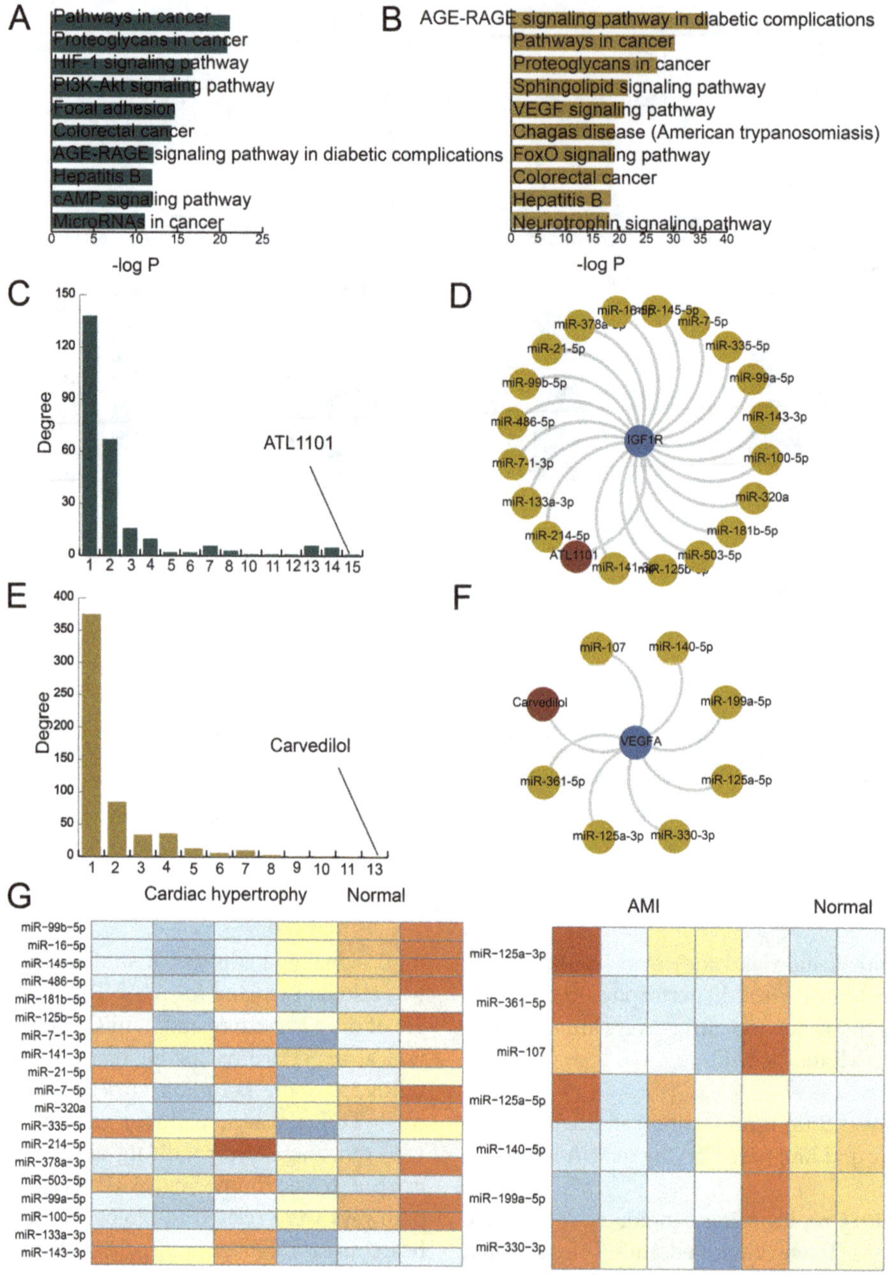

Fig. 4 Functional analyses and construction of a miRNA-mediated subnetwork. **a** The KEGG pathway enrichment results for all genes in the dysregulated MGDTs in the cardiac hypertrophy network ranked by – log10(*P*) are presented as bar plots. **b** The KEGG pathway enrichment results for all genes in the dysregulated MGDTs in the AMI network ranked by – log10(*P*) are presented as bar plots. **c** A bar plot showing the degrees of drugs in the cardiac hypertrophy network. **d** The IGFR1-centered subnetwork of the cardiac hypertrophy network. **e** A bar plot showing the degrees of drugs in the AMI network. **f** The VEGFA-centered subnetwork in the AMI network. **g** The heat maps show miRNA expression in the two subnetworks

Our results suggested that ATL1101 could be a candidate drug for cardiac hypertrophy based on the computational drug repurposing method.

Discussion

Cardiac hypertrophy and AMI are two common heart diseases worldwide. However, cardiac hypertrophy often carries a poor prognosis due to an increased risk of arrhythmia [26] and the development of congestive heart failure. Research into the underlying mechanisms and the development of novel drugs for cardiac hypertrophy and AMI are essential. Drug repurposing is an effective, time-saving, and cost-saving method to study novel drugs for heart disease. Here, we developed a comprehensive and computational approach to perform drug repurposing for cardiac hypertrophy and AMI by

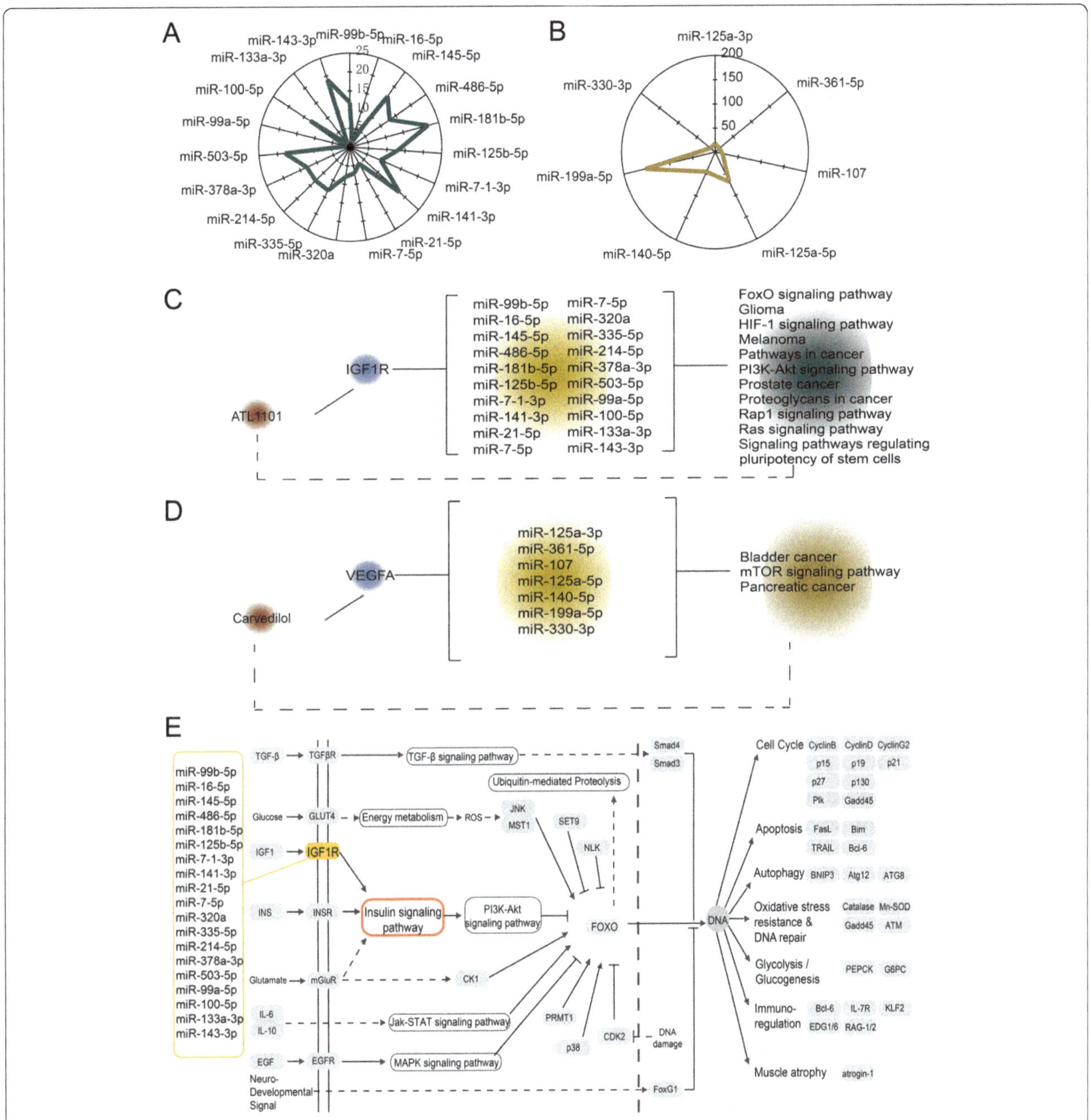

Fig. 5 Drug repurposing candidates for cardiac hypertrophy and AMI based on miRNA-regulated drug-pathway. **a, b** The radar diagrams show the numbers of target genes for each miRNA in the two subnetworks. **c** The miRNA-regulated drug-pathway relationship in the cardiac hypertrophy network. **d** The miRNA-regulated drug-pathway relationship in the AMI network. **e** The FOXO signaling pathway is shown

integrating heart disease-associated genes, experimentally verified miRNA-gene interactions, drug-gene interactions, mRNA and miRNA expression profiles, and pathway annotation data. A global MGDT network was constructed and characterized, and cardiac hypertrophy- and AMI-specific MGDTs were identified. These specific MGDTs were important candidates for drug repurposing analyses. This comprehensive computational approach identified some significantly dysregulated MGDTs, and a KEGG pathway enrichment was performed by the target genes of miRNAs. Some candidate drugs were considered had common and unknown mechanisms of action by shared common targets of miRNA and pathways. Thus, the comprehensive computational approach could realize drug repurposing.

In our analysis, we discovered that ATL1101 was an effective drug candidate for cardiac hypertrophy. ATL1101 is an antisense compound targeting insulin-like growth factor 1 receptor, or IGF1R. Karina Huynh et al. suggested that overexpression of insulin-like growth factor 1 receptor prevented diabetes-induced cardiac fibrosis and diastolic dysfunction. Knezevic et al. demonstrated the existence of a negative feedback loop between miR-378, IGF1R, and IGF1R that was associated with postnatal cardiac remodeling and regulation of cardiomyocyte survival during stress [27]. Here, we suggested that IGF1R influenced cardiac hypertrophy through the FOXO signaling pathway by interacting with a series of miRNAs. In addition, other candidate drugs, such as Insulin Human, Insulin Lispro, and Insulin Pork which were all investigational or approved insulin-related drugs, were identified in our analysis as drug repurposing candidates for cardiac hypertrophy. The computational approach for drug repurposing provided novel insights into mechanistic and drug candidate research in cardiac hypertrophy and AMI.

miRNAs regulate gene expression through translational repression and degradation of mRNAs and significantly contribute to post-transcriptional regulation of drugs [28]. Downregulation of miR-455-3p could be linked to proliferation and drug resistance of pancreatic cancer cells via targeting TAZ [29]. Lopez-Riera et al. indicated that steatotic drugs induced a common set of hepatic miRNAs that could be used in drug screening during preclinical development for fatty liver disease [30]. In our analyses, we also considered the essential role of miRNAs in drug repurposing. We constructed miRNA-mediated drug and pathway regulatory relationship networks for cardiac hypertrophy and AMI and identified enriched pathways based on miRNA target genes. Our results suggested that integrating miRNA interactions and expression was essential for drug repurposing. Well-designed experiments or clinical trials should be conducted in future works to determine whether these repurposing candidate drugs were applicable for the treatment of cardiac hypertrophy and AMI.

Conclusions

In summary, we constructed a miRNA-gene-drug network and analyzed its topological features based on heart disease-associated genes and experimentally verified gene-miRNA and gene-drug interactions. We also presented a computational and integrated approach to identify candidate risk MGDTs, followed by mRNA and miRNA expression profiles, in cardiac hypertrophy and AMI. The candidate risk MGDTs had specific and strong activity score profiles in the cardiac hypertrophy and AMI networks. The IGFR1-related subnetwork in cardiac hypertrophy and the VEGFA-related subnetwork in AMI were extracted for analysis. Finally, we explored the underlying mechanisms and identified candidate drugs for cardiac hypertrophy and AMI based on common pathways of target genes for all miRNAs in the subnetworks. Collectively, our results contributed to a better understanding of the relationships among genes, miRNAs, pathways, and drugs and identified promising drug repurposing candidates for cardiac hypertrophy and AMI.

Methods

Collection of high-throughput miRNA and gene data

We downloaded expression profiles for cardiac hypertrophy and AMI from the Gene Expression Omnibus database (www.ncbi.nlm.nih.gov/geo). The two relevant studies included both miRNA and gene expression profiles from the same sample. A total of three disease samples and three control samples for cardiac hypertrophy were obtained from GSE60291 [31], and four disease samples and one control sample for AMI were obtained from GSE24591 (unpublished data).

Cardiovascular disease-associated genes

We downloaded cardiovascular disease-associated genes from DisGeNET, which integrates disease-associated genes and variants from expert-curated repositories, GWAS catalogs, animal models, and the scientific literature [32]. We extracted keywords for diseases named "heart" or "cardiac". Finally, we found 2293 cardiovascular disease-associated genes and their corresponding risk scores for subsequent analysis.

Experimentally validated miRNA-gene and gene-drug interactions

We downloaded the gene-miRNA associations from the public database miRTarBase 7.0, which accumulated more than three hundred and sixty thousand miRNA-gene interactions [33]. We only extracted experimentally validated miRNA-gene interactions. Then, we obtained gene-drug interaction data from DrugBank, which is a web-enabled database containing comprehensive molecular information about drugs, their mechanisms, their interactions, and their targets [34]. We constructed a MGDT network based on these experimentally validated interactions used Cytoscape 3.0 (http://www.cytoscape.org/).

Dissecting topological characteristics of the MGDT network

We used the degree distributions and topological coefficients to assess the entire MGDT network for all nodes. All analyses were performed using Cytoscape 3.0 (http://www.cytoscape.org/).

Identification of cardiac hypertrophy- and AMI-specific MGDTs based on expression data

We designed an integrative and computational approach to identify specific MGDTs in cardiac hypertrophy and AMI that used the MGDT regulatory networks and the miRNA and mRNA expression data. First, we used Student's t test to compare differences in mRNA and miRNA expression between patients with disease (cardiac hypertrophy and AMI) and the corresponding controls for each MGDT. Second, we calculated Pearson's correlation coefficients (PCCs) for mRNA and miRNA interactions for each MGDT in the disease and control samples. We calculated the significant difference between the disease and control samples. The absolute difference in the PCCs between the disease and control samples was obtained for the subsequent analysis. We presented three comprehensive scores (S_{risk}, S_P, and S_{PCC}) to evaluate the dysregulated levels for each MGDT in cardiac hypertrophy and AMI. The equations were as follows:

$$S_{risk} = \text{risk} - \text{score}$$
$$S_P = P_{mRNA}{}^{*}P_{miRNA}$$
$$S_{pcc} = \mid D_{pcc} - C_{pcc} \mid$$

In the three equations, S_{risk} represents the verified level between the disease and genes. P_{mRNA} and P_{miRNA} represent the P values of mRNAs and miRNAs, respectively, for each MGDT derived from the above t test. S_P is the difference between the expression level of the MGDT between the samples with disease and the corresponding controls. D_{pcc} and C_{pcc} refer to the PCCs of the mRNA-miRNA interaction pairs for the disease and control samples, respectively. S_{pcc} is the absolute distinction of the PCC score between the disease and control samples in each MGDT. We used an equally weighted approach to rank all MGDTs following the above three comprehensive scores [35]. We obtained three ranked lists, and the ranking positions in the three lists were used to calculate the last ranking score list for each MGDT in the cardiac hypertrophy and AMI networks. Higher ranking scores referred to stronger dysregulated MGDTs between the disease and control samples. The permutation-based final ranking scores were generated by randomly disturbing all sample labels in the expression profiles 1000 times. We compared each final ranking score of a MGDT with the permutation-based final ranking score to obtain significant P values ($P < 0.05$). All analyses were performed using the R software (version 3.2.3; https://www.r-project.org/).

Pathway enrichment analysis

We used the Database for Annotation, Visualization, and Integrated Discovery (DAVID) to annotate enriched pathways for the genes [36]. We extracted enriched pathways using the Kyoto Encyclopedia of Genes and Genomes (KEGG) with a P value cutoff of 0.05. Then, we used the target gene sets of miRNAs to identify miRNA-associated pathways. Finally, we constructed relationships, including drugs, pathways, genes, and miRNAs.

Abbreviations

AMI: Acute myocardial infarction; GEO: Gene Expression Omnibus; KEGG: Kyoto Encyclopedia of Genes and Genomes; MGDTs: miRNA-gene-drug triplets; miRNAs: microRNAs; PCCs: Pearson correlation coefficients

Acknowledgements

Not applicable.

Funding

Heilongjiang Provincial Department of Health (2011-032).

Authors' contributions

SJT and LN conceived and designed the experiments. YJM and CJ analyzed the data. DX and SJT wrote the manuscript. All authors read and approved the final manuscript.

Consent for publication

Not applicable.

Competing interests

The authors declare that they have no competing interests.

Author details

[1]Department of Cardiology, the First Affiliated Hospital, Harbin Medical University, Harbin, Heilongjiang, People's Republic of China. [2]Department of Obstetrics, the Second Affiliated Hospital, Harbin Medical University, 246 XueFu Road, Harbin 150086, Heilongjiang, People's Republic of China.

References

1. Roth GA, Johnson C, Abajobir A, Abd-Allah F, Abera SF, Abyu G, Ahmed M, Aksut B, Alam T, Alam K, Alla F, Alvis-Guzman N, Amrock S, Ansari H, Arnlov J, Asayesh H, Atey TM, Avila-Burgos L, Awasthi A, Banerjee A, Barac A, Barnighausen T, Barregard L, Bedi N, Belay Ketema E, Bennett D, Berhe G, Bhutta Z, Bitew S, Carapetis J, Carrero JJ, Malta DC, Castaneda-Orjuela CA, Castillo-Rivas J, Catala-Lopez F, Choi JY, Christensen H, Cirillo M, Cooper L Jr, Criqui M, Cundiff D, Damasceno A, Dandona L, Dandona R, Davletov K, Dharmaratne S, Dorairaj P, Dubey M, Ehrenkranz R, El Sayed Zaki M, Faraon EJA, Esteghamati A, Farid T, Farvid M, Feigin V, Ding EL, Fowkes G, Gebrehiwot T, Gillum R, Gold A, Gona P, Gupta R, Habtewold TD, Hafezi-Nejad N, Hailu T, Hailu GB, Hankey G, Hassen HY, Abate KH, Havmoeller R, Hay SI, Horino M, Hotez PJ, Jacobsen K, James S, Javanbakht M, Jeemon P, John D, Jonas J, Kalkonde Y, Karimkhani C, Kasaeian A, Khader Y, Khan A, Khang YH, Khera S, Khoja AT, Khubchandani J, Kim D, Kolte D, Kosen S, Krohn KJ, Kumar GA, Kwan GF, Lal DK, Larsson A, Linn S, Lopez A, Lotufo PA, El Razek HMA, Malekzadeh R, Mazidi M, Meier T, Meles KG, Mensah G, Meretoja A, Mezgebe H, Miller T, Mirrakhimov E, Mohammed S, Moran AE, Musa KI, Narula J, Neal B, Ngalesoni F, Nguyen G, Obermeyer CM, Owolabi M, Patton G, Pedro J, Qato D, Qorbani M, Rahimi K, Rai RK, Rawaf S, Ribeiro A, Safiri S, Salomon JA, Santos I, Santric Milicevic M, Sartorius B, Schutte A, Sepanlou S, Shaikh MA, Shin MJ, Shishehbor M, Shore H, Silva DAS, Sobngwi E, Stranges S, Swaminathan S, Tabares-Seisdedos R, Tadele Atnafu N, Tesfay F, Thakur JS, Thrift A, Topor-Madry R, Truelsen T, Tyrovolas S, Ukwaja KN, Uthman O, Vasankari T, Vlassov V, Vollset SE, Wakayo T, Watkins D, Weintraub R, Werdecker A, Westerman R, Wiysonge CS, Wolfe C, Workicho A, Xu G, Yano Y, Yip P, Yonemoto N, Younis M, Yu C, Vos T, Naghavi M, Murray C. Global, regional, and national burden of cardiovascular diseases for 10 causes, 1990 to 2015. *J Am Coll Cardiol.* 2017;70(1):1–25.
2. Frey N, Olson EN. Cardiac hypertrophy: the good, the bad, and the ugly. *Annu Rev Physiol.* 2003;65:45–79.
3. Anderson JL, Morrow DA. Acute myocardial infarction. N Engl J Med. 2017; 376(21):2053–64.

4. Yuan J, Liu H, Gao W, Zhang L, Ye Y, Yuan L, Ding Z, Wu J, Kang L, Zhang X, Wang X, Zhang G, Gong H, Sun A, Yang X, Chen R, Cui Z, Ge J, Zou Y. MicroRNA-378 suppresses myocardial fibrosis through a paracrine mechanism at the early stage of cardiac hypertrophy following mechanical stress. Theranostics. 2018;8(9):2565–82.
5. Diniz GP, Lino CA, Guedes EC, Moreira Ldo N, Barreto-Chaves ML. Cardiac microRNA-133 is down-regulated in thyroid hormone-mediated cardiac hypertrophy partially via type 1 angiotensin II receptor. Basic Res Cardiol. 2015;110(5):49.
6. Wei L, Yuan M, Zhou R, Bai Q, Zhang W, Zhang M, Huang Y, Shi L. MicroRNA-101 inhibits rat cardiac hypertrophy by targeting Rab1a. J Cardiovasc Pharmacol. 2015;65(4):357–63.
7. Ai J, Zhang R, Li Y, Pu J, Lu Y, Jiao J, Li K, Yu B, Li Z, Wang R, Wang L, Li Q, Wang N, Shan H, Yang B. Circulating microRNA-1 as a potential novel biomarker for acute myocardial infarction. Biochem Biophys Res Commun. 2010;391(1):73–7.
8. Zhang L, Chen X, Su T, Li H, Huang Q, Wu D, Yang C, Han Z. Circulating miR-499 are novel and sensitive biomarker of acute myocardial infarction. J Thorac Dis. 2015;7(3):303–8.
9. Yang X, Qin Y, Shao S, Yu Y, Zhang C, Dong H, Lv G, Dong S. MicroRNA-214 inhibits left ventricular remodeling in an acute myocardial infarction rat model by suppressing cellular apoptosis via the phosphatase and Tensin homolog (PTEN). Int Heart J. 2016;57(2):247–50.
10. Das A, Samidurai A, Salloum FN. Deciphering non-coding RNAs in cardiovascular health and disease. Front Cardiovasc Med. 2018;5:73.
11. Jeong MH, Lee JS, Kim DH, Park WJ, Yang DK. Identification of novel microRNAs negatively regulating cardiac hypertrophy. Biochem Biophys Res Commun. 2012;428(1):191–6.
12. Yang KC, Ku YC, Lovett M, Nerbonne JM. Combined deep microRNA and mRNA sequencing identifies protective transcriptomal signature of enhanced PI3Kalpha signaling in cardiac hypertrophy. J Mol Cell Cardiol. 2012;53(1):101–12.
13. Santana ET, Feliciano RD, Serra AJ, Brigidio E, Antonio EL, Tucci PJ, Nathanson L, Morris M, Silva JA Jr. Comparative mRNA and MicroRNA profiling during acute myocardial infarction induced by coronary occlusion and ablation radio-frequency currents. Front Physiol. 2016;7:565.
14. Ashburn TT, Thor KB. Drug repositioning: identifying and developing new uses for existing drugs. Nat Rev Drug Discov. 2004;3(8):673–83.
15. Donner Y, Kazmierczak S, Fortney K. Drug repurposing using deep embeddings of gene expression profiles. Mol Pharm. 2018.
16. Athauda D, Foltynie T. Drug repurposing in Parkinson's disease. CNS Drugs. 2018.
17. Datta A, Kim H, McGee L, Johnson AE, Talwar S, Marugan J, Southall N, Hu X, Lal M, Mondal D, Ferrer M, Abdel-Mageed AB. High-throughput screening identified selective inhibitors of exosome biogenesis and secretion: a drug repurposing strategy for advanced cancer. Sci Rep. 2018;8(1):8161.
18. Amaral LA, Scala A, Barthelemy M, Stanley HE. Classes of small-world networks. Proc Natl Acad Sci U S A. 2000;97(21):11149–52.
19. Cao Y, Wang P, Ning S, Xiao W, Xiao B, Li X. Identification of prognostic biomarkers in glioblastoma using a long non-coding RNA-mediated, competitive endogenous RNA network. Oncotarget. 2016;7(27):41737–47.
20. Simos T, Georgopoulou U, Thyphronitis G, Koskinas J, Papaloukas C. Analysis of protein interaction networks for the detection of candidate hepatitis B and C biomarkers. IEEE J Biomed Health Inform. 2015;19(1):181–9.
21. Sano M, Minamino T, Toko H, Miyauchi H, Orimo M, Qin Y, Akazawa H, Tateno K, Kayama Y, Harada M, Shimizu I, Asahara T, Hamada H, Tomita S, Molkentin JD, Zou Y, Komuro I. p53-induced inhibition of Hif-1 causes cardiac dysfunction during pressure overload. Nature. 2007;446(7134):444–8.
22. Evans-Anderson HJ, Alfieri CM, Yutzey KE. Regulation of cardiomyocyte proliferation and myocardial growth during development by FOXO transcription factors. Circ Res. 2008;102(6):686–94.
23. Ni YG, Berenji K, Wang N, Oh M, Sachan N, Dey A, Cheng J, Lu G, Morris DJ, Castrillon DH, Gerard RD, Rothermel BA, Hill JA. Foxo transcription factors blunt cardiac hypertrophy by inhibiting calcineurin signaling. Circulation. 2006;114(11):1159–68.
24. McMullen JR, Shioi T, Huang WY, Zhang L, Tarnavski O, Bisping E, Schinke M, Kong S, Sherwood MC, Brown J, Riggi L, Kang PM, Izumo S. The insulin-like growth factor 1 receptor induces physiological heart growth via the phosphoinositide 3-kinase(p110alpha) pathway. J Biol Chem. 2004;279(6): 4782–93.
25. Laustsen PG, Russell SJ, Cui L, Entingh-Pearsall A, Holzenberger M, Liao R, Kahn CR. Essential role of insulin and insulin-like growth factor 1 receptor signaling in cardiac development and function. Mol Cell Biol. 2007;27(5): 1649–64.
26. Nakagami H, Takemoto M, Liao JK. NADPH oxidase-derived superoxide anion mediates angiotensin II-induced cardiac hypertrophy. J Mol Cell Cardiol. 2003;35(7):851–9.
27. Knezevic I, Patel A, Sundaresan NR, Gupta MP, Solaro RJ, Nagalingam RS, Gupta M. A novel cardiomyocyte-enriched microRNA, miR-378, targets insulin-like growth factor 1 receptor: implications in postnatal cardiac remodeling and cell survival. J Biol Chem. 2012;287(16):12913–26.
28. Nakano M, Nakajima M. Current knowledge of microRNA-mediated regulation of drug metabolism in humans. Expert Opin Drug Metab Toxicol. 2018;14(5):493–504.
29. Zhan T, Huang X, Tian X, Chen X, Ding Y, Luo H, Zhang Y. Downregulation of MicroRNA-455-3p links to proliferation and drug resistance of pancreatic cancer cells via targeting TAZ. Mol Ther Nucleic Acids. 2018;10:215–26.
30. Lopez-Riera M, Conde I, Tolosa L, Zaragoza A, Castell JV, Gomez-Lechon MJ, Jover R. New microRNA biomarkers for drug-induced steatosis and their potential to predict the contribution of drugs to non-alcoholic fatty liver disease. Front Pharmacol. 2017;8:3.
31. Aggarwal, P.; Turner, A.; Matter, A.; Kattman, S. J.; Stoddard, A.; Lorier, R.; Swanson, B. J.; Arnett, D. K.; Broeckel, U., RNA expression profiling of human iPSC-derived cardiomyocytes in a cardiac hypertrophy model. PLoS One 2014, 9, (9), e108051.
32. Pinero J, Bravo A, Queralt-Rosinach N, Gutierrez-Sacristan A, Deu-Pons J, Centeno E, Garcia-Garcia J, Sanz F, Furlong LI. DisGeNET: a comprehensive platform integrating information on human disease-associated genes and variants. Nucleic Acids Res. 2017;45(D1):D833–9.
33. Chou CH, Shrestha S, Yang CD, Chang NW, Lin YL, Liao KW, Huang WC, Sun TH, Tu SJ, Lee WH, Chiew MY, Tai CS, Wei TY, Tsai TR, Huang HT, Wang CY, Wu HY, Ho SY, Chen PR, Chuang CH, Hsieh PJ, Wu YS, Chen WL, Li MJ, Wu YC, Huang XY, Ng FL, Buddhakosai W, Huang PC, Lan KC, Huang CY, Weng SL, Cheng YN, Liang C, Hsu WL, Huang HD. miRTarBase update 2018: a resource for experimentally validated microRNA-target interactions. Nucleic Acids Res. 2018;46(D1):D296–302.
34. Wishart DS, Feunang YD, Guo AC, Lo EJ, Marcu A, Grant JR, Sajed T, Johnson D, Li C, Sayeeda Z, Assempour N, Iynkkaran I, Liu Y, Maciejewski A, Gale N, Wilson A, Chin L, Cummings R, Le D, Pon A, Knox C, Wilson M. DrugBank 5. 0: a major update to the DrugBank database for 2018. Nucleic Acids Res. 2018;46(D1):D1074–82.
35. Aerts S, Lambrechts D, Maity S, Van Loo P, Coessens B, De Smet F, Tranchevent LC, De Moor B, Marynen P, Hassan B, Carmeliet P, Moreau Y. Gene prioritization through genomic data fusion. Nat Biotechnol. 2006;24(5): 537–44.
36. Dennis G Jr, Sherman BT, Hosack DA, Yang J, Gao W, Lane HC, Lempicki RA. DAVID: database for annotation, visualization, and integrated discovery. Genome Biol. 2003;4(5):P3.

18

Mixture models for gene expression experiments with two species

Yuhua Su[1*], Lei Zhu[2], Alan Menius[2] and Jason Osborne[3]

Abstract

Cross-species research in drug development is novel and challenging. A bivariate mixture model utilizing information across two species was proposed to solve the fundamental problem of identifying differentially expressed genes in microarray experiments in order to potentially improve the understanding of translation between preclinical and clinical studies for drug development. The proposed approach models the joint distribution of treatment effects estimated from independent linear models. The mixture model posits up to nine components, four of which include groups in which genes are differentially expressed in both species. A comprehensive simulation to evaluate the model performance and one application on a real world data set, a mouse and human type II diabetes experiment, suggest that the proposed model, though highly structured, can handle various configurations of differential gene expression and is practically useful on identifying differentially expressed genes, especially when the magnitude of differential expression due to different treatment intervention is weak. In the mouse and human application, the proposed mixture model was able to eliminate unimportant genes and identify a list of genes that were differentially expressed in both species and could be potential gene targets for drug development.

Keywords: Orthology, Drug development, Drug response prediction, Type II diabetes

Introduction

Background

Pharmaceutical medicine is an industry with huge upfront investment for rewards that may or may not come years later. A complete drug development process, including drug discovery, preclinical research (on animals) and clinical trials (on humans), is lengthy, expensive, and risky. Determined by the US Food and Drug Administration (FDA) [1], the average total cost per drug development is about \$1.9 billion. The typical development time is 10 to 15 years. The overall attrition rate of a drug compound from first-in-man to registration is approximately 80%–90% [2,3].

FDA [1] calls the preclinical and clinical research together as the 'critical path' development phase, where most investment required for a successful drug launch occurs. Currently, this development phase is inherently inefficient. The goal of preclinical research is to assess how a drug is absorbed, distributed, metabolized, and excreted in animals, and to use the findings to determine potential human outcomes before starting clinical trials. Yet the rate of success after a drug candidate enters Phase I is undesirably low. As mentioned in FDA [1] and Kola and Landis [3], animal models with poor clinical relevance may be accountable for this perplexity. Hence, improving translation between two species to increase the predictive power of animal models to human studies is of tremendous value to drug discovery and development.

Homology and multiple species gene expression analysis in drug development

Microarrays are tools for gene expression analysis and can be potentially useful for investigating the mechanism of drug activities that translates across species. The utility of microarray information in the drug development process is reviewed by Braxton and Bedilion [4] who embraced the idea that gene expression analysis can be a surrogate marker for the interaction between compounds and cells and should yield information about efficacy. Debouck and Goodfellow [5] believed that microarrays can be used to generate clues to patterns of gene

*Correspondence: yhsejo@gmail.com
[1] Dr. Su's Statistics & Department of Human Nutrition, Food, and Animal Sciences, University of Hawaii at Manoa, Honolulu, HI 96822, USA
Full list of author information is available at the end of the article

function that can help improve the efficiency of drug development.

As stated before, one key challenge of drug development is to successfully translate the results of preclinical findings in animal models to human beings in the clinic. Pre-clinical experiments assume that the effect of the drug tested on animals is comparable to that on humans, which can only be true if a functional equivalent of the human drug target exists in the experimental species. Orthology [6-8] is a strong indication of functional conservation and therefore provides the best functional annotation of experimentally undetermined genes across species. Holbrook and Sanseau [9] remarked that the use of orthologs has the potential to improve the understanding of biological differences between species (animals and humans).

Many of the successful applications of cross-species microarray gene expression analysis involve orthology [10-13]. Additionally, over the past decade, researchers have tried to use orthology and gene expression data to do cross-species comparison in order to understand how genes interact to perform particular biological processes [14,15]. These studies support the idea that orthologs could be a useful tool for researchers to link experiments between species in drug development. Note that orthologous relationships can be one-to-one, one-to-many, or many-to-many [8].

The rest of the paper is structured as follows: Section 'Joint modeling across species' describes the proposed bivariate mixture model across species. Section 'Simulation' describes a simulation study undertaken to investigate the effects of different experimental designs on the power to detect important genes and on misclassification rates. Section 'Application: the mouse and human type II diabetes experiment' illustrates the methodology using an application to data collected in a mouse/human experiment. Section 'Concluding remarks' concludes.

Joint modeling across species

Let $X_{a_{ij}}$ and $X_{h_{il}}$ denote gene expression measurements from the ith orthologous gene pair for the jth animal and the lth human. The following independent linear models describe the association between gene expression and treatment:

$$X_{a_{ij}} = \beta_{0a_i} + \beta_{1a_i} T_{a_j} + e_{a_{ij}}, \quad (1)$$

$$X_{h_{il}} = \beta_{0h_i} + \beta_{1h_i} T_{h_l} + e_{h_{il}}, \quad (2)$$

where T_{a_j} and T_{h_l} are $\{0, 1\}$ treatment indicators, and $e_{a_{ij}}$ and $e_{h_{il}}$ are independent $N(0, \sigma_a^2)$ and $N(0, \sigma_h^2)$ random variables. σ_a^2 and σ_h^2 are variances for $e_{a_{ij}}$ and $e_{h_{il}}$, respectively. In drug development, the animal research and human experiments are conducted independently - one's results do not affect the other's. However, the treatment effects are expected to have some kind of association between the two species. This results in our choice of using two independent models for the two species to capture the effects of treatment on gene expression.

A nine-component bivariate mixture model for two species experiments

β_{1a_i} and β_{1h_i} quantify the differential expression of the ith orthologous animal and human genes due to a treatment intervention. A given gene can be classified as non-differentially expressed (NDE) - showing no signs of treatment effects, positively differentially expressed (pDE) - showing positive treatment effects, or negatively differentially expressed (nDE) - showing negative treatment effects. Therefore, for a human and animal gene pair, there are nine possibilities for categorizing this pair of genes. Further, dependency is assumed between differentially expressed orthologs, i.e., existence of association posited only for $(\beta_{1a_i}, \beta_{1h_i})^T$ in categories (1, 2, 3, 4) and zero correlation presumed for $(\beta_{1a_i}, \beta_{1h_i})^T$ in categories (0, 5, 6, 7, 8). Table 1 illustrates the nine possible categories of $(\beta_{1a_i}, \beta_{1h_i})^T$. $(\mu_{\beta_{1a_i}}, \mu_{\beta_{1h_i}})^T$ is the vector of population means of $(\beta_{1a_i}, \beta_{1h_i})^T$ under each category.

In consequence of these possible patterns of $(\beta_{1a_i}, \beta_{1h_i})^T$, mixture models [16,17] are adopted to deal with the correlation and distribution of each subgroup of genes across species. An additional advantage of mixture models is that, after prior weights for the components are specified, estimates of the posterior probabilities of population membership can be formed for each observation to give a probabilistic clustering. As a result, the pooling of information for genes across species can be exploited to better understand the underlying rela-

Table 1 Possible categories of $(\beta_{1a_i}, \beta_{1h_i})^T$

Category	$(\beta_{1a_i}, \beta_{1h_i})$	$(\mu_{\beta_{1a_i}}, \mu_{\beta_{1h_i}})$	Corr $(\beta_{1a_i}, \beta_{1h_i})$
0	(NDE,NDE)	(0, 0)	0
1	(pDE,pDE)	(+, +)	ρ_1
2	(nDE,nDE)	(−, −)	ρ_2
3	(pDE,nDE)	(+, −)	ρ_3
4	(nDE,pDE)	(−, +)	ρ_4
5	(NDE,pDE)	(0, +)	0
6	(NDE,nDE)	(0, −)	0
7	(pDE,NDE)	(+, 0)	0
8	(nDE,NDE)	(−, 0)	0

tionship between the treatment intervention for both species.

Tailoring the mixture model to two-species experiments with restrictions on the parameters made according to Table 1 and assuming that the treatment effects for non-differentially expressed genes are deterministically zero, i.e., $(\beta_{1a_i}, \beta_{1h_i})^T = (0,0)^T$, the following bivariate normal mixture model is adopted as the prior distribution of the vector $(\beta_{1a_i}, \beta_{1h_i})^T$:

$$\begin{aligned}\begin{pmatrix}\beta_{1a_i}\\ \beta_{1h_i}\end{pmatrix} &\sim \pi_0 N\left(\begin{pmatrix}\mu_{a0}\\ \mu_{h0}\end{pmatrix}, \begin{pmatrix}\eta_{a0}^2 & \rho_0\eta_{a0}\eta_{h0}\\ \rho_0\eta_{a0}\eta_{h0} & \eta_{h0}^2\end{pmatrix}\right)\\
&+\pi_1 N\left(\begin{pmatrix}\mu_{a1}\\ \mu_{h1}\end{pmatrix}, \begin{pmatrix}\eta_{a1}^2 & \rho_1\eta_{a1}\eta_{h1}\\ \rho_1\eta_{a1}\eta_{h1} & \eta_{h1}^2\end{pmatrix}\right)\\
&+\pi_2 N\left(\begin{pmatrix}\mu_{a2}\\ \mu_{h2}\end{pmatrix}, \begin{pmatrix}\eta_{a2}^2 & \rho_2\eta_{a2}\eta_{h2}\\ \rho_2\eta_{a2}\eta_{h2} & \eta_{h2}^2\end{pmatrix}\right)\\
&+\pi_3 N\left(\begin{pmatrix}\mu_{a3}\\ \mu_{h3}\end{pmatrix}, \begin{pmatrix}\eta_{a3}^2 & \rho_3\eta_{a3}\eta_{h3}\\ \rho_3\eta_{a3}\eta_{h3} & \eta_{h3}^2\end{pmatrix}\right)\\
&+\pi_4 N\left(\begin{pmatrix}\mu_{a4}\\ \mu_{h4}\end{pmatrix}, \begin{pmatrix}\eta_{a4}^2 & \rho_4\eta_{a4}\eta_{h4}\\ \rho_4\eta_{a4}\eta_{h4} & \eta_{h4}^2\end{pmatrix}\right)\\
&+\pi_5 N\left(\begin{pmatrix}\mu_{a5}\\ \mu_{h5}\end{pmatrix}, \begin{pmatrix}\eta_{a5}^2 & \rho_5\eta_{a5}\eta_{h5}\\ \rho_5\eta_{a5}\eta_{h5} & \eta_{h5}^2\end{pmatrix}\right)\\
&+\pi_6 N\left(\begin{pmatrix}\mu_{a6}\\ \mu_{h6}\end{pmatrix}, \begin{pmatrix}\eta_{a6}^2 & \rho_6\eta_{a6}\eta_{h6}\\ \rho_6\eta_{a6}\eta_{h6} & \eta_{h6}^2\end{pmatrix}\right)\\
&+\pi_7 N\left(\begin{pmatrix}\mu_{a7}\\ \mu_{h7}\end{pmatrix}, \begin{pmatrix}\eta_{a7}^2 & \rho_7\eta_{a7}\eta_{h7}\\ \rho_7\eta_{a7}\eta_{h7} & \eta_{h7}^2\end{pmatrix}\right)\\
&+\pi_8 N\left(\begin{pmatrix}\mu_{a8}\\ \mu_{h8}\end{pmatrix}, \begin{pmatrix}\eta_{a8}^2 & \rho_8\eta_{a8}\eta_{h8}\\ \rho_8\eta_{a8}\eta_{h8} & \eta_{h8}^2\end{pmatrix}\right),\end{aligned} \tag{3}$$

where π_k is the probability that an observation belongs to the kth component, with $\sum_{k=0}^{8}\pi_k = 1$ and $\pi_k \geq 0$. The following restriction of the parameter space is imposed: $\mu_{a0} = 0$, $\mu_{h0} = 0$, $\mu_{a1} \geq 0$, $\mu_{h1} \geq 0$, $\mu_{a2} \leq 0$, $\mu_{h2} \leq 0$, $\mu_{a3} \geq 0$, $\mu_{h3} \leq 0$, $\mu_{a4} \leq 0$, $\mu_{h4} \geq 0$, $\mu_{a5} = 0$, $\mu_{h5} \geq 0$, $\mu_{a6} = 0$, $\mu_{h6} \leq 0$, $\mu_{a7} \geq 0$, $\mu_{h7} = 0$, $\mu_{a8} \leq 0$, $\mu_{h8} = 0$, $\eta_{a0} = 0$, $\eta_{h0} = 0$, $\eta_{a5} = 0$, $\eta_{a6} = 0$, $\eta_{h7} = 0$, $\eta_{h8} = 0$, $\rho_0 = 0$, $\rho_5 = 0$, $\rho_6 = 0$, $\rho_7 = 0$, and $\rho_8 = 0$.

According to the theory of least squares, the marginal distribution of $(\hat\beta_{1a_i}, \hat\beta_{1h_i})^T$, the parameter estimates, has means equal to the prior means of $(\beta_{1a_i}, \beta_{1h_i})^T$ and variances involving contributions from the prior distribution of $(\beta_{1a_i}, \beta_{1h_i})^T$ and the conditional distribution of $(\hat\beta_{1a_i}, \hat\beta_{1h_i})^T$ given $(\beta_{1a_i}, \beta_{1h_i})^T$. The marginal distribution of $(\hat\beta_{1a_i}, \hat\beta_{1h_i})^T$ is as follows:

$$\begin{aligned}\begin{pmatrix}\hat\beta_{1a_i}\\ \hat\beta_{1h_i}\end{pmatrix} &\sim \pi_0 N\left(\begin{pmatrix}0\\ 0\end{pmatrix}, \begin{pmatrix}\sigma_{a0}^2 & 0\\ 0 & \sigma_{h0}^2\end{pmatrix}\right)\\
&+\pi_1 N\left(\begin{pmatrix}\mu_{a1}\\ \mu_{h1}\end{pmatrix}, \begin{pmatrix}\sigma_{a1}^2 & \rho_1\sigma_{a1}\sigma_{h1}\\ \rho_1\sigma_{a1}\sigma_{h1} & \sigma_{h1}^2\end{pmatrix}\right)\\
&+\pi_2 N\left(\begin{pmatrix}\mu_{a2}\\ \mu_{h2}\end{pmatrix}, \begin{pmatrix}\sigma_{a2}^2 & \rho_2\sigma_{a2}\sigma_{h2}\\ \rho_2\sigma_{a2}\sigma_{h2} & \sigma_{h2}^2\end{pmatrix}\right)\\
&+\pi_3 N\left(\begin{pmatrix}\mu_{a3}\\ \mu_{h3}\end{pmatrix}, \begin{pmatrix}\sigma_{a3}^2 & \rho_3\sigma_{a3}\sigma_{h3}\\ \rho_3\sigma_{a3}\sigma_{h3} & \sigma_{h3}^2\end{pmatrix}\right)\\
&+\pi_4 N\left(\begin{pmatrix}\mu_{a4}\\ \mu_{h4}\end{pmatrix}, \begin{pmatrix}\sigma_{a4}^2 & \rho_4\sigma_{a4}\sigma_{h4}\\ \rho_4\sigma_{a4}\sigma_{h4} & \sigma_{h4}^2\end{pmatrix}\right)\\
&+\pi_5 N\left(\begin{pmatrix}0\\ \mu_{h5}\end{pmatrix}, \begin{pmatrix}\sigma_{a5}^2 & 0\\ 0 & \sigma_{h5}^2\end{pmatrix}\right)\\
&+\pi_6 N\left(\begin{pmatrix}0\\ \mu_{h6}\end{pmatrix}, \begin{pmatrix}\sigma_{a6}^2 & 0\\ 0 & \sigma_{h6}^2\end{pmatrix}\right)\\
&+\pi_7 N\left(\begin{pmatrix}\mu_{a7}\\ 0\end{pmatrix}, \begin{pmatrix}\sigma_{a7}^2 & 0\\ 0 & \sigma_{h7}^2\end{pmatrix}\right)\\
&+\pi_8 N\left(\begin{pmatrix}\mu_{a8}\\ 0\end{pmatrix}, \begin{pmatrix}\sigma_{a8}^2 & 0\\ 0 & \sigma_{h8}^2\end{pmatrix}\right),\end{aligned} \tag{4}$$

An EM algorithm is developed to accomplish the nontrivial likelihood maximization, along with methodology for handling singular covariance matrices that arise during the implementation of the algorithm. (See the Appendix for details). Gene membership is determined according to the maximum posterior probability that an observation $(\hat\beta_{1a_i}, \hat\beta_{1h_i})^T$ comes from the kth component of the mixture.

Simulation

The following Monte Carlo simulation studies investigated the performance of the proposed mixture model using information across two species in comparison to the traditional microarray method using just one-species information when identifying genes associated with treatment stimulus under several different scenarios.

Several factors influence the sampling properties of the estimated treatment effects $(\hat\beta_{1a_i}, \hat\beta_{1h_i})^T$ using the mixture model were considered in the simulation:

- Replicates (number of arrays) per treatment for each species: n_a and n_h for animals and humans, respectively.
- Number of orthologous genes in each category: n_k, $k = 0, \ldots, 8$, the kth category.

- Array noise: $e_{a_{ij}}$ and $e_{h_{ij}}$ in (1) and (2). Also recall that, by assumption, $e_{a_{ij}}$ and $e_{h_{il}}$ are independent $N(0, \sigma_a^2)$ and $N(0, \sigma_h^2)$ random variables.
- Parameters in (3) by which the sampling distribution of $(\hat{\beta}_{1a_i}, \hat{\beta}_{1h_i})^T$ is determined.

With so many variables, it is impractical to study the sampling properties of the fitted model without fixing some variables. That is, an experimental design for the simulation in which these factors are completely considered is not feasible. The simulation study instead focused on three aspects. First, although high-density microarrays provide useful genome-wide data, they are often associated with a substantial amount of experimental noise that could affect the performance of the analysis. Hence, it is of interest to investigate how the array noise would affect the model efficiency on gene identification across species.

Second, the sample size of cross-species experiment is likely to be different, and may be one of the deciding factors of the power associated with the modeling approach. In particular, the efficiency of gene identification, whether the proposed model gains power over one-species experiments through pooling information across species, should be examined carefully, especially when the sample size of the experiments is small.

Third, over-fitting may be of concern. The proposed mixture model is, by its nature, highly structured and data driven. If the data are not driven by all nine categories as the model suggests, will the mixture model fail? Is the proposed model flexible enough to handle different types of data structure? To examine the model performance systematically and to test if the proposed model will fail when too many components are used to fit the data where there are actually fewer clusters, two types of data were generated: all nine categories non-empty (case I) and some of the nine components empty (case II).

In simulation studies case I and case II, two methods of gene identification were implemented: the proposed mixture model, utilizing information across two different species, and the traditional t statistics adjusting for multiple comparisons based on single-species data. Five hundred data sets were generated for each different scenario under each simulation study.

Parameter determination and data generation

Theoretically, the number of genes in category 0 (non-differentially expressed in both species) should dominate others, and every other category may comprise some genes. Orthology information from HomoloGene of the National Center for Biotechnology Information (NCBI) (http://www.ncbi.nlm.nih.gov/homologene) and Mouse Genome Informatics (MGI) of Jackson Laboratory [18] and the practical experience gained from analysis of two-species gene expression experiments at GlasoSmithKline (GSK) was used as reference to determine a reasonable number of genes in each category.

The vectors of the number of genes in each category $(n_0, n_1, \ldots, n_8)^T$ determined for simulation studies case I and case II are categories $(6,000, 30, 30, 30, 30, 100, 100, 100, 100)^T$ and categories $(6,000, 30, 30, 0, 0, 100, 0, 100, 0)^T$, respectively. For experiments across species, sample sizes may differ. Considering that this proposed bivariate method could benefit from pooling information across species, especially when the sample size is small, and the practical situation, two scenarios were implemented: the number of replicates per treatment for each species is equal and small, and the number of replicates per treatment for animals is greater than humans. In addition, to evaluate how robust the proposed method is against array noise, two situations were considered: the two experiments are equally noisy and the human data are noisier than the animal's. Furthermore, values of parameters in (3) for the sampling distribution of $(\hat{\beta}_{1a_i}, \hat{\beta}_{1h_i})^T$ were predetermined. Variances of $(\beta_{1a_i}, \beta_{1h_i})^T$ in each component were assumed to be the same: $\eta_{a1}^2 = \eta_{a2}^2 = \eta_{a3}^2 = \eta_{a4}^2 = \eta_{a7}^2 = \eta_{a8}^2 = \eta_{h1}^2 = \eta_{h2}^2 = \eta_{h3}^2 = \eta_{h4}^2 = \eta_{h5}^2 = \eta_{h6}^2 = 0.25$. The correlation between $(\beta_{1a_i}, \beta_{1h_i})^T$ in categories $(1, 2, 3, 4)$ was assumed to be 0.9, i.e., $\rho_1 = \rho_2 = \rho_3 = \rho_4 = 0.9$. Nonzero component means $(\mu_{ak}, \mu_{hk})^T$, $k = 0, \ldots, 8$, were determined so that $|\mu/\eta| = 0.5$ or 1.5. The combination of these parameters resulted in eight different scenarios for each case as presented in Table 2. Note that $|\mu_{\beta_{1a_i}}|$ and $|\mu_{\beta_{1h_i}}|$ represent the absolute value of the mean vector of $(\beta_{1a_i}, \beta_{1h_i})^T$.

After generating $(\beta_{1a_i}, \beta_{1h_i})^T$ accordingly, the next step is to simulate the two species gene expression data X_a and X_h based on linear models (1) and (2). Note that β_{0a_i} and β_{0h_i} are independent $N(8, 1)$ random variables for differentially expressed genes and deterministically 0 for non-differentially expressed genes.

Simulation results

It is of interest to compare how effective the mixture model is on gene identification using information across two species with the conventional one-species approach. The conventional two-sample t test for gene selection was performed using just single species data (animals or humans) and a multiplicity adjustment was made according to the procedure proposed by Benjamini and Hochberg [19].

The results are presented in Table 3. The first section of Table 3, categories (1, 2, 3, 4, 5, 6), manifests the number of genes classified into categories (1, 2, 3, 4, 5, 6) using the the mixture model (Mixture) and the number of genes selected using human data only (Human only), with the corresponding nominal FDR controlled at FDR_I. For

Table 2 Combination of parameters for simulation studies case I and case II

Case I	sim1	sim2	sim3	sim4	sim5	sim6	sim7	sim8
n_a	10	10	10	10	100	100	100	100
n_h	10	10	10	10	10	10	10	10
$\lvert\mu_{\beta_{1a_i}}\rvert$	0.25	0.75	0.25	0.75	0.25	0.75	0.25	0.75
$\lvert\mu_{\beta_{1h_i}}\rvert$	0.25	0.75	0.25	0.75	0.25	0.75	0.25	0.75
σ_a^2	0.1	0.1	0.1	0.1	0.1	0.1	0.1	0.1
σ_h^2	0.1	0.1	0.3	0.3	0.1	0.1	0.3	0.3
Case II	sim9	sim10	sim11	sim12	sim13	sim14	sim15	sim16

each simulated data set, FDR_I was calculated as (number of genes that are erroneously classified into categories (1, 2, 3, 4, 5, 6))/(total number of genes classified into categories (1, 2, 3, 4, 5, 6)). This was to ensure a fair comparison between the mixture model and the conventional one-species method. FDR_{II} was calculated in the same fashion. Avg FDR_I and Avg FDR_{II} are simply the averaged values of FDR_I and FDR_{II} across the 500 simulated data sets. When the estimated nominal FDR $= 0$, i.e., the mixture model did not falsely categorize any genes, the nominal FDR for the single-species method was controlled at 0.0001. The second section of Table 3, categories $(1, 2, 3, 4, 7, 8)$, represents the number of genes classified into categories $(1, 2, 3, 4, 7, 8)$ using the mixture model (Mixture) and number of genes selected using animal data alone (Animal only). Beneath each set of eight simulation cases is Tukey's Honestly Significant Difference (HSD) for a familywise error rate of 0.05 for the results obtained using the proposed mixture model. Tukey's HSD was calculated as $q_{0.05}(8, 3, 992) \times (\text{MS(Error)}/500)^{1/2}$, since there were eight simulation cases (500 simulated data sets in each situation) in each simulation study (case I and case II) and the error degree of freedom was 3,992. MS(Error) denotes the error mean square (= Error sum of squares/Error degree of freedom, see Table 4). $q_{0.05}(8, 3, 992) = 4.29$.

The effect of array noise on the mixture model can be easily seen from the column of Avg FDR_I and by comparing the results of sim1 vs. sim3, sim5 vs. sim7, sim9 vs. sim11, and sim13 vs. sim15. These are the cases

Table 3 The number of genes selected based on (a) bivariate mixture model, (b) conventional one-species approach

	Categories (1,2,3,4,5,6)			Categories (1,2,3,4,7,8)		
	Mixture	Avg FDR_I	Human only	Mixture	Avg FDR_{II}	Animal only
sim1	132	0.034	100(0.070)	129	0.029	96(0.063)
sim2	224	0.003	145(0.021)	223	0.012	188(0.016)
sim3	113	0.246	85(0.318)	135	0.048	109(0.073)
sim4	166	0.050	115(0.043)	222	0.012	188(0.016)
sim5	132	0.028	98(0.041)	234	0.004	238(0.012)
sim6	227	0.011	194(0.021)	289	0.003	289(0.007)
sim7	112	0.235	78(0.282)	241	0.011	246(0.020)
sim8	167	0.048	124(0.065)	288	0.002	288(0.007)
Tukey's HSD	30.908	0.021		52.958	0.016	
sim9	92	0.126	81(0.296)	88	0.129	75(0.307)
sim10	118	0.033	104(0.048)	118	0.036	99(0.061)
sim11	141	0.470	109(0.670)	80	0.128	70(0.214)
sim12	103	0.116	68(0.118)	118	0.049	102(0.088)
sim13	84	0.140	67(0.169)	180	0.349	167(0.407)
sim14	120	0.023	88(0.023)	152	0.022	151(0.101)
sim15	119	0.480	99(0.636)	168	0.358	157(0.369)
sim16	96	0.093	57(0.105)	147	0.020	148(0.061)
Tukey's HSD	3.947	0.011		2.337	0.004	

Under simulation studies case I and case II. Numbers in parentheses are the observed FDRs. Averaged over the 500 simulated datasets. Tukey's HSD for an α level of 0.05 is included beneath each set of eight simulation cases.

Table 4 ANOVA table to quantify variability

			Categories (1, 2, 3, 4, 5, 6)	Categories (1, 2, 3, 4, 7, 8)
	Source of variation	*df*	Sum of squares	Sum of squares
Case I	Replicates	1	1,141(0.006)	7,319,401(0.408)*
	Mean magnitude	1	5,415,341(11.560)*	4,982,736(0.252)*
	Array noise	1	1,561,198(15.950)*	6,353(0.042)
	Replicates × Mean magnitude	1	1,197(0.032)	392,099(0.122)*
	Replicates × Array noise	1	697(0.012)	351(0.011)
	Mean magnitude × Array noise	1	400,720(7.021)*	16,601(0.043)*
	Replicates × Mean magnitude × Array noise	1	145(0.002)	214(0.010)
	Error	3,992	1,689,667(12.887)	592,184(1.817)
	Total	3,999	9,070,107(47.471)	13,309,941(2.706)
Case II	Replicates	1	73,917(0.006)	3,676,664(2.888)
	Mean magnitude	1	6(56.346)	22,274(2.830)
	Array noise	1	130,794(43.770)*	865,448(0.001)*
	Replicates × Mean magnitude	1	37,277(0.190)	36,778(1.038)
	Replicates × Array noise	1	34,404(0.015)	5,065(0.049)
	Mean magnitude × Array noise	1	929,915(17.537)	19,128(0.043)
	Replicates × Mean magnitude × Array noise	1	1,467(0.004)	58(0.000)
	Error	3,992	103,604,971(47.182)	304,161,196(27.427)
	Total	3,999	104,812,751(165.052)	308,786,610(34.276)

ANOVA was performed independently for simulation studies case I and case II to quantify the variability among the results (gene counts and observed FDRs). Numbers in parentheses are the sum of squares for the observed FDRs. For gene counts, *indicates which sources of variability could be declared significant at level $\alpha = 0.05$.

with smaller means and variances for humans which change from 0.1 to 0.3 for each pair of comparisons. The differences between the observed FDRs for these four groups were at least 0.2 and 0.3 for case I and case II, respectively. In contrast, when means were larger, changes of variances did not seem to affect the results in the sense that the corresponding observed FDRs had barely changed while the variances of human increased. The observed FDRs for animals were not as sensitive to the array noise on humans as the observed FDRs for humans.

Under both simulation studies case I and case II, increasing the number of replicates in the animal experiment helped the gene identification for animals: more animal genes were identified for sim5 to sim8 than for sim1 to sim4, and for sim13 to sim16 than for sim9 to sim12. The corresponding FDRs were also lower for sim5 to sim8 and sim13 to sim16. In contrast, increasing the number of replicates in the animal experiment did not significantly improve the results of gene identification for humans.

Table 4 is the summary of a three-way analysis of variance (ANOVA). Three factors, each with two levels, were used in the analysis: replicates ($(n_a, n_h)^T = (10, 10)^T$ or $(100, 10)^T$), mean magnitude ($((|\mu_{\beta_{1a_i}}|, |\mu_{\beta_{1h_i}}|)^T = (0.25, 0.25)^T$ or $(0.75, 0.75)^T$), and array noise ($(\sigma_a^2, \sigma_h^2)^T = (0.1, 0.1)^T$ or $(0.1, 0.3)^T$). This analysis, performed independently, quantifies the variability among the results (gene counts and observed FDRs) obtained using the proposed mixture model in Table 3 for the 16 different simulated situations under simulation studies case I and case II.

Throughout the 16 simulation cases, with nominal FDR controlled at FDR_I, the bivariate mixture model outperformed the single-species method for human gene identification by always recognizing more genes with lower observed FDRs. For the animal part, the mixture model performed at least as well as the single-species method on gene selection by identifying at least as many genes. Notice that selecting genes related to humans (categories (1, 2, 3, 4, 5, 6)) seemed to be associated with higher false discovery rate than selecting genes related to animals (categories (1, 2, 3, 4, 7, 8)). Furthermore, the observed FDRs were lower for case I than for case II, regardless of the type of genes interested (differentially expressed for humans or animals).

The comprehensive simulation study suggested that the proposed model, though highly structured, offered advantages over single-species analyses, especially when the magnitude of differential expression due to different treatment intervention was weak.

Application: the mouse and human type II diabetes experiment

Background introduction

A systems biology study was completed by GlaxoSmithKline (GSK) to study the efficacy of type II diabetes drugs in both preclinical (mice) and clinical (humans) experiments. The mouse and human data were collected and preprocessed using Affymetrix MAS 5.0 at the probe set level on Affymetrix MOE430A array and Human Genome U133 Plus 2.0 array, respectively. For mice, the total number of probe sets was 22,690. Mice were fed a diet enriched in fat (58% kcal from fat) for 8 weeks prior to treatment. Most of the mice of this susceptible strain developed obesity and mild hyperglycemia and hyperinsulinemia. Control mice on an 11% low fat diet remained normal. The mouse treatment arm consisted of a diabetes drug at multiple dose levels with vehicle controls over a 2-week period. The study was a full factorial design, where 40 animals in high fat diet and 40 animals in low fat diet were randomized to receive either placebo, or different dosages of the type II diabetes drug (low, medium or high). Note that the results for mice were measured at one time point, the end of the study. For simplicity, only integration results on animals treated with placebo (10 mice) or high dose of the drug (9 mice) were demonstrated.

On the other hand, there were 54,676 probe sets in the human data set and all 59 subjects were type II diabetes patients. The gene expression measurements for human subjects were collected twice during the experiment, one at baseline before the treatment started (week 0) and the other one at the completion of the study (week 8). Among the 59 subjects, 14 only had data for only one time point and hence were not included in further data analysis. Subjects in the clinical trial were treated by either placebo, or three other type II diabetes drugs, including the one given to the mice. Titrated dosing was implemented to ensure that each person received his/her dose based on his/her body profile. Human subjects treated with placebo (number of subjects = 11) and the same type II diabetes drug given to mice (number of subjects = 13) were used in this analysis. Besides being measured at two time points, other information contained in the human data and used in the data analysis included: prior therapy (four categorical levels) and concomitant medication status (two categorical levels).

Data for both species were logarithmic transformed (base equal to 2). Methods for combining information from multiple probe sets that were not identical have been discussed in many publications [20,21]. A gene-level transcript value in order to pair the mouse and human genes through orthology was obtained by averaging probe sets across a gene. This resulted in 13,483 and 20,252 genes for mouse and human, respectively. Missing values were replaced with array means in both data sets.

The mouse and human orthology information, MGI release 4.32, was used to map the mouse and human orthologous genes. Human and mouse orthologs (17,834) were included in release 4.32. Combining the information among MGI release 4.32 and mouse and human genes from the GSK data gave a total of 11,922 orthologs.

In addition to the measurements of gene expression for both mice and humans, different efficacy endpoints, such as blood glucose, insulin, hemoglobin A1c (HbA1c), and others were also measured during the preclinical and clinical experiments by GSK in order to evaluate the effect of treatment intervention on both species.

The purpose of this data analysis was to evaluate the capability of the proposed mixture model, an approach utilizing the information across two species, to identify genes that may help scientists reveal the biological similarity between two species (ex: mouse and human), essentially genes in categories $(1, 2, 3, 4)$, and so to improve the efficiency of drug development by decreasing the compound attrition rate from preclinical trials to clinical trials.

Data analysis

The estimated treatment effects for mice and humans are obtained by the following independent simple linear models:

$$X_{a_{ij}} = \beta_{0a_i} + \beta_{1a_i} T_{a_j} + e_{a_{ij}}, \tag{5}$$

$$X_{h_{il}}^{week8} = \beta_{0h_i} + X_{h_{il}}^{week0} + \beta_{1h_i} T_{h_l} + \boldsymbol{\beta}_{2h_i}\,\text{PriorTherapy} + \beta_{3h_i}\,\text{ConMed} + e_{h_{il}}, \tag{6}$$

where $i = 1, \ldots, 11{,}922$ (number of orthologs); $j = 1, \ldots, 19$ (number of mice); $l = 1, \ldots, 24$ (number of humans). $X_{a_{ij}}$, $X_{h_{il}}^{week0}$ and $X_{h_{il}}^{week8}$ are gene expressions from the ith orthologous gene for the jth mouse, gene expression from the ith orthologous gene for the lth human before treatment intervention, and gene expression from the ith orthologous gene for the lth human at the completion of the clinical experiment, respectively. T_{a_j} and T_{h_l} are $\{0, 1\}$ treatment indicators, and $e_{a_{ij}}$ and $e_{h_{il}}$ are independent $N(0, \sigma_a^2)$ and $N(0, \sigma_h^2)$ random variables. Additionally, there are two more covariates in the human model: PriorTherapy (a four-level categorical variable indicating patients' therapy prior to the clinical trial) and ConMed (a two-level categorical variable for concomitant medication status).

Equation (4) was used to model the distribution of the estimated treatment effects. Genes in categories (1, 2, 3, 4) are believed to be potential biomarkers that can greatly improve the design of the process of drug development as these orthologous genes interact with drugs in a way that shows some relationship between two different species (in this case, human and mouse) and so studying the behavior of these genes in preclinical trials might help scientists better understand the mechanism of drug activities in clinical trials.

Results

Parameter estimation

The maximum likelihood estimates of the parameters in the bivariate normal mixture model using the EM algorithm are given in Table 5. The estimated mixture weight for category 0 was $\hat{\pi}_0 = 0.889$ indicating approximately 10,599 ($11,922 \times 0.889$) pairs of uninteresting mouse and human orthologs. $(\mu_a, \mu_h)^T$ denotes the mean vector of each mixture component. The estimated treatment effect means of mice were in general larger than that of humans, indicating that the magnitude of the difference of expression in genes due to treatment intervention in mice tended to be larger than in genes where differential expression is exhibited in humans. The estimated variance for mice $\widehat{\sigma}^2_{ak}$ tended to be larger than that for humans $\widehat{\sigma}^2_{hk}$, suggesting that overall, the variability in the mouse data set was larger than the human data set. The estimated correlation coefficients between the treatment effects for both species were $(-0.531, 0.380, -1, 0.102)$ for categories $(1, 2, 3, 4)$, respectively. The estimated correlation for category 3 was based on only two observations. Standard errors of the parameter estimates from the two-species experiment were obtained by bootstrapping with 1,000 bootstrap replicates. Based on the bootstrap standard errors, there was little evidence of bias for the parameter estimates.

Gene identification

The vector of the number of genes identified for each category was $(\hat{n}_0, \hat{n}_1, \ldots, \hat{n}_8)^T$ = (10,814, 41, 12, 2, 20, 168, 578, 12, 275)^T. Figure 1 displays the scatter plots of $(\hat{\beta}_{1a_i}, \hat{\beta}_{1h_i})^T$ before and after gene membership identification, including the scatter plot of $(\hat{\beta}_{1a_i}, \hat{\beta}_{1h_i})^T$ for all orthologs, orthologs after eliminating the uninteresting ones (orthologs not in category 0), and orthologs reacting to the treatment stimulus for both species (orthologs in categories (1, 2, 3, 4)).

Based on the bivariate mixture model, among the 11,922 pairs of orthologs, 10,814 pairs did not react to the drug treatment for either species, 75 pairs of orthologs (sum of the gene counts in categories 1 through 4) showed evidence of differentiation between treatments for both species. Genes in categories $(5, 6, 7, 8)$ are also potential candidates for further investigation to improve the process of drug development since studying these genes might uncover the myth of the overall high attrition rate of a drug compound from preclinical trials to clinical trials.

In comparison, an attempt was made to identify differentially expressed human genes using solely the human data, i.e., traditional t statistics were used to test whether or not $\beta_{1h_i} = 0$ and the approach of Benjamini and Hochberg [19] was used to adjust for multiple comparisons. With the nominal FDR controlled at 0.01, 0.1, 0.5, and 0.9, this single-species method failed to identify any differentially expressed human genes at any levels of FDR. With the p values histograms in Figure 2 showing an obvious difference between the observed significance of differential expression for mice and humans, specifically, the p values were nearly uniformly distributed for humans, the result was not surprising.

Concluding remarks

This research was motivated by a fundamental yet still not well-understood problem in the drug development process. The results obtained in preclinical animal trials do not seem to translate well enough to make inferences for human clinical trials, resulting in an undesirably high attrition rate in human experiments. A bivariate mixture model which utilizes information across two species was proposed to identify genes that exhibit similar patterns of expression across species, with the hope that studying

Table 5 Parameter estimates of the bivariate mixture model

	Parameter estimates					
Category	$\widehat{\pi}_k$	$\widehat{\mu}_{ak}$	$\widehat{\mu}_{hk}$	$\widehat{\sigma}^2_{ak}$	$\widehat{\rho_k\sigma_{ak}\sigma_{hk}}$	$\widehat{\sigma}^2_{hk}$
0	0.889(0.013)	NE	NE	0.117(0.002)	NE	0.052(0.001)
1	0.002(0.001)	1.440(0.190)	0.139(0.203)	0.112(0.064)	−0.070(0.040)	0.154(0.061)
2	0.001(0.001)	−1.174(0.228)	−0.853(0.128)	0.156(0.132)	0.033(0.053)	0.048(0.039)
3	0.000(0.001)	2.104(0.319)	−1.231(0.361)	0.006(0.124)	−0.005(0.078)	0.003(0.111)
4	0.002(0.001)	−1.047(0.081)	0.660(0.128)	0.027(0.018)	−0.005(0.023)	0.087(0.047)
5	0.021(0.001)	NE	0.669(0.003)	0.144(0.000)	NE	0.050(0.006)
6	0.049(0.002)	NE	−0.787(0.001)	0.149(0.000)	NE	0.055(0.004)
7	0.003(0.008)	1.528(0.310)	NE	0.543(0.201)	NE	0.084(0.022)
8	0.034(0.009)	−1.038(0.146)	NE	0.225(0.051)	NE	0.055(0.006)

Bootstrap ($B = 1,000$) standard errors in parentheses. NE, not estimated.

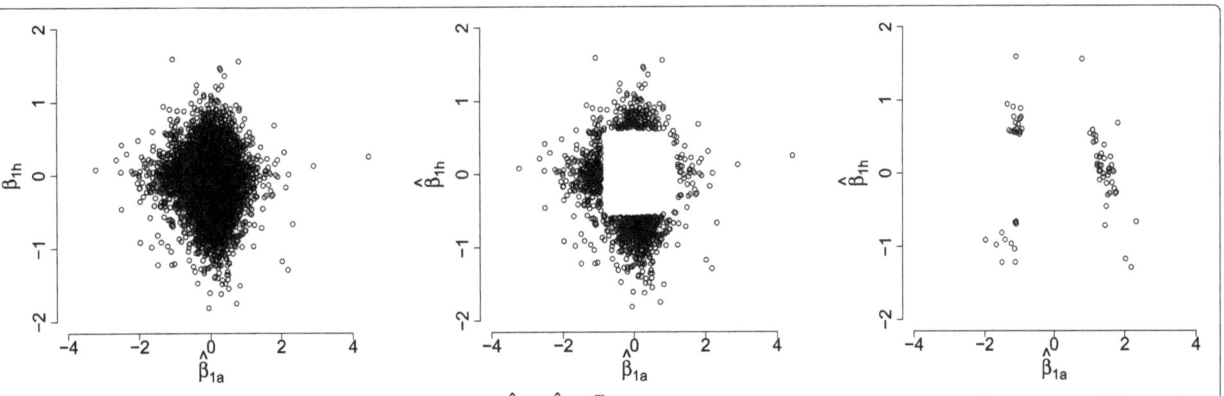

Figure 1 Scatter plots of the estimated treatment effects $(\hat{\beta}_{1a_i}, \hat{\beta}_{1h_i})^T$ before and after gene membership identification. From left to right: all orthologs, orthologs differentially expressed in either species (categories (1, 2, 3, 4, 5, 6, 7, 8)), and orthologs differentially expressed in both species (categories (1, 2, 3, 4)).

genes could help understand biological differences across species at the molecular level and ultimately help reduce attrition in drug development. It is also of great interest to identify genes active in animal, but not in human since studying this group of genes might lead to answers that explain why some drug trials fail in translation to humans. The comprehensive simulation study suggested that the proposed model, though highly structured, can accommodate various configurations of differential gene expression, especially when the magnitude of differential expression due to different treatment intervention was weak.

In the application of the bivariate mixture model on the GSK type II diabetes experiment, the mixture model was able to separate differentially expressed genes from non-differentially expressed genes. A potential multi-gene predictor may be developed according to the genes identified by the bivariate mixture model to benefit patients in therapeutic decision making.

The mixture model is highly structured, with strong but somewhat simplifying assumptions. The grouping of all genes for which the expression difference is positive in both species into a single category parameterized by a single bivariate mean may be somewhat of a simplistic approach. In practice, the data may not be normally distributed or be comprised by exactly nine groups and lead to bias and inefficiency. Forcing the normality assumption and the grouping may be inefficient. However, by modeling the least squares estimates of the expression differences as bivariate realizations from a distribution with a single mean vector, some flexibility in the model is retained. It is perhaps less important to precisely quantify the magnitude of the expression difference than to determine whether it is positive or negative and whether or not the direction is preserved across species.

Using the proposed mixture model for gene identification is completely data-driven. The simulation study in Section 'Simulation' indicated that the mixture model at times report a poor observed false discovery rate due to large variability in measurement of expression. Currently, gene membership classification is determined by maximizing the posterior probability that observation y_i belongs to the kth cluster. It is possible to choose costs to attach weight to different types of misclassification and then choose a classification rule to minimize expected

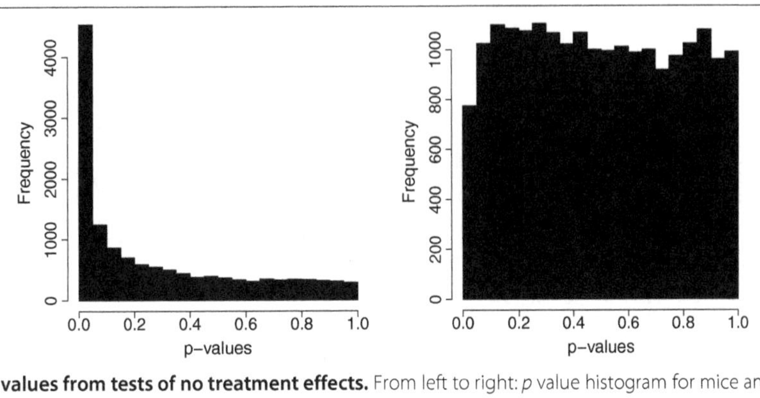

Figure 2 Histograms of p values from tests of no treatment effects. From left to right: p value histogram for mice and p value histogram for humans.

cost. This rule may lead to a more desirable list that can better accommodate goals for future research.

The mixture model currently only handles data with two treatments/cancer types/drugs, i.e., data containing only two-level variables. In practice, it is often the case that an experiment is run under multiple conditions. An extension of the model to handle experiments with factors with three-or-more levels is an important future work.

This approach focuses on identifying orthologs that show same/opposite mechanism between two species. However, genes identified by the bivariate mixture model (genes in categories (1, 2, 3, 4)) may not lead to the most powerful model for prediction of cancer types/response status for either one of the species. The most powerful model may be based on those human genes that lie in categories 5 and 6. For those genes, the corresponding animal genes show no signs of differential expression. Hence, incorporating prediction ability into the model or developing a prediction model that can help utilize the genes selected by the mixture model is of great interest and is an obvious candidate for future research.

Appendix

Mixture models and the EM algorithm

Estimating the parameters in (4) is nontrivial. Redner and Walker [22] offer an excellent review of estimating the parameters which determine a mixture density. In particular, the paper is devoted to a particular iterative procedure for numerically approximating maximum likelihood estimates (MLE) of the parameters in mixture densities. This method was formalized by Dempster et al. [23] and termed the *EM (Expectation-Maximization) algorithm*, and is used for numerically approximating the maximum likelihood estimates for (4).

The EM algorithm with no constraints

For a finite mixture model with C components, given data $\mathbf{y}$ with independent multivariate observations $\mathbf{y}_1, \ldots, \mathbf{y}_g$, each $\mathbf{y}_i$ is taken to be a realization of the mixture probability density function,

$$f(\mathbf{y}_i|\boldsymbol{\Psi}) = \sum_{k=1}^{C} \pi_k f_k(\mathbf{y}_i|\boldsymbol{\theta}_k),$$

where $\boldsymbol{\Psi} = (\boldsymbol{\theta}_1, \ldots, \boldsymbol{\theta}_C, \pi_1, \ldots, \pi_C)^T$, a vector of unknown parameters. f_k and $\boldsymbol{\theta}_k$ are the density and parameters of the kth component in the mixture, respectively. π_k is the probability that an observation arises from the kth component. Note that $\pi_k \geq 0$ and $\sum_{k=1}^{C} \pi_k = 1$. For classification purpose and to achieve minimum misclassification rates, $\mathbf{y}_i$ is assigned to the population (category) for which the posterior probability that $\mathbf{y}_i$ belongs to the kth cluster (the kth component of the mixture) is maximized. The posterior probability is given by

$$\tau_k(\mathbf{y}_i; \boldsymbol{\Psi}) = \frac{\pi_k f_k(\mathbf{y}_i|\boldsymbol{\theta}_k)}{\sum_{h=1}^{C} \pi_h f_h(\mathbf{y}_i|\boldsymbol{\theta}_h)}.$$

In summary, the EM algorithm may be implemented to maximize the likelihood of a multivariate normal mixture model by following these two steps:

E-step: *The E-step on the (j+1) iteration takes the conditional expectation of the complete-data log likelihood, given the observed data* $(Q(\boldsymbol{\Psi}|\boldsymbol{\Psi}^{(j)}))$.

At the $(j+1)$ iteration, the E-step results in

$$Q(\boldsymbol{\Psi}|\boldsymbol{\Psi}^{(j)}) = \sum_{i=1}^{g}\sum_{k=1}^{C} \tau_k(\mathbf{y}_i; \boldsymbol{\Psi}^{(j)})(\log \pi_k + \log f_k(\mathbf{y}_i|\boldsymbol{\theta}_k)), \tag{7}$$

where $f_k(\mathbf{y}_i|\boldsymbol{\theta}_k) = (2\pi)^{-\frac{p}{2}}|\boldsymbol{\Sigma}_k|^{-\frac{1}{2}} e^{-\frac{1}{2}(\mathbf{y}_i-\boldsymbol{\mu}_k)^T\boldsymbol{\Sigma}_k^{-1}(\mathbf{y}_i-\boldsymbol{\mu}_k)}$

and $\tau_k(\mathbf{y}_i; \boldsymbol{\Psi}^{(j)}) = \dfrac{\pi_k^{(j)} f_k(\mathbf{y}_i|\boldsymbol{\theta}_k^{(j)})}{\sum_{h=1}^{C} \pi_h^{(j)} f_h(\mathbf{y}_i|\boldsymbol{\theta}_h^{(j)})}$.

M-step: *The M-step on the (j+1) iteration requires the global maximization of* $Q(\boldsymbol{\Psi}|\boldsymbol{\Psi}^{(j)})$ *with respect to* $\boldsymbol{\Psi}$ *over the parameter space to give the updated estimate* $\boldsymbol{\Psi}^{(j+1)}$.

$$\hat{\pi}_k^{(j+1)} = \frac{\sum_{i=1}^{g} \tau_k(\mathbf{y}_i; \boldsymbol{\Psi}^{(j)})}{g}; \tag{8}$$

$$\hat{\boldsymbol{\mu}}_k^{(j+1)} = \frac{\sum_{i=1}^{g} \tau_k(\mathbf{y}_i; \boldsymbol{\Psi}^{(j)})\mathbf{y}_i}{\sum_{i=1}^{g} \tau_k(\mathbf{y}_i; \boldsymbol{\Psi}^{(j)})}; \tag{9}$$

$$\hat{\boldsymbol{\Sigma}}_k^{(j+1)} = \frac{\sum_{i=1}^{g} \tau_k(\mathbf{y}_i; \boldsymbol{\Psi}^{(j)})(\mathbf{y}_i - \boldsymbol{\mu}_k)^T(\mathbf{y}_i - \boldsymbol{\mu}_k)}{\sum_{i=1}^{g} \tau_k(\mathbf{y}_i; \boldsymbol{\Psi}^{(j)})}. \tag{10}$$

The iterations of the EM algorithm continue until some stopping criterion is met, such as the difference of the conditional expectation of the complete-data log likelihood at the $(j+1)$ step and the conditional expectation of the complete-data log likelihood at the j step is sufficiently small, i.e.,

$$Q(\boldsymbol{\Phi}^{(j+1)}|\boldsymbol{\Phi}^{(j)}) - Q(\boldsymbol{\Phi}^{(j)}|\boldsymbol{\Phi}^{(j)}) \leq \epsilon.$$

Throughout this research, $\epsilon = 0.0001$.

The EM Algorithm with constraints

With constraints on the parameter space, the EM algorithm derived in Section 'The EM algorithm with no constraints' cannot be used directly. To accommodate the restricted parameter space introduced for (4), first note that (4) is a bivariate normal mixture with nine components and the density for each component can be written as

$$f_k\left(\mathbf{y}_i|\boldsymbol{\theta}_k\right) = \frac{e^{-\frac{1}{2}\frac{1}{\sigma_{a_k}^2\sigma_{h_k}^2\left(1-\rho_k^2\right)}\left(\sigma_{h_k}^2\left(y_{a_i}-\mu_{a_k}\right)^2-2\rho_k\sigma_{a_k}\sigma_{h_k}\left(y_{a_i}-\mu_{a_k}\right)\left(y_{h_i}-\mu_{h_k}\right)+\sigma_{a_k}^2\left(y_{h_i}-\mu_{h_k}\right)^2\right)}}{2\pi\sqrt{\sigma_{a_k}^2\sigma_{h_k}^2\left(1-\rho_k^2\right)}},$$

where $\mathbf{y}_i = (y_{a_i}, y_{h_i})^T = (\hat{\beta}_{1a_i}, \hat{\beta}_{1h_i})^T$ and $\boldsymbol{\theta}_k = (\mu_{a_k}, \mu_{h_k}, \sigma_{a_k}^2, \sigma_{h_k}^2, \rho_k)^T$.

The solution for the E-step remains the same. The membership probability $\tau_k(\mathbf{y}_i; \mathbf{\Psi}^{(j)})$ can be obtained by taking the conditional expectation of the complete-data log likelihood, given the observed data.

As for the M-step, the MLE for π_k remains the same, $\hat{\pi}_k^{(j+1)} = \frac{\sum_{i=1}^{g}\tau_k(\mathbf{y}_i;\mathbf{\Psi}^{(j)})}{g}$. However, the MLEs for $\boldsymbol{\mu}_k$ and $\mathbf{\Sigma}_k$ need to be modified according to the constrained parameter space for each mixture component.

Essentially, the MLEs on the $(j+1)$ iteration for $(\mu_{ak}, \mu_{hk})^T, k = 1, \ldots, 4$, are

$$\hat{\mu}_{a1}^{(j+1)} = \begin{cases} \frac{\sum_{i=1}^{g}\tau_1(\mathbf{y}_i;\mathbf{\Psi}^{(j)})y_{a_i}}{\sum_{i=1}^{g}\tau_1(\mathbf{y}_i;\mathbf{\Psi}^{(j)})} & \text{if } \sum_{i=1}^{g}\tau_1(\mathbf{y}_i;\mathbf{\Psi}^{(j)})y_{a_i} \geq 0; \\ 0 & \text{otherwise.} \end{cases}$$

$$\hat{\mu}_{h1}^{(j+1)} = \begin{cases} \frac{\sum_{i=1}^{g}\tau_1(\mathbf{y}_i;\mathbf{\Psi}^{(j)})y_{h_i}}{\sum_{i=1}^{g}\tau_1(\mathbf{y}_i;\mathbf{\Psi}^{(j)})} & \text{if } \sum_{i=1}^{g}\tau_1(\mathbf{y}_i;\mathbf{\Psi}^{(j)})y_{h_i} \geq 0; \\ 0 & \text{otherwise.} \end{cases}$$

$$\hat{\mu}_{a2}^{(j+1)} = \begin{cases} \frac{\sum_{i=1}^{g}\tau_2(\mathbf{y}_i;\mathbf{\Psi}^{(j)})y_{a_i}}{\sum_{i=1}^{g}\tau_2(\mathbf{y}_i;\mathbf{\Psi}^{(j)})} & \text{if } \sum_{i=1}^{g}\tau_2(\mathbf{y}_i;\mathbf{\Psi}^{(j)})y_{a_i} \leq 0; \\ 0 & \text{otherwise.} \end{cases}$$

$$\hat{\mu}_{h2}^{(j+1)} = \begin{cases} \frac{\sum_{i=1}^{g}\tau_2(\mathbf{y}_i;\mathbf{\Psi}^{(j)})y_{h_i}}{\sum_{i=1}^{g}\tau_2(\mathbf{y}_i;\mathbf{\Psi}^{(j)})} & \text{if } \sum_{i=1}^{g}\tau_2(\mathbf{y}_i;\mathbf{\Psi}^{(j)})y_{h_i} \leq 0; \\ 0 & \text{otherwise.} \end{cases}$$

$$\hat{\mu}_{a3}^{(j+1)} = \begin{cases} \frac{\sum_{i=1}^{g}\tau_3(\mathbf{y}_i;\mathbf{\Psi}^{(j)})y_{a_i}}{\sum_{i=1}^{g}\tau_3(\mathbf{y}_i;\mathbf{\Psi}^{(j)})} & \text{if } \sum_{i=1}^{g}\tau_3(\mathbf{y}_i;\mathbf{\Psi}^{(j)})y_{a_i} \geq 0; \\ 0 & \text{otherwise.} \end{cases}$$

$$\hat{\mu}_{h3}^{(j+1)} = \begin{cases} \frac{\sum_{i=1}^{g}\tau_3(\mathbf{y}_i;\mathbf{\Psi}^{(j)})y_{h_i}}{\sum_{i=1}^{g}\tau_3(\mathbf{y}_i;\mathbf{\Psi}^{(j)})} & \text{if } \sum_{i=1}^{g}\tau_3(\mathbf{y}_i;\mathbf{\Psi}^{(j)})y_{h_i} \leq 0; \\ 0 & \text{otherwise.} \end{cases}$$

$$\hat{\mu}_{a4}^{(j+1)} = \begin{cases} \frac{\sum_{i=1}^{g}\tau_4(\mathbf{y}_i;\mathbf{\Psi}^{(j)})y_{a_i}}{\sum_{i=1}^{g}\tau_4(\mathbf{y}_i;\mathbf{\Psi}^{(j)})} & \text{if } \sum_{i=1}^{g}\tau_4(\mathbf{y}_i;\mathbf{\Psi}^{(j)})y_{a_i} \leq 0; \\ 0 & \text{otherwise.} \end{cases}$$

$$\hat{\mu}_{h4}^{(j+1)} = \begin{cases} \frac{\sum_{i=1}^{g}\tau_4(\mathbf{y}_i;\mathbf{\Psi}^{(j)})y_{h_i}}{\sum_{i=1}^{g}\tau_4(\mathbf{y}_i;\mathbf{\Psi}^{(j)})} & \text{if } \sum_{i=1}^{g}\tau_4(\mathbf{y}_i;\mathbf{\Psi}^{(j)})y_{h_i} \geq 0; \\ 0 & \text{otherwise.} \end{cases}$$

The MLEs of $\mathbf{\Sigma}_k$, $k = 1, \ldots, 4$, at the $(j+1)$ M-step remain unchanged as in (10).

The MLEs on the $(j+1)$ iteration for $(\mu_{ak}, \mu_{hk})^T, k = 5, \ldots, 8$, are

$$\hat{\mu}_{h5}^{(j+1)} = \begin{cases} \frac{\sum_{i=1}^{g}\tau_5(\mathbf{y}_i;\mathbf{\Psi}^{(j)})y_{h_i}}{\sum_{i=1}^{g}\tau_5(\mathbf{y}_i;\mathbf{\Psi}^{(j)})} & \text{if } \sum_{i=1}^{g}\tau_5(\mathbf{y}_i;\mathbf{\Psi}^{(j)})y_{h_i} \geq 0; \\ 0 & \text{otherwise.} \end{cases}$$

$$\hat{\mu}_{h6}^{(j+1)} = \begin{cases} \frac{\sum_{i=1}^{g}\tau_6(\mathbf{y}_i;\mathbf{\Psi}^{(j)})y_{h_i}}{\sum_{i=1}^{g}\tau_6(\mathbf{y}_i;\mathbf{\Psi}^{(j)})} & \text{if } \sum_{i=1}^{g}\tau_6(\mathbf{y}_i;\mathbf{\Psi}^{(j)})y_{h_i} \leq 0; \\ 0 & \text{otherwise.} \end{cases}$$

$$\hat{\mu}_{a7}^{(j+1)} = \begin{cases} \frac{\sum_{i=1}^{g}\tau_7(\mathbf{y}_i;\mathbf{\Psi}^{(j)})y_{a_i}}{\sum_{i=1}^{g}\tau_7(\mathbf{y}_i;\mathbf{\Psi}^{(j)})} & \text{if } \sum_{i=1}^{g}\tau_7(\mathbf{y}_i;\mathbf{\Psi}^{(j)})y_{a_i} \geq 0; \\ 0 & \text{otherwise.} \end{cases}$$

$$\hat{\mu}_{a8}^{(j+1)} = \begin{cases} \frac{\sum_{i=1}^{g}\tau_8(\mathbf{y}_i;\mathbf{\Psi}^{(j)})y_{a_i}}{\sum_{i=1}^{g}\tau_8(\mathbf{y}_i;\mathbf{\Psi}^{(j)})} & \text{if } \sum_{i=1}^{g}\tau_8(\mathbf{y}_i;\mathbf{\Psi}^{(j)})y_{a_i} \leq 0; \\ 0 & \text{otherwise.} \end{cases}$$

The MLE for $\mathbf{\Sigma}_k, k = 0, 5, 6, 7, 8$, on the $(j+1)$ iteration is

$$\widehat{\mathbf{\Sigma}}_k = \begin{pmatrix} \frac{\sum_{i=1}^{g}\tau_k(\mathbf{y}_i;\mathbf{\Psi}^{(j)})y_{a_i}^2}{\sum_{i=1}^{g}\tau_k(\mathbf{y}_i;\mathbf{\Psi}^{(j)})} & 0 \\ 0 & \frac{\sum_{i=1}^{g}\tau_k(\mathbf{y}_i;\mathbf{\Psi}^{(j)})y_{h_i}^2}{\sum_{i=1}^{g}\tau_k(\mathbf{y}_i;\mathbf{\Psi}^{(j)})} \end{pmatrix}.$$

Regularized covariance matrices in the EM algorithm

The component covariance matrices of a mixture model may be singular or near singular in the EM iterative process. When the covariance matrices corresponding to one or more components are ill-conditioned (singular or near singular), the EM algorithm breaks down. Particularly, applying the EM algorithm for a mixture model with large numbers of components when there are actually fewer groups often results in the failure of the EM algorithm due to ill-conditioning [24,25]. Indeed, this break-down of the EM algorithm may imply that clusters contain insufficient observations and too many components are used to fit the data set where there are actually fewer clusters, or clusters contain points that are of very little variation compared to other clusters. Hence, an intuitive solution to this is to decrease the number of the mixture components. However, this immediately leads to another question: how many clusters are needed. Though an active area of research, it is beyond the scope of this study. Nonetheless, various approaches have been proposed to generate numerically non-singular covariance matrices [26-33]. Among such, the regularization method proposed by Sato and Ishii [32] has been adopted to obtain numerically non-singular covariance matrices throughout this research. In Sato and Ishii [32], the regularized covariance matrix for the kth mixture component in the $(j+1)$ M-step is

$$\mathbf{\Sigma}_{Rk}^{(j+1)} = \mathbf{\Sigma}_{k}^{(j+1)} + \alpha \frac{\mathrm{tr}(\mathbf{\Sigma}_{k}^{(j+1)})}{p} I_p, \quad (11)$$

where $0 \leq \alpha \leq 1$ is a small constant and I_p is a p-dimensional identity matrix. If $\mathbf{\Sigma}_{k}^{(j+1)}$ equals 0, then $\mathrm{tr}(\mathbf{\Sigma}_{k}^{(j+1)})$ is set to be a small threshold value (0.0001 in this research).

Competing interests

The authors declare that they have no competing interests.

Authors' contributions

YS, LZ, AM and JO have participated in the development of the proposed model. YS has drafted the manuscript. All authors read and approved the final manuscript.

Acknowledgements

The authors thank GlaxoSmithKline for sponsoring the systems biology study and collaborating in the data analyses.

Author details

[1]Dr. Su's Statistics & Department of Human Nutrition, Food, and Animal Sciences, University of Hawaii at Manoa, Honolulu, HI 96822, USA. [2]Biomarker and Predictive Analytics, GlaxoSmithKline, 5 Moore Drive, Research Triangle Park, NC 27709, USA. [3]Department of Statistics, North Carolina State University, Raleigh, NC 27695, USA.

References

1. FDA: **Innovation and stagnation: challenge and opportunity on the critical path to new medical products.** *FDA White Paper* 2004.
2. Bolten B, DeGregorio T: **Trends in development cycles.** *Nat Rev Drug Discov* 2002, **1:**335–336.
3. Kola I: **Landis J: Can the pharmaceutical industry reduce attrition rates?** *Nat Rev Drug Discov* 2004, **3:**711–715.
4. Braxton S, Bedilion T: **The integration of microarray information in the drug development process.** *Curr Opin Biotechnol* 1998, **9:**643–649.
5. Debouck C, Goodfellow P: **DNA microarrays in drug discovery and development.** *Nat Genet* 1999, **21:**48–50.
6. Koonin E: **An apology for orthologs - or brave new memes.** *Genome Biol* 2001, **2**(4):1005.1–1005.2.
7. Sonnhammer E, Koonin E: **Orthology, paralogy and proposed classification for paralog subtypes.** *Trends Genet* 2002, **18:**619–620.
8. Theiben G: **Secret life of genes.** *Nature* 2002, **415:**741.
9. Holbrook J, Sanseau P: **Drug discovery and computational evolutionary analysis.** *Drug Discov Today* 2007, **12:**826–832.
10. Grigoryev D, Ma S, Irizarry R, Ye S, Quackenbush J, Garcia J: **Orthologous gene-expression profiling in multi-species models: search for candidate genes.** *Genome Biol* 2004, **5:**R34.1–R34.13.
11. Batzoglou S, Pachter L, Mesirov J, Berger B, Lander E: **Human and mouse gene structure: comparative analysis and application to exon prediction.** *Genome Res* 2008, **10:**950–958.
12. Taher L, Rinner O, Garg S, Sczyrba A, Morgenstern B: **AGenDA: gene prediction by cross-species sequence comparison.** *Nucleic Acids Res* 2004, **1:**W305–W308.
13. Ogorek B: **Orthology-based multilevel modeling of differentially expressed mouse and human gene pairs.** *PhD thesis* 2008.
14. Lelandais G, Vincens P, Badel-Chagnon A, Vialette S, Jacq C, Hazout S: **Comparing gene expression networks in a multi-dimensional space to extract similarities and differences between organisms.** *Bioinformatics* 2006, **22:**1359–1366.
15. Park D, Park J, Park S, Park T, Choi S: **Analysis of human disease genes in the context of gene essentiality.** *Genomics* 2008, **92:**414–418.
16. McLachlan G, Basford K: *Mixture Models: Inference and Applications to Clustering.* New York: Marcel Dekker, Inc.; 1988.
17. McLachlan G, Peel D: *Finite Mixture Models.* New York: Wiley; 2000.
18. Blake J, Richardson J, Bult C, Kadin J: **Eppig J, the Mouse Genome Database Group: The Mouse Genome Database (MGD): the model organism database for the laboratory mouse.** *Nucleic Acids Res* 2002, **30:**113–115.
19. Benjamini Y, Hochberg Y: **Controlling the false discovery rate: a practical and powerful approach to multiple testing.** *J Roy Stat Soc B* 1995, **57:**289–300.
20. Li C, Wong W: **Model-based analysis of oligonucleotide arrays: expression index computation and outlier detection.** *Proc Natl Acad Sci USA* 2001, **98:**31–36.
21. Li C, Zhu D, Cook M: **A statistical framework for consolidating sibling probe sets for Affymetrix GeneChip data.** *BMC Genomics* 2008, **9:**188.
22. Redner R, Walker H: **Mixture densities, maximum likelihood and the EM algorithm.** *J Soc Ind Appl Math* 1984, **26**(2):195–239.
23. Dempster A, Laird N, Rubin D: **Maximum likelihood from incomplete data via the EM algorithm.** *J Roy Stat Soc B* 1977, **39:**1–38.
24. Fraley C, Raftery A: **How many clusters? Which cluster method? Answer via model-based cluster analysis.** *Comput J* 1998, **41**(8):578–588.
25. Fraley C, Raftery A: **Model-based clustering, discriminant analysis, and density estimation.** *J Am Stat Assoc* 2002, **97**(458):611–631.
26. Robotka Z, Zempleni A, Hajas C, Seres C, Balazs S: **Genetic algorithms and grid technologies in clustering, an example: clustering of images.** *Qual Reliab Eng Int* 2008, **24:**693–703.
27. Vlassis N, Likas A: **A greedy EM algorithm for Gaussian mixture.** *Neural Process Lett* 2002, **15:**77–87.
28. Hsieh P, Landgrebe D: **Statistics enhancement in hyperspectral data analysis using spectral-spatial labeling, the EM algorithm, and the leave-one-out covariance estimator.** In *SPIE International Symposium on Optical Science, Engineering, and Instrumentation.* Denver, Colorado; 1999:19–24.
29. Snoussi H, Mohammad-Djafari A: **Penalized maximum likelihood for multivariate Gaussian mixture.** In *AIP Conference Proceedings*; 2002:36–46.
30. Mao J, Jain A: **A self-organizing network for hyperellipsoidal clustering (HEC).** *IEEE Trans Neural Netw* 1996, **7:**16–29.
31. Archambeau C, Verleysen M: **Fully nonparametric probability density function estimation with finite gaussian mixture models.** In *Fifth International Conference on Advances in Pattern Recognition. 10-13 Dec 2003.* Calcultta, India; 2003:81–84.
32. Sato M, Ishii S: **On-line EM algorithm for the normalized Gaussian network.** *Neural Comput* 2000, **12:**407–432.
33. Lee K: **A new, EM algorithm for resource allocation network.** In *Pattern Recognition and Data Mining.* Berlin: Springer; 2005.

19

A tissue-specific gene expression template portrays heart development and pathology

Amy Rodemoyer[1], Nataliya Kibiryeva[2,3], Alexis Bair[2,3], Jennifer Marshall[2,3], James E O'Brien Jr[2,3] and Douglas C Bittel[2,3*]

Abstract

Congenital heart defects (CHD) are the most common cause of death in children under the age of 1. Tetralogy of Fallot (TOF) is a severe CHD that results from developmental defects in the conotruncal outflow tract. Recently, a tissue-specific gene expression template (GET) was derived from microarray data that accurately characterized multiple normal human tissues. We used the GET to examine spatial, temporal, and a pathological condition (TOF) within a single organ, the heart. The GET, as previously defined, generally identified temporal and spatial differences in the cardiac tissue. Differences in the stoichiometry of the GET reflected the severe developmental disturbance associated with TOF. Our analysis suggests that the homoeostatic equilibrium assessed by the GET at the inter-organ level is generally maintained at the intra-organ level as well.

Keywords: Gene expression template, Congenital heart defect, Tetralogy of Fallot

Background

With the advent of tools for whole transcriptome analysis, there has been great interest in defining the gene expression profile of normal tissues as well as pathological states in order to understand the genetic regulation of development and identify potential therapeutic targets [1-5]. These studies have produced insight into the complexity of temporal and spatial regulation of gene expression. They also illustrate the interconnected nature of genes, forming pathways that are themselves interconnected.

Congenital heart defects (CHD) are the most common birth defect and are the highest cause of mortality in children under the age of 1. Tetralogy of Fallot (TOF) is a severe constellation of defects that results from a disruption of the communication pathways between the first and second heart fields at about 20 days of gestation. A multitude of genes and genetic networks contribute to the spatial and temporal specification required for proper embryological heart formation [6-11]. Variation in the expression of cardiac genes or genes involved in network buffering, variation in the expression of microRNAs, and/or methylation differences or differences in gene transcript processing, could all cause shifts in pathway function leading to failure of the tight control of cell lineage specification required for normal heart development. However, even with the sophisticated tools that allow whole genome analysis, we still know relatively little about the genetic causes of TOF, as is the case for most CHDs.

The complexity of the cardiac regulatory system controlling heart development is challenging, but it was recently shown that a gene expression template (GET) containing only 56 genes could be used as a molecular signature to accurately specify at least 24 different disease-free tissues [12], including the heart. Hwang et al. [12] suggested that tissues preserve normal functioning and morphology by maintaining specific stoichiometry among genes and genetic networks. The state of the biochemical tissue-specific stoichiometry can be portrayed by the expression pattern of a compact set of representative genes that may reflect the status of key regulatory pathways. The pattern of expression of the 56 genes in the GET could uniquely identify 24 distinct tissue types. Interestingly, they looked at the developmental behavior of the GET by analyzing expression in cultured cells and two embryonic tissues, the lung and skin. These analyses suggested that embryonic tissues have a distinct GET stoichiometry that progresses to the terminal equilibrium as the developmental stage

* Correspondence: dbittel@cmh.edu
[2]The Ward Family Heart Center, Children's Mercy Hospitals and Clinics, Kansas City, MO 64108, USA
[3]University of Missouri-Kansas City School of Medicine, 5100 Rockhill Rd, Kansas City, MO 64110, USA
Full list of author information is available at the end of the article

progresses. Moreover, it would be expected that the significant deviation from normal stoichiometry, as assessed by the GET, would result in malfunction or abnormal growth of cells and tissues. They demonstrated that their GET model could be used to differentiate a pathologic state (cancer) from the normal tissue. Therefore, they concluded that the change in the expression pattern of the 56 genes that comprise their GET reflected the deviation in biochemical stoichiometry resulting in abnormal growth.

We wondered if the expression pattern of the 56 genes comprising the GET defined by Hwang et al. [12] would produce expression patterns that were unique to the different regions of the heart, or to different time points in development of the heart, or to a pathological state (TOF). Therefore, using this set of 56 genes, we examined temporal and spatial changes in expression in normally developing heart tissue and the expression pattern in the right ventricular tissue from children with TOF. The significant variation seen in the pathologic tissue demonstrates that the GET can be used to characterize tissue-specific pathologic states as well as temporal and spatial differences in normally developing cardiac tissue.

Results and discussion

Hwang et al. [12] used Affymetrix gene expression arrays (Affymetrix Inc., Santa Clara, CA, USA) to derive tissue-specific expression patterns that could distinguish at least 24 distinct tissues using as few as 56 genes, creating a GET. We previously used whole genome expression microarrays to analyze right ventricular tissue from infants with TOF, normally developing-age-matched infants and three fetuses at approximately 90 days of gestation [13]. In addition, the Gene Expression Omnibus contained gene expression microarray data for adult left and right ventricles and the sigmoid colon, which we downloaded (see Additional file 1: Table S1 for a complete listing of the original array data, as well as the source). We extracted the expression levels for these 56 genes from our cardiac expression data [13] and the cardiac array data downloaded from the Gene Expression Omnibus (GEO) to assess the GET in different regions of the heart, at different time points during heart development, and in a pathological condition, tetralogy of Fallot (TOF).

Of the 56 genes used by Hwang et al., we were able to identify 54 containing core probes on the exon arrays (genes are listed in Additional file 2: Table S2). The two genes that did not have core probes on our arrays were HLC-A and MOBP, and we chose not to include them in the clustering analysis as they were inadequately sampled on any of the arrays. We used the remaining 54 genes to generate an unsupervised hierarchical dendrogram of the data derived from the heart tissue (Figure 1, clustering was based on a complete linkage algorithm, see Section 'Methods' for explanation). Next, we looked at the statistically significant changes in gene expression (*t* test with Benjamini-Hochburg correction for multiple testing) in pairwise assessments among groups in order to determine what genes and/or pathways were driving divergence among sets of tissues (Additional file 2: Table S2). Three genes, PRKCB, TFPI2, and CA2, did not have significant changes in expression in any of the comparisons we made. Regardless, the dendrogram was generated using all 54 genes from the GET derived by Hwang et al. [12].

As seen in Figure 1, the GET produced a dendrogram in which individuals were assembled into groups that reflected the temporal and spatial characteristics of each group. The temporal stage (mature vs. young) was the most important component in clustering the samples as mature right ventricle (RV) and left ventricle (LV) clustered more closely together compared to fetal or infant LV. The TOF samples also clustered independently indicating that pathology was an important component in generating the dendrogram. We also included the expression pattern of genes from the colon as an outgroup comparison due to its different embryological origin from that of cardiac tissue (Additional file 3: Figure S1). As expected, there was a distinct difference in clustering between the heart tissue and the colon tissue. Organ type was a much greater clustering component than either spatial or pathological differences in expression of the GET.

Each tissue from within the heart clustered according to spatial, temporal, or pathological conditions, supporting the theory of tissue/cell type specificity previously set forth by Hwang et al. We had a single exception to this, which was one sample from an infant with TOF that clustered with the group of normal infant RV. The medical record of this infant did not indicate any unusual differences compared to the other infants with TOF which might have explained the deviation in expression pattern. The GET pattern in this infant likely reflects less perturbation in the GET than that seen in the other infants with TOF.

In addition, principal component analysis (PCA) clearly demonstrated that the variability between the tissues (colon vs. heart) was greater than the intra-tissue variability (Figure 2A). The PCA produced a clear grouping of cardiac tissue according to common origin. In the adult tissues examined, adult RV and adult LV were more closely related to each other than to infant or fetal tissues, again indicating that age (mature vs. fetal or infant tissue) influenced expression of the GET to a greater extent than did spatial origin. PCA placed the samples from infants with TOF clustered graphically between the adult and infant tissues.

We analyzed ten randomly assembled groups of 54 genes to determine if their expression pattern might also reflect group differences. We saw no discernible pattern in the dendrograms generated from the random sets of genes and none of the groups were appropriately clustered (data not shown). Thus, the sensitivity of the

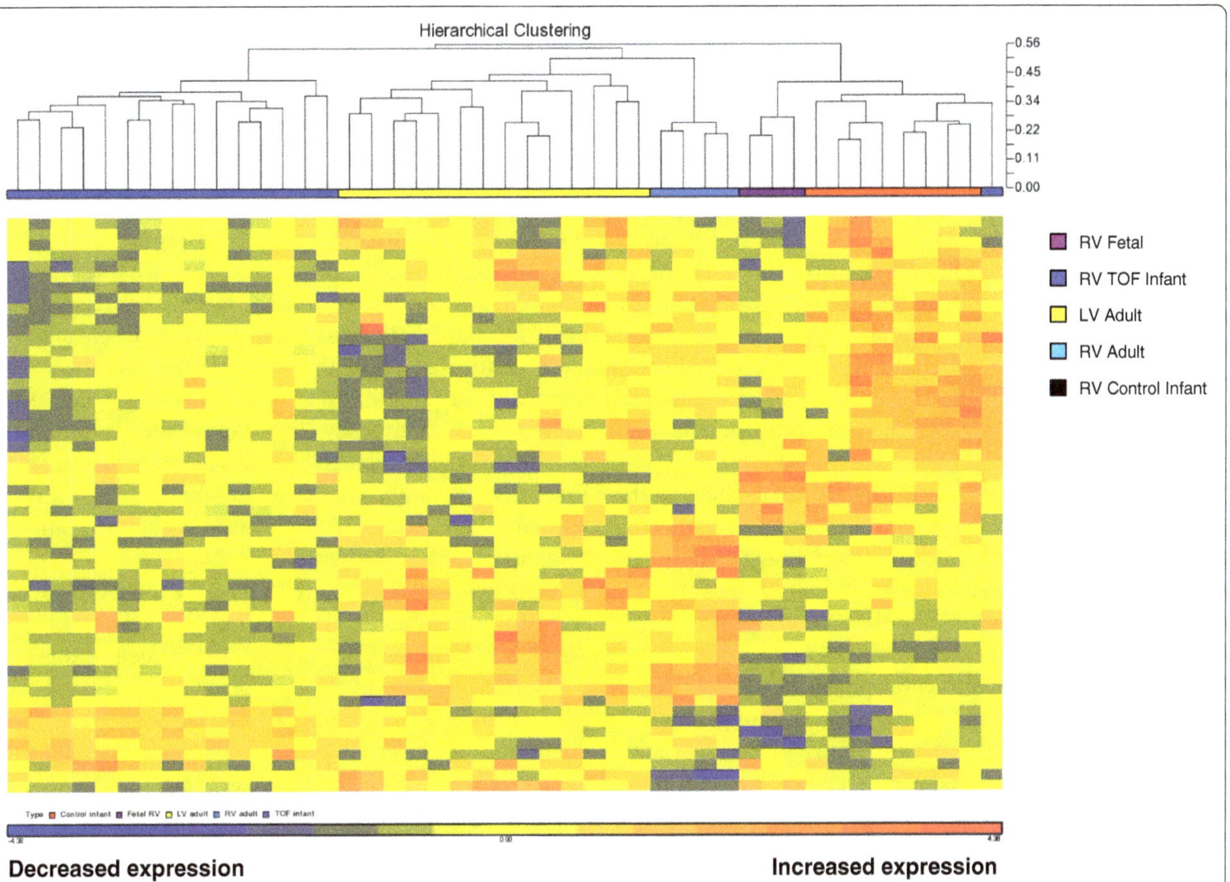

Figure 1 Hierarchical clustering based on 54 genes of the gene expression template (GET). The clustering algorithm used the complete linkage algorithm (i.e., point-to-point distance of furthest neighbors). Changes in expression are based on comparisons to the average values from samples from the normally developing infants.

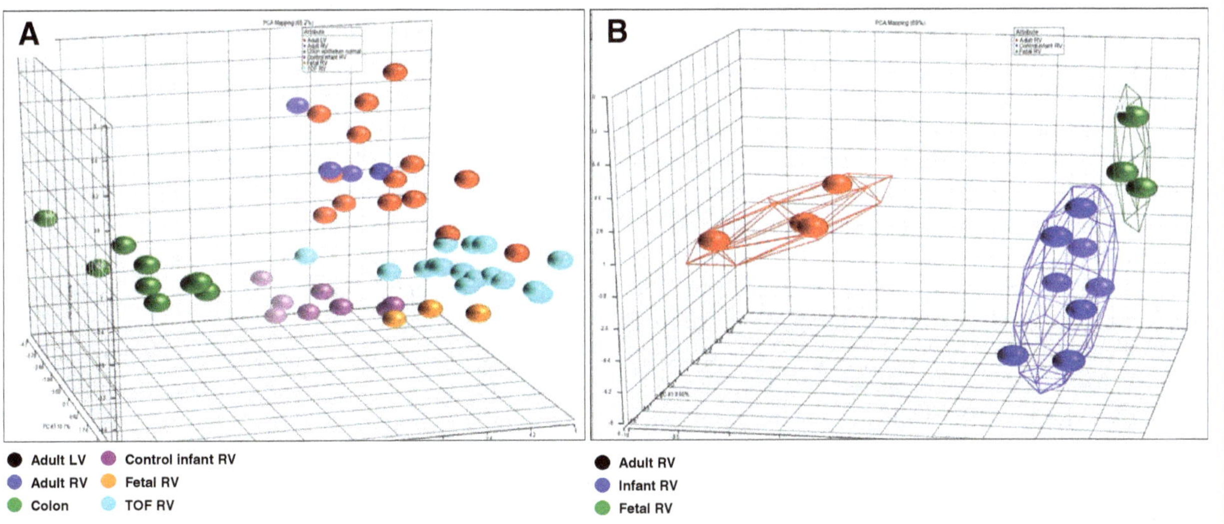

Figure 2 Principal component analysis of the expression pattern of the GET within. (A) All groups examined. **(B)** Fetal, infant, and adult right ventricular tissues (all normally developing with no known defects). The *colored connected lines* form a cloud around the group at two standard deviations.

previously derived GET to reflect tissue specificity and pathological conditions appears to also discriminate anatomically distinct regions within the heart.

Spatial pattern

We compared the expression of the GET between adult RV and adult LV. There were just 18 genes with significant changes in expression between the two tissues (Additional file 2: Table S2). We used Ingenuity Pathway Analysis (IPA, Ingenuity Systems, Redwood CA, USA) to assess the biological roles of these 18 genes. IPA is a bioinformatic software that identifies functional and network relationships that are significantly overrepresented within gene lists. The most significant network function represented by these 18 genes was organ morphology, suggesting that the subset of genes from the GET with changed expression between the right and left ventricles was involved in developing and maintaining structural integrity within the heart.

Temporal pattern

We examined the temporal development of the right ventricle using fetal tissue (approximately 90 days of gestation), normally developing infant right ventricular tissue, and adult right ventricular tissue. The clustering algorithm accurately placed the right ventricular samples into their appropriate groups (Figure 1). The fetal RV and infant RV samples were more closely associated with each other than to any other samples, suggesting the GET was strongly influenced by maturity of the tissue. In looking at individually significant changes in gene expression, there were 11 genes with altered expression between the fetal RV and infant RV. There were 25 genes that differed in expression between the infant and adult RV, suggesting the homoeostatic patterns reflected by the GET differed much more between the adult and infant RV as compared to the infant and fetal RV. This is reflected in the PCA analysis shown in Figure 2B. The primary component of separation appeared to be related to age, mature vs. young. In addition, the groups had no members that overlapped within two standard deviations, demonstrating the clear discrimination by the GET among groups.

Taken together, there were 32 genes that differed in expression in at least one of the comparisons among the three different normally developing RV datasets (Additional file 2: Table S2). Ontological analysis (using IPA) of these 32 genes revealed the highest associations with the network functions of cell movement, cell death and survival, and molecular transport. The top canonical pathways associations were inhibition of angiogenesis and regulation of actin-based motility. Since these genes represent the stoichiometric changes in the GET during the fetal to adult maturation of the right ventricle, it is perhaps not surprising that the regulation of cell movement and cell survival are predominant categories represented by these 32 genes.

Pathological pattern

The patterns from the right ventricular tissue from infants with TOF all grouped together with the exception of one sample that clustered most closely with the group of control infant RV (discussed above). Interestingly, the TOF RV tissues were more closely associated with adult LV and RV than to the age-matched controls. The TOF tissue was distinctly different from similarly aged, normally developing RV with 33 of the 54 genes examined having a statistically significant change in expression (Additional file 2: Table S2). This is perhaps not surprising for a tissue with developmental disarray resulting in dramatically different physiological conditions compared to structurally normal tissue.

The most closely clustered group to the TOF patients was the normal adult LV. The right ventricle of infants with TOF is typically hypertrophic. Our gene expression clustering suggests the pathophysiological conditions experienced by the RV resulting from TOF may influence gene expression stoichiometry in a way that similarly mimics the physiological conditions of the adult ventricle.

There were 19 GET genes with statistically significant changes in expression between TOF RV and normally developing infant RV but were unchanged between TOF RV and adult LV (marked with an 'x' in Additional file 2: Table S2). We reasoned that these genes might represent networks functioning in common between TOF and adult LV which might suggest a physiological explanation for the clustering pattern. The most statistically significant functional network identified using IPA (see 'Methods' for explanation of bioinformatic assessment) contained 10 of the 19 GET genes and formed an interactive network involved broadly in gene expression, cell signaling, and cell growth. More specifically, several members of this network are known to be involved in cardiac development, myogenesis, and cardiac hypertrophy (Figure 3). These comparisons specifically substantiate the hypothesis that pathological conditions are associated with the significant deviation from normal biochemical stoichiometry which can be represented by the expression patterns of a small number of key genes.

As mentioned above, the 54 genes we used for hierarchical clustering placed one TOF sample with the control infant RV group and the rest of the subjects with TOF clustered as a single group. With respect to the GET correctly predicting the pathological condition, this represents 94% sensitivity (correct grouping of the defect).

Based on our analysis, the GET can be applied to pathologic tissues as well as normal tissues with great accuracy. Most interesting is the difference between the TOF RV and

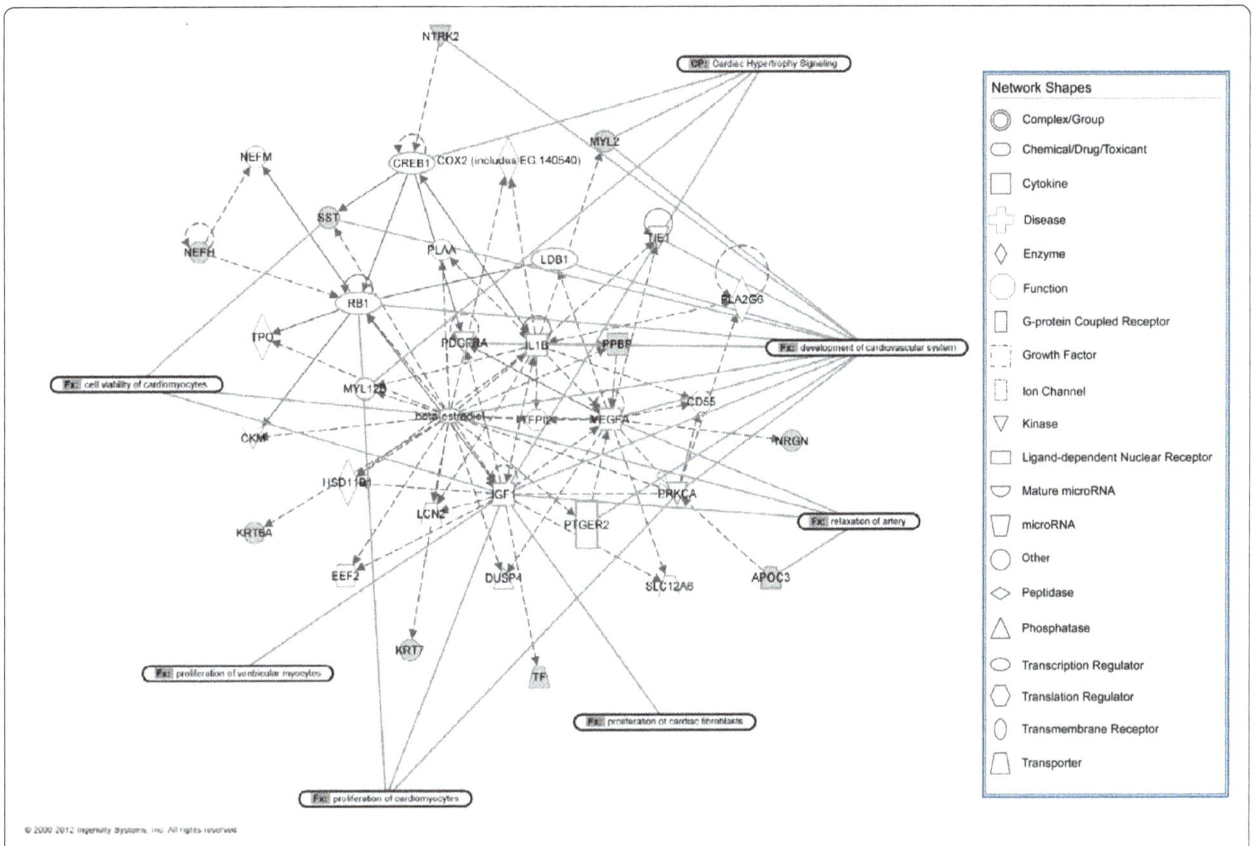

Figure 3 Interactive network of GET genes with shared expression patterns between TOF RV and adult LV. Interactive network of genes associated with the GET with shared expression patterns in TOF and adult LV compared to normally developing infant RV. Genes in *gray* are from the GET.

control-matched infant RV. This comparison has the most genes in the GET with a significant change in expression (33 genes, see Additional file 2: Table S2) and directly reflects how the GET can model pathologic tissues. This undoubtedly reflects the consequences of the failure of correct cardiac development in infants with TOF. Furthermore, it may signal the presence of genetic variants that collectively destabilized developmental networks leading to the heart defect. This warrants additional research as it may provide insight for the current difficulty in identifying the genetic basis for most CHDs.

Conclusions

Our results suggest that even at the intra-organ level, cells differentiate and maintain a biochemical stoichiometry that is reflected in the expression of a small representative sample of genes which likely represents functional networks required for homeostasis. Perhaps not surprisingly, in the pathophysiological conditions resulting from the failure of proper development, homeostatic imbalance is reflected in the disruption of the stoichiometry of the GET. The GET reflects key genetic pathways, whose disturbance may have contributed to the heart defect and/or its physiological consequences. The perturbations in the GET suggest a possible genetic signature that might aid in prognosis and genetic counseling and, with additional study, might contribute to improved therapy.

Methods

The Children's Mercy Hospitals and Clinics' institutional review board approved this research protocol. The parents of all subjects provided written consent for participation after reading the consent document and having their questions answered.

Our subjects were children less than 1 year of age with TOF requiring surgical reconstruction. The diagnosis and anatomy were obtained by echocardiography and angiography and confirmed at the time of surgery. All microarray analyses were run on samples from sixteen infants with TOF who had normal chromosomes (i.e., without 22q11.2 deletions, as determined by comparative genomic hybridization and/or *in situ* hybridization by the clinical cytogenetics lab at Children's Mercy Hospital), eight infants with normally developing hearts, and three fetal samples (Additional file 1: Table S1). The comparison tissues from the eight normally developing infants (three males, five females) were obtained from LifeNet Health (http://www.lifenethealth.org; Virginia Beach, VA, USA). LifeNet Health is a non-profit regenerative medicine company that provides bioimplants and organs for transplantation. The comparison samples were matched for age to the study population, and all control subjects expired due to non-cardiac related causes as described in detail previously [13]. We obtained three fetal hearts (approximately 90 days of gestation) through the National Institute of Child Health and Human Development-supported tissue retrieval program from the Central Laboratory for Human Embryology at the University of Washington (Seattle, WA, USA). The fetal hearts were dissected by one of the surgeons who also performed many of the reconstructions of the conotruncal defects (JEO) to ensure that the tissue analyzed was from a similar location as the tissues removed during surgery (as described previously [13]).

In addition, exon array data was downloaded from the GEO derived from the right ventricular tissue of 4 adult subjects [14] and the left ventricular tissue of 14 adult subjects [15]. As an outgroup comparison, exon array data was downloaded from nine noncancerous colon samples [16]. Sex and age of the subjects and GEO accession numbers for all arrays are presented in Additional file 1: Table S1.

Microarrays

We generated exon array data for this study using RNA extracted from the right ventricular tissue from 16 infants with tetralogy of Fallot, right ventricle from 8 typically developing age- and sex-matched comparison infants, and right ventricle from three fetal hearts (gestational age 90 days as described above). The exon arrays were all Affymetrix HuEx-1_0-st-v2 and gene expression levels were generated as a mean of all probes within the coding sequence of the gene. The raw data from our arrays have been deposited in the GEO (accession number to be supplied upon acceptance). Our arrays were run at the University of Kansas Medical Center-Microarray Facility (KUMC-MF) according to the manufacturer's protocols. The KUMC-MF is supported by the Kansas University-School of Medicine, KUMC Biotechnology Support Facility, the Smith Intellectual and Developmental Disabilities Research Center (HD02528), and the Kansas IDeA Network of Biomedical Research Excellence (RR016475). All of our array data has been deposited in the GEO and will be available after July 2014. However, we make the data available prior to this date upon request.

Statistical analysis

All statistical analyses of expression patterns were performed using the statistical software: Partek Genomics Suite software version 6.6. Study arrays were uploaded to Partek, and quality assessment and RMA background correction and quantile normalization were applied to ensure unbiased downstream analysis. Unsupervised hierarchical clustering was utilized within the Partek software to group subjects with similar expression patterns based on the set of genes from the gene expression template described by Hwang et al. [12]. No *a priori* grouping was applied. We tested several algorithms for accuracy in clustering: average linkage with squared euclidian distance (averaged point-to-point distances to define cluster to cluster distance), complete linkage without squared euclidian distance (furthest neighbor clustering algorithm uses the furthest distance between points to derive the groups), and single linkage (point-to-point distance of closest neighbors). The complete clustering algorithm without squaring the euclidian distance produced the best dendrogram, accurately reflecting group relationships with only one TOF sample associated with the normal infant RV. The average linkage algorithm correctly clustered most of the groups, but split the LV samples into two subgroups, one group with ten samples that were most closely associated with the TOF samples and four samples that were most closely associated with the RV samples. Adding colon samples also had the effect of causing separation of the LV samples regardless of the clustering algorithm (Additional file 3: Figure S1). This obviously reflects subtle underlying structure within the data. The single linkage clustering algorithm produced no clear pattern among the samples.

Differences in expression were determined using *t* test with significance set at $p \leq 0.05$ after using the Benjamini-Hochberg correction for multiple testing based on the entire set of genes in an array, as we have done previously [13,17]. Likewise, principal component analysis was performed within Partek using the set of 54 genes for partitioning.

Network and pathways analysis was done using the bioinformatic software IPA which allows statistical assessment of functional associations within gene lists derived from comparative expression analysis.

Additional files

Additional file 1: Table S1. Sample demographic data.

Additional file 2: Table S2. Significant changes in expression among heart tissues (fold change).

Additional file 3: Figure S1. Hierarchical clustering based on 54 genes of the gene expression template (GET). The clustering algorithm used a complete linkage algorithm without squaring the euclidian distance to establish the dendrogram.

Competing interests

The authors declare that they have no competing interests.

Authors' contributions

AR participated in the study design, analysis of data and drafting of the manuscript. NK participated in the study design, microarray analysis, generation of GET data, and review of the manuscript. AB participated in analysis of data and review of the manuscript. JM participated in study design, sample collection and review of the manuscript. JEO participated in study design, sample collection and review of the manuscript. DCB participated in the study design, generation and analysis of data and drafting of the manuscript. All authors read and approved the final manuscript.

Author details

[1]Kansas City University of Medicine and Biosciences, Kansas, MO 64106, USA. [2]The Ward Family Heart Center, Children's Mercy Hospitals and Clinics, Kansas City, MO 64108, USA. [3]University of Missouri-Kansas City School of Medicine, 5100 Rockhill Rd, Kansas City, MO 64110, USA.

References

1. Ge X, Yamamoto S, Tsutsumi S, Midorikawa Y, Ihara S, Wang SM, Aburatani H: **Interpreting expression profiles of cancers by genome-wide survey of breadth of expression in normal tissues.** *Genomics* 2005, **86**:127–141.
2. Hsiao LL, Dangond F, Yoshida T, Hong R, Jensen RV, Misra J, Dillon W, Lee KF, Clark KE, Haverty P, Weng Z, Mutter GL, Frosch MP, MacDonald ME, Milford EL, Crum CP, Bueno R, Pratt RE, Mahadevappa M, Warrington JA, Stephanopoulos G, Stephanopoulos G, Gullans SR: **A compendium of gene expression in normal human tissues.** *Physiol Genomics* 2001, **7**:97–104.
3. Su AI, Wiltshire T, Batalov S, Lapp H, Ching KA, Block D, Zhang J, Soden R, Hayakawa M, Kreiman G, Cooke MP, Walker JR, Hogenesch JB: **A gene atlas of the mouse and human protein-encoding transcriptomes.** *Proc Natl Acad Sci USA* 2004, **101**:6062–6067.
4. Shyamsundar R, Kim YH, Higgins JP, Montgomery K, Jorden M, Sethuraman A, van de Rijn M, Botstein D, Brown PO, Pollack JR: **A DNA microarray survey of gene expression in normal human tissues.** *Genome Biol* 2005, **6**:R22.
5. Yu K, Ganesan K, Tan LK, Laban M, Wu J, Zhao XD, Li H, Leung CH, Zhu Y, Wei CL, Hooi SC, Miller L, Tan P: **A precisely regulated gene expression cassette potently modulates metastasis and survival in multiple solid cancers.** *PLoS Genet* 2008, **4**:e1000129.
6. Bruneau BG: **The developmental genetics of congenital heart disease.** *Nature* 2008, **451**:943–948.
7. Bentham J, Bhattacharya S: **Genetic mechanisms controlling cardiovascular development.** *Ann N Y Acad Sci* 2008, **1123**:10–19.
8. Huang JB, Liu YL, Sun PW, Lv XD, Du M, Fan XM: **Molecular mechanisms of congenital heart disease.** *Cardiovasc Pathol* 2009, **19**:e183–193.
9. Kalsotra A, Wang K, Li PF, Cooper TA: **MicroRNAs coordinate an alternative splicing network during mouse postnatal heart development.** *Genes Dev* 2010, **24**:653–658.
10. Thum T, Catalucci D, Bauersachs J: **MicroRNAs: novel regulators in cardiac development and disease.** *Cardiovasc Res* 2008, **79**:562–570.
11. Wessels MW, Willems PJ: **Genetic factors in non-syndromic congenital heart malformations.** *Clin Genet* 2010, **78**:103–123.
12. Hwang PI, Wu HB, Wang CD, Lin BL, Chen CT, Yuan S, Wu G, Li KC: **Tissue-specific gene expression templates for accurate molecular characterization of the normal physiological states of multiple human tissues with implication in development and cancer studies.** *BMC Genomics* 2012, **12**:439.
13. O'Brien JE Jr, Kibiryeva N, Zhou XG, Marshall JA, Lofland GK, Artman M, Chen J, Bittel DC: **Noncoding RNA expression in myocardium from infants with tetralogy of Fallot.** *Circ Cardiovasc Genet* 2012, **5**:279–286.
14. Gupta S, Halushka MK, Hilton GM, Arking DE: **Postmortem cardiac tissue maintains gene expression profile even after late harvesting.** *BMC Genomics* 2012, **13**:26.
15. Kong SW, Hu YW, Ho JW, Ikeda S, Polster S, John R, Hall JL, Bisping E, Pieske B, dos Remedios CG, Pu WT: **Heart failure-associated changes in RNA splicing of sarcomere genes.** *Circ Cardiovasc Genet* 2010, **3**:138–146.
16. Mojica W, Hawthorn L: **Normal colon epithelium: a dataset for the analysis of gene expression and alternative splicing events in colon disease.** *BMC Genomics* 2010, **11**:5.
17. Bittel DC, Butler MG, Kibiryeva N, Marshall JA, Chen J, Lofland GK, O'Brien JE Jr: **Gene expression in cardiac tissues from infants with idiopathic conotruncal defects.** *BMC Med Genomics* 2011, **4**:1.

20

K-Map: connecting kinases with therapeutics for drug repurposing and development

Jihye Kim[1], Minjae Yoo[1], Jaewoo Kang[2] and Aik Choon Tan[1*]

Abstract

Protein kinases play important roles in regulating signal transduction in eukaryotic cells. Due to evolutionary conserved binding sites in the catalytic domain of the kinases, most inhibitors that target these sites promiscuously inhibit multiple kinases. Quantitative analysis can reveal complex and unexpected interactions between protein kinases and kinase inhibitors, providing opportunities for identifying multi-targeted inhibitors of specific diverse kinases for drug repurposing and development. We have developed K-Map—a novel and user-friendly web-based program that systematically connects a set of query kinases to kinase inhibitors based on quantitative profiles of the kinase inhibitor activities. Users can use K-Map to find kinase inhibitors for a set of query kinases (obtained from high-throughput 'omics' experiments) or to reveal new interactions between kinases and kinase inhibitors for rational drug combination studies.

Availability and implementation: K-Map has been implemented in python scripting language and the website is freely available at: http://tanlab.ucdenver.edu/kMap.

Introduction

Protein kinases represent one of the largest 'druggable' and well-studied families in the human genome [1]. This class of proteins (kinome) plays a key role as regulators and transducers of signaling in eukaryotic cells. There is an estimated >500 members of the human kinome which can be classified into seven different kinase families based on their conserved catalytic domain sequences [2]. Kinases are relatively easy to target with small molecules and have been extensively studied at the biochemical, structural, and physiological levels. In cancer cells, some kinases are mutated and acquire oncogenic properties to drive tumorgenesis. Small molecules that inhibit these oncogenic kinases can effectively kill cancer cells, as demonstrated by the success story of imatinib (Gleevec®, Novartis, Basel, Switzerland) in inhibiting the activity of *BCR-ABL* in chronic myelogenous leukemia [3]. Imatinib also inhibits *KIT* and *PDGFRA*, which are commonly dysregulated in gastrointestinal stromal tumors [4]. The imatinib example illustrates that small-molecule kinase inhibitors interact with multiple protein kinase family members (*BCR-ABL*, *KIT*, *PDGFRA*), and understanding these complex interactions between kinases and inhibitors could be useful for drug repurposing and development. These complex interactions could only be revealed by systematic interrogation of the small molecules across a large panel of kinases using quantitative assays (kinase activity profiles). Here, we have developed K-Map—a novel and user-friendly web-based program that systematically connects a set of query kinases to kinase inhibitors based on quantitative profiles of the kinase inhibitor activities. K-Map is motivated by the 'connectivity map' concept [5] where gene expression changes could be used as the 'universal language' to connect between biological systems, genes, and drugs. Instead of gene expression signatures, we used the kinase activity profiles as the 'language' for connecting kinases and small molecules in K-Map to reveal the complex interactions of kinases and inhibitors.

* Correspondence: aikchoon.tan@ucdenver.edu
[1]Translational Bioinformatics and Cancer Systems Biology Laboratory, Division of Medical Oncology, Department of Medicine, University of Colorado Anschutz Medical Campus, Aurora, CO 80045, USA
Full list of author information is available at the end of the article

K-Map methods and features

Quantitative kinase inhibitor selectivity data sources

Two recently published comprehensive analyses of kinase inhibitor selectivity [6,7] were used to construct the K-Map reference database (kinase activity profiles). The first study systematically interrogates 178 commercially available inhibitors against a panel of 300 protein kinases using a radiometric phospho-transfer method to assess the percent kinase inhibition (IC_{50}) [6]. The second study measures inhibitor selectivity and potency of 72 inhibitors across 442 kinases using direct binding affinities between inhibitors and kinases (K_d) [7]. These kinase activity profiles were converted into rank-ordered lists according to their inhibitions and potencies against the kinases and used as the K-Map reference profiles for matching query kinases. For each study, the kinase activity profiles for individual drugs were converted into rank-ordered lists according to their inhibitions and potencies against the kinases. As a result, we generated two K-Map reference databases from these two studies: one for IC_{50} and the other one are for K_d. Both databases will be used to connect the query kinases and return the drugs in K-Map.

Pattern matching strategy

We implemented the K-Map pattern matching strategy based on the Kolmogorov-Smirnov (KS) statistics. The KS test is a nonparametric, rank-based pattern matching approach implemented in the connectivity map [5]. The query is a list of kinases, and the goal of the algorithm is to correlate kinase inhibitor that enriches the same kinases based on kinase inhibition profiles. For every inhibitor in the reference database, the KS statistic is computed and a connectivity score is defined.

Similar to the connectivity map approach [5], to compute the connectivity score, let N be the number of kinases in the reference database and M be the number of query kinases. For every drug in the reference database, we can compute the rank-ordered list R for all kinases (1, 2, ..., N) based on the drug inhibitions and potencies against the kinases. For a list of query kinases of j, where j = 1, 2, ..., M, compute the following two values for each drug i in the reference database:

$$a = \max_{j=1}^{M}\left[\frac{j}{M}-\frac{R(j)}{N}\right]$$

and

$$b = \max_{j=1}^{M}\left[\frac{R(j)}{N}-\frac{(j-1)}{M}\right]$$

Let KS^i be the KS score for drug i,

$$KS^i = \begin{cases} a, & \text{if } a > b; \\ -b, & \text{if } b > a. \end{cases}$$

Finally, to compute the connectivity score (S^i) for drug i in a reference database, let $P = \max(KS^i)$ and $Q = \min(KS^i)$,

$$S^i = \begin{cases} \dfrac{KS^i}{P}, & \text{if } KS^i > 0; \\ -\left(\dfrac{KS^i}{Q}\right), & \text{if } KS^i < 0. \end{cases}$$

The connectivity score (S^i) for every drug is reported as the 'Score' in the results page. A positive score represents that the inhibitor has a similar rank order as the query kinases, indicating that the inhibitor is more specific in inhibiting the query kinases. A negative score represents that the inhibitor has a reverse rank order as the query, hence not specific in inhibiting the query kinases. Connectivity scores for each inhibitor were normalized to yield a score ranging 0 to 1, and inhibitors were ranked based on this normalized score. We also computed the running sum of the connectivity score for each inhibitor. The maximum value of the running sum is equivalent to the connectivity score of each inhibitor. Since the query kinases are unitless, K-Map can be applied to any technology platform.

Computing the permutation p value

To estimate the p value for each drug i, we perform a permutation test by randomly selecting the number of M instances from the rank-ordered drug i kinase profiles. Let t = 1, 2, ..., T trials; the same procedure as computing the KS^i for drug i is performed T times and is denoted as KS_t^i. Let KS_0^i denote the actual KS^i for drug i. Count the number of times f where

$$\left[\left|KS_t^i\right| \geq \left|KS_0^i\right|\right]_{t=1}^{T}$$

is true. The frequency of this event (f/T) is estimated as a (two-sided) p value. This procedure is similar to the implementation of permutation test by the connectivity map [5]. The p value reported in the results page of K-Map is computed by 500 permutations.

Query features

K-Map implements three query functions: users can (1) directly enter query kinases in the query text box or upload a list of query kinases (Figure 1 (A)) in the K-Map tab, (2) select kinases from the kinase family (Figure 1 (B)) in the K-Map (by family) tab, or (3) query a set of kinases involved in certain biological processes according to Gene Ontology (Figure 1 (C)) in the K-Map (by GO) tab. Users also need to define which database they would like their query kinases to connect with (IC_{50} or K_d). All inhibitors available in the K-Map could be browsed under the Drug Info tab (Figure 1 (D)). Under the Download tab, users can search and download kinase-inhibitor relationships. The Help tab provides user guide to query and navigate the K-Map. The user manual for K-Map is available at http://tanlab.ucdenver.edu/kMap.

Connectivity results and linking features

The output of K-Map is a rank-ordered list of inhibitors based on the normalized connectivity scores, accompanied by p values and running sum plots. The 2D drug structure is viewable by scrolling through the drug name. Kinase

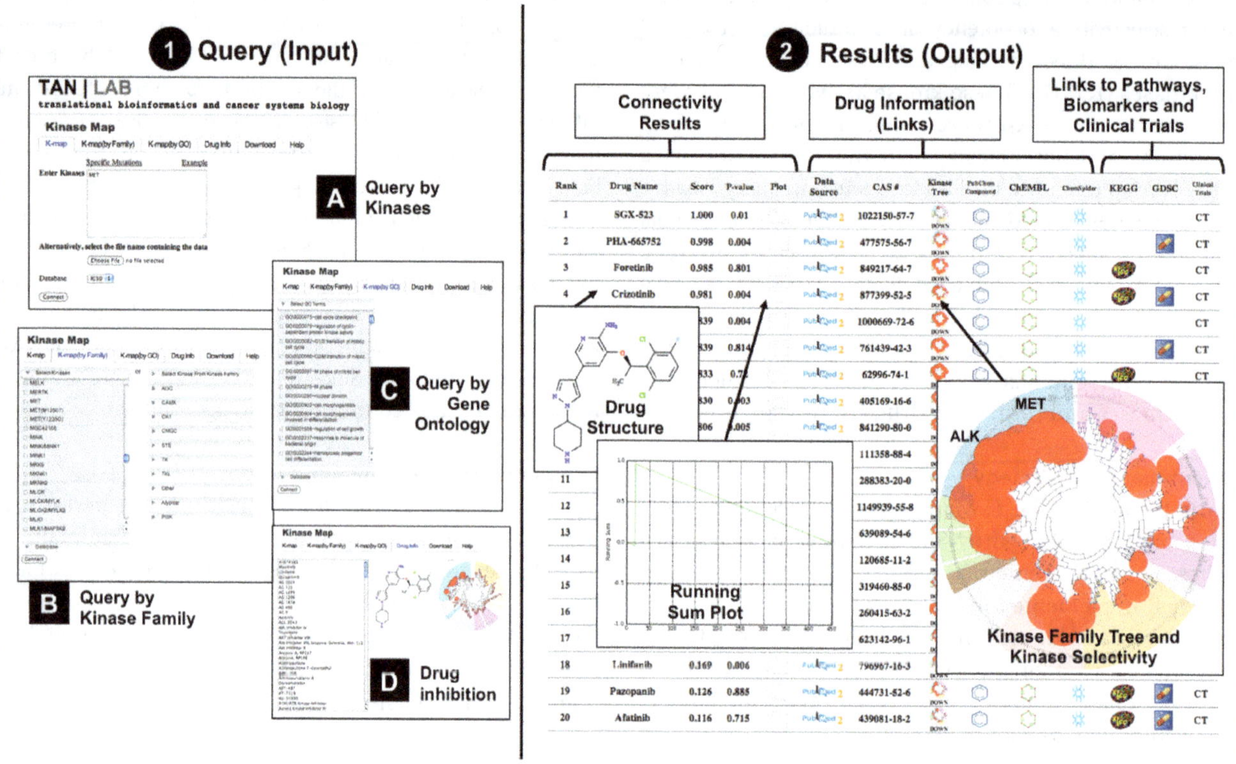

Figure 1 Query and results of the K-Map. Left, query features. K-Map could be queried by: **(A)** direct input or directly uploading a list of kinases in the K-Map tab, **(B)** by selecting kinases from the kinase family, or **(C)** querying by Gene Ontology Biological Processes. All drug information is available in the Drug Info tab **(D)** and could be downloaded in the Download tab. Right, connectivity results. Query kinases were connected to the inhibitors and sorted by normalized connectivity scores. Link-out features include PubMed, PubChem, ChEMBL, and ChemSpider for drug sources and information. K-Map also provides links to pathway, biomarker, and clinical trial information for each drug via KEGG, GDSC, and ClinicalTrials.gov databases, respectively.

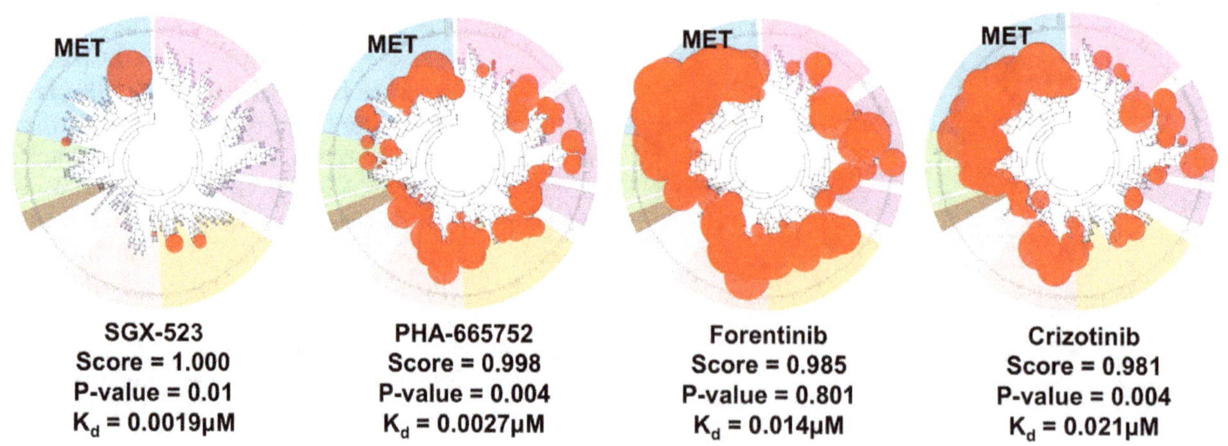

Figure 2 Query results for *MET* using K$_d$ database. These four compounds were returned with connectivity score >0.9, indicating that these compounds were highly specific in inhibiting *MET*. SGX-523 is ranked #1 and is a specific *MET* inhibitor, with K$_d$ = 0.0019 μM as illustrated in the kinase family tree. PHA-665752 is ranked #2 with K$_d$ = 0.0027 μM against *MET*. These two compounds (SGX-523 and PHA-665752) were preclinical compounds and have not moved into clinical trials. Forentinib is an FDA-approved drug that inhibits *MET* and *KDR* (K$_d$ = 0.014 μM against *MET*) and is ranked #3; however, the *p* value is high (*p* = 0.801). Crizotinib is also an FDA-approved drug that inhibits *ALK*, and this compound has K$_d$ = 0.021 μM against *MET* (*p* value = 0.004). Crizotinib was validated in *in vitro* experiments and showed synergistic effects when combined with Nutlin-3 in p53wild-type cancer cell lines [13].

inhibitor specificity within the kinase family tree is generated under KinaseTree column where the red circles indicate degrees of inhibition. Linking features are available for data source of the kinase inhibition assay (via PubMed) and three major chemical databases (PubChem [8], ChEMBL [9], and ChemSpider (www.chemspider.com)). Additional links to drug pathway and drug biomarkers are available through the Kyoto Encyclopedia of Genes and Genomes (KEGG) [10] and Genomics of Drug Sensitivity in Cancer (GDSC) [11] databases, respectively. K-Map also provides link-out to ClinicalTrials.gov for ongoing or completed clinical trials of these inhibitors in various diseases. We plan to update the K-Map database every quarter to keep up with the new data and link-out information.

Implementation

K-Map is implemented in python (v2.6) and CGI script. The kinase family tree map and 2D drug structure are generated by the E.T.E. software (v2.0) and Open Babel (v2.3.1) [12], respectively. The K-Map website is freely available at: http://tanlab.ucdenver.edu/kMap.

K-Map application: case study

We have recently performed a genome-wide functional genetic screen to identify synthetic lethality genes for Nutlin-3 (p53 inhibitor) in p53 wild-type cancer cell lines [13]. From this screening, we identified *MET* as a synthetic lethal gene with Nutlin-3 in killing cancer cell. By querying *MET* in the K-Map using K_d database (Figure 1 (A)), four compounds were returned with connectivity score >0.9 (Figure 1,right side). All four compounds are specific in inhibiting *MET* with $K_d \leq 0.025$ μM (Figure 2). Interestingly, crizotinib, a recently FDA-approved *ALK* inhibitor is ranked #4 (p value = 0.004). As we demonstrated, treating p53 wild-type cancer cells with Nutlin-3 and crizotinib inhibits proliferation and enhances cell killing in *in vitro* experiments [13]. This supports the finding that the K-Map could reveal new inhibition of kinase inhibitor (Figure 1, kinase family tree indicates that crizotinib shows the highest selectivity in inhibiting *ALK* and *MET*).

Summary

K-Map is a novel and user-friendly web-based tool for connecting kinases with drugs based on quantitative profiles of the kinase inhibitor activities. Many kinase inhibitors could promiscuously inhibit multiple kinases due to conserved sequence similarity among kinase family members; we have exploited these complex and unexpected interactions between kinases and inhibitors as opportunities for drug repurposing and development. Users can use K-Map to search kinase inhibitors for a set of query kinases (obtained from high-throughput 'omics' experiments) or to reveal new interactions between kinases and kinase inhibitors for rational combination studies. In the future, we plan to extend K-Map by including more kinase inhibitor profiles. In summary, we believe that K-Map will be a valuable bioinformatics tool in connecting altered/mutated genes identified by next-generation sequencing with therapeutics, accelerating the process of personalized medicine.

Competing interests

The authors declare that they have no competing interests.

Authors' contributions

The authors wish it to be known that, in their opinion, the first two authors should be regarded as joint first authors. JK carried out the K-map studies, participated in the method implementation, and drafted the manuscript. MY prepared the dataset and implemented all web version of K-map. JK participated in the design of the study. ACT conceived of the study, participated in its design and coordination, and wrote the final manuscript. All authors read and approved the final manuscript.

Acknowledgements

We gratefully thank Drs. Subhajyoti De and Tzu Phang, and the Tan Lab members for the constructive suggestions and discussion. We also like to thank the comments and suggestions from the two reviewers that have helped to improve the presentation of this manuscript. Part of this work was supported by the Cancer League of Colorado (JK and ACT), the Department of Defense Award W81XWH-11-1-0527 (ACT), and Institutional start-up fund (ACT).

Author details

[1]Translational Bioinformatics and Cancer Systems Biology Laboratory, Division of Medical Oncology, Department of Medicine, University of Colorado Anschutz Medical Campus, Aurora, CO 80045, USA. [2]Data Mining and Information Systems Laboratory, Department of Computer Science and Engineering, Korea University, Seoul 136-713, South Korea.

References

1. Cohen P: **Protein kinases—the major drug targets of the twenty-first century.** *Nat Rev Drug Discov* 2002, **1**(4):309–315.
2. Manning G, Whyte DB, Martinez R, Hunter T, Sudarsanam S: **The protein kinase complement of the human genome.** *Science* 2002, **298**(5600):1912–1934.
3. Druker BJ, Talpaz M, Resta DJ, Peng B, Buchdunger E, Ford JM, Lydon NB, Kantarjian H, Capdeville R, Ohno-Jones S, Sawyers CL: **Efficacy and safety of a specific inhibitor of the BCR-ABL tyrosine kinase in chronic myeloid leukemia.** *N Engl J Med* 2001, **344:**1031–1037.
4. Demetri GD, von Mehren M, Blanke CD, Van den Abbeele AD, Eisenberg B, Roberts PJ, Heinrich MC, Tuveson DA, Singer S, Janicek M, Fletcher JA, Silverman SG, Silberman SL, Capdeville R, Kiese B, Peng B, Dimitrijevic S, Druker BJ, Corless C, Fletcher CD, Joensuu H: **Efficacy and safety of imatinib mesylate in advanced gastrointestinal stromal tumors.** *N Engl J Med* 2002, **347:**472–480.
5. Lamb J, Crawford ED, Peck D, Modell JW, Blat IC, Wrobel MJ, Lerner J, Brunet JP, Subramanian A, Ross KN, Reich M, Hieronymus H, Wei G, Armstrong SA, Haggarty SJ, Clemons PA, Wei R, Carr SA, Lander ES, Golub TR: **The connectivity map: using gene-expression signatures to connect small molecules, genes and disease.** *Science* 2006, **131**(5795):1929–1935.
6. Anastassiadis T, Deacon SW, Devarajan K, Ma H, Peterson JR: **Comprehensive assay of kinase catalytic activity reveals features of kinase inhibitor selectivity.** *Nat Biotechnol* 2011, **29**(11):1039–1045.
7. Davis MI, Hunt JP, Herrgard S, Ciceri P, Wodicka LM, Pallares G, Hocker M, Treiber DK, Zarrinkar PP: **Comprehensive analysis of kinase inhibitor selectivity.** *Nat Biotechnol* 2011, **29**(11):1046–1051.
8. Bolton E, Wang Y, Thiessen PA, Bryant SH: **PubChem: Integrated platform of small molecules and biological activities.** In *Annual Reports in Computational Chemistry.* 4th edition. Washington, DC: American Chemical Society; 2008.
9. Gaulton A, Bellis LJ, Bento AP, Chambers J, Davies M, Hersey A, Light Y, McGlinchey S, Michalovich D, Al-Lazikani B, Overington JP: **ChEMBL: a large-scale bioactivity database for chemical biology and drug discovery.** *Nucleic Acids Res* 2011, **40**(Database issue):D1100–1107.

10. Kanehisa M, Goto S, Sato Y, Furumichi M, Tanabe M: **KEGG for integration and interpretation of large-scale molecular datasets.** *Nucleic Acids Res* 2012, **40**:D109–D114.
11. Yang M, Soares J, Greninger P, Edelman EJ, Lightfoot H, Forbes S, Bindal N, Beare D, Smith JA, Thompson IR, Ramaswamy S, Futreal PA, Haber DA, Stratton MR, Benes C, McDermott U, Garnett MJ: **Genomics of Drug Sensitivity in Cancer (GDSC): a resource for therapeutic biomarker discovery in cancer cells.** *Nucleic Acids Res* 2013, **41**(Database issue):D955–961.
12. O'boyle NM, Banck M, James CA, Morley C, Vandermeersch T, Hutchison GR: **Open Babel: an open chemical toolbox.** *J Cheminform* 2011, **3**:33.
13. Sullivan KD, Padilla-Just N, Henry RE, Porter CC, Kim J, Tentler JJ, Eckhardt SG, Tan AC, DeGregori J, Espinosa JM: **ATM and MET kinases are synthetic lethal with nongenotoxic activation of p53.** *Nat Chem Biol* 2012, **8**(7):646–654.

21

Screening *in silico* predicted remotely acting *NF1* gene regulatory elements for mutations in patients with neurofibromatosis type 1

Stephen E Hamby[1,3], Pablo Reviriego[2], David N Cooper[2], Meena Upadhyaya[2] and Nadia Chuzhanova[1*]

Abstract

Neurofibromatosis type 1 (NF1), a neuroectodermal disorder, is caused by germline mutations in the *NF1* gene. NF1 affects approximately 1/3,000 individuals worldwide, with about 50% of cases representing *de novo* mutations. Although the *NF1* gene was identified in 1990, the underlying gene mutations still remain undetected in a small but obdurate minority of NF1 patients. We postulated that in these patients, hitherto undetected pathogenic mutations might occur in regulatory elements far upstream of the *NF1* gene. In an attempt to identify such remotely acting regulatory elements, we reasoned that some of them might reside within DNA sequences that (1) have the potential to interact at distance with the *NF1* gene and (2) lie within a histone H3K27ac-enriched region, a characteristic of active enhancers. Combining Hi-C data, obtained by means of the chromosome conformation capture technique, with data on the location and level of histone H3K27ac enrichment upstream of the *NF1* gene, we predicted *in silico* the presence of two remotely acting regulatory regions, located, respectively, approximately 600 kb and approximately 42 kb upstream of the *NF1* gene. These regions were then sequenced in 47 NF1 patients in whom no mutations had been found in either the *NF1* or *SPRED1* gene regions. Five patients were found to harbour DNA sequence variants in the distal H3K27ac-enriched region. Although these variants are of uncertain pathological significance and still remain to be functionally characterized, this approach promises to be of general utility for the detection of mutations underlying other inherited disorders that may be caused by mutations in remotely acting regulatory elements.

Keywords: NF1, Neurofibromatosis type 1, Gene mutation, Hi-C data, Histone H3K27ac, Enhancer

Background

Germline mutations of the *NF1* gene cause the tumour predisposition syndrome, neurofibromatosis type 1 (NF1), which affects 1/3,000–4,000 individuals worldwide. The *NF1* gene, spanning 283 kb on chromosome 17q11.2, contains 61 exons that give rise to a 12-kb mRNA transcript encoding neurofibromin [1,2]. The 327-kDa (2,818-amino acid) protein product, neurofibromin, is expressed in most tissues.

Neurofibromin is a tumour suppressor protein, reflecting its role as a key negative regulator of the cellular Ras signalling pathway (reviewed by Bennett et al. [3]). More specifically, it is a Ras-specific GTPase-activating protein (GAP), with strong structural and sequence homologies to the GAP superprotein family [4]. It functions by downregulating Ras, thereby resulting in an overall reduction in cellular mitogenic signalling via the Ras pathway. Thus, any *NF1* gene mutation that serves to inactivate neurofibromin function may be expected to increase cellular levels of active Ras-GTP significantly, leading to uncontrolled cell growth and, potentially, tumorigenesis [5]. Germline mutations in the *SPRED1* gene have previously been detected in individuals with clinical features overlapping those of NF1 patients [6].

Consistent with Knudson's two-hit hypothesis, NF1 patients harbouring a heterozygous germline *NF1* mutation develop neurofibromas upon somatic mutation of the second wild-type *NF1* allele. The somatic loss of the second *NF1* allele in the progenitor cell (either the Schwann cell or its precursor), combined with haploinsufficiency in a variety

* Correspondence: nadia.chuzhanova@ntu.ac.uk
[1]School of Science and Technology, Nottingham Trent University, Clifton Lane, Nottingham NG11 8NS, UK
Full list of author information is available at the end of the article

of supporting cells [2,7], is then required for tumour formation. The mutation rate at the *NF1* locus is one of the highest reported in any human disorder [8]; almost 50% of all NF1 patients exhibit a *de novo NF1* mutation. The *NF1* mutational spectrum is shaped in large part, and often in remarkably predictable ways, by the local DNA sequence environment [9]. Nearly 1,300 different inherited mutations of the *NF1* gene have been reported as a cause of NF1; these vary in size from deletions spanning more than a megabase to subtle single base-pair substitutions that alter an encoded amino acid or the function of a splice junction [9]. In classical NF1 patients, *NF1* gene mutations are detectable in 50% to 95% of individuals depending upon the mutation detection techniques employed and the source of tissue used for analysis [2,10]. In our own study, the underlying pathogenic *NF1* mutation was detected in approximately 92% of NF1 patients despite sequencing the exons, splice junctions, untranslated regions and proximal promoter region of the *NF1* gene, and screening for gross gene deletions and rearrangements as well as subtle lesions [11-13]. The undetected mutations in such patients could in principle reside within a remote regulatory element at some distance from the *NF1* gene.

In the human genome, not all regulatory elements occur immediately 5′ to the genes that they regulate; indeed, some are located at considerable distances from their cognate genes. A variety of micro-lesions causing human inherited disease have been found to occur >10 kb 5′ upstream of the corresponding disease genes [14]. These include a total of eight mutations within a 1-kb region (termed the long-range or limb-specific enhancer, ZRS) approximately 979 kb 5′ to the transcription initiation site of the sonic hedgehog (*SHH*) gene [15]. Far upstream polymorphic variants that influence gene expression and impact on disease have also been documented. Thus, for example, the C>T functional single nucleotide polymorphism (SNP) 14.5 kb upstream of the interferon regulatory factor 6 (*IRF6*) gene, which is associated with cleft palate, alters the binding of transcription factor AP-2α [16]. Similarly, a T>C functional SNP approximately 6 kb upstream of the α-globin-like *HBM* gene serves to create a binding site for the erythroid-specific transcription factor GATA1 and interferes with the activation of the downstream α-globin genes [17]. Finally, a T>G functional SNP approximately 335 kb upstream of the *MYC* gene increases the risk of colorectal and prostate cancer by altering the binding strength of transcription factors TCF4 and/or TCF7L2 within a transcriptional enhancer [18]. On the basis of these findings in a number of different genes, we postulated that remotely acting regulatory elements might be present far upstream of the *NF1* gene and that these could be mutated in NF1 patients in whom no pathogenic mutations had been detected.

The *NF1* gene contains a TATA-less promoter within a classic CpG island that extends from the proximal promoter into exon 1, and a 454-bp 5′ untranslated region [19]. The CpG island is normally unmethylated, and the gene is actively transcribed in all tissues so far examined. Despite the high degree of conservation of the proximal regulatory sequences in rodent orthologs [20,21], the distal upstream sequence, potentially harbouring additional regulatory elements, diverges quite significantly between different mammalian species.

Histone H3K27ac serves to distinguish active enhancers from inactive ones [22]. Information on various functional elements, including regions enriched in histone H3K27ac, encoded by the human genome, have recently become available through the ENCODE project resources (ENCODE Project Consortium 2011 [23]; http://genome.ucsc.edu/index.html), a comprehensive collection of experimental data produced using biochemical assays mapped to human genome data. Using a variety of high-throughput techniques for identifying features characteristic to enhancers (e.g. specific histone modifications), up to 1.4 million putative enhancers have been identified in the human genome [23,24].

It has long been hypothesized that communication between widely spaced genomic elements is facilitated by the spatial organization of chromosomes that brings genes and their cognate regulatory elements into close spatial proximity [25]. The development of 'chromosome conformation capture' techniques has led to the discovery of many long-range interactions, both intra- and inter-chromosomal (reviewed in [26]). Recently, Lieberman-Aiden et al. [27] employed a novel approach, based on chromosomal conformation capture techniques, and termed Hi-C, to probe the 3D architecture of the entire human genome by coupling proximity-based ligation with massively parallel sequencing to produce a catalogue of approximately 8.4 million inter- and intra-chromosomal interacting fragments. Approximately 6.7 million of these fragments were found to be of long range (>20 kb apart). A genome-wide matrix of DNA-DNA interactions (also known as a contact map), created by dividing the genome into 1-Mb regions and counting the number of interactions between these 1-Mb regions [27], was subsequently analyzed by Yaffe and Tanay [28] to eliminate various biases in experimental procedure.

In this study, we postulated that remotely acting regulatory elements might occur within DNA fragments that interact with the DNA fragment containing the *NF1* gene, and further that these elements might be located within an H3K27ac-enriched region. We first combined long-range DNA-DNA interaction data and ENCODE resources to predict *in silico* the location of novel remotely acting regulatory regions upstream of the *NF1* gene. Finally, we screened these regions for mutation in those

NF1 patients in whom no mutations had been found in either the *NF1* or *SPRED1* genes. Germline mutations in the *SPRED1* gene have previously been detected in individuals with clinical features overlapping those of NF1 patients [6].

Results and discussion

The Hi-C data indicated that a 1-Mb fragment of chromosome 17, starting at position 29,000,000 and ending at position 29,999,999, termed the *NF1*-containing fragment since it contained the entire *NF1* gene (positions 29,421, 945–29,709,134), was found to interact most strongly with the adjacent 1-Mb fragment on chromosome 17 (703 and 255 intra-chromosomal interactions with the *NF1*-containing fragment recorded in *Hind*III- and *Nco*I-maps, respectively) which occupies positions 28,000,000–28,999, 999 upstream of the *NF1*-containing fragment (Figure 1). The ENCODE data indicated the presence of an H3K27 ac-enriched region somewhere between positions 28,846, 790 and 28,847,790 in the interacting fragment (region A in Figure 1). This region is distal (approximately 600 kb upstream) to the *NF1* gene. Another peak in H3K27ac enrichment was observed within the *NF1*-containing fragment (region B between positions 29,378,421 and 29,379,750) which is proximal (approximately 42 kb) to the *NF1* gene. The level of enrichment was higher in the distal region A than in the proximal region B. ENCODE data also revealed the presence in region A of three overlapping binding sites for the transcription factors, *p300* (positions 28,846,840–28,847,158), *c-Fos* (28,846,815–28, 847,158) and *c-Jun* (28,846,819–28,847,094), all of which were identified by *in vitro* ChIP-seq assay (http://genome.ucsc.edu/index.html).

Two sets of primers (Table 1) were designed using Primer3 software [29]. These were used for the polymerase chain reaction (PCR) amplification and sequencing of the two regions of interest: region A (positions 28,846, 790–28,847,790) and region B (positions 29,378,421–29, 379,750), from the genomic DNA of 47 NF1 patients as described in the 'Methods' section.

Three sequence variants were identified in the distal region, the region that corresponds to the highest level of histone H3K27ac enrichment. DNA sequencing revealed the presence of a heterozygous novel C>T variant at position 28,846,793 in two NF1 patients. This variant is not present in the dbSNP database (http://www.ncbi.nlm.nih.gov/sites/entrez?db=snp). Two other variants, rs78190160 (position 28,847,605) and rs71372224 (position 28,846,883), were detected each in three different patients. Both of these variants are listed in dbSNP as being of unknown clinical significance; minor allele frequency/minor allele count based on 1000 Genomes Project data was 0.007/16, indicating that they are rare variants. Unfortunately, no linkage disequilibrium data (HapMap Project; http://hapmap.ncbi.nlm.nih.gov/) were available for this region. The rs71372224 SNP was however found to occur within the three overlapping binding sites for transcription factors *p300*, *c-Fos* and *c-Jun*. Recent studies [30] have shown that enhancer elements have a high propensity to be bound by *p300*, an enhancer-binding transcription factor. One may therefore speculate that a mutation in this putative enhancer element could influence the expression of the *NF1* gene in a spatially specific manner. No variants were found in the H3K27ac-enriched region (region B) lying proximal to the *NF1* gene region and corresponding to the lower level of H3K27ac enrichment.

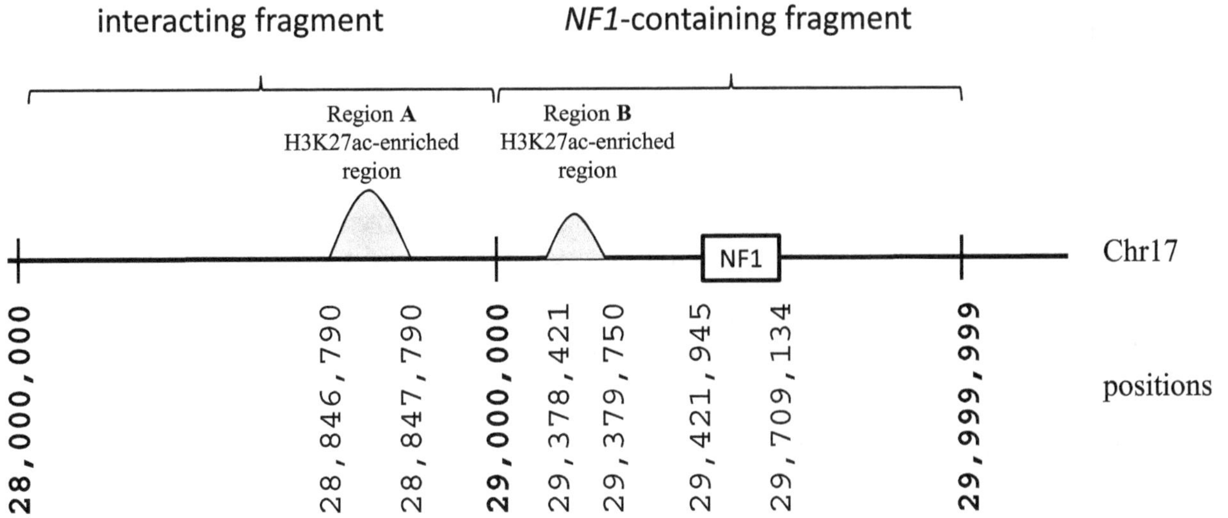

Figure 1 Schematic of the occurrence and level of H3K27ac enrichment within interacting and NF1-containing DNA fragments. The level of enrichment is shown by the *height of the curves* (not to scale).

Table 1 List of primers used to amplify and sequence DNA regions A (28,846,790–28,847,790) and B (29,378,421–29,379,750)

Primer ID	Sequence (5'>3')
chr17_28846841_1F	GCAAACATAGGAAGTGGCTTAC
chr17_28846841_2F	GAGGGGAGAAGTGTCTGTGTG
chr17_28846841_3F	TTTTCCCATTTAGAGATAAGTCAGTG
chr17_28846841_1R	TTCTGAGGTGCAGTCTTTTAGG
chr17_28846841_2R	GGTTACAACAAACAAGTGGAGAATG
chr17_28846841_3R	TACTTAGGGTGACAAGGCAAG
chr17_29387421_1F	TCTCCCTATGATGTCCAGGC
chr17_29387421_2F	TGCAGCAATAGGTGACTAAAACAC
chr17_29387421_3F	AGGTCCAAATGCAGGTGTG
chr17_29387421_4F	TCTGGAAGCTCTGCTTGG
chr17_29387421_1R	AATTGTTGGCATGAAAACTGG
chr17_29387421_2R	AGATGTGTACCCTGCGGAAG
chr17_29387421_3R	ACGAAGAGATGTGGTTTCCC
chr17_29387421_4R	AACATCCCCTTCCAATTTCC

Conclusions

This pilot study has shown that a combination of long-range DNA sequence interaction data and information about the location of functional elements available from ENCODE allows us to predict the possible location of novel regulatory regions that may act at distance from the genes whose expression they might influence. Mutations in these regions may in turn modulate the expression of their cognate target gene(s) that are spatially close to these regions. Although the functional ascertainment of these variants far upstream of the *NF1* gene has not yet been performed, the type of *in silico* analysis described here served to guide the mutation screening procedure, allowing us to detect sequence variants in five unrelated patients in whom no pathogenic mutations had previously been found in either the *NF1* gene or the *SPRED1* gene [6]. Even if eventually none of the detected sequence variants turn out to be of pathogenic significance, the Hi-C data indicate that several other 1-Mb fragments have a high number of interactions with the *NF1*-containing fragment and could potentially harbour remotely acting regulatory elements. Among them are two 1-Mb fragments occurring 1 Mb (positions 31,000,000–31,999,999) and 2 Mb (positions 32,000,000–32,999,999) downstream of the *NF1*-containing fragment that have, respectively, 699 and 150 intra-chromosomal interactions with the *NF1*-containing fragment in the *Nco*I-map and, respectively, 222 and 59 interactions in the *Hind*III-map. Another, albeit weaker, inter-chromosomal interaction (21 interactions in the *Nco*I-map) was recorded between the *NF1*-containing fragment and a 1-Mb fragment on chromosome 1 (positions 1–1,999,999). Hence, applicability of this approach is not only confined to *cis*-acting regulatory elements but could also be employed with *trans*-acting regulatory elements. The use of additional information that recently became available through the ENCODE resources, i.e. on the occurrence of CTCF binding factors linked to a range of gene regulatory functions including enhancer-blocking activity of insulator elements; DNase I hypersensitive sites characterizing open chromatin conformations, etc., may help to improve the *in silico* prediction of remotely acting regulatory elements. This approach therefore promises to be of potential utility in investigating those other disorders in which mutations could occur in remotely acting regulatory elements.

Methods

Patient samples

A sample of 47 unrelated NF1 patients (out of a total of 624 NF1 patients studied in our diagnostic centre), who tested negative for *NF1* (and *SPRED1*) point mutations and intra-genic insertions/deletions, was selected for this study. This project was approved by the local Ethics committee. Informed consent for sample collection was obtained according to the protocols approved by this committee.

Bioinformatics analysis

Long-range chromosomal DNA sequence interaction data were downloaded from http://compgenomics.weizmann.ac.il/tanay/?page_id=283. These data comprised the Hi-C contact maps [27], normalized to eliminate various biases associated with the experimental procedure [28]. Two matrices of interactions between 1-Mb fragments, each combining the results obtained using, respectively, the restriction enzymes *Hind*III and *Nco*I in the experimental procedures, were available. Henceforth, these contact maps will be termed, respectively, the *Hind*III- and *Nco*I-maps. Information on the genome-wide occurrence of one particular functional element, the histone H3K27ac-enriched region, was downloaded from the ENCODE database available at http://genome.ucsc.edu/index.html.

The *NF1* gene, spanning positions 29,421,945–29,709,134 from pter of chromosome 17 (NCBI build 37, UCSC HG18 and Ensembl GRCh37), occurs almost in the middle of a 1-Mb DNA fragment that starts at position 29,000,000 and ends at position 29,999,999. This 1-Mb fragment will henceforth be termed the *NF1*-containing fragment. Two of the contact maps described above were searched for DNA fragments, whether occurring on the same chromosome or on different chromosomes that had the most interactions with the *NF1*-containing fragment.

Data on the occurrence and level of H3K27ac enrichment (as measured by the ChIP-seq assay) within the 1-Mb fragment that had the strongest interaction with the *NF1*-containing fragment were downloaded from the ENCODE database. H3K27ac data were also downloaded for the *NF1*-containing fragment. For each of these two 1-Mb fragments (i.e. the fragment that had the strongest interaction with the *NF1*-containing fragment and the *NF1*-containing fragment itself), relatively short regions, corresponding to the highest level of H3K27ac enrichment, termed regions A and B, respectively, were selected for DNA sequencing in 47 NF1 patients in whom no pathogenic mutations had been found by screening both the *NF1* and *SPRED1* genes.

PCR and sequencing

Two sets of primers for regions A and B, selected as described above, were designed using Primer3 software [29] and purchased from Eurogentec (Southampton, UK). Specificity was confirmed by BLAST analysis.

The genomic DNA isolated from the peripheral blood cells of the NF1 patients was subjected to PCR and Sanger sequencing as described [31]. PCR reaction mixtures of 25 μl contained 5 μl of genomic DNA (6 ng/μl), 5 pmol each of the forward and reverse primers, 0.25 U AmpliTaq Gold polymerase, 3 mM $MgCl_2$, PCR buffer and 0.125 mM each dNTP. PCR cycling conditions were 95°C for 10 min followed by 40 cycles of 95°C × 30 s, 60°C × 30 s, 72°C × 30 s with a final extension step of 72°C for 10 min. PCR fragments were confirmed by gel electrophoresis in 1.5% agarose gels and visualized with ethidium bromide staining. The sequencing of the PCR products was performed with BigDye Terminator v3.1 Cycle Sequencing Kits and run on an ABI 3730 genetic analyzer. The obtained sequences were analyzed using Sequencher software version 4.7 (Gene Codes Corp., Ann Arbor, MI, USA). All reagents were purchased from Life Technologies Ltd, Paisley, UK.

Competing interests

The authors declare that they have no competing interests.

Authors' contributions

NC conceived the approach. SEH performed the *in silico* analysis. MU and PR performed the PCR and sequencing. NC, PR and DNC interpreted the results. NC drafted the manuscript. All authors participated in the preparation of the manuscript, and read and approved the final manuscript.

Author details

[1]School of Science and Technology, Nottingham Trent University, Clifton Lane, Nottingham NG11 8NS, UK. [2]Institute of Medical Genetics, School of Medicine, Cardiff University, Heath Park, Cardiff CF14 4XN, UK. [3]Current address: Department of Cardiovascular Sciences, University of Leicester, Glenfield Hospital, Leicester LE3 9QP, UK.

References

1. Upadhyaya M, Chuzhanova N, Cooper DN: **The somatic mutational spectrum of the *NF1* gene.** In *Neurofibromatosis Type 1: Molecular and Cellular Biology.* Edited by Upadhyaya M, Cooper DN. Heidelberg: Springer; 2012:211–233.
2. Upadhyaya M: **Neurofibromatosis type 1: diagnosis and recent advances.** *Expert Opin Med Diagn* 2010, **4**(4):307–322.
3. Bennett E, Thomas N, Upadhyaya M: **Neurofibromatosis type 1: its association with the Ras/MAPK pathway syndromes.** *J Paediatr Neurol* 2009, **7**:105–115.
4. Scheffzek K, Ahmadian MR, Wiesmuller L, Kabsch W, Stege P, Schmitz F, Wittinghofer A: **Structural analysis of the GAP-related domain from neurofibromin and its implications.** *EMBO J* 1998, **17**(15):4313–4327.
5. Scheffzek K, Welti S: **Neurofibromin: protein domains and functional characteristics.** In *Neurofibromatosis Type 1: Molecular and Cellular Biology.* Edited by Upadhyaya M, Cooper DN. Heidelberg: Springer; 2012:305–326.
6. Brems H, Chmara M, Sahbatou M, Denayer E, Taniguchi K, Kato R, Somers R, Messiaen L, De Schepper S, Fryns JP, Cools J, Marynen P, Thomas G, Yoshimura A, Legius E: **Germline loss-of-function mutations in *SPRED1* cause a neurofibromatosis 1-like phenotype.** *Nat Genet* 2007, **39**(9):1120–1126.
7. Cichowski K, Jacks T: ***NF1* tumor suppressor gene function: narrowing the GAP.** *Cell* 2001, **104**(4):593–604.
8. Kehrer-Sawatzki H, Cooper DN: **Mosaicism in sporadic neurofibromatosis type 1: variations on a theme common to other hereditary cancer syndromes?** *J Med Genet* 2008, **45**(10):622–631.
9. Cooper DN, Upadhyaya M: **The germline mutational spectrum in neurofibromatosis type 1 and genotype-phenotype correlations.** In *Neurofibromatosis Type 1: Molecular and Cellular Biology.* Edited by Upadhyaya M, Cooper DN. Heidelberg: Springer; 2012:115–134.
10. Messiaen L, Wimmer K: **NF1 mutational spectrum.** In *Monographs in Human Genetics. Volume 16.* Edited by Kaufmann D. Basel: Karger; 2008:63–77.
11. Cowley GS, Murthy AE, Parry DM, Schneider G, Korf B, Upadhyaya M, Harper P, MacCollin M, Bernards A, Gusella JF: **Genetic variation in the 3' untranslated region of the neurofibromatosis 1 gene: application to unequal allelic expression.** *Somat Cell Mol Genet* 1998, **24**(2):107–119.
12. Osborn M, Cooper DN, Upadhyaya M: **Molecular analysis of the 5'-flanking region of the neurofibromatosis type 1 (NF1) gene: identification of five sequence variants.** *Clin Genet* 2000, **57**(3):221–224.
13. Horan MP, Osborn M, Cooper DN, Upadhyaya M: **Functional analysis of polymorphic variation within the promoter and 5' untranslated region of the neurofibromatosis type 1 (NF1) gene.** *Am J Med Genet A* 2004, **131**(3):227–231.
14. Cooper DN, Chen JM, Ball EV, Howells K, Mort M, Phillips AD, Chuzhanova N, Krawczak M, Kehrer-Sawatzki H, Stenson PD: **Genes, mutations and human inherited diseases at the dawn of the age of personalized genomics.** *Hum Mutat* 2010, **31**(6):631–655.
15. Gordon CT, Tan TY, Benko S, Fitzpatrick D, Lyonnet S, Farlie PG: **Long-range regulation at the *SOX9* locus in development and disease.** *J Med Genet* 2009, **46**(10):649–656.
16. Rahimov F, Marazita ML, Visel A, Cooper ME, Hitchler MJ, Rubini M, Domann FE, Govil M, Christensen K, Bille C, Melbye M, Jugessur A, Lie RT, Wilcox AJ, Fitzpatrick DR, Green ED, Mossey PA, Little J, Steegers-Theunissen RP, Pennacchio LA, Schutte BC, Murray JC: **Disruption of an AP-2α binding site in an *IRF6* enhancer is associated with cleft lip.** *Nat Genet* 2008, **40**(11):1341–1347.
17. De Gobbi M, Viprakasit V, Hughes JR, Fisher C, Buckle VJ, Ayyub H, Gibbons RJ, Vernimmen D, Yoshinaga Y, de Jong P, Cheng JF, Rubin EM, Wood WG, Bowden D, Higgs DR: **A regulatory SNP causes a human genetic disease by creating a new transcriptional promoter.** *Science* 2006, **312**(5777):1215–1217.
18. Pomerantz MM, Ahmadiyeh N, Jia L, Herman P, Verzi MP, Doddapaneni H, Beckwith CA, Chan JA, Hills A, Davis M, Yao K, Kehoe SM, Lenz HJ, Haiman CA, Yan C, Henderson BE, Frenkel B, Barretina J, Bass A, Tabernero J, Baselga J, Regan MM, Manak JR, Shivdasani R, Coetzee GA, Freedman ML: **The 8q24 cancer risk variant rs6983267 shows long-range interaction with *MYC* in colorectal cancer.** *Nat Genet* 2009, **41**(8):882–884.
19. Li H, Wallace MR: **NF1 gene: promoter, 5' UTR, and 3'UTR.** In *Neurofibromatosis Type 1: Molecular and Cellular Biology.* Edited by Upadhyaya M, Cooper DN. Heidelberg: Springer; 2012:105–134.
20. Bernards A, Snijders AJ, Hannigan GE, Murthy AE, Gusella JF: **Mouse neurofibromatosis type 1 cDNA sequences reveals high degree of conservation of both coding and non-coding mRNA segments.** *Hum Mol Genet* 1993, **2**(6):645–650.
21. Hajra A, Martin-Gallardo A, Tarlé SA, Freedman M, Wilson-Gunn S, Bernards A, Collins FS: **DNA sequences in the promoter region of the *NF1* gene are highly conserved between human and mouse.** *Genomics* 1994, **21**(3):649–652.
22. Creyghton MP, Cheng AW, Welstead GG, Kooistra T, Carey BW, Steine EJ, Hanna J, Lodato MA, Frampton GM, Sharp PA, Boyer LA, Young RA, Jaenisch R: **Histone H3K27ac separates active from poised enhancers and predicts developmental state.** *Proc Natl Acad Sci U S A* 2010, **107**(50):21931–21936.

23. Dunham I, Kundaje A, Aldred SF, Collins PJ, Davis CA, Doyle F, Epstein CB, Frietze S, Harrow J, Kaul R, Khatun J, Lajoie BR, Landt SG, Lee BK, Pauli F, Rosenbloom KR, Sabo P, Safi A, Sanyal A, Shoresh N, Simon JM, Song L, Trinklein ND, Altshuler RC, Birney E, Brown JB, Cheng C, Djebali S, Dong X, Dunham I, ENCODE Project Consortium, *et al*: **An integrated encyclopedia of DNA elements in the human genome.** *Nature* 2012, **489**(7414):57–74.
24. Thurman RE, Rynes E, Humbert R, Vierstra J, Maurano MT, Haugen E, Sheffield NC, Stergachis AB, Wang H, Vernot B, Garg K, John S, Sandstrom R, Bates D, Boatman L, Canfield TK, Diegel M, Dunn D, Ebersol AK, Frum T, Giste E, Johnson AK, Johnson EM, Kutyavin T, Lajoie B, Lee BK, Lee K, London D, Lotakis D, Neph S, *et al*: **The accessible chromatin landscape of the human genome.** *Nature* 2012, **489**(7414):75–82.
25. van Steensel B, Dekker J: **Genomics tools for unraveling chromosome architecture.** *Nat Biotechnol* 2010, **28**(10):1089–1095.
26. Sexton T, Bantignies F, Cavalli G: **Genomic interactions: chromatin loops and gene meeting points in transcriptional regulation.** *Semin Cell Dev Biol* 2009, **20**(7):849–855.
27. Lieberman-Aiden E, van Berkum NL, Williams L, Imakaev M, Ragoczy T, Telling A, Amit I, Lajoie BR, Sabo PJ, Dorschner MO, Sandstrom R, Bernstein B, Bender MA, Groudine M, Gnirke A, Stamatoyannopoulos J, Mirny LA, Lander ES, Dekker J: **Comprehensive mapping of long-range interactions reveals folding principles of the human genome.** *Science* 2009, **326**(5950):289–293.
28. Yaffe E, Tanay A: **Probabilistic modeling of Hi-C contact maps eliminates systematic biases to characterize global chromosomal architecture.** *Nat Genet* 2011, **43**(11):1059–1065.
29. Rozen S, Skaletsky H: **Primer3 on the WWW for general users and for biologist programmers.** *Methods Mol Biol* 2000, **132**:365–386.
30. Hwang YC, Zheng Q, Gregory BD, Wang LS: **High-throughput identification of long-range regulatory elements and their target promoters in the human genome.** *Nucleic Acids Res* 2013, **41**(9):4835–4846.
31. Thomas L, Kluwe L, Chuzhanova N, Mautner V, Upadhyaya M: **Analysis of *NF1* somatic mutations in cutaneous neurofibromas from patients with high tumor burden.** *Neurogenetics* 2010, **11**(4):391–400.

Permissions

All chapters in this book were first published in JNI, by BioMed Central; hereby published with permission under the Creative Commons Attribution License or equivalent. Every chapter published in this book has been scrutinized by our experts. Their significance has been extensively debated. The topics covered herein carry significant findings which will fuel the growth of the discipline. They may even be implemented as practical applications or may be referred to as a beginning point for another development.

The contributors of this book come from diverse backgrounds, making this book a truly international effort. This book will bring forth new frontiers with its revolutionizing research information and detailed analysis of the nascent developments around the world.

We would like to thank all the contributing authors for lending their expertise to make the book truly unique. They have played a crucial role in the development of this book. Without their invaluable contributions this book wouldn't have been possible. They have made vital efforts to compile up to date information on the varied aspects of this subject to make this book a valuable addition to the collection of many professionals and students.

This book was conceptualized with the vision of imparting up-to-date information and advanced data in this field. To ensure the same, a matchless editorial board was set up. Every individual on the board went through rigorous rounds of assessment to prove their worth. After which they invested a large part of their time researching and compiling the most relevant data for our readers.

The editorial board has been involved in producing this book since its inception. They have spent rigorous hours researching and exploring the diverse topics which have resulted in the successful publishing of this book. They have passed on their knowledge of decades through this book. To expedite this challenging task, the publisher supported the team at every step. A small team of assistant editors was also appointed to further simplify the editing procedure and attain best results for the readers.

Apart from the editorial board, the designing team has also invested a significant amount of their time in understanding the subject and creating the most relevant covers. They scrutinized every image to scout for the most suitable representation of the subject and create an appropriate cover for the book.

The publishing team has been an ardent support to the editorial, designing and production team. Their endless efforts to recruit the best for this project, has resulted in the accomplishment of this book. They are a veteran in the field of academics and their pool of knowledge is as vast as their experience in printing. Their expertise and guidance has proved useful at every step. Their uncompromising quality standards have made this book an exceptional effort. Their encouragement from time to time has been an inspiration for everyone.

The publisher and the editorial board hope that this book will prove to be a valuable piece of knowledge for researchers, students, practitioners and scholars across the globe.

List of Contributors

Angus J Clarke and David N Cooper
Institute of Medical Genetics, School of Medicine, Cardiff University, Cardiff, Wales CF14 4XN, UK

Michael Krawczak
Institute of Medical Informatics and Statistics, Christian-Albrechts University Kiel, Brunswiker Straße 10, Kiel 24105, Germany

Chris Tyler-Smith
The Wellcome Trust Sanger Institute, Wellcome Trust Genome Campus, Hinxton, Cambridgeshire CB10 1SA, UK

Helen M Wallace
GeneWatch UK, 60 Lightwood Rd, Buxton SK17 7BB, UK

Andrew O M Wilkie
Weatherall Institute of Molecular Medicine, John Radcliffe Hospital, University of Oxford, Headington, Oxford OX3 9DS, UK

Frances Lucy Raymond
Department of Medical Genetics, Cambridge Institute for Medical Research, University of Cambridge, Cambridge CB2 0XY, UK

Ruth Chadwick
Cesagen, 6 Museum Place, Cardiff University, Cardiff, Wales CF10 3BG, UK

Nick Craddock
Department of Psychological Medicine, Cardiff University School of Medicine, Heath Park, Cardiff CF14 4XN, UK

Ros John
Cardiff School of Biosciences, Cardiff University, Cardiff, Wales CF10 3AX, UK

John Gallacher
Clinical Epidemiology, School of Medicine, Cardiff University, Cardiff, Wales CF14 4XN, UK

Mathias Chiano
GlaxoSmithKline Medicines Research Centre, Gunnels Wood Road, Stevenage, Hertfordshire SG1 2NY, UK

I-Chun Tsai
Center for Human Disease Modeling, Duke University, 300 North Duke Street, Durham, NC 27701, USA

Georgios Kellaris
Center for Human Disease Modeling, Duke University, 300 North Duke Street, Durham, NC 27701, USA
Department of Medical Genetics, University of Athens Medical School, Aghia Sophia Children's Hospital, 11527 Athens, Greece

Kamal Khan
Human Molecular Genetics Laboratory, Health Biotechnology Division, National Institute for Biotechnology and Genetic Engineering (NIBGE), Faisalabad 38000, Pakistan

Shahid M. Baig
Human Molecular Genetics Laboratory, Health Biotechnology Division, National Institute for Biotechnology and Genetic Engineering (NIBGE), Faisalabad 38000, Pakistan

Paul Ruggieri
Imaging Institute, Cleveland Clinic, 9500 Euclid Avenue, Cleveland, OH 44195, USA

Marvin R. Natowicz
Pathology and Laboratory Medicine and Genomic Medicine Institutes, Cleveland Clinic, Cleveland, OH 44195, USA

Francisca Millan Zamora
GeneDx, 207 Perry Parkway, Gaithersburg, MD 20877, USA

Nicholas Katsanis
Center for Human Disease Modeling, Duke University, 300 North Duke Street, Durham, NC 27701, USA
Imaging Institute, Cleveland Clinic, 9500 Euclid Avenue, Cleveland, OH 44195, USA

Saumya Shekhar Jamuar
Genetics Service, Department of Paediatrics, KK Women's and Children's Hospital, Singapore, Singapore
Paediatrics Academic Clinical Programme, SingHealth Duke-NUS Graduate Medical School, Singapore, Singapore

Ene-Choo Tan
Paediatrics Academic Clinical Programme, SingHealth Duke-NUS Graduate Medical School, Singapore, Singapore
KK Research Centre, KK Women's and Children's Hospital, 100 Bukit Timah Road, 229899 Singapore, Singapore

Izabela Krupska
Department of Cell Biology, Downstate Medical Center, Brooklyn, NY 11203, USA
Department of Ophthalmology, Downstate Medical Center, Brooklyn, NY 11203, USA

Elspeth A. Bruford
HUGO Gene Nomenclature Committee, European Molecular Biology Laboratory, European Bioinformatics Institute, Wellcome Genome Campus, Hinxton, Cambridge CB10 1SD, UK

Brahim Chaqour
Department of Cell Biology, Downstate Medical Center, Brooklyn, NY 11203, USA
Department of Ophthalmology, Downstate Medical Center, Brooklyn, NY 11203, USA
State University of New York (SUNY) Eye Institute Downstate Medical Center, 450 Clarkson Avenue, MSC 5, Brooklyn, NY 11203, USA

Claudia Pisanu, Donatella Congiu and Alessio Squassina
Section of Neurosciences and Clinical Pharmacology, Department of Biomedical Sciences, University of Cagliari, SP8 Km. 0,700, 09042 Monserrato (CA), Italy

Stefano Caproni, Ilenia Corbelli and Paola Sarchielli
Neurologic Clinic, University of Perugia, Perugia, Italy

Letizia M. Cupini
Headache and Cerebrovascular Diseases Center, Ospedale S. Eugenio, Rome, Italy

George P. Patrinos
Department of Pharmacy, University of Patras, School of Health Sciences, Patras, Greece

Maria Del Zompo
Section of Neurosciences and Clinical Pharmacology, Department of Biomedical Sciences, University of Cagliari, SP8 Km. 0,700, 09042 Monserrato (CA), Italy
Institute of Neuroscience, CNR, Cagliari, Italy

Paolo Calabresi
Neurologic Clinic, University of Perugia, Perugia, Italy
IRCCS Fondazione "S. Lucia", Rome, Italy

Eileen C. P. Lim, Maggie Brett and Siew-Peng Lee
KK Research Centre, KK Women's and Children's Hospital, 100 Bukit Timah Road, Singapore 229899, Singapore

Ene-Choo Tan
KK Research Centre, KK Women's and Children's Hospital, 100 Bukit Timah Road, Singapore 229899, Singapore
Paediatrics Academic Clinical Programme, SingHealth Duke-NUS Graduate Medical School, Singapore 169857, Singapore

Angeline H. M. Lai, Ee-Shien Tan, Saumya S. Jamuar and Ivy S. L. Ng
Genetics Service, Department of Paediatrics, KK Women's and Children's Hospital, Singapore 229899, Singapore
Paediatrics Academic Clinical Programme, SingHealth Duke-NUS Graduate Medical School, Singapore 169857, Singapore

Li An and Yingxiang Lin
Beijing Key Laboratory of Respiratory and Pulmonary Circulation Disorders, Beijing Institute of Respiratory Medicine, Department of Respiratory and Critical Care Medicine, Beijing Chao-Yang Hospital, Capital Medical University, Beijing 100020, China

Ting Yang
Department of Respiratory and Critical Care Medicine, China-Japan Friendship Hospital, Beijing 100029, China

Sherry G. Clendenon and James A. Glazier
Biocomplexity Institute and Department of Intelligent Systems Engineering, Indiana University, Bloomington, IN 47405, USA

Lin Hua
School of Biomedical Engineering, Capital Medical University, Beijing 100069, China
Beijing Key Laboratory of Fundamental Research on Biomechanics in Clinical Application, School of Biomedical Engineering, Capital Medical University, Beijing 100069, China

Rita M. C. de Almeida
Biocomplexity Institute and Department of Physics, Indiana University, Bloomington, IN 47405, USA
Instituto de Física and Instituto Nacional de Ciência e Tecnologia, Universidade Federal do Rio Grande do Sul, 91501-970 Porto Alegre, RS, Brazil

William G. Richards, Michael Boedigheimer and Michael Damore
AMGEN Inc., One Amgen Center Drive, Thousand Oaks, CA 91320-1799, USA

Sandro Rossetti and Peter C. Harris
Division of Nephrology, Mayo Clinic, 200 First Street SW, Rochester, MN 55905, USA

Britney-Shea Herbert
Department of Medical and Molecular Genetics, Indiana University School of Medicine, Indianapolis, IN 46202, USA

Wei Min Xu and Robert L. Bacallao
Division of Nephrology, Department of Medicine, Richard Roudebush VAMC and Indiana University School of Medicine, Indianapolis, IN 46202, USA

Angela Wandinger-Ness
Department of Pathology MSC08-4640 and Cancer Research and Treatment Center, University of New Mexico Health Sciences Center, Albuquerque, NM 87131, USA

Heather H. Ward
Division of Nephrology, Department of Medicine, University of New Mexico Health Sciences Center, Albuquerque, NM 87131, USA

Kuo Wang, Mingyue Yang and Xiaosong Wang
Institute of Translational Medicine, the First Hospital of Jilin University, Changchun 130061, China

Genhong Cheng
Institute of Translational Medicine, the First Hospital of Jilin University, Changchun 130061, China
Department of Microbiology, Immunology and Molecular Genetics, University of California Los Angeles, Los Angeles, CA 90095, USA

Fanzheng Meng, Deli Li, Ruihua Lu, Yan Wang, Huadong Zhuang and Man Gao
Department of Pediatrics, the First Hospital of Jilin University, Changchun 130021, China

Mengyao Li
Institute of Translational Medicine, the First Hospital of Jilin University, Changchun 130061, China
Bethune Medical School of Jilin University, Changchun 130021, China

Khalid Mahmood, Chol-hee Jung, Gayle Philip, Peter Georgeson, Jessica Chung, Bernard J. Pope and Daniel J. Park
Melbourne Bioinformatics, The University of Melbourne, Melbourne, Australia

Lidiia Zhytnik
Department of Traumatology and Orthopedics, University of Tartu, Puusepa 8, 51014 Tartu, Estonia

Katre Maasalu and Aare Märtson
Department of Traumatology and Orthopedics, University of Tartu, Puusepa 8, 51014 Tartu, Estonia
Clinic of Traumatology and Orthopedics, Tartu University Hospital, Puusepa 8, 51014 Tartu, Estonia

Ene Reimann and Sulev Kõks
Centre of Translational Medicine, University of Tartu, Ravila 14a, 50411 Tartu, Estonia
Department of Pathophysiology, University of Tartu, Ravila 19, 50411 Tartu, Estonia

Ele Prans
Department of Pathophysiology, University of Tartu, Ravila 19, 50411 Tartu, Estonia

Vasiliki Chondrou, Vlasia Kastrinou and Theodora Katsila
Department of Pharmacy, School of Health Sciences, University of Patras, University Campus, Rion, GR-265 04 Patras, Greece

Petros Kolovos
Biotech Research and Innovation Centre (BRIC), University of Copenhagen, Copenhagen, Denmark

Argyro Sgourou
Hellenic Open University, Patras, Greece

Alexandra Kourakli and Argiris Symeonidis
Hematology Division, Department of Internal Medicine, Faculty of Medicine, University of Patras, Patras, Greece

Alexia Pavlidaki
Department of Pharmacy, School of Health Sciences, University of Patras, University Campus, Rion, GR-265 04 Patras, Greece
Institut de Génétique et de Biologie Moléculaire et Cellulaire IGBMC/CNRS/INSERM/UDS, 67404 ILLKIRCH, BP 10142 CU de Strasbourg, France

Anne John
Department of Pathology, College of Medicine & Health Sciences, United Arab Emirates University, Al-Ain, United Arab Emirates

Bassam R. Ali
Department of Pathology, College of Medicine & Health Sciences, United Arab Emirates University, Al-Ain, United Arab Emirates
Zayed Bin Sultan Center for Health Sciences, United Arab Emirates University, Al-Ain, United Arab Emirates

Adamantia Papachatzopoulou
Laboratory of General Biology, Faculty of Medicine, University of Patras, Patras, Greece

George P. Patrinos
Department of Pharmacy, School of Health Sciences, University of Patras, University Campus, Rion, GR-265 04 Patras, Greece
Department of Pathology, College of Medicine & Health Sciences, United Arab Emirates University, Al-Ain, United Arab Emirates
Zayed Bin Sultan Center for Health Sciences, United Arab Emirates University, Al-Ain, United Arab Emirates

Kushani Jayasinghe
Department of Nephrology, Monash Medical Centre, Melbourne, Australia
KidGen Renal Genetics Flagship, Australian Genomic Health Alliance, elbourne, Australia

Cathy Quinlan
KidGen Renal Genetics Flagship, Australian Genomic Health Alliance, elbourne, Australia
Murdoch Children's Research Institute, Melbourne, Australia
Department of Paediatric Nephrology, Royal Children's Hospital, Melbourne, Australia

Zornitza Stark
KidGen Renal Genetics Flagship, Australian Genomic Health Alliance, elbourne, Australia
Murdoch Children's Research Institute, Melbourne, Australia
Department of Pediatrics, University of Melbourne, Melbourne, Australia

Chirag Patel
KidGen Renal Genetics Flagship, Australian Genomic Health Alliance, elbourne, Australia
Genetic Health Queensland, Royal Brisbane and Women's Hospital, Brisbane, Australia

Matthew G. Sampson
Department Of Pediatrics-Nephrology, University of Michigan School of Medicine, Ann Arbor, USA

Moin Saleem
Bristol Renal, Bristol Medical School, University of Bristol, Bristol, UK

Andrew J. Mallett
KidGen Renal Genetics Flagship, Australian Genomic Health Alliance, elbourne, Australia
Faculty of Medicine, The University of Queensland, Brisbane, Australia
Kidney Health Service and Conjoint Renal Research Laboratory, Royal Brisbane and Women's Hospital, Butterfield Street, Herston, Brisbane, Queensland 4029, Australia

Suleyman Vural, Richard Simon and Julia Krushkal
Computational and Systems Biology Branch, Biometric Research Program, Division of Cancer Treatment and Diagnosis, National Cancer Institute, 9609 Medical Center Dr, Rockville, MD 20850, USA

Magnus Ingelman-Sundberg, Souren Mkrtchian, Yitian Zhou and Volker M. Lauschke
Department of Physiology and Pharmacology, Section of Pharmacogenetics, Karolinska Institutet, SE-171 77 Stockholm, Sweden

Vasiliki Chondrou, Eleana F. Stavrou and Argyro Sgourou
School of Science and Technology, Biology Laboratory, Hellenic Open University, Patras, Greece

Georgios Markopoulos
Faculty of Medicine, Biology Laboratory, University of Ioannina, Ioannina, Greece

Alexandra Kouraklis-Symeonidis
Thalassemia and Hemoglobinopathies Unit, Hematology Division, Department of Internal Medicine, General University Hospital of Patras, Patras, Greece

Vasilios Fotopoulos
School of Science and Technology, Digital Systems and Media Computing Laboratory, Hellenic Open University, Patras, Greece

Argiris Symeonidis
Medical School, Hematology Division, Department of Internal Medicine, University of Patras, Patras, Greece

Efthymia Vlachaki
Thalassemia Unit, "Hippokrateio" General Hospital of Thessaloniki, Thessaloniki, Greece

Panagiota Chalkia
Thalassemia and Sickle Cell Unit, AHEPA University General Hospital of Thessaloniki, Thessaloniki, Greece

George P. Patrinos
School of Health Sciences, Department of Pharmacy, Laboratory of Pharmacogenomics and Individualized Therapy, University of Patras, Patras, Greece

Adamantia Papachatzopoulou
Medical Faculty, Laboratory of General Biology, University of Patras, Patras, Greece

Jiantao Sun, Jiemei Yang, Jing Chi and Xue Ding
Department of Cardiology, the First Affiliated Hospital, Harbin Medical University, Harbin, Heilongjiang, People's Republic of China

Nan Lv
Department of Obstetrics, the Second Affiliated Hospital, Harbin Medical University, 246 XueFu Road, Harbin 150086, Heilongjiang, People's Republic of China

Yuhua Su
Dr. Su's Statistics & Department of Human Nutrition, Food, and Animal Sciences, University of Hawaii at Manoa, Honolulu, HI 96822, USA

Lei Zhu and AlanMenius
Biomarker and Predictive Analytics, GlaxoSmithKline, 5 Moore Drive, Research Triangle Park, NC 27709, USA

Jason Osborne
Department of Statistics, North Carolina State University, Raleigh, NC 27695, USA

Amy Rodemoyer
Kansas City University of Medicine and Biosciences, Kansas, MO 64106, USA

Nataliya Kibiryeva, Alexis Bair, Jennifer Marshall, James E O'Brien Jr and Douglas C Bittel
The Ward Family Heart Center, Children's Mercy Hospitals and Clinics, Kansas City, MO 64108, USA
University of Missouri-Kansas City School of Medicine, 5100 Rockhill Rd, Kansas City, MO 64110, USA

Jihye Kim, Minjae Yoo and Aik Choon Tan
Translational Bioinformatics and Cancer Systems Biology Laboratory, Division of Medical Oncology, Department of Medicine, University of Colorado Anschutz Medical Campus, Aurora, CO 80045, USA

Jaewoo Kang
Data Mining and Information Systems Laboratory, Department of Computer Science and Engineering, Korea University, Seoul 136-713, South Korea

Nadia Chuzhanova and Stephen E Hamby
School of Science and Technology, Nottingham Trent University, Clifton Lane, Nottingham NG11 8NS, UK
Department of Cardiovascular Sciences, University of Leicester, Glenfield Hospital, Leicester LE3 9QP, UK

Pablo Reviriego, David N Cooper and Meena Upadhyaya
Institute of Medical Genetics, School of Medicine, Cardiff University, Heath Park, Cardiff CF14 4XN, UK

Index